OCCUPATIONAL HEALTH IN AMERICA

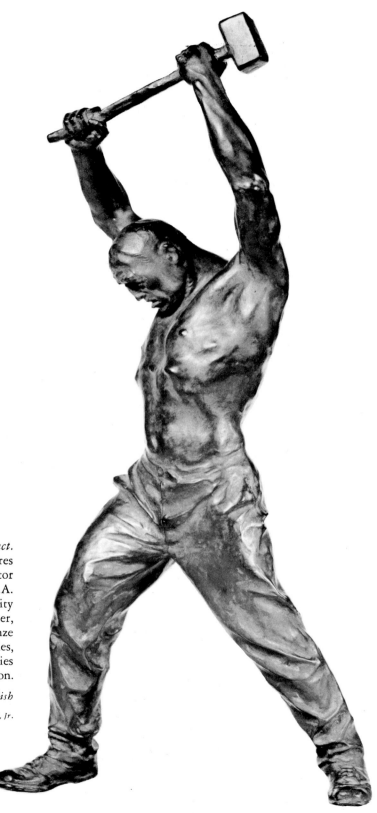

1. *Impact.*
One of a group of figures
by the noted American sculptor
Max Kalish, A.N.A.
His statues, dedicated to the dignity
of man-the-worker,
have caught in imperishable bronze
the play of tensed muscles,
the grace and rhythm of bodies
glorying in action.

—*By permission of Mrs. Max Kalish*

Photo, Joseph Klima, Jr.

OCCUPATIONAL HEALTH IN AMERICA

by Henry B. Selleck

in collaboration with Alfred H. Whittaker, M.D., F.A.C.S.

THIS BOOK WAS PREPARED UNDER THE DIRECTION OF
THE HISTORY COMMITTEE OF THE INDUSTRIAL MEDICAL ASSOCIATION
ALFRED H. WHITTAKER, M.D., CHAIRMAN

*OTTO P. GEIER, M.D. | JAMES I. ROBERTS, M.D. | *ROBERT T. LEGGE, M.D.

*LOYAL A. SHOUDY, M.D. | MCIVER WOODY, M.D.

**ARTHUR J. VORWALD | **EDWARD C. HOLMBLAD

**GEORGE ROSEN

*Deceased   **Appointed to replace deceased member.

1962
Wayne State University Press   Detroit

*Grateful acknowledgement is made to the McGregor Fund of Detroit
and to the Industrial Medical Association for financial assistance
making possible the publication of this book.*

THIS VOLUME is respectfully dedicated to those pioneering doctors who laid, upon the bedrock of their personal integrity, the foundation stones of the Industrial Medical Association. By their vision, courage, crusading spirit, and devotion to Hippocratic ideals, they not only reflected great honor upon their profession but contributed immeasurably to the advancement of industrial medicine and of the organization which guides its destinies in this era of momentous social, scientific, and economic change.

FOR PERMISSION TO QUOTE, GRATEFUL ACKNOWLEDGEMENT IS MADE TO THE FOLLOWING:

The American Association of Industrial Nurses, Inc., for quotations from Evelyn Johnson (September 1956 and from Sara P. Wagner (July 1956), in the *A. A. I. N. Journal.*

The American College of Surgeons, for quotations from Gaylord Hess, *Medical Service in Industry* (1946).

The American Dental Association, for quotations from the "Report of the Committee on Economics" in the *Journal of the American Dental Association* (January 1943).

The American Medical Association, for quotations from Earl F. Lutz, "The Relationship Between the General Practitioner and the Industrial Physician," in the *A.M.A. Archives of Industrial Hygiene and Occupational Medicine* (October 1953).

The American Public Health Association, Inc., for quotations from Robert T. Legge, "Progress of American Industrial Medicine in the First Half of the Twentieth Century," in the *American Journal of Public Health* (August 1952).

Appleton-Century-Crofts, Inc., for quotations from E. F. Humphrey, *An Economic History of the United States* (1931).

The College of Physicians of Philadelphia, for a quotation from the *Transactions of the College of Physicians of Philadelphia* (2:65, 1934).

Alice Hamilton, for quotations from her book, *Exploring the Dangerous Trades* (Little, Brown and Co., 1943).

Harcourt, Brace and Company, for quotations from Matthew Josephson, *The Robber Barons* (1934).

Harper & Brothers, for quotations from Stuart Chase, *The Proper Study of Mankind* (1948); and from Earl Chapin May, *Principio to Wheeling* (1945).

Industrial Medicine and Surgery, for the use of the many references from this journal.

J. B. Lippincott Company, for quotations from C. O. Sappington, *Essentials of Industrial Health* (1943).

Francis D. Moore, for quotations from his "Endocrine Changes after Anesthesia, Surgery, and Un-anesthetized Trauma, in Man," published in *Recent Progress in Hormone Research* (13:511–82, 1957).

The New England Journal of Medicine, for quotations from Daniel L. Lynch, "Industrial Health and War," in the *Journal* (227:209–16, 1942).

W. B. Saunders Company, for quotations from Harry E. Mock, *Industrial Medicine and Surgery* (1919).

The University of Michigan School of Public Health, for quotations from *Proceedings of the Fourth Discussional on Industrial Health Programs* (1952).

PREFACE

THIS volume has been many years in the making. The stages of planning, preparation and production have covered nearly two decades, for reasons that will soon be apparent.

Just when the idea for such a story first suggested itself—and to whom—no one knows: but available records show that a history of some sort was officially discussed by the (then) American Association of Industrial Physicians & Surgeons in the very early 1940's. And older members had talked about the project among themselves long before that time.

The members urging immediate action on the plan included several from the little group that had, by sheer determination, blazed the way to a historic new era in American occupational medicine—during the founding and formative years of the association. Uppermost in their minds was the thought that, unless a detailed account of that period were preserved in printed form, personalities, ideas and events would fade from memory or remain buried in dusty files and scattered periodicals. Thus, material of widespread interest and historical significance would be lost.

At the annual business meeting of the association in April 1942, Dr. E. C. Holmblad voiced a hope that "next year there will be appointed a committee for the purpose of preparing a history, which should go down in the annals of medicine."

That hope was realized sooner than expected, for the incoming president, Dr. John J. Wittmer, promptly appointed Dr. Loyal A. Shoudy as chairman of a committee on history, and soon afterward Drs. Otto P. Geier and Frank L. Rector were named to serve with him.

Among active supporters of the project was A. D. Cloud, publisher of the association journal, *Industrial Medicine.* He too thought that work on the book should be started at once, fearing that the identification of men and movements might "all too soon be blotted out from living recollection." In June 1942, he wrote Shoudy to that effect, and offered his services in gathering and organizing material, checking facts, and assembling related data.

In the following months Cloud interviewed many of the "old-time" members and sent questionnaires to many more, collecting numerous official publications, professional papers, letters and documents—the nucleus of long and exhaustive research. Frequently encountered in correspondence of the period are the names of Volney S. Cheney, Harry E. Mock, Emery R. Hayhurst, R. D. Mudd, Andrew M. Harvey, William A. Sawyer, C. O. Sappington, and other pioneers in the industrial medical field.

At that time, leaders of the association could view in close perspective the first quarter-century of its history, but they could not possibly have imagined the momentous developments soon to come in industrial-medical affairs. Nevertheless, it quickly became evident that a simple narrative of the origin and growth of the organization would not accomplish what its proponents had in mind. Indeed, a story of such limited scope would merely add another statistical work to the voluminous, and growing, literature in this field.

A time less opportune than the early forties could scarcely have been selected for planning and producing a history of sufficient breadth and depth to meet the desired objectives. America was at war—a fact which placed a tremendous burden upon the entire medical profession and created an acute medical crisis in industry. The nation's doctors, *making* history, had no time for *writing* it.

Planning continued, however, and some progress was made. Shoudy thought it advisable to broaden the content of the proposed book, but he also realized that to do so would call for considerably more basic research. "It is going to take time," he told the Board of Directors in the autumn of 1943, "but I think we have made a good start. We are going to have a history, and when we get through with it we will have the story of industrial medicine."

This idea—of a history reflecting the association's influence on the progress of occupational medicine—appealed strongly to the membership. Nor did there then seem to be any valid reason why the project could not be carried out promptly and effectively, in spite of wartime handicaps.

It is now evident, however, that any history purporting to cover truly *modern* health care in industry would necessarily have been incomplete and inconclusive, if written and produced in the middle or late forties. It would have left many important questions unanswered, and hence would have fallen short of its objectives.

Doctor Shoudy himself, again reporting to the Board early in 1944, unwittingly put his finger on one factor that contributed to this unsatisfactory situation. "It is interesting," he remarked, "to look over our old programs and note that we discussed twenty-five years ago some of the same things we have been discussing to-night. And we are still bringing up and talking about some of the problems we thought we had solved twenty years ago."

It was true at the time of this comment that several controversial issues, after a quarter-century of maneuver and debate, were still unresolved. Although the association was enjoying a remarkable growth in membership and influence, it had not yet won general recognition as the official organization representing occupational medicine in America. And although the special nature of industrial practice was becoming better understood, certification of the specialty was still only a distant hope.

The fact is that during the 1940's the scope and character of industrial practice itself were undergoing changes of far-reaching consequence. Great advances in science, medicine and technology were on the way, all of which were to affect profoundly the future of health conservation in industry. As a guest of the American Association of Industrial Physicians & Surgeons (IMA) in 1945, Dr. Raymond Hussey, the dean of the Wayne University School of Medicine, talked of one aspect of these changing conditions. He told the Board of Directors:

> This field certainly has medical engineering relations that differ from practically any other field of medicine. It has a relationship with management of industry, and medical-management relationships that are distinctly different from other branches of medicine.
>
> It also has a physician-employee relationship which, in principle, is the same as the physician-patient relationship. It is similar not only in principle but in attitude, but it is different in several important aspects, and it has a responsibility for administrative procedure that is dissimilar to any other branch of medicine.

The ultimate pattern of these in-plant relationships was still unclear at the end of the forties. Time was needed to settle the issues involved as well as other human relations problems. Thus, in retrospect, it is apparent that a conclusive and significant story of modern occupational medicine had to await decisive events that did not occur until after 1950.

Very early, in its consideration of subject matter, Shoudy's History Committee faced the problem of where to start. Little that even remotely resembled modern medical practice in American industry existed before the 1900's. But efforts in the right direction were made well before the turn of the century, in the "company" medicine of railoads and mines. Indeed, it was from these small and ineffectual experiments that later thinking evolved.

If, however, we acknowledge industrial medicine's debt to the nineteenth century, why not carry the chronology back to the remote past? The temptation is hard to resist, but the task is endless. One who sets out to trace occupational health hazards, and counter measures, to their very beginnings must be prepared to go back to antiquity and beyond—reconstructing events that occurred long before the dawn of recorded history.

When Dr. Alfred H. Whittaker became a member of the association's History Committee in 1943, he made available for reference and research his own private library of occupational medicine—a collection of several thousand volumes which dated back to the earliest printed works of Aristotle, and covered subsequent periods down to modern times. This rich store of source material suggested many attractive possibilities for a history built upon this ancient foundation; but the immediate task was to assemble all pertinent data on health care in industry in the first two or three decades of the twentieth century.

Ironically, detailed and reliable information on that colorful and exciting formative period in the story of industrial medicine proved to be less readily accessible than suitable background material from far older times. Records were scanty and scattered. Important activities had to be reconstructed, in many instances, from the memory of participants.

This must not be taken to mean that there was a dearth of writers or writings in the field. The period from 1910 to 1940 produced a rapidly growing volume of significant literature relating to occupational health; but by far the greater part of it was devoted to the medical and scientific aspects of industrial practice. Necessarily missing from this body of professional books and papers was a thread of connected narrative tracing the evolution of present-day occupational medicine against a background of social, economic and technological change.

In a broad sense, preparation of a history that would bridge this important gap was the primary aim of the association. And the work of gathering and correlating relevant material went on through the 1940's and into the 1950's as rapidly as the time of busy professional men permitted.

From 1943 to 1950 the project was under the direction of Shoudy, Geier and Whittaker—though C. F. N. Schram (association president 1929–30), served briefly on the committee in 1943, and C. O. Sappington (lecturer, consultant and editor of *Industrial Medicine*), in 1949 and 1950. In August, 1947, Whittaker was appointed chairman by President Henry S. Brown, and has continued in that capacity to the present writing.

It is worthy of note that Loyal Shoudy, Otto Geier and Robert Legge gave unstintingly of their time and effort to the history as long as their health permitted, and that they remained actively interested to the end of their lives.* In recognition of their devotion and contributions to this purpose, their names remain in the final list of committee members.

Soon after Shoudy's death, the History Committee was augmented by the appointment of William A. Sawyer (Eastman Kodak Company), James B. McConnaughy (Aluminum Company of America), and H. G. Murray (Dennison Manufacturing Company). About a year later, in the fall of 1951, major revision of personnel was made, by the appointment of the following members, under Whittaker's chairmanship:

* Shoudy died August 30, 1950; Geier, February 28, 1954; Legge, March 21, 1960.

Robert T. Legge—educator, bibliophile and historian; one of the founders' group of the Industrial Medical Association, with more than fifty years of active service in occupational medicine.

McIver Woody—a former professor of surgery, with an avid interest in medical history; president of the association, 1939–1940, and for many years medical director of the Standard Oil Company (New Jersey).

James I. Roberts—a medical consultant for New England public utilities, with experience in the publishing field; a district counselor of the Industrial Medical Association, and chairman of the important Committee on Medical Care (1954–55).

From the very earliest discussions of this history down to its publication, the association has been fortunate in counting among its members an exceptionally large group of experienced doctors having an understanding of medical history and an appreciation of historical values. Officers, directors and committees have been consistently sympathetic toward the concept of a book in which strictly medical interest would be subordinated to a story of the specialty and the association in all their complex professional and public relationships. Departures from that central theme have been few, and of minor importance.

Very early in the 1950's it was apparent that every branch of medical science was in the midst of an era of great change. Each year, each month, brought dramatic, and climactic, developments—which gave new meaning to all that had gone before.

This volume, therefore, has taken shape as an account of the men, the events and the times responsible for the emergence of occupational medicine from its formative stage, and the application, in the twentieth century, of its protective and preventive technics to a major segment of our entire society. It has been a most significant transition—a giant stride in man's conquest of the environment in which he works and earns his livelihood.

Because of time required for preparation and production, it is not possible in this narrative to follow the mainstream of events and activities much beyond the middle 1950's. It will be noted, however, that tabulated matter in some appendices covers several more recent years. This method of handling makes it possible to include useful reference data without delaying publication.

* * *

For source material bearing on the early history of the Industrial Medical Association, we are deeply indebted to a large group of founders and other members who were most active from about 1910 to the 1930's. Their names recur again and again in this text and they are quoted liberally on many subjects, to assure authenticity.

Emphasis on that period and on those personages has been deliberate—for it is doubtful that the association could have survived in its present form without their influence and activity. So close is their world of yesterday that, to hundreds of members now at the height of their careers, it is still peopled by old and intimate friends whom memory clothes with warm and vivid personalities.

Special note is made of the fine cooperation of the association's History Committee. Both as a body, officially, and individually, they have done all that could be done to achieve the objectives sought—through policy decisions, professional counsel in medical matters, constructive suggestions as to content, and a thorough and careful reading of text. The same spirit and attitude have also prevailed among the officers and directors of the Industrial Medical Association through successive administrations down to the present.

Inevitably, material covering so many diverse subjects and activities must be gathered from widely scattered sources. Space forbids a detailed listing here, but we are particularly indebted—for help given through personal interviews and correspondence—to C. D. Selby, Carey P. McCord, H. E. Mock, W. A. Sawyer, H. W. Lawrence, H. G. Gardiner, and W. J. Fulton.

Further acknowledgment is made both to individuals and to organizations for help in assembling information on special subjects of various kinds. These sources include: among medical educators, T. Lyle Hazlett and A. J. Vorwald; personnel of the American Association of Industrial Nurses; representatives of the American Association of Industrial Dentists; casualty insurance companies; suppliers to industrial medicine.

Readers will note that published books and papers of the industrial medical profession are extensively quoted throughout this volume. This policy has been followed for three purposes: to cite authority for any information or comment on strictly medical subjects; to preserve and give due credit for the best thinking of leaders in the profession; to preserve excerpts from important works for convenient reference.

Owing to the fact that a great deal of this source material has been taken from letters, conversations and private records—and that much information has been obtained from reprints that are not paged and frequently bear no date—some reference notes in this text are of necessity, incomplete. Every effort has been made, however, to validate all footnotes. In this work of verification we are indebted to Mrs. Fanny Anderson, of the medical library staff of Wayne State University, for valuable assistance.

Despite the emphasis on personalities in this narrative, omissions far outnumber inclusions—doing an injustice to hundreds of doctors who have performed important duties in the field, particularly in recent years.

Nevertheless, something of all of them—their thinking, their work, their accomplishments—is reflected in this volume, although recognition must take the form of a blanket acknowledgement of the splendid cooperation that has made possible the success of association programs.

HENRY B. SELLECK

FOREWORD

To ASK one to write a foreword to these significant pages on the history of industrial medicine is to suggest a somewhat superfluous undertaking. Nevertheless the temptation to comply with the request of my colleagues cannot be resisted, since it affords me the opportunity to record wholeheartedly my endorsement of the entire project and its text.

Would that Otto Geier, Tom Crowder, and Loyal Shoudy were here with their eloquence to express our appreciation to the History Committee and to the author for recording in strong and accurate terms the growth of the American Association of Industrial Physicians & Surgeons, or, as we know it now, the Industrial Medical Association.

The association was blest in 1916 in choosing as the organizing group approximately 125 members who were imbued with a spirit of idealism—who believed in their cause, were enthusiastic workers, and, furthermore, were strengthened by a certain amount of adverse criticism from the rank and file of their medical fraternity.

We were fortunate in the early years of our new organization in attracting new members who added to, and elevated, the standards of our specialty. Their work in the field furnished new examples of its value; their teachings and writings lifted our banners ever higher. It is noteworthy that the association's object, stated at its first annual meeting, has remained unchanged and still stands as the guiding spirit of the membership.

At this first meeting a committee, consisting of Thomas R. Crowder (chairman),

C. G. Farnum and Andrew M. Harvey, was appointed to draw up the final draft of the constitution and bylaws. Their report was adopted, and it is noteworthy that, with only a few minor changes, this draft remains unchanged.

Then Otto Geier, the man who, most of us thought, deserved the honor of being our first president, rose to his feet and nominated J. W. Schereschewsky for that office. Otto's oratory is well remembered. With his prophecy of what he expected this new association to accomplish and his review of what the great "Scherry" had already done for preventive medicine (as a senior official of the United States Public Health Service) he so thrilled the audience that, bylaws or no bylaws, "Scherry's" election as our first president became unanimous.

Before the meeting closed that afternoon, there was a dramatic moment when Frank Billings, of Chicago, a past president of the American Medical Association and one of the stalwarts of organized medicine, asked permission to address the gathering. He had been present at most of our organizational meetings, as had Joseph C. Bloodgood of Johns Hopkins Hospital, and Victor Vaughan, dean of the University of Michigan Medical School. Billings said that he and Vaughan had just returned from a meeting of the House of Delegates of the American Medical Association, and he wanted to tell us of an important announcement he had made to the delegates. "I told them," he said, "that a husky new baby had just been born to the ranks of organized medicine, the American Association of Industrial Physicians & Surgeons. Its parents, forming this association, are only 125, but I predict that this baby will grow in numbers, strength and usefulness until within a few years it will become a most valuable component part of organized medicine."

This talk, and the unofficial recognition of such leaders in the American Medical Association as Billings, Vaughan and Bloodgood, aroused great enthusiasm, and stands as one of the greatest stimulants ever administered to a newly-arrived infant.

The birth of a new century ushered in a new era. As a young nation we had been prodigal of all our resources, including our manpower. Not until World Wars I and II came upon us, with their terrible destruction, was public attention focused upon this wastefulness. These wars stimulated and abetted the spirit of conservation typical of the new era. Hand in hand with our need for preparedness and civil defense, industrialization moved swiftly forward, and conservation of our industrial army became a necessity, as did efforts to conserve all our resources.

Change is slow among conservative men and women. Progress is slow and irksome to those who first see the light. For example, consider the handful of men and women who, in 1921, organized the "Safety First" movement. Thousands of converts have since been added to the rolls of the National Safety Council, and it is still growing.

One can visualize the disappointments and heartaches of the leaders in accident prevention as the death rate from automobile injuries has risen year after year. Yet our safety engineers and the other advocates of safety can point with satisfaction to their accomplishments in our homes, on our farms, and in our plants—the "working homes" of industry. Progress is slow, but who would give up the Safety First movement?

Consider "rehabilitation." We were less than a year in World War I when the words "physical reconstruction" and "rehabilitation" entered our nomenclature.

Today, less than fifty years later, the language of rehabilitation of the handicapped is well understood and fluently used by thousands of physicians and laymen alike. There is an increasing number of rehabilitation centers, crippled children's schools, and allied movements for reclaiming those who either are born handicapped or become disabled by accidents or disease. The terminology is new, yet centuries of manpower and brainpower had to be wasted before this country, and others, awoke to the need and began to obey the call of conservation.

Consider the overcrowding and the accompanying insanitary conditions of both the living and "working" homes of the majority of factory workers at the turn of the century. Slum clearance and the flow of new homes from congested areas to the suburbs were only dreams in 1907, when the City Club of Chicago formed its first housing committee, and when similar committees in other major cities started to study the problem in the early 1900's. True, many pioneers in other decades and other centuries had cried out and worked for these reforms, and many others will have to continue the fight before the ideal is approached.

Consider the municipal tuberculosis associations—the numerous chapters that make up the National Tuberculosis Association—and consider the effect that doctors like Theodore Sachs and E. L. Trudeau had on our thinking. Consider the employment of school doctors and school nurses, the formation of milk commissions, the inspections and surveys of penal institutions, insane asylums, almshouses and other state and federal institutions, and the reforms and improvements that resulted. This was the period when young medical men began to think of entire groups rather than of individuals as their patients. The various industries, with their few hundred to several thousand employees under one roof, constituted a veritable human laboratory wherein the doctor could test these new ideas of health, life, and limb conservation.

The time was ripe for an industrial association.

In 1919 when the infant organization was three years old, the trustees of the American Medical Association chose it to take charge of the meeting of the Miscellaneous Section of the American Medical Association program. A comprehensive program was presented, including some twelve papers, followed by the usual discussions. Again, Frank Billings and Victor Vaughan attended all the sessions of the sectional meeting. At the concluding session, Vaughan gave a talk that was the second stimulant received by the association. He said: "I have listened attentively to these addresses and discussions, and it seems to me that the text for all the papers was undoubtedly chosen from the Thirteenth Chapter of First Corinthians. You members of the new industrial medical association are preaching and practicing 'brotherly love.' I predict a great and glorious future for your association." It is interesting to note that Vaughan referred to the organization by the name which it later adopted.

This June (1957) the Industrial Medical Association reached its forty-first birthday and some 3,500 members, a significant growth from its organizing membership of 125 in 1916!

Not until the 1940's did the association reach a financial situation that enabled it to afford a full-time managing director. It chose Edward C. Holmblad for this important and exacting position. Because of well coordinated effort among officers and directors and because of the solid foundation on which they built, the Industrial Medical Association can point thus far to accomplishments of which the organizing members, were they all still with us, could well be proud.

We have been fortunate in having noted medical historians among our members. Robert T. Legge—a pioneer industrial physician early in the century and a prolific contributor to the literature of industrial medicine—serves on our History Committee.

Alfred H. Whittaker, whose private collection teems with books and data dating back many centuries prior to this organization, is the committee's chairman. Because we were able to secure one so qualified both as an historian and as an active member of the Industrial Medical Association to "spark" the enterprise, this history of industrial medicine was made possible. And the selection of a gifted interpretive writer, Henry B. Selleck, as author, insures it as a work that will live in medical literature.

HENRY E. MOCK, M.D., September, 1957

CONTENTS

PART ONE

THE BACKDROP

PART TWO

THE ASSOCIATION IS BORN

PART THREE

A NEW SPECIALTY

PART FOUR

TRENDS

PART FIVE

THE TURBULENT TWENTIES

PART SIX

TRIAL BY DEPRESSION

PART SEVEN

THE ATOMIC AGE

APPENDICES

ILLUSTRATIONS

PART ONE

THE BACKDROP

MODERN INDUSTRY AND MEDICINE
VIEWED AGAINST THE BACKGROUND OF THE
SCIENTIFIC REVOLUTION

The tree of knowledge grows slowly and is slow to yield its fruit

I

LABOR AND HEALTH

IN NINETEENTH-CENTURY ENGLAND

THIS is a book about *Man: the Worker.* In it is a bit of his dreams and aspirations, more than a bit about his struggle toward an unknown destiny, something of his present problems, much more about the miracles of accomplishment we have witnessed in this, the twentieth century.

Man: the Worker! He is man, the inventor, builder, creator of wealth, consumer, user of the goods he makes. He is MAN, inheritor of the earth!

Our story deals mainly with his health—the hazards of his occupations and environments. For without health, life loses its savor, productivity declines, and there can be no future.

But this is not a book about medicine as such—nor social science, nor any of the sciences. These intrude only because health is everybody's business, because accident and disease affect the lives of everyone, and because all human resources must be mobilized for their effective control.

Specifically, we are concerned with the work of those men and women in medicine, science, business, and industry who have taken up the gage of battle against the ills of body and mind that stem from industrial occupations and thrive in complex modern societies.

Upon victory in this battle, survival of our industrial civilization depends. Thus, the subject is of interest and import to all who work with body, or brain, or both. Doctors and scientists. Teachers and students. Capital and labor. Employers and employed.

The history of occupational disease dates back to dim and distant centuries. But

3

the problems of our day have their origin in the dawn of the machine age, which in the beginning was an age of steam. For steam is power. Power is machinery. Machinery is production.

And production as we know it is the source of all the real wealth in the world—a wealth of consumption goods and mechanical servants that have eased man's back, lifted his eyes to the sun, given him the means and the leisure to enjoy the fruits of his labor.

So, since this is a story of modern times, we pick it up in England—less than two centuries ago. It was then and there that the first thread in the fabric of today's industrial system was spun. . . .

How many thousands, perhaps millions, of Americans remember from the schoolbooks of childhood the story of James Watt and the birth of the steam-driven engine? It is a bit of standard educational lore—immortal as the legend of George Washington and the cherry tree.

In those half-forgotten texts, hurrying along to cram world history into convenient capsule form for juvenile minds, the tale is simply and forthrightly told. It conjures up a picture of the precocious young Scot, chin cupped in hands, staring intently at a singing teakettle on the hearth before him—as its popping lid transmitted to his agile mind the idea that steam, properly harnessed and applied, could be turned to man's use and advantage. No child, scanning the story of Watt and the kettle, could be blamed for concluding that the youth, under the spell of his inspiration, leaped to his feet shouting, "Eureka," and promptly invented the steam engine—full-blown and equipped with all the maze of parts and gadgets that make it today one of the most useful servants of civilization.

Adults do not need to be reminded that science does not work that way. Science does not span great gaps, from basic principles to perfected products, in a matter of days, or months, or years. It progresses by the slow, painstaking accumulation of knowledge, and its even more leisurely application to the needs of the society of its time. Its path is littered with disappointment, error, social and economic tragedy.

This fact is pertinent; it may be a warning not to expect too much too soon from the major scientific discoveries of our day, a warning not to grow impatient because Utopia is not yet here, and will be a long time in coming.

In this age of speed—of countless scientific wonders—it is easy to overlook the fact that the tree of knowledge grows slowly and is slow to yield its fruit in tangible benefits to society. No invention, however revolutionary, is of practical value except in relation to the general knowledge and culture of its time.

Stuart Chase points out that "even if Leonardo had evolved the laws of an aeroplane in flight, it could never have flown (except as a glider) because no engine had been invented light enough to power it."[1] One might add that even if there had been such an engine, the airplane would have remained an idle anachronism in a fifteenth century society which lacked the technology to build it in quantity, the gasoline to fuel it, and the host of adjuncts necessary for its successful use in transportation.

Watt was born in 1736 and died in 1819 at the age of eighty-three. His chief contributions to the steam engine were rotary action and a condensing chamber, incorporated in his improved model patented in 1781. This practical, workable engine found ready acceptance, for it came at a time when England's expanding textile industry was eagerly awaiting a power unit to drive spinning and weaving machinery where water power was not available.

Watt is a towering figure in the annals of engineering, but many other men, far less well known, had patiently experimented with steam, laying the groundwork for his accomplishments. And a great many were to follow him before steam power reached its present stage of perfection.

Legend has it that Hero, an ancient Greek scholar, not only was aware of the power of steam but also had some idea of how to apply it. As early as 130 B.C. he is supposed to have contrived an immense globe of metal, which the steam from heated water revolved slowly upon its axis. This was the forerunner, in principle at least, of the turbine.

More than a thousand years later Roger Bacon (1214–94) confidently predicted: "We shall be able to construct machines which will propel large ships with greater speed than a whole garrison of rowers and which will need only one pilot to direct them."

That day was long in coming. From time to time throughout the eighteenth century, steam-powered vessels appeared in German and British waters. But all failed, for one reason or another. John Fitch, an American engineer, built and demonstrated two small steamers, but skepticism and ridicule were his only reward. He took his own life because he could not raise funds to carry on his promising experiments. His first crude craft (1786) antedated Fulton's successful *Clermont* by more than twenty years.

For the purpose of this work we are interested in the invention of the steam engine not as an engineering triumph (which it surely was), but because its consequences and its implications are of vast importance for a proper understanding of all subsequent history.

The development of steam power parallels the pattern of progress in practically every other major field—the chemical and electrical industries; communication by telegraph, telephone and radio; atomic and electronic science. All these industries have many things in common. All had their origin in the discovery of basic natural laws. All had to wait through long periods of experiment before these laws were translated into practical products.

Invariably, man's ingenuity outruns his foresight. Intent upon discovery and invention, he thinks in terms of the advantages of a new product or process—but rarely realizes either its ultimate possibilities or its full impact upon the established order. Hence, the dislocations in industry and society that have so often followed periods of great inventive progress.

Lest we dismiss these facts too lightly, let us note that historians have tended to charge the advent of "the machine" with full responsibility for the plight of British labor in the nineteenth century. The inference is that labor-saving machinery *per se* has been a bane, rather than a blessing, to the workers whose physical labor it has so largely supplanted.

Even now, beyond the middle milestone of the twentieth century, such arguments are a stock-in-trade of those who declare that the American system of competitive enterprise is basically unsound, and blame the personal-incentive and profit motives for all the shortcomings of our present industrial society.

As late as 1933 the so-called "technocrats," led by a group of engineers, loudly proclaimed the imminent arrival of a day when machines would almost wholly replace human skill—creating universal unemployment and bringing about the complete collapse of our manufacturing and distributing system.

The persistence of such pessimistic thinking is significant to us because similar criticism is directed today against the basic philosophy underlying the American system of medical care, including the field of industrial medicine, which, though far from perfect, has made more progress within a few decades than in all preceding time.

Critics of that kind ignore many factors other than machine production—the social, economic, political and sanitary factors—that contributed to the ills that afflicted British society in the 1800's and are still to be reckoned with in our present highly industrialized civilization. Those critics are likewise prone to underemphasize the sweeping improvements that have come about, and are steadily gathering momentum, in every aspect of both public and industrial health and well being. This rapid progress is the reward of a new kind of teamwork—a pooling of knowledge and plans—by medical, industrial, social, and governmental groups.

When man first harnessed power to serve his needs, he found the golden key that made him master of the earth and its infinite resources. Power *plus* wheels equals land transportation in its many forms. Power *plus* hulls equals dominion over the seas. Power *plus* wings equals travel and transport by air. And power *plus* tools equals the machinery of manufacture.

The invention of practical steam engines in Watt's time represented the first widespread application of mechanical power to replace brawn in doing man's heavy work. Seen in the perspective of the ages, this event looms as a gigantic step in a process that has been going on since man first walked erect in a hostile world.

The consequences of that step are beyond computation. Industry requires, above everything else, the close association of people in large numbers. Association, in turn, draws the line of difference between civilization and savagery. Human contacts have made the world what it is, and have dictated the type of society in which we live. As Collis points out: "The statement may be made that the intelligence of the human race is measured by its industry, and that the *raison d'être* of industry is safety and health. In other words industry is the means human intelligence employs to insure the existence of the race."[2]

History shows that once a civilization commits itself to an economy based on industry, the road must be followed to its end. There can be no turning back, no reversion to any other type of society. This means acceptance in full of the consequences of such a change, including the physical and social ills and problems that invariably accompany it.

Early man could not have had the slightest notion of the mammoth evolution that lay locked in the future. He was engaged in a day-to-day struggle for bare survival against human and animal enemies, cold, starvation, and great convulsions of nature.

Thanks to the reasoning mind that sets him apart from the beasts, man is the only animal to win mastery over, and relative independence from, his environment. His life, from the beginning, has been spent in an endless effort to know his world and conquer it. And his one weapon in this battle has been (and still remains) invention. Thus considered, the invention of power machinery becomes one incident in the onsweep of a tide of scientific inquiry and discovery that had been rising steadily for two centuries or more and was soon to engulf the civilized world.

The important fact is that those first crude engines "triggered" the advent of the Machine Age, much as the first successful internal combustion engines launched the Automobile Age in our century. Steam power also set in motion forces that brought about, or at least greatly accelerated, the so-called Industrial Revolution.

Friedrich Engels is credited with originating the term "industrial revolution," and it was popularized in the English speaking world by Arnold Toynbee. The phrase today is generally regarded as a misnomer. More accurately, the process was a *scientific* revolution—or, more broadly still, a phase of a societal evolution that brought about radical changes not only in industry, but in all the sciences and arts, including medicine.

The Scientific (Industrial) Revolution had its roots in the economic life and commercial expansion of the sixteenth and seventeenth centuries. It gained impetus in England as cotton textile manufacture began to flourish about 1733. It leaped the Atlantic to America late in the same century. It spread to continental Europe, and to Germany in particular, after 1840, expanding rapidly after the Franco-Prussian War.

Of the Scientific Revolution Herbert Butterfield declares: "It outshines everything since the rise of Christianity, and reduces the Renaissance and Reformation to the rank of mere episodes."[3]

The same author warns that we can no longer use the old "periodization" of European history in discussing the Scientific Revolution. He places its origin back even beyond the Sixteenth Century, in the beginnings of a scientific approach that "overthrew the authority" of older science and philosophy.

We can better understand the impact of this gigantic movement upon the lives and destinies of humans if we follow the stages of man's progress from savagery to what we call civilization.

In the beginning there were untold ages of absolute independence and individualism, with every man against every other man in the struggle for survival. Then came forms of rudimentary cooperation, with families and tribes, largely nomadic, wandering together over the continents in a search of friendly climates and sufficient food.

Not until man turned to agriculture do we find anything like settled civilizations and a relatively dependable source of food. This new stability enabled the landed classes to turn to manufacture, trade, and commerce as a means of amassing wealth and securing power.

Each of these major transitions brought about great changes in man's relationship to men. Each saw a lessening of his independence as an individual and a corresponding increase of interdependence within the society of which he was a member. The skyrocketing of industry over the past two hundred and fifty years has speeded up the trend immeasurably. And the world situation today indicates that it has not yet reached its peak.

Slavery was a deeply rooted institution in all ancient civilizations of any importance. Slaves worked the quarries of Egypt and built its pyramids. Slaves dug mineral wealth from Europe's mines at untold cost in misery and human lives. At the height of "the glory that was Greece" Athens boasted some hundred thousand slaves. Life in the Roman Empire followed the same pattern. Slavery, in modified form, persisted through medieval times. Naturally, there was less incentive to invention and industrial development in such societies than among free peoples.

"Before the eighteenth century," Collis observes, "industry as we know it did not exist in England."[4] In much the same way as other nations, Britain had followed a leisurely path of progress—from slave labor (or its equivalent), to domestic production, to handicraft, to simple forms of factory production. For some five-and-a-half centuries there had been no appreciable change in the living conditions of the people.

It was upon this scene of semi-somnolence that the Scientific Revolution suddenly intruded, exploding as if by chain reaction. The speed of invention in England's textile industry is well illustrated by the following chronology in this field: John Kay's fly shuttle, 1733; Wyatt's spinning machine, 1738; Hargreave's spinning jenny, 1765; Arkwright's water frame, 1787; Crompton's mule, 1779; Cartwright's power loom, 1785.

By the end of the eighteenth century, cotton was highly industrialized in England; but, though Watt's steam engine had been on the scene for several years, the use of steam power made slow progress until after 1860. In 1810 only about five thousand steam engines were operating in England and some two hundred in France.[5]

There is an old English proverb to the effect that "the foot of the sheep turns sand into gold." The reference, obviously, is to fertilization of the soil for agricultural use. The sheep also has a fleece of gold, but the industrialization of wool lagged behind that of cotton, not only because of the agricultural tradition, but also because the first crude machines were not well adapted to wool processing.

Nevertheless, the ubiquitous sheep became a factor of some consequence to England's dietary habits and its social revolution. When woolen textiles came into their own, arable land on a large scale was turned into pasture, a process which displaced the residents of villages and materially reduced the production of needed cereal foods.

What we may call a "factory system" of sorts sprang up in Italy in the fifteenth and sixteenth centuries with the manufacture of silk and woolen goods. Cloth, carpet, arms and porcelain industries grew rapidly in sixteenth-century France. And there was a similar progress in Holland and Germany in the production of sugar, gold and silver work, dyes and textiles.[6]

The rapid rise of cotton manufacture in England, before the day of steam power, brought about what is commonly known as the "cottage system" of production, in which one weaver, working at home, usually kept three women busy at their spinning wheels in order to supply him with thread.

Historians have been inclined to paint this period as a sort of golden age, an idyllic prelude to the unspeakable misery and want that followed as the factory system spread across the English and Scottish countryside. It is easy to picture sturdy, well-fed families happily engaged the day long at productive work in their tidy rose-covered cottages. Facts tragically belie the fiction. The cottage was often a hut, with a minimum of comfort. The workers had little or no education; they toiled in semi-darkness and breathed foul air. Drunkenness, depravity, pauperism, squalor—the inevitable companions of ignorance—were common.

As the use of steam power became more and more widespread, the cottage method was replaced by a combined system of home handicraft and factory manufacture under a directing head. Cottage production was not long in disappearing from the British scene as an economic or social factor.

As textile manufacture gained momentum, factories naturally gravitated to areas where labor was cheap and plentiful. There ensued mass migrations of working populations, which marked the real beginning of mechanization in the textile and other industries.

Hard as was the lot of British labor under older regimes, conditions that followed in many factory centers were infinitely worse. It is not for us to discuss in detail the philosophies of conflicting schools of social and economic thought. However, some brief examination of causes and effects is in order, since the merits of the machine are still bitterly debated in our world and our time.

A tremendous literature has been written dealing with the dark and terrible dawn of the Scientific Revolution in England. W. E. H. Lecky paints a picture of conditions in the nineteenth century that is both concise and typical:

The sanitary neglect, the demoralization, the sordid poverty, the acute and ago-nizing want prevailing among great sections of the population of our (British) manufacturing towns during the fifty or sixty years that followed the inventions of Arkwright and Crompton, can hardly be exaggerated. Human nature has seldom shown itself in a more unlovely form than in those crowded and pestilential alleys, in that dark, sulphurous atmosphere.

Transitions from one industry to another, the violent fluctuations of wages and of work, sudden disruptions of old ties and habits and associations, the transfer of thousands of female spinners from their country homes to the crowded factory, the vast masses of ignorance and pauperism that were attracted to the towns by vague prospects of employment, have all led to a misery and demoralization of an extreme character.

The transitions of industry are all painful, but very few transitions have been so much so as in the closing years of the eighteenth century.[7]

In areas where large groups of textile workers were concentrated the whole pe-riod was one of social upheaval. Violence flared. Rioting and sabotage were com-mon. This was the workers' protest against the machine which they regarded as a satanic invention designed to take away their jobs. Those who had work found the conditions of their employment no less intolerable than the sordid surroundings in which they were obliged to live. Hours were long; adjustment to the monotonous routine was difficult for people used to rural and village life.

Sir Thomas Oliver, in his book *Occupations,* points out that a "new kind of fa-tigue" made its appearance in British factories—the result of work in crowded, over-heated, moist and poorly ventilated rooms. It is interesting to note that, even then, the the noise of machinery was a factor to be reckoned with.[8]

Lecky, while detailing the gross social injustices of the period, makes this pointed comment: "Human progress rarely means more than a surplus of advantages over evils."[9] The evils, unfortunately, were an immediate by-product of the Machine Age; only time could demonstrate the advantages. It is not strange that British workers re-garded their unhappy lot as heralding a new slavery to the machine, and not as the birth pains of a new freedom for man.

In 1833 Philip Gaskell, a medical man, observed that the wages of cotton operatives, "with proper economy and forethought, would enable them to live comfortably, nay, in comparative luxury."[10] But who could expect economy and foresight from ignorant, impoverished people unused to anything more than the bare necessities of existence?

Later writers, from a longer perspective of time, have deplored the tendency of some "reform" advocates to blame the profit system for all the ills that have plagued, and continue to plague, modern society. In *Capitalism and the Historians,* F. A. Hayek declares:

There is . . . one supreme myth which more than any other has served to dis-credit the economic system to which we owe our present-day civilization. . . . It is the legend of the deterioration of the working classes in consequence of the rise of "capitalism.". . . The widespread emotional aversion to "capitalism" is closely connected with this belief that the undeniable growth of wealth which the competitive order has produced was purchased at the price of depressing the standard of life of the weakest elements in society.[11]

A few key comments from the same work, describing the condition of workmen in nineteenth-century England, pointedly summarize Hayek's findings:

> Economic suffering both became more conspicuous and seemed less justified, because general wealth was increasing faster than ever before. . . . While there is every evidence that great misery existed, there is none that it was greater or even as great as it was before. . . .
>
> Though the rapid growth of the industrial centers created sanitary problems with which the people had yet slowly and painfully to learn to cope, statistics leave little doubt that even general health was on the whole benefited rather than harmed.

And, later in the same discussion: "The very claims and ambitions of the working classes were and are the result of the enormous improvement of their position which capitalism brought about."[12]

These statements are cited not in justification of the inhumanity that prevailed during those dark years, but merely to point out that such conditions were part and parcel of their times, and were only accentuated by the difficult transition to a machine economy. Humaneness, as a social concept, was conspicuous by its absence; callousness and indifference to the welfare of the masses were the rule.

It may be noted that conditions as bad, or worse, still exist in many parts of the world—and in countries which, while they seek to destroy capitalism, continue to employ, to the limits of their capacity, the latest productive techniques developed by capitalistic societies.

What applies to the general condition of British labor two hundred years ago applies equally to the exploitation of children in the same period. Their story is a blot on English history, as it has been elsewhere. They were recruited in large numbers from London workhouses and other institutions. They were employed at tender ages (seven, eight, and nine years) and for long hours (twelve or more per day) because their labor was readily available, and because it was cheap.

"The greater part of the children," says W. Hunt in his *Political History of England*, "were pauper apprentices bound by parochial authorities to the mill owners; others, the children of very poor or callous parents."[13]

J. L. and B. Hammond, among a multitude of other writers, dwell on the substandard physical condition of young textile workers. They were commonly undersized, undernourished, pallid, listless—easy prey to the diseases associated with poverty and neglect. "These cotton mills," say the Hammonds, "crowded with overworked children, were hotbeds of what was called putrid fever,"[14] which often assumed epidemic proportions. Yet these same writers are careful to point out that

11

child labor was not a discovery of the industrial revolution, but the new industry provided infinite scope for the labor of children, and drove the workmen to rely upon them.

Continued oppression of whole races or classes of people, whatever the source of the tyranny, eventually leads to revolt—to public outcry, and to remedial action of one sort or another. It seems that human society must be driven by disaster, or glaring abuses, to examine itself and set its machinery in balance.

So it was in England. Workmen publicly branded their condition as slavery, and the factories as slaughter houses. The youthful population of Manchester in 1833 was described as "worn out before manhood." Authorities declared that "the average age of the laboring classes was only twenty-two years, as compared with forty-four years among the upper classes."[15]

From the beginning of the nineteenth century the condition of labor was thoroughly aired, both in Parliament and in the literature of the time. There was strong and organized opposition to legislative reforms. There were bitter debates which, beyond doubt, were often colored by political bias, and in which charges and counter-charges unsupported by valid evidence were freely bandied about. The net result was a series of laws, and many amendments, only a few of which were of major importance:

In 1802 the Factory Health and Morals Act, the first act to regulate labor in factories. Among other things it limited apprentices to a twelve-hour day, provided for some education and one suit of clothes per year, and prescribed a form of factory inspection. It is recorded that employers found the inspection "irksome," and that free child labor gradually replaced apprentices from the workhouses.

In 1819 an act limiting the age of employment to nine years or more and providing that no one under sixteen could be worked more than twelve hours a day.

In 1825 an act reducing the work day in textile mills by one and one-half hours and limiting labor to nine hours on Saturdays. Sir Thomas Oliver comments that "to enable some factories to close earlier on Saturday, work had to be begun at five o'clock in the morning."[16]

In 1833 an act prohibiting night work for persons under eighteen years, and broadening the authority of inspectors.

In 1847 an act giving the working classes a basic ten-hour day.

Viewed from our time this legislation—won as it was at great cost in misery and want—seems pathetically primitive and inadequate. And it may be noted that the question of compensation for accident and disease is nowhere raised. There was no compensation. Not until 1901 did England pass her first modern workshop act for the protection of the health of workers.

If there is one lesson above others to be learned from the early years of the Scientific Revolution in England it is that its recorded history must be interpreted with caution. Often ignored is the fact that social progress in any period is limited by the science and culture of its time and that the betterment of mass standards of living has ever been a slow and painful evolution.

It has remained for our century to realize that if discovery and invention are to bear their fruit, social, political and medical planning must advance hand in hand with the progress of industry and production.

II

MILESTONES IN INDUSTRIAL MEDICINE

PROGRESS of the physical sciences since the fifteenth century has been so heavily accented by many historians that achievements in other fields are often overshadowed, and given less than their rightful share of recognition.

Actually, the chain of great discoveries and inventions that harnessed machine power, and changed the face of the globe, was only part of a larger process. The Scientific Revolution, from its very dawn, was marked by an insurgence of new thought in every sphere of human endeavor. Throughout Europe the arts, the sciences, and the crafts flourished as never before.

It was an era in which men of genius in all walks of life shook their minds clear of dogmas of the past and embarked on uncharted paths. And while physicists, chemists, and engineers were constructing a new material world and a new type of society, other men of like stature were revolutionizing medicine by equally significant discoveries.

A simple listing of important milestones in medical history indicates how tremendous was the progress in knowledge of the human body, and of the diseases to which it is subject, during this amazing period of liberation from ancient thinking.

Paracelsus (1493–1541) defied the authorities who had been followed blindly up to his time. He made firsthand studies of the Tyrolese miners; described minutely the diseases of foundry and smelter workers, caused by inhaling metallic fumes; and greatly advanced pharmacy by the introduction of chemicals in the treatment of disease. His independence of thought was perhaps of more moment than his observations on disease and curative medicine.

Georg Agricola (1494–1555), German scholar and scientist, is generally regarded as the founder of modern minerology. His *De re metallica,* a classic on mining and metallurgy, was translated from the Latin by Herbert and Mrs. Hoover in 1912.

Vesalius (1514–1564), a brilliant Flemish doctor, pioneered under the most difficult conditions imaginable in exploring the mysteries of human anatomy. His work in dissection laid bare secrets unknown to anyone up to his time, and by teaching his pupils to dissect he laid the groundwork for a modern approach to the study of anatomy. While his views were greeted by derision on every hand, time has made his fame secure. The anatomical sketches which illustrate existing editions of his *De fabrica humani corporis* (1543) are marvels of completeness and accuracy, considering the period in which they were made.

William Harvey (1578–1657) demonstrated the circulation of the blood and the functions of the heart in its movement. His findings, detailed in a series of lectures in 1616, were both revolutionary and conclusive. The work of this distinguished English physician is considered to have had a greater influence on medicine than that of any other man of this time except Vesalius.

Thomas Sydenham (1624–1689), a London practitioner, preached throughout his career a return to the Hippocratic idea that observation should take precedence over theory. "Study the patient!" was the essence of his message. Noted for his discussions of epidemic and endemic diseases, Sydenham has justly been called the founder of modern clinical medicine.

Bernardino Ramazzini (1633–1714), universally accepted as the father of industrial medicine, was the first to recognize the importance of occupations in the etiology of disease. A worshiper of Hippocrates, whom he called "our inspired teacher," he invariably asked of a patient "what occupation does he follow?"[1] It is safe to say that few if any industrial physicians or surgeons of today have not been influenced to some degree by Ramazzini's thinking and writings.

G. Morgagni (1682–1771) was an intimate friend, follower, and biographer of Ramazzini. He followed up the work of the master by demonstrating the relation of symptoms to pathological changes in the body, and was beyond doubt the greatest pathological anatomist of his period.

Herman Boerhaave (1668–1738), eminent Dutch physician, for many years taught medicine at the bedside of his patients in Leyden. His methods, closely followed by others of his school, set the pattern for modern clinical diagnosis, and, in essence, are part of the basic training of medical students in the hospitals of our day.

John Hunter (1728–1793) made surgery an experimental science, realizing that its scope could be broadened and its techniques improved only through continued practice by bold but competent men. This was his sage advice to surgeons of his time: "Don't think, try; be patient, be accurate."

Edward Jenner (1749–1823) demonstrated the prevention of smallpox by vaccination, and thus launched the first practical work in immunizing human and animal bodies against disease, by inoculation.

Crawford W. Long (1815–1878), an American physician, in 1842 removed a small tumor from the neck of a patient under the influence of ether, after noting accidentally the anesthetic effects of the drug. Two years later another American, William Thomas Green Morton (1819–1868), successfully used ether in filling a tooth, and published the results of his experiment before Long's work became widely known. In October, 1846, two historic surgical operations performed in Massachusetts General Hospital at Morton's behest confirmed the success of ether anesthesia, and established his fame as its co-discoverer.

Rudolf Virchow (1821–1902), a German physician and lecturer, conducted brilliant studies in the pathology of tissues. He was one of the leading pathologists of his time, and his work in sanitation and epidemic control contributed significantly to the world's knowledge of those fields.

Louis Pasteur (1822–1895) revolutionized the science of bacteriology through his discovery that many human and animal diseases were the result of bacterial infection. He developed the method of inoculation with a weak culture of bacteria, which induced a mild attack of the disease and left the subject immune. His work in the control of cattle anthrax, chicken cholera, rabies, and other diseases armed modern preventive medicine with one of its most potent weapons. Pasteur is regarded by many as the greatest of them all.

Joseph Lister (1827–1912) was the founder of antiseptic surgery. A student of Pasteur, he noted the high death rate from surgical complications due to infection of various types. His use of carbolic acid and other antiseptic agents amply demonstrated the soundness of his theories, from which today's aseptic surgery has evolved.

Robert Koch (1843–1910) stands beside Pasteur as a towering figure in the field of bacteriology. He isolated the bacillus of anthrax in 1876 and the tubercle bacillus in 1882. Modern progress in the conquest of tuberculosis and other communicable diseases has been largely shaped by his findings.

So, in many countries and over a period of four busy centuries, men of genius have led the search for medical truth. Scores of major discoveries and a host of distinguished figures in research have been omitted from the chronology, since this cannot be a history of medicine or a discussion of its technical aspects.

Nevertheless, this brief and arbitrary listing serves to emphasize the reluctance with which Nature gives up her secrets—the slowness of the pace at which man proceeds from the unknown to the known. Science must work that way, each period leaning upon the period before, adding its own bit of hard-won new knowledge and passing the aggregate along as an heritage for the future.

The progress of medicine throughout the Scientific Revolution paralleled exactly the progress of the physical sciences. Both followed the same methodology, using observation as the springboard to conjecture and insisting on proof to establish the validity of their findings.

Vesalius was close upon the heels of that lonely genius of a dozen arts and

16

sciences, Leonardo da Vinci, whose work in military engineering, hydraulics, architecture, and even aeronautics, places him far, far ahead of his time. It has been said that his was the "greatest of all brains."

While Harvey, in England, was demonstrating the circulation of the blood, Galileo in Italy abandoned the teachings of his idol, Aristotle, espoused the Copernican theory of the universe, and conducted gravitational experiments with falling objects. He faced the Inquisition for his heresies.

"Aristotle," says the psychologist Kurt Lewin, "was concerned with the properties of stones; Galileo, on the contrary, concerned himself with the relations of stones to environment."[2] A modern concept, as applicable to medicine as it is to physics.

In the Renaissance Sir Francis Bacon, one of the most learned men of his time, preached his basic creed: "Go to nature, study it first hand." His approach was characteristic of the scientific spirit of his age; it inspired countless men to inquire, discover, demonstrate, invent.

Contemporary with Sydenham, Ramazzini, and Morgagni in the field of medicine was Sir Isaac Newton. In the world of physics he has been called the greatest universal genius the world has ever produced. Roughly a century after Galileo's experiments he propounded his law of gravitation: in turn, our own century has seen the overthrow of much of Newton's physics.

So the parallel march of the sciences continued into the eighteenth century, which saw Hunter and Jenner blaze new trails in medicine, while Watt and a galaxy of engineering geniuses raised the curtain on the machine age in Britain. There is, however, one great and basic difference between the problems and procedures of the physical scientist and those of the medical pioneer. It should not be overlooked.

Mechanical invention, as a rule, moves in a relatively straight line to its objectives —from an understanding of certain fundamental principles, through a period of experiment, to construction of a machine, an instrument, or a "gadget." The inventor can build, tear down, correct his mistakes, make model after model until he gets one that will work.

Watt's first practical engine at best was crude, inefficient, uncomplicated. Were it on display at a museum today it would be viewed with amused tolerance. The same is true of the prototypes of the printing press, telegraph, telephone, automobile, radio, airplane. These arrived at their present perfection, and complexity, by a long process of slow, patient improvement. We wonder whether Watt or Stephenson, given the completely disassembled parts of a modern locomotive weighing hundreds of tons, could put it together again and make it run.

The human body stands in awesome contrast to these man-made contrivances. It is and ever has been the most intricate, most delicately balanced, most mysterious of machines. Man can "disassemble" the human machine, at the cost of life itself. He cannot reassemble it, cannot start it again after it has stopped running, cannot build or replace the simplest of its vital parts. Man can only patch and repair the human body: nurse it, feed it the fuel that keeps it going, counteract by medicine and surgery some of its ailments, and leave the rest to Nature. For all our knowledge of its structure and the elements of which it is made, there is much more that we do not know about the "whys" and "hows" of the body's functioning.

Human bodies, basically, have been as they are since the beginning of recorded history. The earliest physicians faced much the same enigma of disease and maladjustment that we face today, but without benefit of any but primitive science and in almost total ignorance of the processes of life and death.

The marvel is not that medicine has progressed so slowly, but that it has accomplished so much in a span of centuries which are but drops in the bucket of time.

Disease, on our planet, appears to be as old as life itself. Science tells us this, and offers evidence from geological formations so ancient that their age until very recently, could often be estimated only in round millions, or tens of millions, of years.

By the magic of microscope and test tube, science discloses that even the most primitive living organisms, struggling instinctively to survive and multiply, were hosts to other organisms which destroyed life that they, too, might live. Life preyed upon life then, as it does today.

The great medical historian, Henry E. Sigerist, mentions the presumptive existence of periostitis, osteitis, and osteomyelitis in very ancient times. He finds some evidence of tumors and sarcoma, but declares it is not conclusive, and remarks that even now, eons later, we do not know all there is to know about the etiology of cancer.[3]

Primitive man must have learned his primitive medicine by watching Nature at work. Arthur Selwyn-Brown notes that what animals, when ill, did by instinct, men were quick to adopt as good medical practice. By way of illustration he quotes this paragraph from Cornelius Agrippa:

"The sick magpie puts a bay leaf into her nest and is recovered. The lion, if he is feverish, is recovered by the eating of an ape. By eating the herb dittany, a wounded stag, or goat, expels the dart out of its body. Cranes medicate themselves with bulrushes, leopards with wolf's bane, boars with ivy; for between such plants and animals there is an occult friendship."[4]

Early man could observe, but he could not explain. And what he could not explain he naturally attributed to evil spirits or angry gods. Remnants of these ancient superstitions and beliefs have persisted down to modern times in witchcraft, the "hex" and the evil eye, hypnotic power, the divining rod, alchemy, voodoo, dream books, astrology, and many more.

"The medical errors of one century constitute the popular faith of the next," said Dr. Alonzo Clark. And science has discovered more than one grain of medical truth in old folk lore. A brew containing foxglove was used in treating dropsy long before an English physician, in 1785, discovered the essential ingredient—digitalis.

Cobwebs were applied to wounds, for no demonstrable reason. Then, one day, came penicillin.

Few medical men, in the early part of the new scientific age, gave much attention to occupational diseases as such. The reasons are not hard to find. Not only was the body an almost unexplored continent, but industry on a large scale did not exist, and the diseases associated with it were a negligible factor in society as a whole.

Says Sigerist: "We must not forget . . . that ancient technology was mostly small-scale technology. The artisans frequently worked in the open air, as they still do in the Orient, so that hazards were infinitely less than in later centuries after technology had assumed larger proportions."[5]

The first printed thesis dealing with occupational health, of which we have record, was written by Ulrich Ellenbog, a fifteenth-century doctor of medicine. It dealt with "poisons and the evil vapors of smoke and of metals, such as silver, quicksilver, lead, and others which the worthy trade of the goldsmith and other workers were compelled to use. How they should conduct themselves concerning these matters and how to dispel the poison."[6]

This work is of more interest as a literary curiosity than as a medical treatise. Only two copies of the text are extant, one in the University Library at Munich, the other in the library of Dr. Alfred H. Whittaker, of Detroit.

The great Ramazzini was the first physician in history to take as his province a specialized study of industry and its diseases, with the aim of protecting the worker from the hazards of his trade. In his master work, *De morbis artificum,* he recognizes and describes in detail the diseases of some forty types of tradesmen, among them miners, gilders, potters, painters, glass blowers, chemists, metal workers, cleaners of privies and cesspits. Anent the last named, he quotes Hippocrates: "For a doctor must inspect the unseemly and handle the horrible."

In the dedication of his work, Ramazzini modestly explained its purpose as follows: "I believed it would benefit the commonwealth of mankind if I should examine carefully the special diseases of workers and prescribe suitable remedies, a task that no one had undertaken hitherto."[7]

That the master recognized the limitations of his own science is evidenced in this passage: "So many and so inexplicable are the mixtures of metals confined in the bowels of the earth that it is almost impossible to determine precisely what injurious element is present in this or that mine and how it is that one part rather than another is affected."[8]

Dr. Robert T. Legge, one of the founders of the Industrial Medical Association and an authority on Ramazzini, quotes from *De morbis artificum:* " 'It is but a poor profit which is achieved by the destruction of health.' " Commenting, Legge continues: "What a satisfaction fate has bestowed upon our calling by applying our science and skills to the humanizing of industry. Labor and capital both profit, the span of life has been increased, and wealth and happiness have been amplified for the world's workers. Thus Ramazzini's challenge has been proudly met."[9] His fame rests solidly upon his attitude toward the health and well being of the worker rather than upon the value of the remedies he prescribes.

While Ramazzini was endowed with the curiosity and imagination that mark the true scientist, he was little influenced by Galileo, Bacon, and Harvey, who preceded him. He clung, rather, to the scholasticism of Hippocrates. How, we wonder, would his nimble mind have reacted to the discoveries of Boerhaave, Jenner, Virchow, Pasteur, and Koch, who were to follow him?

General medicine, it may be said, advanced spasmodically during the eighteenth and nineteenth centuries in Europe and elsewhere. Each great basic discovery was greeted by feverish interest and activity, followed by comparative lulls while the profession consolidated its gains and awaited new scientific light from the fresh discoveries which punctuated those centuries.

Naturally, the greatest emphasis was upon diseases that menaced the public health, rather than on those of specifically industrial or occupational origin. Man's most devastating enemies were cholera, yellow fever, smallpox, malaria, tuberculosis, and the other great plagues that scourged big cities and sometimes decimated populations. Upon such enemies science turned its heaviest guns.

Malaria was well known in ancient Greece, but it did not receive what may be its *coup de grace* until World War II. Tuberculosis, also of distant origin, is still a major target in the war on disease. Despite Jenner and vaccination, smallpox was a foe to be reckoned with in this country well into the twentieth century.

According to Dr. Legge, a tick the bite of which induced relapsing fever was found in Africa by David Livingston in 1837, and the infective organism was discovered in 1868, yet Legge himself cast an entirely new light on the etiology of this disease as late as 1933.[10]

These examples are cited as illustrations of the costly and destructive time lag that invariably occurs between the acquisition of new knowledge and its application on a broad scale for the betterment of society. The chief problem of organized medicine, even today, is how to bring a larger fraction of its benefits to a larger fraction of the people.

New legislation in the interest of public health was passed periodically in Britain in the eighteenth and nineteenth centuries. It was a step in the right direction, but by our standards was pitifully inadequate. Basic improvement of public health had to await not only a more modern concept of sanitation and hygiene, but also a will on the part of society to purge itself of the filth and squalor in which disease breeds and flourishes.

There are those who blandly blame industrialization for all or most of the ills that afflicted Britain in the flowering years of the Scientific Revolution; we have the counterpart of such pessimists among critics of our present industrial system in America. Their conclusions are hard to justify.

Actually, it is impossible to measure accurately the direct effect of mechanization on general health in England during that revolution. Statistics are fragmentary and unreliable. And there were many other factors that influenced mortality and morbidity, among them the rapid growth of population, major shifts of workers to towns and cities, and the lack of ordinary sanitary safeguards.

Conditions as bad or worse have characterized big cities in every country and every age, and industry could not be blamed for them, because there was no industry of any consequence.

Nevertheless, where we have industry we have large concentrations of people; and where we have these we have overcrowding, with its inseparable companions—poverty, squalor, disease. So it was in England, as families migrated in large numbers to new centers of manufacture in search of work and higher wages.

Writing of this, Collis declares: "Industry, apart from agriculture, had no appreciable influence upon the health of the nation, and England down to the beginning of the eighteenth century was overwhelmingly, and as late as 1770 mainly, devoted to agriculture."[11]

In a letter to the English poet Southey in 1816, one John Rickman commented: "Human comfort is to be estimated by human health, and that by the length of human life. Since 1780 life has been prolonged by five to four—and the poor are too large a portion of society to be excluded from this effect; rather, they are the main cause of it; for the upper classes had food and cleanliness abundant before."[12]

As British manufacture grew, in volume and in concentration, it naturally brought about a steady increase in diseases directly traceable to occupation. Of these, some were old familiar enemies; but many other hazards, new at least to English industry, made their appearance. As a result, more and more doctors and scientists turned their attention to the study of causes, effects, and possible remedies.

Poisoning by lead and other metals offers a good example of ancient occupational maladies that have plagued mankind through the ages. Ramazzini and his followers wrote exhaustively on this subject. Early students, however, were hopelessly handicapped by a lack of basic knowledge of tissue structures, and of opportunity for first-hand analysis.

Dissection, a *sine qua non* in pathological research, was often forbidden by religious taboos. Denied this tool, the student could go little beyond conjecture, and until the bans were lifted there could be no modern pathology.

Galen tells of finding a robber's body, picked by birds of prey, and says: "As regards yourself, even if you do not have the luck to see anything like this, still you can dissect an ape, and learn each of the bones from it, by carefully removing the flesh."[13]

Centuries later, in a far more enlightened era, we find a thriving black market in cadavers in Edinburgh, Scotland. And in America, in the late 1800's, a body stolen from a Detroit cemetery was found in the Michigan College of Medicine.

Not everywhere nor always, however, was the gate to knowledge barred by prejudice. In France, between 1831 and 1841, Tanquerel des Planches made brilliant contributions to the literature on lead. He shared the spotlight with other lesser figures—Chevreul, Devergie, Orifla, Merat, Grissoli, and Dehaen.

Of Tanquerel, Dr. Legge makes particular note that in Tanquerel's etiological studies "he made numerous experiments on animals and performed many autopsies on deceased patients who had succumbed to lead disease."[14]

In England Sir George Baker (1722–1809) relied on a keen clinical knowledge of disease, as well as the shrewd deductions of a trained scientist, in solving the famous mystery of the Devonshire Colic, which he traced to leaden joints in the troughs through which cider flowed.

John A. Paris (1785–1856), a Cambridge physician, found horses and cows suffering from "cancerous infections" after grazing near copper melting works and rightly ascribed their condition to arsenical fumes. Paris green was so named in his honor. He also investigated the tin mines of Cornwall, and invented a safety bar to prevent the premature explosion of blasting powder.

In his monumental work, *Occupations,* Sir Thomas Oliver tells of ducks para-lyzed in the polluted waters of a pond near a zinc and lead smeltery, of animals killed by lead and arsenic deposited on their pasturage, of cattle dying of anthrax beside a woolen factory.[15]

Sir Thomas, however, declares: "The greatest enemy of a worker in any trade is dust."[16] His work covers skin, eye, nose and throat infections, tuberculosis, and carbon dioxide and other direct poisons from manufacturing processes.

According to K. Neville Moss, English scientists have been concerned with the physics, chemistry, and physiology of mining since the sixteenth century. He finds a reference to choke damp in shallow coal pits as early as 1550, and notes that miners waved cloths or jackets to blow it out.[17]

In Agricola's time, deaths from such gases were attributed to "a blast of breath from a subterranean demon." In seventeenth-century England they were recognized for what they were, but safety measures remained primitive. To rid a mine of ex-plosive fire damp, a miner soaked his clothing, crawled into the pit, raised a lighted candle on a pole to burn off the gas. This hazardous process was still carried on in a few mines as late as 1847, thirty years after the introduction of Davy's safety lamp.[18]

A towering figure in England in the latter part of the nineteenth century was Sir Thomas Morison Legge. An authority on public health, he served as secretary of the Royal Commission on Tuberculosis and as senior medical inspector of factories and workshops. His contributions to the literature of lead, arsenic, and mercurial poisoning; occupational diseases of the nose, mouth, and throat; anthrax and glass blowers' cataract, were many and significant.[19]

These are but a few in a long list of greats who laid the foundation of modern industrial medicine in eighteenth-century England. They were the living spirit of the Scientific Revolution. Their work is important to us because the spark that kindled it leaped the Atlantic to inspire an age of even greater accomplishment in both in-dustry and medicine.

Bringing the picture closer to our time, Oliver declares: "There is not the least doubt that social welfare of the workers has not received in our country [England] the attention it has received on the other side of the Atlantic."[20] He also comments: "In large iron works, and in collieries and large textile factories there should be a small hospital with two or three beds. At one of the collieries close to Newcastle there is such a building. It has to my knowledge served a useful end and been the means of averting much suffering, if not saving life."[21]

The idea seems rather rudimentary, in view of the time of its publication (1916); but the fact remains that our own progress in the same direction was almost equally tardy up to that date—which, by chance, marks the greatest of all milestones in the history of American industrial medicine.

III

INDUSTRY IN THE NEW WORLD

Migration to America in the seventeenth century may fairly be considered an offshoot of the Scientific Revolution. Notably in New England and Pennsylvania, the early colonists came in quest of political, religious, and economic freedom. Their revolt was one more step in a long-drawn struggle against the harsh authority of church and state that had held Europe in subjection during medieval times.

It was an English tradition and an English civilization that the early settlers brought to the new land. With the exception of the Dutch, who ruled briefly in Manhattan and along the Hudson, they were almost wholly of British origin. In fact, of 2,600,000 inhabitants of the thirteen colonies in 1776, an overwhelming majority were Englishmen, with Scotch and Irish next in numbers.

Life in the colonies was naturally shaped by this British heritage. Laws were English; customs, crafts and culture followed the pattern of society in the homeland. These influences persisted through a century and a half of British rule and far beyond; it left an indelible mark upon American place names, architecture, laws, morals, institutions, and industries.

Scientists were few, indeed, among those first immigrants. There was little or nothing for science to do. Food, shelter, and safety were a first consideration. The need was for farmers, tradesmen, artisans in many crafts. Industry, even in the English sense, did not exist; the colonists were without capital, without machinery, without many basic materials needed in manufacture.

The first settlements were but toeholds on a rugged and inhospitable coast. Behind them lay a dark continent; the colonists could not even have guessed its true extent, or dreamed of the wealth in natural resources it contained. The story of its conquest is a saga without parallel in history.

Importation, even of tools and household goods, was rigorously restricted in that early period by distance, cost, and lack of cargo space. The settlers, of necessity, hewed their own lumber, fashioned their own nails, built their own homes and much of their furniture, spun their own cloth and made their clothing.

Nevertheless, the pioneers brought with them from England the spirit and outlook of the new scientific age—its freedom of thought and action, its resourcefulness and inventive genius. Once the hardships of bare existence had been overcome, cities and towns flourished, governments were stabilized, populations moved slowly inland, and industries sprouted with amazing speed.

Agricultural products, for both consumption and export, were the mainstay of the colonial economy and were to remain so down to modern times. Yet the agriculture of that period was primitive: methods were slovenly, implements crude. Farming, like other industry, had to wait upon invention before it could attain its full stature.

"The agricultural methods of the seventeenth century," says W. E. Woodward, "were almost precisely the same as those of the seventh century. For a thousand years—or, better, two thousand—there had been no improvement of any importance in the cultivation of the soil. The modern plow, the reaper, the mechanical thresher, the cotton gin—all these originated in the nineteenth century."[1]

In New England the first colonists found the climate severe in winter, the soil stony and infertile, but they were used to poverty and content to win a fairly comfortable existence from the soil. Timber was abundant, and the crafts were well represented by skilled cabinet makers, joiners, weavers, potters, sawyers, carpenters, shipwrights, coopers, tanners, iron workers and edge-toolmakers.

Much of the unskilled labor in all the northern colonies was performed by indentured servants, bound to their masters for long terms to work out the cost of their passage to America. By contrast, slavery thrived in New York for more than a century. It is recorded that nearly one-fifth of New York's 13,000 inhabitants in 1750 were Negro slaves.

In matters of administration, the Puritans were hard taskmasters. Themselves austere, deeply religious, dissenters, they sought to regulate every detail of life for the governed. The Puritan code made fetishes of hard work and piety and imposed severe penalties on idleness and frivolity. It is strange that men, once they have fled one form of intolerance, should so meekly submit to another.

Class distinctions were sharply marked among the people in their new land. It was a Puritan leader, John Cotton, who wrote in 1636: "Democracy I do not conceive that ever God did ordain as a fit government either for church or commonwealth. If the people be governor who shall become governed? As for monarchy and aristocracy, they are both of them clearly approved and directed in scripture."[2] This, in a country that was so soon to become the standard bearer of democracy for the entire world!

For its young men, early New England offered almost nothing in the way of intellectual careers except in schoolteaching and the ministry. Lawyers were social pariahs. Doctors were few and far between, and medical practices were at least as backward as in England during the same period. In this spacious land, with little or no industry, the diseases associated with overcrowding, squalor, and poverty were, obviously, absent.

Typical of the primitive *materia medica* of the time was the standard treatment for diphtheria, then known as "throat distemper." Poultices of pepper, mustard, and bark of the elder tree, pounded into a paste, were applied to the necks of children; and these were supplemented with copious draughts of "snail water," a nauseous compound of snails and earthworms, ground and boiled with garden vegetables.[3] A favorite remedy, in this era, for measles or any other common ailment of children was "Venice treacle," an equally repulsive nostrum made by boiling the pounded bodies of snakes with white wine and a mixture of twenty herbs—and adding a small amount of opium.[4]

Writing of this period, Woodward mentions that there were no physicians in Sudbury, and since the nearest apothecary was in Boston, all girls were trained before marriage to make "palsey drops, mithridate, Venice treacle, snail water and poke-berry plaster, besides a long list of other salves and potions."[5] Every wife her own doctor—an economical, if somewhat precarious, arrangement.

On the whole they got along well, these Puritans, by dint of hard work and largesse of the soil and sea. Handicrafts flourished; artisans who had labored for journeymen's wages in England learned that they could make substantial profits by selling the products of their family enterprises to new settlers, or by exporting them to the mother country.

Shipbuilding started early in heavily forested New England, and spread quickly along the coast. The colonists built hulls for a substantial intercolonial and overseas trade. They exported skins, furs, lumber and other products, and brought back manufactured goods from England for their own use.

In Virginia and the other southern colonies, wealth was centered almost entirely in the hands of a landed aristocracy. The Virginians were planters by nature and training, and with an entrenched system of slave labor they were content to grow tobacco on a large scale, and leave manufacturing to others. Tobacco found a ready market abroad; despite violent fluctuations in price, its culture brought wealth to the growers, and gave them the means of importing clothing and luxuries of all sorts from the homeland.

From the very beginning of emigration to the colonies, England saw the value of the New World as a market for British products and as a source of raw materials. Its rulers shrewdly sought to shape trade in both directions to their own advantage— determined that the settlers should buy goods of British manufacture and should not compete with the mother country in world markets.

In the 1650's the English government imposed heavy export duties on woolen broadcloth and forbade entirely the exportation of sheep, wool and woolen yarns from England.[6] In the Navigation Act of 1660, the British listed products which could be exported only to England by the colonies. These included sugar, tobacco, cotton wool, indigo, and dye woods.

Such oppressive measures were typical of the economic clamps which England continued to tighten upon the vigorous young colonies for more than a century of its rule. They led, as everyone knows, to Revolution—and Liberty.

It is remarkable that a people representing many ethnic strains, many diverse political and religious faiths could ever agree upon and vote into effect two such amazing documents as the Declaration of Independence and the Constitution of the United States. But they did unite—aristocrats and commoners, Whigs and Tories, intellectuals and illiterates, Puritans in New England, Dutch in New York, Quakers and Germans in Pennsylvania, men of a dozen sects and denominations. They had one thing in common: the vision of freedom and unlimited opportunity that seeped through to them from the awesome expanse of land at their backs.

Under the Treaty of Paris the United States came into possession of something more than 800,000 square miles of territory, roughly bounded by the Canadian border on the north, Florida on the south, and the Mississippi on the west. In 1803–05, acquisition of the Louisiana and Oregon territories more than doubled these holdings, and by 1867 the new nation stretched from coast to coast, and south to Mexico. With Alaska, it was more than four times its original area.[7]

A fabulous land, this America, fabulous beyond imagining, with climates ranging from temperate to sub-tropical. Thousands of miles of coast, pitted by natural, ice-free ports. Great rivers and the largest body of inland fresh water in the world. Endless forests and giant watersheds. Towering mountains and vast plains teeming with game. Areas of heavy rainfall and/or arid desert. Its store of mineral and other natural resources is still beyond accurate estimate. Gold, silver, uranium, lead, zinc, copper, aluminum, iron, cement, sulphur, coal, oil, gas. Soil favorable to growing almost any agricultural crop that can be named. Never, anywhere, has such treasure trove been laid at the feet of any people.

At the end of the Revolutionary War, cotton had not yet come into its own. It was indigenous to the southern states; its culture was easy; and it was planted on a moderate scale in the early 1600's. But the problem of cleaning cotton seemed insurmountable. One slave, working an entire day, could pick the seeds from only five pounds. Even with free labor it was impossible to process large crops and make them pay.

Then came a Connecticut lad to visit friends on a Georgia plantation. He listened to talk of tobacco and cotton, and idly plucked the lint from a handful of cotton bolls. It is said that within a week he had built a small cotton gin, "not much bigger'n a hat box," to do the work mechanically. Eli Whitney's first crude model enabled one man to clean fifty pounds of cotton in a day.[8] It was the first notable invention to appear in colonial America.

England, zealously fostering its infant textile industries, lacked cotton, but looked to India rather than to America for its supply. Whitney's invention, in 1793, had earth-shaking consequences. Cotton soon supplanted tobacco as the main money crop of the south. Despite patents, blacksmiths copied Whitney's designs and built cotton gins at their forges to meet the demand.

The colonies, on the other hand, lacked machinery for spinning and weaving. The English, fighting American competition to the last ditch, used every means to block the use of spinning machinery on this side of the Atlantic. In a series of Parliamentary acts they prohibited the export of all engines, tools, machines, parts, and even designs, which could be utilized for textile manufacture. Penalties were severe; supervision was rigid.[9]

These acts applied not only to the early inventions of Hargreaves and Arkwright but also to Cartwright's power loom, invented in 1785. Smuggle, or invent. That was the challenge to the colonies. Samuel Slater, an English textile expert, chose the first course. In 1789 he embarked for America, carrying in his head a mass of design details of English equipment. A year later, he and Moses Brown, of Providence, Rhode Island, started the first American textile mill, with machinery built from memory. Slater has gone down in history as "the father of American cotton manufacture." He can rightly be called the father of American industry, since the production methods he introduced set the pattern for manufacture in many other fields.

Steam power came to America almost as early as it did to England. Steam freed the colonies from dependence on water power. It started the development of vast iron resources. No longer did the new country need to smuggle either ideas or machinery. Yankee inventive genius, released in a treasure house of raw materials, eagerly set about the conquest of distance, and the conversion of natural wealth into useful products.

Our people looked at their new country as a land of boundless opportunity, a vast empire to be taken by the bold and venturesome. They were descended from men who had been hungry and ill clad. They were driven by idealism of a sort, and they recognized religious dicipline. But they had tasted political freedom—and the urge to acquisition was strong in them. In the machine, these men saw the means of multiplying production, reducing labor and cost. They were followers of Franklin and others who exemplified the spirit of the new age. In their eyes the business of life was the business of applying the results of science to their use and profit. That persisting viewpoint has brought into being our present trade and commerce, our industry, and our medicine.

So the Machine Age came to America. Distance and transportation were, in the last analysis, the chief barriers to its progress. Until freed from dependence on stage coach and barge, men could tap only a tiny fraction of the wealth of mines, forests, or fields; and in a land so immense, the pace of conquest was necessarily slow.

Jefferson, while President, declared it would be a thousand years before the great northwest could be settled. But he could not foresee the coming of the railroads or any of the other great inventions that were irrevocably to mechanize America's economy. Railroads were the key to westward expansion. Their routes were to determine the movements of population, its concentration in great cities-to-be, the living conditions of masses of workers. And those factors, in turn, were to create the first real need for industrial health care as a phase of medicine.

Practical locomotives were built in America as early as 1804, but in 1830 only twenty-three miles of railroad were in operation. In the next ten years, 9,000 miles of track were laid, and by 1860, the mileage had jumped to 30,000—with the great Pacific lines still to come.

At the close of the Civil War, with a million men returning to peaceful occupations, the need for opening up new land became acute. Writing of that period, Matthew Josephson comments on "the immensity of the tasks to be done, the new machinery to be created—banks, mines, furnaces, shops, powerhouses—if the new Americans were to make their continent habitable."[10]

"They had no time for thought," says Henry Adams, "save for that single fraction called a railway system. . . . The generation between 1865 and 1895 was already mortgaged to the railways and no one knew it better than the generation itself."[11]

The quickest way to settle a continent was to dangle the incentive of profit before the people. Lincoln's Homestead Act resulted in enormous grants of land for railroad rights of way, along with stone and timber grants, and huge cash subsidies. America went railroad-mad, and in the van of the movement a group of shrewd men, driving rail lines through the sparsely populated west, netted huge fortunes by their manipulations. This was the real dawn of our capitalistic age, in a nation not yet a hundred years old.

Still remembered by the people of America was the pronouncement of President Jefferson that little was needed for happiness and prosperity beyond "a wise and frugal government which shall restrain men from injuring one another, which shall leave them otherwise free to regulate their own pursuits of industry and improvement, and shall not take from the mouth of labor the bread it has earned. This is the sum of good government, and this is needed to close the circle of our felicities."

Long before the coming of the railroads, the eyes of all America had turned to the west and the undiscovered wealth of plains, forests, and mineral deposits. Each year had seen frontiers pushed deeper and deeper into the wilderness. The discovery of gold in California touched off a stampede to the coast. The inpouring of the Forty-Niners soon made a shambles of San Francisco and other quiet towns, and where there were no towns, new shambles sprang up overnight.

When Drake tapped oil in Pennsylvania in 1859, the scene was repeated, though the chief market then, and for nearly a half-century afterward, was for illuminating oils and naphtha. Even the most visionary of promoters could not have foreseen the part that petroleum products were to play in the world economy of our time.

That half-century was an era of unbridled exploitation of natural resources of all kinds—silver and gold in Nevada, Colorado and Montana; iron in Pennsylvania and New York; copper in Michigan; great stands of timber in the north and west.

We have seen later parallels in the twentieth century scramble for oil and for uranium and other vitally needed minerals.

The Civil War, probably the most terrible of tragedies in American history, brought urgent demands for raw materials and manufactured products in vast quantities. Sadly, it also invited speculation, which sent prices soaring and fattened the purses of those manipulators who could, and would, exploit the national crisis for private gain.

The Bessemer process, developed in 1859, gave tremendous impetus to industry of every type. During the war and in the decades that followed, the cry was for coal, steel, oil, lumber, machinery—for more and still more of everything that could contribute to agricultural and industrial expansion.

"In this 'War Between the States,'" says Josephson,

all the fullest energies of the long-retarded industrial revolution were liberated. Whether it sensed it or not, the war party headed by Lincoln hastened miraculously a transfer of power to the emergent groups of large-scale capitalism. Under Lincoln, after the Homestead Act, began the distribution of the public domain, which the federal government owned, in favor of its citizenry of free farmers and artisans; half the present area of the United States, or a billion acres of land, with all its subsoil. In a hurried partition, for nominal sums or by cession, this benevolent government handed over to its friends or to the astute first comers, the daring undertakers, all those treasures of coal and oil, of copper and gold and iron, the land grants, the terminal sites, the perpetual rights of way—an act of largesse which is still one of the wonders of history.[12]

In this land, freedom had room in which to grow, unhampered. Its people had never known rule by feudal lords, by prelates of the church, or by armies. Land was to be had almost for the asking. There was little or no governmental control over business. Wealth came easily to those who were bold and clever enough to take it. It is not strange that the public should look with complaisance, and some admiration, upon the operations of conniving politicians and newly made capitalists. From liberty to license is, after all, only a step.

Above all other needs, in this period of expansion, was the need for population. The young republic could not hope, by birth rate alone, to produce the workers necessary for a gigantic development. Immigration was the answer. In 1820, the first year for which statistics are available, something over 8,000 foreigners entered the country. Between 1840 and 1854 the incoming tide rose to nearly 350,000 annually. Still, the need was not met.

The Statue of Liberty, gift of the French people on the centennial anniversary of America, became not only the symbol of freedom but also a voice of welcome to the workers of the Old World. Standing with its back to the land of plenty, it sent its invitation out across the Atlantic:

Give me your tired, your poor, your huddled
masses yearning to breathe free. . . .

The population of continental United States passed the fifty million mark in 1880. Up to that time immigration had been chiefly from northern and western Europe: the British Isles, Germany and the Scandinavian countries, whose ethnological backgrounds were similar to those of colonial America. "The old immigration," it has been called.

Suddenly the trend shifted. From 1881 to 1890 newcomers of Slavic, Italian, and Oriental origin poured in from southern and eastern Europe at an annual rate of more than 400,000. These were the workers who dug the ditches, drove the railway spikes, manned the steel mills and, seeking homes, spilled out over the farm lands. This "new immigration" continued unchecked well into the twentieth century; in 1915 it accounted for 79 percent of all new arrivals. For the first time in its history America faced the problem not only of assimilating peoples of such widely different racial characteristics but also of competing with cheap labor and low living standards.

Not, however, until the restrictive legislation of 1917, 1921 and 1924 was passed did the government take into its own hands determination of the size and character of immigration to be allowed. The effectiveness of those acts is indicated by the fact that whereas in 1910 one of every seven United States inhabitants was foreign-born, by 1950 the ratio was only one to every fifteen.[13]

Exploitation of workers was as characteristic of the late 1800's as exploitation of national resources. Labor was cheap, and submissive. Hours were long, wages low, living conditions for the most part substandard. And remedial legislation was slow to come in the United States, as it was in England.

Speaking of expansion in America, William T. Gossett has said:

> It is not easy to recognize at once the significance of any process of evolution; but there is one which seems to be clearly characteristic of our times, one which deserves special attention. That is bigness—bigness in all aspects of human affairs. The bigness that seems to go with progress is everywhere around us—big governments, big international, political and economic organizations. But, of course, size is not a new preoccupation of Americans.
>
> Industrial enterprise developed in an extremely favorable atmosphere in this country. With our Jeffersonian idea that no government was better than too much government, industry was encouraged as a promising child. By protective tariffs, subsidies and gifts, impressive results were obtained. As early as 1860, the output of our mills and shops found the United States fourth in manufacturing, and by 1890 we were first, with volume exceeding that of Great Britain and Germany combined.[14]

During that period of phenomenal expansion, punctuated by depressions, industry had little inclination and no necessity for thinking in terms of human values or human security. Labor, as an entity, had no standing, no means of enforcing its basic rights. And the big corporations, intent upon consolidating their power and extending their holdings, were of no mind to stir up the issue.

But, says Gossett: "The American people began to fear this concentration of power. Then, as now, people saw that unchecked power inevitably sucks away the vitality of freedom, and by legislative action the nation began to take counter measures. In 1884 an anti-monopoly party appeared, and in 1888 both major political parties condemned the trusts." [15] The many laws that have since been passed, to curb the powers of "big business," are well known to every student.

Very early in the nineteenth century, the voice of labor began to be heard in America, a whisper that later became a clamor, for recognition, for better working conditions, a higher standard of living, a bigger share of the fruits of production. The whole movement was part of a struggle covering all civilized history down to our day.

Results came slowly. Between 1825 and 1850 there were abortive reform movements in New York and New England, but little was accomplished. In 1874 Massachusetts passed the first legislation establishing ten hours as a normal working day for women and children. Other acts followed, providing for factory inspection and the adoption of various safety and sanitary measures.

Massachusetts set the pattern for significant reforms by individual states in the ensuing years. Alabama, in 1825, passed the first act making employers liable for injury to a worker hurt through the carelessness of another worker. An eight-hour day was established for the United States services in 1892, and in the following year safety appliances were installed on the nation's railroads. These were milestones in progress toward the complex liability and safety codes of our day.

Labor, long before, had learned that its only hope lay in organization. The interests of handicraft workers—originally a family affair and later represented by the guilds—were now under the jurisdiction of the trade unions. The tailors had a trade union as far back as 1806. As the years passed, the hatters, shipwrights, carpenters, printers, and workers and scores of other trades followed suit with similar organizations. These were the forerunners of the three big unions which dominated the American scene at the turn of the twentieth century: the Knights of Labor (1869), the American Federation of Labor (1881), and the American Railway Union (1893).

The A.F. L. did not assume its present name until 1886, when Samuel Gompers opened his first office with an old kitchen table and a soap box as its only chair. In less than ten years it had an estimated membership of half a million. Gompers, one of the greatest of all American labor leaders, was to prove a friend indeed to the young American Association of Industrial Physicians & Surgeons (later called the Industrial Medical Association) during the critical days of World War I.

In America, the union movement faced hostility and organized opposition from its very beginnings as it did elsewhere. In England, up to 1824, it was "conspiracy and felony" for workers to unite to get more money or to protect their rights—and early American laws were patterned after the British.

At the trial of journeymen boot and shoemakers in Philadelphia in 1806, the recorder asserted that "a combination of workmen to raise their wages may be considered in a twofold point of view; one is to benefit themselves, the other is to injure those who do not belong to their society. The rule of law condemns *both*."[16]

Merchants and shipowners of Boston, in 1832, declared labor organization would drive trade from their city, and resolved: "We will neither employ any journeyman who at the time belongs to such combinations, nor will we give work to any master mechanic who shall employ them while they continue thus pledged to each other and refuse to work the hours which it has been and is now customary for mechanics to work."[17]

It is a long step indeed from such arbitrary pronouncements to the enlightened conciliation and arbitration procedures of today. Progress has been dearly bought— at the cost of bitterness, violence, and colossal losses of time and money. The nine-teenth century saw the emergence of labor as a power in the national economy; but even greater issues were in the offing, for later generations to resolve.

Carroll Wright's comments on the present era are of more than passing interest, considering they were made in 1895. "We are living," said he, "at the beginning of the age of mind, as illustrated by the results of inventive genius. It is the age of intellect, of brain—for brain is king, and machinery is the king's prime minister."[18]

Again, Wright declares:

> Communism, which means the destruction of labor, cannot coexist with machin-ery. Its use requires too much competition, both social and industrial, to admit of communism. The states, therefore, devoted to industries which require the use of machines to a large extent are safe from the inroads of communism and communistic socialism, for without machinery the world would necessarily retrograde to supersti-tion and to ignorance, and the ingenuity of man would assume its old place among the unused faculties of the mind.[19]

Looking to the future (which is now the past), he says:

> The time is rapidly coming when the community will assert its right to perpetual peace, and so bring to bear upon all parties engaged in industry a great moral influ-ence which will secure all the benefits of voluntary arbitration and render the resort to any compulsory measures unnecessary. Such time will come only when the power of moral forces is recognized as essential in the development and evolution of eco-nomic forces.[20]

We have not reached that Utopian goal, but we are on our way to it. The problems of "big labor" now stand with the problems of "big business." The in-dustrial physicians of America, as we shall see, have played a role of ever increasing importance in their solution and in the progress toward an economic system run by business men with a social conscience and a sense of civic responsibility.

IV

EARLY OCCUPATIONAL MEDICINE
IN AMERICA

STUDENTS who explore the intimate history of the American
colonies for specific references or information relating to occupational diseases will
find little to reward their search. But they will quickly discover the reasons for
ignorance of the subject and a general indifference toward the health and welfare
of working people.

For one thing, there was little or no industry worthy of the name in America
during the colonial period. Manufacturing, on the whole, was limited to home crafts
and the production of small mills and shops—of only local importance. Lacking
anything like a national spirit or outlook, each of the colonies zealously guarded
its own interests and met its individual needs as best it could.

The growing settlements along the Atlantic seaboard desperately needed manufactured products of every type, both for their own use and to maintain a balance
of trade. As we have seen, however, the colonists were thwarted at every turn by
England's stringent laws against the importation of machinery and other means of
production. The new land was sparsely populated; it lacked both the manpower
and the governmental organization needed to develop its vast mineral resources.
These and other factors long delayed the arrival of the Machine Age on this side
of the Atlantic. Not until America had won its liberty and written its immortal
Constitution was it free to work out its own social and economic future.

Even a century after the Mayflower, there was a scarcity of competent doctors
in the colonies. With some outstanding exceptions, they had little formal education
or training. Like physicians of their time the world over, they had only the sketchiest

knowledge of the true etiology of the commonest diseases, let alone the obscure and insidious ailments resulting from occupational causes.

In the early decades of colonial history the mere struggle to survive commanded all the time and energies of the people. Starvation and malnutrition were a constant threat, and exacted an appalling toll of lives. And even when food became more abundant there remained the ever present menace of other, and more vicious, killers.

America escaped the pandemic plagues that scourged Europe intermittently for hundreds of years, but smallpox, diphtheria, cholera, yellow fever, and typhoid ravaged the colonies during the seventeenth and eighteenth centuries, from the cities of the east to remote outposts on the northern, western, and southern frontiers. The persistence of these and other endemic and epidemic diseases, throughout the nineteenth century and down to our time, is important in this history because their continuing prevalence was the spur needed for the introduction of public health services —the starting point of a great crusade for sanitation, hygiene, and preventive medicine in both industrial and general practice.

A century or more ago, the public as well as the medical profession accepted recurring epidemics philosophically, almost casually. In 1850 a Detroit woman wrote: "I judge from the signs that there will be another cholera epidemic this year. We have been most of the winter without snow and mostly warm and pleasant." Her prognosis was not far wrong, for cholera revisited Detroit in 1852 and 1854— the fifth and sixth major outbreaks in a period of twenty-two years. There is a record that cholera attacked an encampment of 1,500 workmen in the winter of 1854, during construction of the first lock of the Soo Ship Canal at Sault Ste. Marie, Michigan. It is said that 250 died of the disease. The bodies were buried secretly at night. The work went on, causing no panic among the men and creating no more than a ripple of excitement elsewhere.

Considering the immature status of medical knowledge in the colonial era, the absence of statistics on mortality, and above all the small scale on which industry operated, it is not strange that recorded colonial history is silent on the subject of occupational diseases for more than a century, and that the literature of industrial medicine is scanty indeed for another hundred years.

There were, beyond doubt, in the colonies many cases of illness traceable to conditions of employment; but they were widely scattered, and their incidence was relatively slight. To a public and a profession preoccupied with far more dangerous diseases, menacing the lives of whole communities, they were of no moment. The very terms "occupational disease" and "industrial medicine" would have been meaningless to people at large, and probably to most physicians.

Writing of that period, in his significant work "Lead and Lead Poisoning in Early America," Dr. Carey P. McCord makes this comment:

> Not until 1750 did American physicians discover that one of their duties to oncoming generations was as medical recorders and reporters. Early physicians saw epidemics but served no whit as epidemiologists or historians. . . . In the midst of so

35

much havoc of human beings, lead poisonings even of epidemic proportions would have attracted no attention as a specific disease. The truth is that not for 150 years could an exact diagnosis have been made, any more than for diabetes or tuberculosis.[1]

Had the doctors chosen to write, they would have set down their experiences and their findings with little hope of recognition or reward, even in professional circles. They had no well stocked medical libraries for reference, no laboratories for research. There were no clinics for discussion of their papers, no journals to circulate and preserve their writings. Thus, our present knowledge of health conditions and medical practice in early America must largely be pieced together from faded diaries and yellowed letters that have survived and found their way into the archives of a history-minded civilization.

As for the working people of colonial times, they were a docile, uncomplaining, and durable breed. They accepted—as the price of employment—a good deal of hardship, many hazards, and even exposure to disabling or fatal disease. Had they raised a chorus of protest, it is doubtful that much would or could have been done to eliminate hazards at their source. The times were not yet ripe.

There seems to exist, in the minds of men, a strange lethargy that leads them to postpone preventive action even when the danger is obvious and the remedy is at hand. They resist change, even for the better. They will repair the leaky roof tomorrow, even though it may rain tonight. History shows that the biggest steps toward protection of life and limb have stemmed from the greatest tragedies—a war, a holocaust, a disaster that rouses human indignation and starts a public clamor for drastic action.

In December, 1903, fire started a stampede in the Iroquois Theater, Chicago, and 600 died in their attempt to reach blocked exits. This horror led to a wholesale revision of safety regulations covering places of public entertainment, and the mandatory installation of asbestos curtains—a simple and obvious safeguard.

In the summer of 1904 nearly 1,000 Sunday School excursionists were burned to death or drowned when flames swept the old steamer *General Slocum,* almost in the shadows of New York's skyscrapers. Most of them were women and children. Investigation disclosed rotten life preservers and lifeboats cleated to the decks, and brought to light graft, corruption, and negligence that had existed for years.

The Triangle shirtwaist factory fire in 1911, resulting in 148 deaths, shocked the nation and promptly brought about the establishment of the New York Investigating Commission, headed by Dr. George M. Price, to conduct studies of health and safety problems in such industries.[2] The investigation exposed insanitary and dangerous conditions of long standing, which had thrived unchecked until an aroused public opinion forced remedial action.

Industry, too, has had its catastrophes—black marks on the pages of its history— but milestones in the progress of industrial medicine. In the aggregate they have cost countless lives. Individually they offer trenchant bits of evidence of man's propensity to bury his head in the sand until public outcry compels him to look horror

36

in the face and do something to mitigate it. Typical of such tragedies is the story of phosphorus necrosis.

Phosphorus poisoning, at least in its industrial manifestations, was unknown in Ramazzini's time, for the reason that a process for extracting phosphorus in commercial quantities from animal bones was not developed until the second quarter of the nineteenth century. From this discovery came the match industry, starting in continental Europe and appearing in Europe and the United States a few years later. "It was with this new trade," writes Curt Proskauer, "that chronic phosphorus poisoning began, the phosphorus necrosis, whose frightful symptoms were a bewildering puzzle. The disease was something entirely new, never having manifested itself before, a fact which in the history of nosology is a rare occurrence indeed."[3] Those symptoms, now well known to every industrial physician, appeared swiftly among workers wherever "lucifers" were impregnated by manual dipping into a syrupy phosphorus mixture. Since practically the same process was in general use in the industry, exposure and poisoning were inevitable, regardless of locale.

The first match factories in Germany and Austria were built around 1833, and almost immediately severe cases of necrosis of the jawbone began to appear in alarming numbers. But more than twelve years elapsed before legal steps were taken to check the spread of the malady. "This delay," says Proskauer," is not to be attributed to the indifference of the civil authorities but rather to the failure of medicine to correlate the disease with the respective occupation of the afflicted."[4]

It was Lorinser, chief surgeon of a suburban Vienna hospital, who first recognized phosphorus fumes as the immediate cause of the necrosis. His findings, published in 1845, led to a decree issued by the provincial government to regulate procedures "during the drying of the matches when there is a free and unhindered circulation of phosphorus fumes in the workrooms without preventive measures." This decree, dated October 7, 1846, covering six closely written pages of German script, prescribed in meticulous detail ventilation and other sanitary provisions intended to minimize exposure to the deadly fumes. It is a notable document in that it represents one of the very first legal steps to be taken by any government aiming at the prevention of a specific industrial disease caused by a specific industrial poison.

The Austrian discoveries and the Austrian ordinance, however, did not signal the end of the phosphorus menace. Far from it. In England, on the continent and in America, the poison had its way with the health and lives of match workers for more than a half-century—unhindered except by ordinary sanitary safeguards.

English producers, with an eye on production costs, hired women and children for the dipping process. Investigations disclosed the fact that "match manufacturers employed boys of the ages of five to seven years for work that exposed the bones of their faces without protection to the horribly disfiguring fumes of phosphorus."[5] According to Sir Thomas Oliver, the death of a London match maker in 1897, and the illness of many other workers, struck the spark that kindled the first real investigation of the industry in England. As a member of the investigating commission, Sir Thomas found that only about 4,000 persons—three fourths of them women—were employed in the industry in Great Britain and Iceland and that of these only about 1,700 were actually engaged in the phosphorous processes. In his opinion less than 1 percent of all match makers in Great Britain suffered from necrosis.[6] It was not the widespread incidence of phosphorus poisoning that aroused public indignation, but its terrible effects on human beings and their deliberate exposure to a known hazard which no amount of sanitary precaution could eliminate.

"The first American case of phosphorus necrosis," says Dr. Alice Hamilton, "was reported in 1851, about fifteen years after the *first patent for the manufacture of lucifer matches was granted to a man in Springfield, Mass., in 1836.*"[7] (The italics are Dr. Hamilton's.) It is safe to assume that in the ensuing half-century the American match industry had its full share of phosphorus poisoning. When Dr. Hamilton first became interested in the disease, in the early 1900's, she was deeply shocked by its pathological aspects but even more disturbed by apparent indifference to the hazard on the part of the industry and the medical profession. In her autobiography she comments:

> Miss [Jane] Addams told me that when she was in London in the 1880's she went to a mass meeting of protest against phossy jaw, and on the platform were a number of pitiful cases, showing their scars and deformities. . . . All this I had learned, but I had been assured by medical men, who claimed to know, that there was no phossy jaw in the United States because American match factories were so scrupulously clean.[8]

Despite this long and socially disgraceful record of disease and suffering, the death warrant of phosphorus poisoning, as a hazard in match manufacturing, was not signed until well after the turn of the twentieth century, even though a harmless substitute, sesquisulphide of phosphorus, had been discovered and was readily available.

In 1900, the International Association for Labor Legislation was organized, with headquarters in Basel, Switzerland, and soon focused its attention on the banishment of the phosphorus hazard from industry. Six years later the governments of France, Italy, Denmark, Luxemburg, Switzerland, the Netherlands, and Germany signed an agreement to prohibit the manufacture, sale, export, and import of poisonous phosphorus matches. These were joined by England in 1908 and Austria in 1909.

By 1912 the International Association had a membership of sixteen nations—all European except the United States. The American Association for Labor Legislation had been organized in 1906 and it was through the efforts of this affiliate, implemented mainly by the studies of its secretary, John B. Andrews, that the poisonous lucifer was finally banished from our shores. The victory, however, was not won without a struggle. In a report to the association at its First National Conference on Industrial Diseases, in 1910, Dr. Andrews declared: "Our American manufacturers, while admitting that the harmless substitute for poisonous phosphorus would make the manufacturers' cost of matches less than 5 percent more,

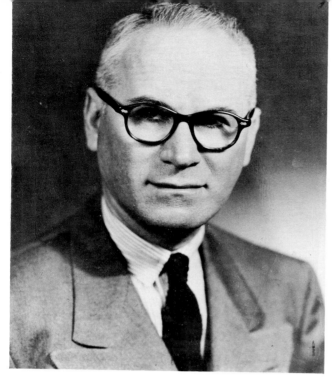

2. *James I. Roberts, M.D.* Medical director, New England Power Service Company, consulting physician for affiliate and associated public utilities in New England; has also served as a consultant for Little-Brown Co., publishers. For four years Roberts was IMA district counselor for the New England states, was certified under the Founders Group of the American Board of Occupational Medicine, is a member of the History Committee, and was chairman, 1954–1955, of the highly important Committee on Medical Care.

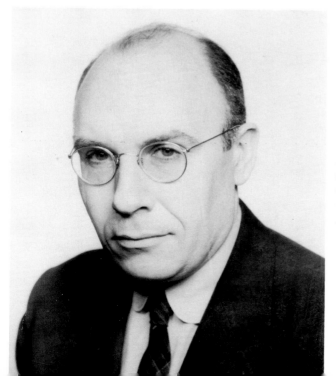

3. *George Rosen, M.D.* Professor of Health Education, Columbia University Faculty of Medicine. In his introduction to the standard English translation of Ramazzini's masterpiece, *De Morbis Artificum,* Dr. Rosen appraised precisely Ramazzini's place in medical history and thereby made an outstanding contribution to the reference literature of occupational medicine. In his own right he is noted for his studies in the field of toxicology and as the author of "History of Miners' Diseases—A Medical and Social Interpretation." Doctor Rosen is a member of the History Committee of the IMA.

5. *Watt's Sun and Planet Steam Engine.* Watt's inventions made steam power workable. Watt patented the first successful condenser in 1769. His sun and planet engine (restored in the Ford Museum), one of the first to employ the rotary principle, was used to operate a pump near Birmingham, England, from 1788 to 1858.

⟶

4. *Arthur J. Vorwald, M.D.* Born in Dubuque, Iowa, Vorwald received a B.A. from Columbia College and a Ph.D. in pathology in 1931, and an M.D. in 1932 from the University of Chicago Medical School. A widely known pathologist and an authority on chest diseases, he did a large part of his early work at Saranac Lake, New York, prior to World War II. There, from 1934 to 1942, he served as a lecturer at the Trudeau School of the Edward L. Trudeau Foundation and as a pathologist at the Trudeau Sanatorium, Saranac Laboratory and the General Hospital of Saranac Lake. Between 1942 and 1947 he was an officer in the Medical Corps, U.S. Naval Reserve, engaged in research, and was a naval medical attache in London. After the war, he returned to Saranac Lake as director of research, director of the Trudeau Foundation and director of the Saranac Laboratory. Since 1954 he has been professor and chairman, Department of Industrial Medicine and Hygiene at Wayne State University College of Medicine. Active for many years in the IMA, he is a member of its History Committee.

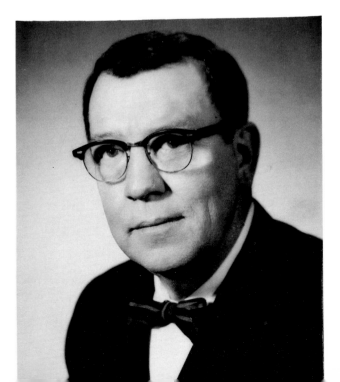

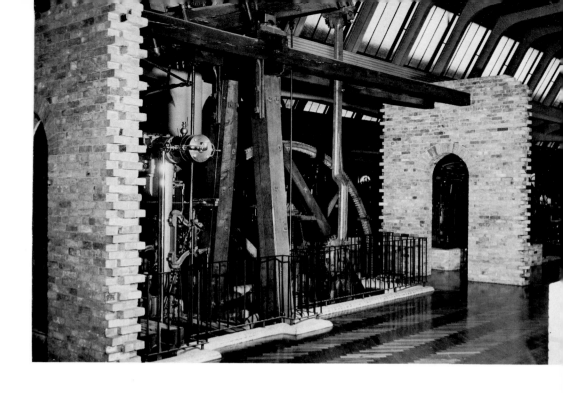

6. *Last of the Coal Burners.* Outmoded, this giant of the rails was retired in the 1950's. Technical progress is banishing the last of the huge
coal burners from American railroads. No. 1601, one of the most powerful
of its type ever built, went to work for the Chesapeake & Ohio Railway in
1941. Locomotive and tender weigh nearly 600 tons and are more than 125
feet in length. How, one wonders, would Watt react to this monster?

—Courtesy of The Henry Ford Museum, Dearborn, Michigan

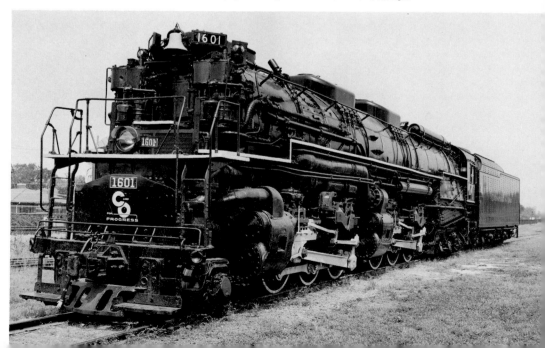

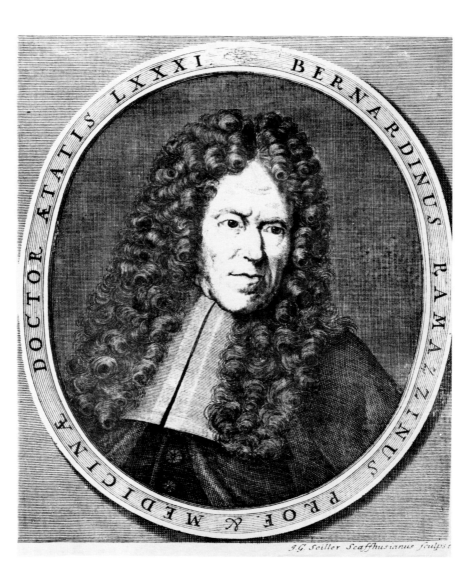

DOCTOR ÆTATIS LXXXI. BERNARDINUS RAMAZZINUS PROF & MEDICINA

J.G. Seiller Scaffhusianus sculps.

7. *Bernardino Ramazzini, 1633–1714.* Commonly considered the father of industrial medicine. He recognized and described some forty types of occupational disease.

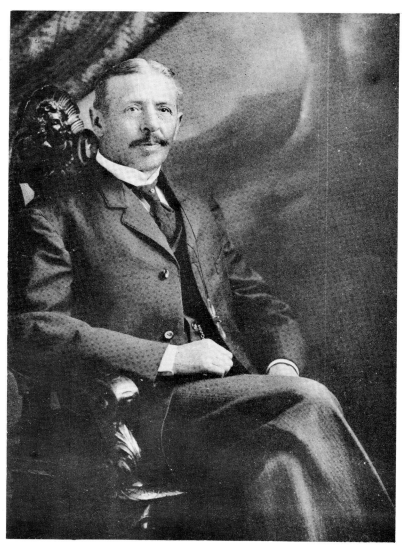

8. *George Martin Kober, M.D., 1850–1931.* A giant of his time
—soldier, scientist, physician, and venerable dean of Georgetown
University Medical School, he greatly stimulated development in
the field of industrial hygiene and contributed to its literature
several books and more than 240 articles.

10. Ramazzini's *De Morbis Artificum.* Bernardino Ramazzini (1633–1714) was a distinguished physician, a professor at the University of Modena, who was called to the famous University of Padua in 1700, the year in which his greatest book, *Of the Diseases of Workers,* was published. It was this work, more than any other factor, that brought him, long afterward, recognition as "the father of occupational medicine." Convinced that occupational diseases played an important part in the life of a community, he read all the literature available on this subject, then went into the shops and mines, talked to the people, and studied the conditions under which they worked. The result was a thorough and authoritative analysis of the health hazards in two-score or more trades and a discussion of the means of curing and/or preventing the diseases involved. Thereafter, Ramazzini declares, he habitually asked every patient what his occupation was, since he considered this information a good starting point in diagnosis.

⟶

9. *George M. Price, M.D.* His investigation of the tragic Triangle Shirtwaist factory fire in 1911 shocked the nation. Two years later he founded the Union Health Center, a model enterprise of its time, which set a pattern for many later industrial health programs.

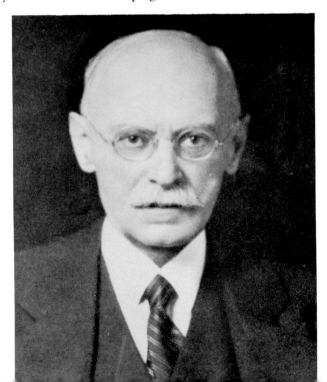

DE
MORBIS ARTIFICUM
DIATRIBA
BERNARDINI RAMAZZINI

IN PATAVINO ARCHI-LYCEO

Practicæ Medicinæ Ordinariæ
Publici Profefforis,

ET NATURÆ CURIOSORUM COLLEGÆ.

Illuftriſs., & Excellentiſs. DD. Ejuſdem

ARCHI-LYCEI
MODERATORIBUS.
D.

MUTINÆ M.DCC.

Typis Antonii Capponi, Impreſſoris Epifcopalis.
Supriorum Conſenſu.

THE
OCCUPATIONAL
DISEASES

THEIR CAUSATION, SYMPTOMS
TREATMENT AND PREVENTION

BY

W. GILMAN THOMPSON, M.D.

PROFESSOR OF MEDICINE, CORNELL UNIVERSITY MEDICAL COLLEGE IN NEW YORK CITY;
VISITING PHYSICIAN TO BELLEVUE HOSPITAL

ILLUSTRATED

NEW YORK AND LONDON
D. APPLETON AND COMPANY

11. *The Occupational Diseases.* Although the literature of occupational medicine gained rapidly in both volume and importance in the latter part of the nineteenth and the early years of the twentieth centuries, *The Occupational Diseases* is generally considered the first really modern work in this highly specialized field. Certainly this book had a considerable effect on the style, subject matter and format of industrial medical literature in the following decades. As the title page indicates, it was broad in scope and authoritative in treatment; and at the same time it reflected the most advanced medical thinking in the rapidly growing industries of America after 1900.

12. *Industrial Health.* Very significant in the mass of industrial medical literature produced in our time is *Industrial Health,* published in 1924 by P. Blackiston's Son & Company, of Philadelphia. A massive volume of nearly 1,200 pages, it might well be called an omnibus of occupational health hazards. It is safe to say that few, if any, single-volume works on this subject give such detailed coverage to such a wide diversity of industrial diseases. To this immense task Kober and Hayhurst summoned the help of thirty-three contributors, each of whom wrote chapters or sections on their specialties. Kober contributed a long and informative historical preface and Hayhurst considerable material for the appendix; both wrote substantial portions of the main text.

INDUSTRIAL HEALTH

EDITED BY

GEORGE M. KOBER, M.D., LL.D.
WASHINGTON, D. C.

AND

EMERY R. HAYHURST, A.M., M.D., Ph.D.
COLUMBUS, OHIO

CONTRIBUTORS

ANDREWS, IRENE OSGOOD, NEW YORK CITY.
ANDREWS, JOHN B., Ph. D., NEW YORK CITY.
APFELBACH, GEORGE L., M. D. CHICAGO, ILL.
ASHFORD, BAILEY K., M. D., SAN JUAN, PORTO RICO.
BLAKE, CLARENCE JOHN, M. D. BOSTON, MASS.
BOWEN, JOHN T., M. D., BOSTON, MASS.
DEVOTO, LUIGI, M. D., MILAN, ITALY
DITTOE, WM. H., C. E., COLUMBUS, OHIO.
ERDMAN, SEWARD, M. D., NEW YORK CITY.
FROTHINGHAM, LANGDON, M. D. V., BOSTON, MASS.
GROENIGER, WM. C. COLUMBUS, OHIO.
HAMILTON, ALICE, M. D., BOSTON, MASS.
HANSON, WM. C., M. D. BOSTON, MASS.
LEE, FREDERICK S., Ph. D., NEW YORK CITY.
LEE, THOMAS S., M. D., WASHINGTON, D. C.
LEGGE, THOMAS M., M. D., LONDON, ENGLAND.
LINENTHAL, HARRY, M. D., BOSTON, MASS.
LOVEJOY, OWEN R. NEW YORK CITY.
OLIVER, SIR THOMAS, M. D., NEWCASTLE-UPON-TYNE, ENGLAND.
ORDWAY, THOMAS, M. D., ALBANY, N. Y.
SAYERS, R. R., M. D., WASHINGTON, D. C.
SCHERESCHEWSKY, J. W., M. D., WASHINGTON, D. C.
SELBY, CLARENCE D., M. D., TOLEDO, OHIO.
SOLOMON, HARRY C., M. D., BOSTON, MASS.
SOUTHARD, ELMER E., M. D., BOSTON, MASS.
TELEKY, LUDWIG, M. D., DÜSSELDORF, GERMANY.
TRASK, JOHN W., M. D., WASHINGTON, D. C.
TRUBY, ALBERT E., M. D., WASHINGTON, D. C.
TYZZER, ERNEST E., M. D., BOSTON, MASS.
WELLS, WALTER A., M. D., WASHINGTON, D. C.
WHIPPLE, GEORGE C., S. B., BOSTON, MASS.
WRIGHT, FLORENCE S, R. N., NEW HAVEN, CONN.
WÜRDEMANN, HARRY V., M. D, SEATTLE, WASH.

WITH ILLUSTRATIONS, REFERENCE TABLES AND APPENDIX

13. *Philippus Aureolus Theophrastus Bombastus von Hohenheim, called Paracelsus (1493–1541),* was one of the most controversial personalities of the world in which he lived, and estimates of the man and his work still vary widely. His outspoken questioning of the old and his advocacy of the new made him many enemies, but he also acquired many followers. His motto *experimenta et ratio* certainly led medicine on the right road. Notable among his works are three books dealing principally with the diseases of miners, catalogued under the overall title *Von der Bergsucht und anderen Bergkrankheiten.* He is regarded by some today as the first modern medical scientist—the precursor of antisepsis, homeopathy, modern wound surgery and other concepts of our time.

The illustration above is reproduced from an engraving of a portrait by Jan van Scorel, which hangs in the Louvre in Paris.

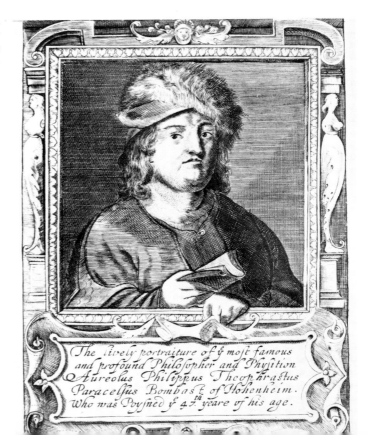

The lively portraiture of ye most famous and profound Philosopher and Physition Aureolus Philippus Theophrastus Paracelsus Bombast of Hohenheim. Who was Poysned ye 47th yeare of his age.

declare that its voluntary use would place them at too great a disadvantage with business competitors."[9]

Uniform prohibitive regulation was the only answer to that objection, but this the American Congress could not force the states to enact. It could, however, use its taxing power to the same end, and in 1912 the Hughes-Esch Act became a law, imposing a prohibitive tax on poisonous phosphorus matches manufactured in the United States after July 1, 1913. Thus, phosphorus necrosis passed from the American scene as a hazard of the match industry.

The story of phossy jaw is significant for several reasons. It typifies the time lag that occurs, through all history, between the acquisition of medical knowledge and its application for the good of society. It emphasizes the impotence of medical science *per se* to translate its findings into progress without public awareness of health hazards and the cooperation of industry, business and government in combating them. Even more important, it points to the need for strong, purposeful organizations, both public and private, dedicated to the conquest of disease and bringing to their cause a viewpoint influenced by political considerations or profit motives. Such organizations are a phenomenon of our day. One after another, they appeared on the medical and social horizon during the first decades of the twentieth century, the result of a birth of new interest in the health and welfare of American workers.

In the van of pioneers in this renaissance was Alice Hamilton (an honorary member of the Industrial Medical Association). A disciple of Osler and Welch and Simon Flexner, she had gone to Chicago to start her career—young, eager, filled with the crusading zeal of Jane Addams and Hull House. Her settlement work naturally brought her in contact with laborers and their wives; from them she learned of the hazards to which working men were exposed and the occupational diseases that commonly afflicted them. Determined to investigate the field of industrial health, Dr. Hamilton promptly visited the Crerar Library to read everything she could find dealing with the subject. "But," she writes in her autobiography,

it was all German, or British, Dutch, Swiss, even Italian or Spanish—everything but American. In those countries industrial medicine was a recognized branch of the medical sciences; in my own country it did not exist. . . .

Everyone with whom I talked assured me that the foreign writings could not apply to American conditions, for our workmen were so much better paid, their standard of living was so much higher, and the factories in which they worked so much finer in every way than the European, that they did not suffer from the evils to which the poor foreigner was subject.[10]

Dr. Hamilton's own findings, however, led her to a far different conclusion. From John Andrews she learned the facts of the phosphorus match controversy. Appointed by Governor Dineen to an Occupational Disease Commission, she was one of a team that conducted the famous Illinois Survey in 1910—the first such survey to be conducted by a state.

"The only poisons we had to cover," she writes, "were lead, arsenic, brass, carbon monoxide, the cyanides, and turpentine. . . . We could not even discover what were the poisonous occupations in Illinois."[11] Her own assignment was the investigation of lead. Among her confreres, Drs. Emery Hayhurst and Peter Bassoe, both important figures in the field of industrial health, undertook, respectively, studies of brass poisoning and caisson disease.

While the Illinois Survey was still in progress Dr. Hamilton was sent to Europe to attend the International Congress on Occupational Accidents and Diseases, in Brussels. Her experience there strengthened her conviction that the United States lagged far behind the older countries in its development of industrial medicine. "It was . . . mortifying," she writes, "to be unable to answer any of the questions put to us: What was the rate of lead poisoning in such and such an industry? What regulations did we have for the dangerous trades? What was our system of compensation? Finally, Dr. Gilbert, of the Belgian Labor Department, dismissed the subject: 'It is well known that there is no industrial hygiene in the United States. *Ça n'existe pas.'* "[12]

There is little doubt that American industries, at the time, suffered by comparison with those of Europe in the matter of organized programs to protect health and regulate industrial procedures. The idea that "it can't happen here" seems to have been widespread among industrialists. Facts, nevertheless, do not justify the bland conclusion that research in the field of occupational disease was at a standstill, that United States physicians were blissfully unaware of the hazards of industry, or that literature on the subject was practically nonexistent.

In a current manuscript Carey McCord thoroughly explodes such assumptions. He declares:

> One of the traditional errors as to occupational health is that in the United States prior to 1900 essentially there were no publications. It is customary to give finality to the matter by stating that the total number of scientific articles did not exceed twenty. Indeed, in those publications in the United States during the first quarter of the century it was customary to draw heavily, as to citations, upon the European literature and usually with the apologetic statement that nothing comparable was available in this country.
>
> Actually, present-day occupational health stems appreciably from publications in our own country prior to 1900. Laying aside large numbers of articles of general nature such as with reference to tuberculosis in industry, hours of labor, need for legislation in worker protection, etc., and adhering strictly to published items precisely directed to occupational diseases or to industrial hygiene, it becomes possible to assemble a substantial listing, all in refutation, that in the United States prior to 1900 occupational health was unknown, or at best little known.[13]

McCord goes on to prove his thesis by citing the titles of some two hundred reports and other articles on occupational health, published in this country before the turn of the century. A substantial percentage of these dealt with industrial poisoning of various types, but on the whole the list is thoroughly representative of the diseases and other health problems of greatest incidence between 1850 and 1900.

Phosphorus offers a case in point. Legal action to reform the match industry, largely as the result of the work of John Andrews and the Association for Labor Legislation, did not come until 1912. But phossy jaw was minutely described in papers published in 1854 and 1856,[14] and several other authoritative articles were published between 1879 and 1898.

Caisson disease did not appear on the American scene until substantial numbers of men were called upon to work under air pressure. Medical literature faithfully reflects the trend. The first American article on the physiological effects of compressed air appeared in 1843.[15] McCord cites a score of papers dealing with this hazard from 1870 to 1896, a period of large-scale activity in bridge and underwater tunnel construction.

Robert Legge, in a chronology of progress in industrial health in the early twentieth century,[16] records that E. W. Moire (in 1904) was the first to use a medical air lock for recompression, in the Hudson River tunnel. New York (in 1909) was the first state to require physical examinations for workers in compressed air; New Jersey followed in 1914. In 1911 Hayhurst organized the Sprague Memorial Foundation which has made important contributions to our knowledge of compressed air, as well as brass and lead poisoning.

Lead—one of the oldest of all industry hazards—has perhaps commanded the greatest attention in research and produced the most extensive literature. McCord cites fourteen publication titles on this subject in the United States up to 1898, and his list does not include many books and reports not appearing in his source material.[17]

In his chronology of industrial medical literature McCord reaches this conclusion: "All considered, it does not appear that any appalling paucity of publications on occupational health characterized the United States prior to 1900 or that this country has need for the apologists who observe backwardness in the inauguration of occupational health measures."

Why, then, the widespread opinions, so frequently expressed, that America was blind if not indifferent to the ravages of occupational diseases in industry and that while medical science abroad was forging ahead physicians in this country were ignoring the entire industrial field?

Discussing his own investigations of industrial poisoning in 1912, Dr. David L. Edsall, of Harvard Medical School, declared: "I have been able to get more information in two or three days from an official introduction in a foreign country than I can get in this country in two or three months. The only difficulty there is that the manufacturers are afraid you are looking into trade secrets; they don't care how much you look into trade health."[18]

Governments in the United States, both federal and state, were indeed dilatory in pressing measures for the control and prevention of industrial diseases. The federal government did not begin to compile even mortality statistics until 1900. Public health services were in their infancy. States rights precluded the application of sweeping regulations to the individual states; it was difficult (as it still is) to obtain anything approaching uniform legislation throughout the country. Early efforts to regulate working hours, and establish the principles of liability and compensation met with stubborn resistance from employers.

There were, in the nineteenth century, relatively few medical societies—hence, few journals to serve as forums for the discussion of either professional problems or public issues. Physicians, by and large, were lone workers; their finest accomplishments received little notice in their time beyond the inner circles of medicine.

American medical science, nevertheless, advanced rapidly in the late 1800's, led by such pioneers as Keen, Welch, the Mayos, Walter Reed, and the great Osler, whose textbook, *Principles and Practice of Medicine*,[19] included chapters on lead poisoning and other industrial hazards. Along with general medical progress, industrial problems began to receive more and more attention from physicians of real stature, who saw in occupational disease the possibilities of an entirely new specialty.

The literature of industrial medicine burgeoned from these beginnings, gaining in volume and variety as interest increased, as new occupational hazards appeared, and as new organizations, devoted to safety and hygiene, came into being. The flood has continued to swell and has not yet reached its peak.

George Martin Kober, among the giants of his time, gave great impetus to study and activity in the field of industrial hygiene. Son of a German revolutionist, Dr. Kober served for many years as a United States Army surgeon and later as dean of the Georgetown University School of Medicine. During his long and fruitful life as soldier, scientist, physician and philanthropist, he wrote several books and more than 240 articles in both German and English, among them significant studies on milk as a factor in the transmission of disease.

In 1907, Kober chanced to meet Dr. E. J. Neisser at the International Congress of Industrial Hygiene in Berlin and was greatly impressed by the German scientist's comments on the dearth of data on health activities in the United States. The meeting was an inspiration for much of his later work. By such commonplace incidents many a recruit was won to the cause of industrial medicine during its early development.

In that same year Kober was appointed by Theodore Roosevelt as chairman of the Committee on Social Betterment of the President's Homes Commission. In 1908 he published his first book, *Industrial and Personal Hygiene*, which he later called "a rather hasty study of the causes of sickness."

A far more comprehensive and significant treatise in this field appeared in 1914 with the publication of *Occupational Diseases*, by Dr. W. Gilman Thompson, of the faculty of Cornell University Medical School in New York City. It was certainly one of the earliest works of its kind in the twentieth century.

The first two decades of this century saw the rise of Emery R. Hayhurst as teacher, writer, authority on industrial poisons, and consultant in the public health services. He contributed chapters to Kober and Hanson's book, *Diseases of Occupation and Vocational Hygiene*[20]; and in 1924, with Kober, he published *Industrial Health*.[21] A voluminous writer, he is credited with more than one hundred articles in periodical publications.

These early pioneers were physicians of real stature as well as gifted writers. They set the pace for a score of others who accomplished much in a short time to offset the deficiency of American data on occupational diseases. At last, industrial medicine—safety, hygiene, sanitation—was on its way to importance as a factor in national health.

The list of contributors to the literature of occupational health during the transition period is a long one, too long for more than a brief highlighting here. It includes Alice Hamilton, with her studies on lead; Thomas R. Crowder, of Chicago, on ventilation; J. W. Schereschewsky, in the United States Public Health Service; and Francis Patterson, in the Pennsylvania Department of Industry and Labor.

There is evidence that, at least by 1910, qualified observers not only were keenly aware of the need for an all-out offensive against industrial hazards and diseases but also realized the size and difficulty of the task that lay ahead. In opening the first National Conference on Industrial Diseases, Professor Henry W. Farnam, of Yale University, president of the American Association for Labor Legislation, declared:

> The present situation of our association is like that of a watchman on a high tower. He does not know exactly how the attack is to be made, but he knows enough to justify him in giving the alarm and in advising that scouts be sent out to ascertain more precisely the strength and position of the foe.
>
> In this warfare against industrial diseases we need the cooperation of many different people, and one of the purposes of this Association is to facilitate this cooperation in order to prevent a waste of energy. This is a warfare in which science, labor, business enterprise, and the government must all unite.[22]

The united front urged by Farnam required, above all else, organized participation by the medical fraternity. And within the next few years he was to get—from a small group of physicians already concerned with industrial health problems—the answer to his call.

V

SETTING THE STAGE

An ALMOST explosive quickening of national life pulsed through America at the turn of the twentieth century, speeding up the tempo of activity on every front. It was as though the country had entered an entirely new era, with new ambitions and objectives. Sir Thomas Oliver wrote in 1902: "The commencement of the twentieth century finds us discussing problems and elaborating plans for amelioration of the life of the people."[1] His words were even more descriptive of America than of Britain.

The glamorous Gay Nineties—hit by a major depression, torn by political strife, and plagued by labor troubles—lay behind. After 1897 big business grew steadily bigger; by 1904 some 5,300 individual plants had been merged into 318 trusts. Theodore Roosevelt's "big stick" was poised for a program of "trust busting."

The Treaty of Paris (1898) formally ended the Spanish-American War, and San Juan Hill and Manila Bay were becoming only memories to a people busy with a multitude of new tasks. The United States—little more than a century away from its colonial childhood—suddenly found itself possessed of important island colonies to administer, police, and protect. The nation was catapulted into world prominence, politically, socially, economically.

America joyously rolled up its sleeves. There was work to be done: the Panama Canal to be dug; skyscrapers to be reared in Manhattan; steel to be poured for the new navy, for new factories, for agricultural and industrial machinery. United States technology, soon to become the best in the world, rode to fame on a flood of Bessemer steel. Production of this material, less than five million tons in 1890, soared to eleven and a half million in 1900 and to more than twenty-nine million in 1910.

Seen in the context of history, the United States was in a uniquely favorable

44

position for the transition from an agricultural to an industrial society. At hand were vast resources to draw upon, vast areas of land to develop. Jobs were plentiful, and so were workers to fill them; immigration took care of that need. In 1905 more than a million were admitted; in 1907 the tide reached a peak of one and a quarter million; the total for the decade was five and six-tenths million.

These and other factors cushioned the impact of growing machine production and made possible a more orderly evolution. This country escaped the unemployment, the suffering and the turmoil that marked the advent of the machine in England. We were to know, later, how violent such changes can be, as in the transition from a peace to a war economy and vice versa.

So the nation went blithely forward on the way to realizing its dreams of industrial and political greatness. Progress scarcely paused for the brief rich man's panic of 1904 and the bankers' panic of 1907. National income rose to new peaks; the purchasing power of the dollar remained high. There was a tingle of expectation in the air, a sense of urgency everywhere. In the melting pot of America the sweat of the Slav in Pittsburgh steel mills mingled with that of the Swedish farmer in Minnesota. The shrewdness of Yankee bankers worked hand in hand with the daring and ingenuity of Midwestern manufacturers. Business became more and more competitive, with rich rewards for those who could survive the battle, and oblivion for those who could not.

But there were apprehensions mingled with the dreams. History shows that the influence and power of races—the progress of civilization—is in direct ratio to their development and application of mathematics and the natural sciences. America had everything required for spectacular advances in science. But the health and well-being of the people are a vital ingredient, more basic than all others. Material gains go for nothing if bought at the cost of sickness and suffering. And, in the welter of other activities, problems of health had been largely neglected in American industry.

Cities become large when industry becomes large. Big industry—requiring the concentration of many people in limited areas, great plants for manufacturing, and the constant movement of materials and products in huge quantities—is the golden egg from which have come not only our wealth and high standards of living but also our problems of overcrowding, slum housing, traffic congestion, squalor, and disease.

Man has no periscope which enables him to see around the corners of the future and appraise the consequences of any trends. Our big industrial centers have grown up haphazardly, without benefit of central planning. The tragedy of the London poor in the eighteenth and nineteenth centuries has its counterpart in every American metropolis. Not until recent years have model industrial communities been designed and built on a new formula. Only now are our older cities—rooted in the fixed pattern of a horse-and-buggy age—being replanned and rejuvenated to meet modern needs.

American factories of the late 1800's and early 1900's were built according to standards already obsolescent. Existing systems of power transmission made them jungles of shafts and belts, with accident hazards overhead, underfoot, at every worker's elbow. They were ill-lighted, poorly ventilated, suited neither to modern production nor to the enforcement of safety and sanitation measures.

In the early twentieth century, four major trends may be singled out as milestones of paramount importance: mass production in industry; new emphasis on health and the growth of organizations dedicated to safety and disease prevention; far-reaching changes in medical education; and legislation designed to protect the worker and better his condition.

Foremost among these factors was the birth of a new type of industry, heralded by the advent of the automobile. It is impossible to measure accurately the impact of the automobile on the world and on the life of its peoples. Not only did it represent a revolutionary advance in the means of transportation, but the ever-widening circles of its influence were to be felt in every phase of every activity around the globe. Industrially, mass production of low-priced cars pointed the way to the use of similar techniques in scores of other manufacturing fields whose output is counted today in billions of dollars annually.

Economically, the automobile tapped a vast new reservoir of purchasing power among the nation's wage earners. Soaring sales, in early years, set the pattern for the now familiar cycle of larger production at lower unit cost, more employment at higher wages, and expanding markets which made possible still bigger production at even lower cost.

Socially, the motor car foreshadowed an end to the isolation of small towns and rural areas, and launched mass migrations of population to industrial centers. The consequences have been enormous in scope and bewildering in complexity.

The Ford Motor Company, generally and justly, is credited with initiating the continuous assembly of stock parts into finished cars on moving production lines. After long experiments the first moving chassis assemblies were started in 1913 at Ford's new Highland Park plant, with rope and windlass as the motive power.

The problem was more than one of quantity output. The great hurdle was the standardization of parts to the point of complete interchangeability. Perfection of these techniques since 1913 has been a task for many industries in many fields. From their combined efforts has come the miracle of American mass production—envied the world over but understood in few foreign countries and matched by none.

The Ford Motor Company, however, was more than a pacemaker in mass production. Henry Ford, the inventor, the builder, the dreamer, saw in his own labor force a great new market for his cars. His announcement in 1914 that even "the commonest laborer who sweeps the floors" would receive five dollars for an eight-hour day burst on the country like a bombshell. Its consequences were momentous. In his relations to labor, Ford was an anomaly. He had unshakable faith in big production, low prices, and high wages as a means to larger sales, widespread employment and general prosperity. Yet he held out implacably against unionization of his shops. When at last he capitulated in 1941, he characteristically gave the union more than it had asked.

Many praised Ford's five-dollars-a-day policy in 1915; some condemned it; a few predicted economic disaster. Nevertheless, it succeeded far beyond expectations. In the following years wages in all industry rose steadily to higher levels. Markets expanded as buying power increased; costs were cut as production soared; wider employment made buyers of new millions.

This is the "American formula" in action. It has brought some seventy million telephones into use in the United States—more than half of all telephones in the world. It has placed television sets in about sixty million households, hospitals, and prisons. It has made "Man, the Worker" the principal buyer of the goods he makes —motor cars, radios, refrigerators, oil and gas furnaces, washing machines, and a host of other commodities.

The history of the automobile business is of more than passing interest in this story of industrial medicine. Mass production of motor vehicles accomplished more toward the industrialization of America in less than fifty years than textile machinery accomplished for English industry in a century and a half. The very size of automotive production, the speed with which it developed, the number of workers employed and the conditions under which they worked—all served to focus attention on industrial hazards and diseases and to hasten measures for their elimination or control.

When Ford was reported to be building a thousand cars a day in 1915, a common comment among people in the East was: "I don't believe it." Yet this figure was soon to be eclipsed by more than one company. The popularity of the automobile increased at a pace never equaled by any other specialty up to that time.

In 1900 only 8,000 motor vehicles were in use in the United States. Ten years later the total was about 468,000; by 1920 it had risen to 26.5 million. Reliable estimates place the number of vehicles on the highways in 1954 at well over 52 million, including about 10 million trucks and buses. In 1938 some 6 million workers were directly employed in the industry; in 1954 the estimated figure was 9.5 million.[2]

Figures on invested capital for the industry are even more staggering. In 1953 the total assets (minus liabilities) of manufacturers of motor vehicles and parts alone were estimated at close to eight billion dollars.[3] These statistics are cited not only to indicate the economic importance of the industry but also to emphasize the magnitude of employer-responsibility for the safety, health, and welfare of the labor force in this and other key industries.

As the automobile swung into mass production many new health hazards appeared, to which large numbers of workers were constantly exposed. Their extent and nature are summed up briefly by Dr. Robert T. Legge:

> In the manufacture of the raw materials and in the fabrication of the automobile alone many occupational diseases resulted, namely, heat exhaustion, asphyxiation by

gases, burns, traumatism, pneumoconiosis, and the ever increasing metallic and solvent toxemias.

The oil industry, from the well to the refinery, produces thousands of by-products, such as petrol, paraffin, oils, solvents, greases, dyes, pigments, insecticides, and pharmaceuticals. All of these are potentially toxic and some are carcinogenic; all affect the physiology of man and require the constant devotion of advanced clinical knowledge, engineering, chemical laboratory research, etc.[4]

In his master work, *Industrial Medicine and Surgery,* Dr. Harry E. Mock, of Chicago, calls attention to the extraordinary susceptibility of immigrant workers to accident and disease in American industry. Quoting liberally from a report of the United States Immigration Commission,[5] he notes that in 1908–1909, almost three-fifths of the total number of wage earners in twenty-one leading industries were of foreign birth. This report points out several vital factors which increased the hazards of employment to the foreign-born and handicapped efforts to enforce safety and preventive measures. Among these were such contributing conditions as illiteracy, inability to speak English, the shifting of Europeans from farm houses to crowded city tenements, drinking habits, and malnutrition due to distaste for American food.

By 1910 the population of the United States was slightly under 93 million; the labor force was estimated at 3.5 million, working an average of fifty hours a week. Production per manhour, however, was increasing rapidly. It was destined by 1950 to total three times the production of 1910—with a forty-hour week and a labor force only one-and-three-fourths times that of 1910.[6] The figures reflect the impact of the new technology upon American productivity.

At the first National Conference on Industrial Diseases in 1910, a report (based on the meager statistics available) was introduced by Frederick L. Hoffman (Prudential Insurance Company of America) to the effect that an estimated 280 million days were lost annually in industry from accident and illness—an average of better than eight days per employee.

Indicative of the lowly status of industrial medicine then is a further statement by Mr. Hoffman at the same conference: "The whole subject of occupational diseases is rather new in this country, and broadly speaking no serious effects of industry have generally been observed except in the case of a comparatively small number of particular trades. In most of these the unfavorable effects of industry on health have been held to be inseparable from industrial processes required for the needs of the community at large."[7]

Very few American physicians, in 1910, were seriously interested in occupational diseases as such, and the majority of those had only the sketchiest knowledge either of the true etiology of common industrial ailments or of effective preventive measures. Even more conspicuous was the absence of statistics on the incidence of specific diseases stemming from specific trades or industrial processes.

Traumatic injuries fell in another category. There, the surgeon was on familiar ground. The causes of accidents were usually obvious; professional treatment, when available, was prompt and efficient. It was only natural that a demand for protective devices and safety education for workers should become the entering wedge which opened the plants of America to the doctor as an industrial specialist.

The menace of tuberculosis came into the industrial limelight at a relatively early date. The crusade to check its inroads, however, was launched as a broad movement in the interest of public health. Though its prevalence in certain industries was recognized as a major factor in case totals, there was little evidence which definitely linked the disease with contributing causes in working environment, materials handled, or processes used.

As industrial production soared and labor forces grew, there was a sharp upturn of interest in the more insidious, but no less destructive, diseases of occupation. Poisoning from toxic materials became more and more prevalent; and these new hazards, one by one, claimed the attention of able research scientists.

Very early in the history of industrial medicine it became apparent that the mere need for legislative measures to protect the health of workers was no guarantee of proper action. The initiative of federal and state agencies alone was not sufficient: the voices of individuals, crying for reform, too often fell upon deaf ears.

In an analysis of medical services in industry, the American College of Surgeons makes this comment:

> Humanitarianism has prompted the existence of very few industrial medical services. It has, of course, permeated a number of medical services in varying degree, but as a motivating force it has exerted a negligible influence. The economic factor has been the prime mover in the organization and growth of industrial medical services —and why not? . . . Humanitarianism without its ultimate economic benefits would be futile no matter what its nature or direction.

The same analysis calls attention to the shocking prevalence of communicable diseases in industry during the early 1900's: "Shortly after the turn of the century a large industrial organization in a Southern state, for instance, reported that its workers and their families were so disabled from malaria, hookworm, typhoid, smallpox, and other communicable diseases that it was necessary to keep five men on the payroll to keep two at work."[8]

The first steps of national importance, dealing with hours and conditions of work, were taken by the federal government with the passage in 1907 of the Hours of Service Act, which limited the services of train employees, and telegraph and signal operators. In 1910 the Bureau of Mines was created. Two years later it inaugurated mine rescue procedures and in 1914 started the use of canaries to aid in the detection of mine gases.

Of far greater significance was the creation in 1913 of the United States Department of Labor, to "foster, promote and develop" the welfare of wage earners. Organization of the Division of Occupational Health of the United States Public Health Service followed in the next year. Its pioneer activities in the fields of safety and hygiene were largely the result of notable work by Joseph W. Schereschewsky and Royd R. Sayers—both of whom played leading roles in the later development of industrial medicine as a specialty.

Meanwhile, progress in accident and disease prevention by the various states followed an irregular pattern. In 1909 the labor laws of only twenty-one states contained sections bearing on industrial safety and health. These dealt largely with factory inspection, ventilation, and sanitation; for the most part they were inadequate and indifferently enforced. Opponents of a ten-hour law for women, passed in Oregon as a health measure, carried it to the United States Supreme Court, where ratification ended the battle in 1910.

Medical services in industry received tremendous impetus in 1913, with the founding of the Union Health Center in the ladies garment industry of New York City. Launched as a result of sensational revelations from an inquiry into sweatshop conditions, it was a pioneer enterprise among union-sponsored health plans. It presently serves approximately 200,000 members.[9]

In early years efforts to establish the principle of compensation of workers for occupational disability met with even more stubborn resistance, from both industries and legislatures, than did measures regulating general safety and hygiene. The federal government, again, set a pattern for efforts in this field by enacting a law in 1908 granting limited benefits to designated classes of public employees. Not until eight years later, with the passage of the first comprehensive federal compensation act, were benefits extended to all government employees under Civil Service.

Progress of the states in framing compensation codes was slow and painful for many years. Early laws—Montana (1909) and New York (1910)—were declared unconstitutional. New York's legislation was the result of shocking revelations in the epoch-making report of the Wainwright Commission, which showed that only one out of eight injured workmen were being awarded compensation and that nearly two-thirds of the amount paid went for legal expenses. This report brought no permanent legal reforms until 1914.

Publication of the report of the Illinois Commission on Workmen's Insurance, including all-important surveys by Hamilton and Hayhurst, stirred prompt action in that state. In 1911 Illinois passed a law providing compensation for industrial diseases caused by poisonous fumes, gases, and dusts, and requiring monthly examinations for workers in industries using lead, zinc, arsenic, brass, mercury, and phosphorus. Many reforms resulted. Employers were forced to insure against possible claims; insurance companies pressed them strongly to improve conditions of employment. Opposition, however, was stubborn. Company attorneys found ways of circumventing many provisions of the first law, and the battle for more decisive legislation dragged on for nearly three decades.

Along with Illinois, nine other states enacted compensation laws in 1911. Steadily, the principle of employer liability for occupational disability gained recognition, as state after state followed suit. By 1940 compensation statutes appeared on the books of forty-seven of the forty-eight state jurisdictions.[10]

Judged by this simple chronology, it might be inferred that the cause of compensation was completely won within a span of thirty years. Such was not the case. Even today, state laws are marked by a serious lack of uniformity. Adding to the confusion are conflicting interpretations of terminology and wide discrepancies in court rulings as to what constitutes valid medical testimony.[11]

Laws, in general, reflect public thinking. They are the product of pressure from the people at large or from groups dedicated to the resolution of specific issues. By 1910, many who espoused the cause of industrial health and safety realized that lone workers, pecking away at the problem, could accomplish little. Only through a powerful and persistent crusade could they attain their ends.

One priceless ingredient was missing—organization. And, to satisfy the need for organizations, they came into being almost as if in response to a signal. This—the second decade of the twentieth century—was a turning point in the story of industrial medicine. Within a half-dozen years, more was done to make this specialty an effective agent in human society than had been previously accomplished in all time.

Early interest in a nationwide safety movement stemmed from independent work by local groups. Progress was made in 1912, when the first Cooperative Safety Congress met in Milwaukee under the auspices of the Association of Iron and Steel Engineers—four doctors appeared on the program to talk of first aid, safety in coal mining, and industrial sanitation.

The following year, after a broad-gauge discussion of industrial safety and welfare at a meeting in New York, the National Safety Council was officially launched. And in Chicago, at its own first convention, the new organization took a momentous step, recorded in the minutes as follows: "In view of the fact that the present campaign for industrial safety has very clearly indicated the close interrelation of the health of workers to the prosperity of industries, the Executive Committee of the National Council for Industrial Safety, at a meeting in Chicago, February 16, 1914, created a Committee for Industrial Hygiene."

Not only have the Council and its committee, in the subsequent years, been a powerful force in the promotion of accident prevention, sanitation and hygiene, but through their cooperation with other industrial health agencies they have greatly furthered the cause of industrial medicine as a special field.

In Washington, in 1912, the foundation was laid for a truly scientific literature in American industrial medicine. The occasion was the Fifteenth International Congress on Hygiene and Demography, with Dr. George M. Kober presiding. At that meeting, in the section devoted to the hygiene of occupation, experts on every phase of the subject contributed sixty-four papers.

Another red-letter year was 1913, which saw the founding of the American

College of Surgeons. Its objectives were to maintain the high standards of character and training in the field of surgery, the betterment of hospitals and of teaching facilities, laws relating to medical practice and privilege, and an "unselfish protection of the public from incompetent medical service."[12]

This organization, through its Committee on Industrial Medicine and Traumatic Surgery, later formulated a Minimum Standard for Medical Service in Industry, and for many years served as the certifying agency for such services.

Management first came into the industrial medical picture under organization auspices as a consequence of the founding, in 1914, of the Conference Board of Physicians in Industrial Practice. This group, one of the first to realize that manpower was the most neglected of all national assets in industry, set forth as its purpose cooperative effort to introduce effective measures for the treatment of industrial injuries and ailments, for the promotion of sanitary conditions in workshops, and for the prevention of industrial diseases.

When, in 1916, the National Industrial Conference Board was established to represent management in the field of industrial health research, the Conference Board of Physicians took over the role of adviser to the new organization, and continued in that capacity until 1937. This cooperative arrangement represented a pioneer step in the coordination of management and medical effort.

The fall of 1914 also saw the establishment of the Industrial Hygiene Section of the American Public Health Association, which added another influential ally to the ranks of the industrial medical movement. Kober and Hayhurst were among the speakers on hygiene at the first section meeting.

Medical education in modern America will be discussed in detail later in this work. Mention at this point, however, is justified by the publication in 1910 of Dr. Abraham Flexner's *Medical Education in the United States and Canada,* at a time when the spotlight was being focused on national health, and industrial medicine was beginning its first real struggle toward recognition. The Flexner report was the result of a survey started in 1908 by the Carnegie Foundation for the Advancement of Teaching. The study was a monumental task. It ruthlessly bared the sad state of medical education in America, and clarified educational needs and problems, with logic that is still pertinent. It was a great turning point in an era of turning points. It was largely responsible for revolutionary changes in the entire system of medical education—with respect to ethics, standards of instruction, fiscal operations of medical schools, and requirements for medical practice.

Early in the century, a few American schools and universities had already recognized industrial and public health and hygiene as promising fields for instruction. Massachusetts Institute of Technology (1905) established a Department of Health and Biology, offering the first formal course in industrial hygiene. The Medical Department of the University of Pennsylvania (1906) offered courses in public health, leading to the degree of Doctor of Public Health. In 1910 Cornell University established, in connection with its medical school in New York City, an outpatient clinic that provided facilities for the study and treatment of occupational diseases—under the direction of W. Gilman Thompson. It was discontinued in 1916. At Harvard, Hugo Münsterberg (1912) applied psychology in industry, using it to test and select motormen for the elevated railroads. At Ohio State College of Medicine (1915) Emery Hayhurst opened a clinic for the study of industrial diseases. Other schools were soon to follow suit.

Thus was the stage set for the future of a new medical specialty. Industrial medicine, it is certain, could not have attained its present stature without such a background of industrial progress, medical research, and organization—or without a renaissance of medical education to insure a succession of able, well-trained medical personnel.

PART TWO

THE ASSOCIATION IS BORN

THE OBJECT of this Association shall be to foster the study and discussion of the problems peculiar to industrial medicine and surgery; to develop methods adapted to the conservation of health among workers in the industries; to promote a more general understanding of the purposes and results of the medical care of employees; and to unite into one organization members of the medical professions specializing in industrial medicine and surgery for their mutual advancement in the practice of their profession.

> *—Application for incorporation of the American Association of Industrial Physicians and Surgeons (revision of 1917).*

If Americans are endowed with any one superlative gift above all others, it is their genius for organizing.

VI

THE FOUNDERS AND THE FOUNDING

THE American Association of Industrial Physicians & Surgeons emerged in the second decade of this century as naturally and inevitably as a plant from the soil or a winged creature from its chrysalis. Everything conspired to bring it into being at the time of greatest need, and under circumstances most favorable for its survival and success.

It should be noted here that the association retained its original unwieldy but descriptive corporate name for thirty-five years. The change to its present name, Industrial Medical Association, was voted by the membership at the annual meeting in April, 1951.

First steps toward organization of the association were inspired by the thinking of a few doctors in scattered industries, who recognized the need for higher standards of industrial health and for a nationwide expansion of medical service to workers. These doctors were encouraged by the activities of other groups already crusading for public health, industrial safety, and hygiene. Their final decision was speeded by the enactment of compensation laws and the slowly awakening social consciousness of employers.

Industry's first reaction to liability laws covering occupational injuries was to reduce the expense of injuries by introducing accident-prevention measures and providing better surgical care. Prior to 1910 there was little in the way of legal compulsion or moral sanctions to force such precautions. Safety was fostered by enlightened, humane employers and neglected by the ignorant and indifferent.

Commenting on conditions at that time, an American College of Surgeons report declares: "Industrial medicine was also given a stimulus by the advent of workmen's compensation laws, but in comparison with the safety movement it has had a slumberous career. The purely repair shop type of surgical service in industry lasted much too long."[1]

The upward surge of American production was attended by serious, often fatal, injuries, which mounted at a scandalous rate; but for many years little of real or lasting benefit was done to reverse the trend. The annual toll was terrifying in typical industries such as steel, mining, railroading.

Here and there, individual doctors did what they could to protect workers on extra-hazardous jobs, but they left almost no records indicating results. A faded clipping from the *Chicago Daily News* reports that Andrew M. Harvey, chief surgeon of the Crane Company, Chicago, provided safety glasses for operators in that plant "as early as 1897." About the same time there is also mention of the use of leather leggings to protect brass molders from molten metal.

"Safety" was a word seldom heard in the steel mills and other ferrous industries of that day—not because employers were indifferent to death and injury, but because high accident ratios were taken for granted as a hazard of such trades. Though industrial employers commonly provided local physicians to care for injured workers, concerted action to reduce the accident toll was still to come. Individual companies, nevertheless, did what they could with the crude protective devices available in the early 1900's. Results were encouraging, and from these small beginnings there developed industry-wide programs calling for the installation of more and more mechanical safeguards, and requiring in-plant treatment of on-the-job injuries.

Within a few years important steel manufacturers were solidly supporting the work of the new National Safety Council, spearheading the crusade for industrial safety. Faced by shocking statistics on accidental deaths and injuries, corporation heads in large industries became ready converts to the cause. Physicians and surgeons, too, in steadily increasing numbers, were attracted to the industrial field.

Results of this attack were soon apparent. Accident curves were halted in their climb—then started to decline. The over-all trend, for the past forty years, has been consistently downward. Citing long-term figures, the *Labor Yearbook* for 1953 points to these significant contrasts: "In coal mining, for example, approximately five miners were killed in work accidents for every million tons of coal mined in 1913. In 1950 the average was down to slightly over one death for each million tons. In railroading, the reduction was even more pronounced. In 1913 one worker in every five hundred employed by the railroads was killed on the job. In 1950 one was killed for every three thousand. These rates are still too high."[2]

Mining appears to have been the first American industry to use the services of physicians on anything like a full-time basis. There is reference to an unnamed doctor who is said to have been employed in a lead mine in 1770. Others are known to have served in mines during the 1800's, though almost all name and place records have vanished with the years.

Appearance of the industrial physician and industrial surgeon, as we know them, is a twentieth century phenomenon. But there was no distinction in the title in early years. On the contrary, men in plant practice were commonly the object of professional scorn—poorly paid, respected neither by management nor by labor. This was to be expected. With notable exceptions the doctor in industry was likely to be a man of mediocre ability, performing routine work acceptably but with little awareness of its potentials. The field, by and large, was uninviting, unrewarding.

Writing of the period around 1910, Alice Hamilton sums up the status of the industrial doctor in these words: "For a surgeon or physician to accept a position with a manufacturing company was to earn the contempt of his colleagues."[3]

It is against this background that the story of the American Association of Industrial Physicians & Surgeons unfolds. In the early years it was a drama of men and of the unusual circumstances that brought them together from all parts of the country. They were for the most part young physicians and surgeons, attracted to industrial practice by the new emphasis on safety, public health, and hygiene. They were exceptions to the rule of mediocrity in plant practice at the time; their stature was the more pronounced because of the scarcity of medical talent in the industrial field. They had in common a conviction that health was the most valuable of all national resources and a belief that the way to conserve it was by concentrating on the accident and disease hazards to which industrial workers were constantly exposed.

Andrew Magee Harvey's introduction of protective goggles for workers in 1897 was a mere incident in the evolution of plant safety. But Harvey, the man, had a double claim to fame. He was perhaps the first American physician to practice modern industrial medicine, and he was a leader in the little group chiefly responsible for the founding of the AAIP&S. Harvey joined the Crane organization in Chicago as medical director in 1896, assuming responsibility for the care of some 18,000 employees. Throughout his career he was a tireless worker in organized medicine, in public health activities, and in the development of the new industrial specialty.

In faraway California Robert Legge joined the select coterie of industrial medical pioneers in 1899. Trauma, at the time, was the main concern of the McCloud River Lumber Company, but Legge, as chief surgeon, soon expanded his work into broader fields—a community health and welfare program, construction of a model hospital, and the successful practice of preventive as well as curative medicine. At McCloud, in 1900, he was the first to employ graduate nurses in industrial service.

An inveterate traveler, he periodically toured the East to attend medical conventions and to visit the great surgical centers and teaching hospitals. On these trips he met many other leaders in the industrial field and through these contacts was drawn into the inner circle of founding fathers of the AAIP&S.

Years later (in 1927) Legge spent an afternoon at Georgetown Medical School with the venerable Dean Kober. To the delight of both, they discovered that McCloud, the scene of Legge's early work, was in the heart of the identical terrain covered by Kober, as a United States Army surgeon, in the Modoc Indian War of 1873–74.

One of the earliest recorded efforts at systematic examination of industrial workers is credited to Frank Fulton, of Providence, Rhode Island, who examined the employees of a large saw company in 1906 as part of a campaign to stamp out tuberculosis in the plant. Other industrial physicians were beginning to realize that physical examinations, both preplacement and periodical, were a fundamental requirement in any effective health program.

Harry E. Mock started the examination of employees of Sears, Roebuck & Company, Chicago, in 1909 to discover and isolate those who were tuberculous. He quickly became convinced of the economic as well as the medical value of thorough examinations and complete case records. Yet these basic procedures, now universally established, remained for many years the source of bitter controversy with both labor and management.

In the period from 1910 to 1915 other medical directors were reporting equal success from similar programs in important industrial plants. These included Irving Clark (Norton Grinding Company, Worcester, Massachusetts); S. M. McCurdy (Youngstown Sheet and Tube Company); Otto P. Geier (Cincinnati Milling Machine Company); Wilbur Post (Peoples' Gas Company, Chicago); C. G. Farnum (Avery Company, Peoria, Illinois); W. G. Hudson (E. I. du Pont de Nemours & Company, Wilmington, Delaware).

Because of its size, the large number of workers it employed, and the new health hazards originating in its manufacturing processes, the automobile industry presented special medical problems from its very beginning. Early in their history, leading companies established medical departments; and the industry has been a potent force in the development of occupational medicine to its present stature.

The first medical director of the Ford Motor Company, James E. Mead, of Detroit, was appointed in 1913 and served the company continuously for twenty-five years. A copy of the *Ford Times* shows that more than 200,000 cases required treatment in the year ending August 31, 1915, about 164,000 of which were handled in the dispensary. Two-thirds of the injuries were received in line of duty and, with few exceptions, were of a minor nature.

In 1916 Mahlon H. Sutton joined Buick as assistant medical director and in 1915 A. Willis Hudson took a post as medical director at Northway Motors, a G. M. subsidiary. They were the first full time physicians employed by General Motors, whose component divisions were in 1954 responsible for the health of some 600,000 workers.

From three men—Mock, Legge, and Otto Geier—we have obtained a great deal of information about events leading directly to the organization of the AAIP&S. Our information has been drawn from personal memories, from reminiscences of chance meetings and conversations, and from correspondence and other scattered records. Without these, along with dates and other basic information relating to events and personalities, some of the most colorful pages in the history of industrial medicine in America would remain, irreparably, a blank.

Harry E. Mock first entertained the idea of industrial practice as the result of a friendship with Jules Gauss, who had served for four years as company doctor with Sears, Roebuck. One day, in 1908, Gauss mentioned to Mock that he was about to resign, his chief reason being that "the Chicago Medical Society had refused his membership because they considered his industrial practice unethical."

Mock, a graduate of Rush Medical College in 1906, was just starting to build a surgical practice in Chicago and was serving as an instructor in gynecology at Rush. Gauss's reasons for believing that the young surgeon would do well to seek a connection as his successor are of interest as a sidelight on the status of industrial medicine at that time.

"He told me," said Mock, "that too many industries, insurance companies, and even railroads were employing full-time doctors who were poorly trained and therefore could be hired for very little money. These doctors found it difficult to compete with the newer type of medical students—with their partial or full college education before four years of medical training, plus internship, and, in an increasing number of cases, postgraduate work as assistants to good men.

"Further, he pointed out that too many industries were invading the field of general medical practice by having their doctors give home treatment to employees at a reduced rate below that usually charged by the profession. The pitfall that had ruined Dr. Gauss's ethical standing was the fact that the Sears Mutual Benefit Association used one-dollar house calls on any member of an employee's family, as an inducement to prospective members.

"Naturally, this practice had aroused the ire of the general practitioners in Chicago, with the result that Dr. Gauss, a Rush man and an intern of Presbyterian Hospital, was classified as unethical. Needless to say, he regained his ethical status, and developed an excellent general practice in Indianapolis."

Armed with Gauss's advice—and his warning—Mock consulted another friend, Frank Billings, an outstanding physician in Chicago at the time. "Why," he asked Mock, "do you want this job?"

Mock had a concise and practical answer: "Because I want to get married, I'm in debt, and I need to make money at once. Furthermore, I consider this a great opportunity."

"I like your last reason best. Just what kind of opportunity do you see at Sears?"

"Well," replied Mock, "here are 15,000 people, men and women, gathered under one roof in a great industry. *This is a great human laboratory.* Think of the opportunity of making a complete physical examination of all these people. We have been trained to examine sick or supposedly sick people, but here I could study average normal workers and could learn what 'normal' as differentiated from 'sick' really is. I could catch the evidence of disease early, and could warn many of these in time to prevent impending trouble.

"In their large packing and shipping rooms, where at least two thousand people are working, they use cut-up paper swept from the floor and contaminated by dirt, for much of their packing. I would try to change this.

"Further, I would examine every man and woman in this department to ascertain how many, if any, had tuberculosis, and thus stop the spread of the disease by ruling them out of this work. And how many of their employees have heart disease and don't know it? Many of these, when found by examination, could be shifted to lighter types of work, and thus could be kept on the job and useful much longer than they might be otherwise.

"Best of all, think of the opportunity this job offers for the prevention of injuries and the teaching of first aid. The more I think of it, the bigger this opportunity grows. I'd like to take the job on a part-time basis only—to have time to develop my private practice and for my teaching. But I want the job."

Seen from a distance of nearly a half century, Mock's thinking and program appear elementary, but in 1908 his was a decidedly advanced viewpoint. Not long before that time the great Bertram Sippy had strongly advised Mock not to think of an industrial career because of the ill repute in which company doctors were held. In Sippy's own work as surgeon for the Anaconda Copper Company there was no attempt at examinations or supervision of the health of employees. And, except for railway surgeons, industrial doctors were usually paid from $150 to $300 per month even for full-time work.

Billings, however, saw the opportunity as Mock pictured it. "That's enough," he said. "I'm sold. You have a great dream there and, I believe, enthusiasm enough to bring it to pass. It will mean working five hours a day longer than your competitors, but I think you can do it.

"Mr. Rosenwald is a great man, and is strong for anything that will better the conditions of mankind. Go and tell him of your dream of a great human laboratory, and I'll bet he'll give you the job. Then play the game fair and square, and I'll guarantee the Chicago Medical Society won't criticize you or claim you are unethical."

By such little things are man's decisions swayed. With the warm approval of Billings, Mock had his conference with Julius Rosenwald, president, and Albert Loeb, vice-president of Sears, Roebuck & Co.

"Doctor," said Loeb, "thus far you haven't seemed very anxious to take this position. Why is this?"

"In the first place, if one carries on under the same arrangement you have with Dr. Gauss, the Chicago Medical Society will call him unethical and ban him from membership. This I wouldn't want. In the second place, you don't pay enough for this work to make a good man want it."

"You think you're a good man, then?"

"Yes, sir," replied Mock.

"Just why," asked Rosenwald, "would you want to accept company work at all if you are as good a man as you say; and under what conditions would you consider it?"

"The only reason I would want it is because your 15,000 employees represent a great human laboratory, where a doctor could practice preventive medicine and surgery."

"Hear that, Julius?" interrupted Loeb. "We have become a great human laboratory. We've had several company doctors, but never before have they thought of us as a human laboratory."

"I rather like the idea," replied Rosenwald.

There was more discussion, but no final decision. Mock was on his honeymoon when, on December 28, 1908, he received a telegram from Loeb: "Your human laboratory idea appeals. We accept your proposition. Start January 2."

Mock's "proposition" included immediate examination of old employees, to check and eliminate infectious diseases—and later, examinations for all job applicants, with the aim not only of raising health standards but also of assigning handicapped men and women to suitable work whenever possible. Mock developed, as the creed of his department, the simple slogan: "Physical qualifications, plus occupational qualifications, equal the job." Much later, during World War I, this slogan became the basis of far-reaching recommendations to the surgeon general of the Army for the assignment of handicapped volunteers and draftees.

Within three years, Mock's dream was well on its way to reality. He had no trouble in maintaining ethical standards at Sears. Cut-rate house calls for employees were ruled out. If they wanted the Sears doctor for illness at home, he would see them as private patients, and charge them standard professional fees.

Then, as Mock described it, came a balmy evening in May, 1912, and another chance conversation. Returning from a medical meeting, Mock drove his friend, Harvey, home in his new Maxwell convertible. The two sat in the open car and discussed their common problems—their work as company doctors. Harvey, with sixteen years' experience in the Crane organization, had built an excellent reputation as a surgeon and administrator of health problems involving both accident and occupational hazards. He had done this without antagonizing the medical profession and had maintained a good ethical standing.

Mock spoke of his new quarters at Sears—twelve rooms staffed by eleven part-time doctors and two full-time nurses. An eye specialist was on duty three days a week, and dental service was available for three and a half hours every day. Mock's enthusiasm, too, had grown with his job. He mentioned that that very day Rosenwald had proudly escorted the president of the Packard Motor Car Company through the department. At the end of the tour the visitor said: "This is all pretty nice, Julius, but I can't see how you can afford to give the most valuable space in your merchandising building to your doctor's office." Rosenwald had replied: "Why, sir, this is the most valuable department we have. It deserves the most valuable space."

So the talk went on, in the convertible at Harvey's door. Around 2:00 A.M. Mock started his motor and prepared to go. Then Harvey broke in:

"Do you know, we ought to organize this company doctor business. It's altogether different from what it was when I went into industrial work. Industrial medicine is here to stay. A lot of good men are doing either part-time or full-time work as company doctors. We ought to get together with those who see a real service in it—both to humanity and to medicine—and form an organization."

There was more discussion before the two men parted to think it over. "So," said Mock, "as far as I know, the first thought of an industrial medical association was wafted in on the balmy spring air on that May night in 1912.

"It was later in that same year that I met Doctor Otto Geier, of Cincinnati. He was a dynamic man, and one of the most likeable personalities I had ever met, with thorough training and ample financial backing that enabled him to select his niche in the medical world and to reach almost any height in his chosen endeavor.

"Geier had organized the first milk commission in Cincinnati and had worked tirelessly for rigid inspection, pasteurization, etc. He came through milk into the field of preventive medicine. His viewpoint was further broadened by other activities in the field of public charities and institutional health, which brought him into contact with the derelicts of society.

"The Geiers had founded and made a great business of the Cincinnati Milling Machine Company. Otto was a prime mover in organizing its first health program, a part-time connection which soon absorbed his entire attention. Hearing of the work we were doing at Sears, he visited our medical department, and left us with many suggestions which enlarged its scope and increased its effectiveness.

"Otto Geier's grasp of the situation and its possibilities in the way of preventive medicine was of the greatest importance in the founding of our association. From the time of his first visit we never lost sight of our ultimate goal—the organization of industrial medicine on a national basis."

From these early contacts and discussions the movement for an association spread rapidly, by chain reaction. Through the efforts of Frank Billings, Thomas R. Crowder was appointed medical director of the Pullman Company. By 1912 he not only was supervising the health of Pullman employees, but also had become a great authority on ventilation, fumigation, and the prevention of contagious diseases by systematic examinations.

Said Mock: "Tom became a wise friend and a man of keen judgment, with a broad vision of the possibilities of industrial medicine and the means by which it could fit itself into the medical world without antagonizing those in the profession who were limiting their work to private practice."

Crowder became familiar with every step in the preorganization thinking of the Chicago group. It was he who wrote the final draft of the constitution of the American Association of Industrial Physicians & Surgeons and set forth its objectives. He later served as its president (1927–1928).

Again, in 1912, Billings recommended the appointment of Wilbur E. Post, a close friend of Crowder and Mock, as medical director of the Peoples Gas Company, of Chicago. Post, in turn, called the attention of the group to Charles G. Farnum, chief surgeon of the Avery Company in nearby Peoria. Farnum had developed a well rounded program of supervision of the health of Avery employees. In this work he was strongly backed by Mr. Avery and with him attended the Chicago convention of the National Safety Council in 1914. It was then that Farnum joined the circle of conferees in their frequent discussions of plans for the new association.

Since the turn of the century William B. Fisk had been chief surgeon of the great and growing International Harvester Company. From a strictly surgical practice he had enlarged the work of his department to include systematic examinations and over-all supervision of health in all company plants. He too became a vital personality in developing association plans.

As time passed, the program took shape. Mock corresponded incessantly with recruits for the cause—important figures in the fields of public health, hygiene, and industrial safety—including Otto Geier, Francis Patterson, Loyal A. Shoudy, Emery R. Hayhurst, and Sir Thomas Oliver. Their replies were encouraging and helped spur immediate action.

On short notice, in October, 1914, Mock called a meeting at his office in the Peoples Gas Building. Only six men were able to answer the call, but they had the backing of many more who could not come to Chicago.

Harvey—Mock—Farnum—Crowder—Fisk—Post. They were the nucleus of the founding group which voted to organize "a National Society of Physicians and Surgeons in Industrial Practice." They constituted themselves an organizing committee, elected Mock secretary, and charged him with the duty of spreading the word among outstanding doctors in all parts of the country.

Mock promptly wrote to a representative group, asking for a show of hands, by mail, on the specific proposal to organize and incorporate. Replies were uniformly favorable. They confirmed the committee's decision that the time was right, and that the new association would receive the initial backing it required, from men whose medical weight would influence others to join.

Mock's personal files yield a partial list of doctors who wired or wrote their emphatic approval. They typify the high caliber of the original membership. Their names recur again and again in the later history of the association. From the start they served as apostles of a new industrial medical creed, which they preached on any and all occasions.

The list included old friends and new. Among the first to reply, and one of the most enthusiastic supporters of the plan, was Otto Geier—as was to be expected. In the East there was Francis Patterson (Pennsylvania Department of Labor and Industry); and in the West, Robert T. Legge, who still held his post at McCloud, California. From Washington came a promise of active support from Joseph W. Schereschewsky, who, until his death, was prominently identified not only with the United States Public Health Service, but also with the early growth of the Association. Among medical directors who added their endorsements were Clarence D. Selby, then serving a number of industrial concerns in Toledo, A. B. George (Packard Motor Car Company), Don B. Lowe (B. F. Goodrich Company), Loyal A.

Shoudy (Bethlehem Steel), Cassius H. Watson (New York Telephone Company), W. Irving Clark (Norton Company), and James E. Mead (Ford Motor Company).

Of the entire group engaged in this voluminous correspondence, no less than six were later to serve as presidents of the Association. Drawing its strength from such diverse sources, and from every section of the country, the association-to-be was assured of truly national representation from the very beginning. Most of its supporters were already members of several organized medical groups concerned with various phases of public health and private practice; yet they rallied behind a new association as the *one* answer to vital industrial problems not yet adequately covered by any existing agency.

Encouraged by this wholesale response, the Organizing Committee met frequently during the winter of 1914–1915. "At each meeting," writes Harry Mock, "there were increasing evidences of approval, ending in agreement to crystallize the movement by formal organization.

"Accordingly, under the friendly auspices of the Illinois Manufacturers Association, a 'meeting of physicians and surgeons in industry' was called in February, 1915, at the Chicago City Club, where the proposal was discussed at length. The unanimous expression was that such an organization would be beneficial to employees and employers, as well as to the physicians specializing in industrial medicine."

At that February meeting a committee was appointed, which, "for the physicians and surgeons engaged in industrial medicine, prepared and executed the documents necessary for a corporation (not for pecuniary profit) to be known as the *American Associational of Industrial Physicians & Surgeons,* under an Act of the General Assembly of the State of Illinois."

So reads the record. Accompanying the application was a formal statement of the corporate purposes—as printed in full at the head of Part Two. Writes Mock: "This statement remains [essentially] unchanged. There has been no occasion to change it. Nothing in the developments of the years since 1915 has been added to the comprehensiveness of its definition of industrial medicine, nor disclosed a facet of the subject which it does not cover."

Spring and summer were gone before charter details had been settled to the satisfaction of the committee. Under date of October 12, 1915, Harvey forwarded to Mock duplicate copies of the application with a letter asking him to get the required signatures "as quickly as possible."

The final document, as notarized and forwarded to the Secretary of State of Illinois, bears the signatures of the Incorporating Committee: J. Chase Stubbs (medical director of the National Malleable Casting Company); A. M. Harvey, H. E. Mock, C. G. Farnum, W. E. Post, and T. R. Crowder, all of Chicago; and S. M. McCurdy, of Cleveland.[4] Stubbs served as chairman.

While the preliminary work of organization was moving slowly ahead, busy doctors elsewhere were taking advantage of every opportunity to win further support for the new association. Many a casual personal contact, at both private and public meetings, became the occasion for a well documented appeal on behalf of the proposed organization. These, trivial in themselves, added up to an impressive total of influence which account in no small measure for the early success and rapid growth of the association. In Mock's words, "They give reason and glamor to its founding."

Otto Geier and Schereschewsky, for example—the one an industrial doctor, the other a surgeon in the USPHS—had become close friends as a result of their common interest in the health and welfare of the working man. At the annual meeting of the National Safety Council in 1914, they raised the question of how far the council intended to go in including sanitation as part of its safety program.

"Does this mean," they wanted to know, *"medical supervision of workers?"* Failing to get a satisfactory answer, they pressed for the creation of a Health Service Section of the council, which was duly voted at the same meeting. The full significance of their cooperative effort, however, did not become apparent until more than a year and a half later.

Schereschewsky's appeals for an entirely new program in occupational medicine were frequent and pointed. In an address to the National Association for the Prevention of Tuberculosis in May, 1914, he declared that the medical examination of employees and the prevention of sickness were the proper foundation of any effective system of industrial insurance.[5] In a paper read before the Section on Industrial Hygiene of the American Public Health Association in October, 1915, he outlined a plan of education for the prevention of occupational diseases and injuries. He estimated that between twenty-five and thirty million workers were exposed to various health hazards and that they were losing eight or nine days per year per worker as a consequence. Noting a great increase in diseases of degeneration, he declared: "It is only too plain that the relation of disease to occupation is regarded as a specialty, and something with which neither the general practitioner nor the specialist in other fields is very closely concerned. Yet industrial workers constitute by far the largest class of medical patients."[6]

On the west coast, in January, 1915, Legge assumed his duties as professor and chairman of the Department of Hygiene at the University of California. One of his earliest activities was the establishment of courses in industrial hygiene for undergraduates. As university physician he also organized a students' health service—requiring vaccination and chest x-rays for all. His system of detailed records, giving the complete medical history of every student, is still regarded as a model.

In June, 1915, Geier made a further contribution of importance to the cause nearest his heart. As chairman of the Section on Preventive Medicine of the American Medical Association, at its first meeting in San Francisco, he organized a symposium at which industrial sanitation, the medical supervision of employees, and health insurance were thoroughly discussed by nationally known speakers.

Such evangelistic efforts, the country over, encouraged national interest in occupational health. Wherever the well-being of working people was discussed professionally, industrial medicine in one or another of its aspects became the topic of the day.

The Incorporating Committee decided to strike the iron while it was hot. The iron, in this case, was the first session of the new Health Service Section of the National Safety Council—scheduled for October 20, 1915, during the annual meeting of the council in Philadelphia. Here was an opportunity to reach, in a single audience, a large and representative number of potential members of the new association.

At a meeting on October 8, only twelve days before the Philadelphia convention, the committee formally adopted the following resolutions:

> That there be extended to all physicians and surgeons engaged in industrial medicine and surgery a most cordial invitation to enroll themselves as charter members of the American Association of Industrial Physicians & Surgeons.

> That the charter be not closed until July 1, 1916, and that all physicians and surgeons becoming members of the association prior to July 1, 1916, be considered, and be, charter members.

> That a meeting of all charter members be held in Detroit, Michigan, during the session of the American Medical Association in June, 1916, on some day hereafter determined by the Incorporating Committee.

> And that physicians and surgeons in attendance at the National Safety Congress be especially invited to enroll themselves as charter members of the American Association of Industrial Physicians & Surgeons and to appoint a committee consisting of seven members to cooperate with the Incorporating Committee in arranging for the meeting at Detroit, Michigan, and to secure charter members prior to that date.

In order to assure a representative showing of Western and Middlewestern doctors on the original charter list, the committee arranged a general dinner meeting at the City Club, Chicago, on October 15. In the invitations for the dinner, issued to a broad but carefully selected list, Mock wrote: "It is very important to have as large a number of men as possible at this meeting, so that we will have at least one hundred names on our charter before it goes east to be presented to the doctors in other parts of the country doing this line of work."

Mock laconically summed up the results of this official session as follows: "The meeting was eminently satisfactory; all previous acts of the Incorporating Committee were approved; and planning for the general meeting in Detroit the following June was begun."

Unfortunately, no written record of the Philadelphia meeting of the Health Service Section of the National Safety Council has survived the years. But Geier and Schereschewsky were on hand—armed with authority to enroll charter members for the AAIP&S, and ready to resume the discussion of the *medical supervision of workers* which they had interjected at the 1914 Safety Congress.

Shortly before his death, Otto Geier commented on results of the session in these words: "With Sherry in his seat as chairman and yours truly as secretary, some two-hundred physicians associated with industry in a more or less loose way showed great interest in our program."

The AAIP&S was born of a great need, which became increasingly apparent, year by year, in the turbulent period preceding the United States' entry into World War I. The association was founded on faith and friendship—faith in the bright future of a new medical specialty and the friendship of men remarkably alike in training, outlook and aspirations.

It was a magnificent accident of chance and circumstance that brought these men together. Seldom, if ever, in any profession, have so many with so much in common united to launch a national movement of equal importance. The pioneers of the association were bound together not only by the traditions and principles of medicine but also by a specialized interest in its many industrial phases.

In the words of Harry Mock: "Friendships formed at our early meetings, and at the first convention, have remained the warmest and closest throughout life—for many of those old-timers are now gone. Beyond doubt, those friendships became the nucleus of effective organization and were mainly responsible for the rapid growth of the association since 1916."

VII

1916—A NEW MILESTONE IN MEDICINE

As AN EVENT in the medical news of 1916, the first national convention of the American Association of Industrial Physicians & Surgeons was almost completely overshadowed by the sixty-seventh annual meeting of the American Medical Association, with which it shared quarters in the stately Hotel Cadillac in downtown Detroit.

The Organization and Incorporating committees of the new association, with practically identical personnel, had done their work quietly, skilfully, thoroughly, but without benefit of headlines or fanfare. In the eyes of many, at the time, this was "just another medical organization." The association had been an official entity since February 11, 1916, when Lewis J. Stephenson, Secretary of State in Illinois, certified it as a legal corporation. The ten-dollar incorporating fee was duly paid the following day.

There was much activity in the ensuing months. Harry Mock recalled that letters, and more letters, were written and favorable replies continued to accumulate right up to the final day. Typical was the response of John J. Moorhead, consulting surgeon for several railways, who wrote on June 2:

> I have yours of the 26th, telling me of the activities of the American Association of Industrial Physicians & Surgeons and of their coming meeting in Detroit. I think the time is ripe to form a national association of this type, and my suggestion would be that each of the respective local organizations might coordinate at an annual meeting, so that unity of purpose and method might be better attained.
>
> You may be sure that our Conference Board of Physicians in Industry will be glad to cooperate in any attempts to standardize this branch of medical and surgical service which is rapidly becoming a definite specialty.

70

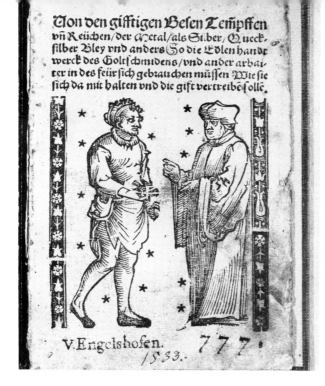

V. Engelshofen.   777.
1533.

14. *A Fifteenth Century Work on Occupational Poisons.* An eight-page booklet, recognized as the first work ever printed on the subject of occupational health. The author, Ulrich Ellenbog, was born in Feldkirch, Austria, in 1440, and died in 1499. His manuscript bears the date August 6, 1473; the booklet was probably printed in 1533.

The title is fully descriptive, as this translation of the six lines of German text above the illustration demonstrates: "Concerning the poisonous biting, vaporizing, and smoking of metals, such as silver, quicksilver, lead and others, which the worthy trade of the goldsmith and other workers are compelled to use. How they should conduct themselves concerning these matters and how to dispel the poison."

Only one original copy of the book is known to be in existence.

15. *The Anatomy of Human Bodies.* This rare and interesting book, printed in 1694, is an English translation of a Latin work by Isbrand de Diemerbroeck, "Professor of Physick and Anatomy" in Utrecht. William Salmon was a London professor of "Physick." Diemerbroeck's work contains many observations that were advanced for their time, not the least of them being his description of the pathology of silicosis. Writing of the lungs of miners removed in an autopsy, he says: "insomuch that I seemed to cut through a heap of sand, so that the vesicles being filled with dust, could not admit the air, which was the occasion of the poor fellow's death."

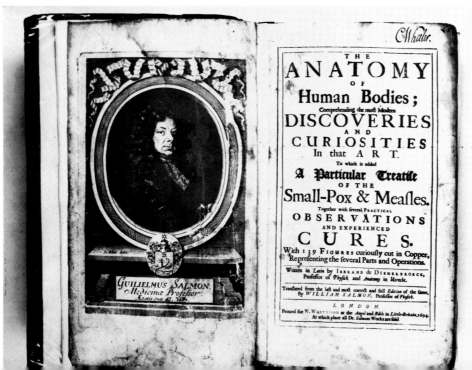

THE
ANATOMY
OF
Human Bodies;
Comprehending the moſt Modern
DISCOVERIES
AND
CURIOSITIES
In that ART.
To which is added
A Particular Treatiſe
OF THE
Small-Pox & Meaſles.
Together with ſeveral PRACTICAL
OBSERVATIONS
AND EXPERIENCED
CURES.
With 139 FIGURES curiouſly cut in Copper,
Repreſenting the ſeveral Parts and Operations.
Written in Latin by ISBRAND de DIEMERBROECK,
Profeſſor of Phyſick and Anatomy in Utrecht.
Tranſlated from the laſt and moſt correct and full Edition of the ſame,
By WILLIAM SALMON, Profeſſor of Phyſick.
LONDON
Printed for W. WHITWOOD at the Angel and Bible in Little-Britain, 1694.
At which place all Dr. Salmon's Works are ſold.

GUILIELMUS SALMON.
Medicinæ Profeſſor.

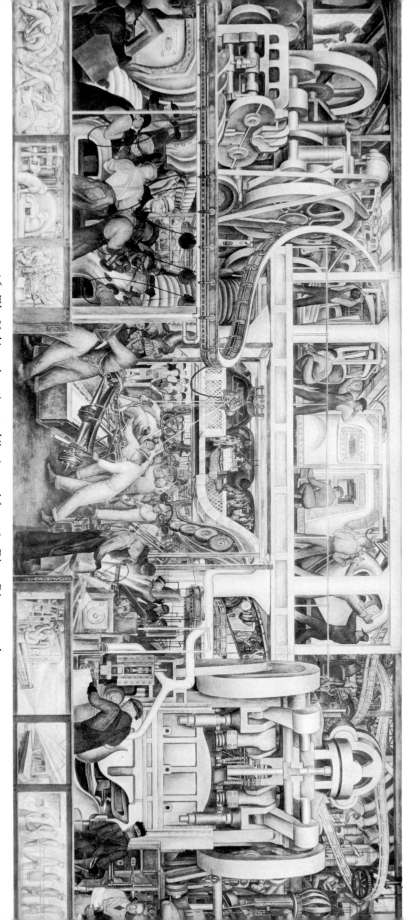

16. *The Making of an Automobile.* A panel from the Diego Rivera murals in the Detroit Institute of Arts, symbolic of world leadership in automobile manufacture.

—*Courtesy of the Detroit Institute of Arts*

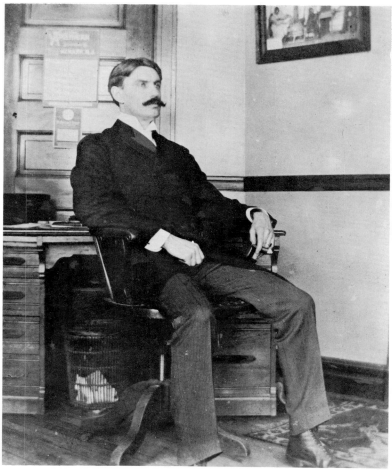

17. *Dr. A. M. Harvey at his Desk in the Old Crane Plant.* Harvey was born in 1868, received B.S. and M.S. degrees at Knox College, studied at the University of Michigan Medical School, got his M.D. degree at University of Illinois College of Medicine, and entered industrial practice in 1896 as medical director of the Crane Company, Chicago, where he was responsible for the health care of 18,000 employees.

—Courtesy of the Crane Company

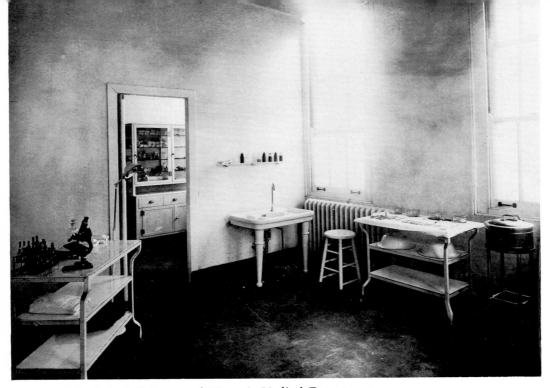

18. *The Principal Rooms of Harvey's Medical Department.*

19. *Shower Baths in the Crane Pipe Mill.* "With individual dressing rooms," says the caption on this print. Such facilities in industry, rough though they were, were rare in their day.

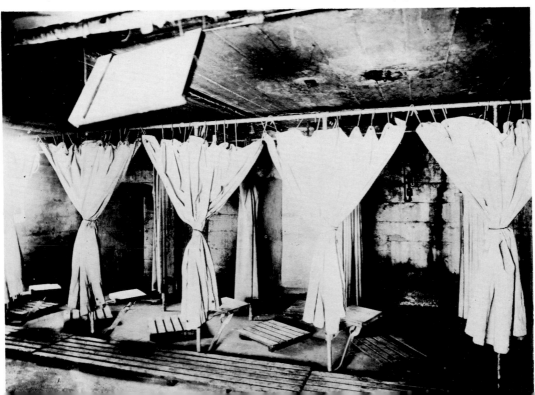

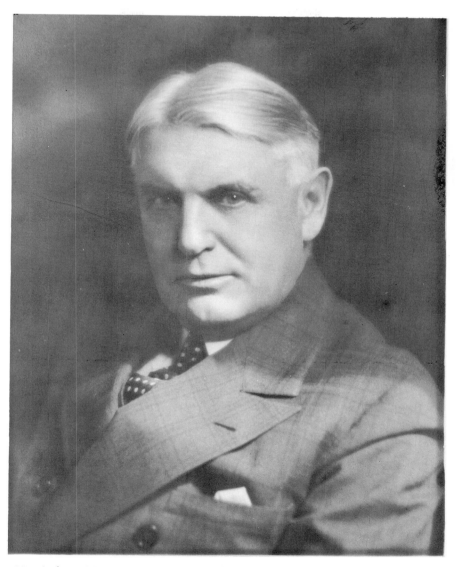

20. *Andrew Magee Harvey, M.D.* A founder of the AAIP&S and perhaps the first American to practice true industrial medicine. His chance remark to Otto Geier, "Perhaps we ought to organize," led to plans for the new organization.

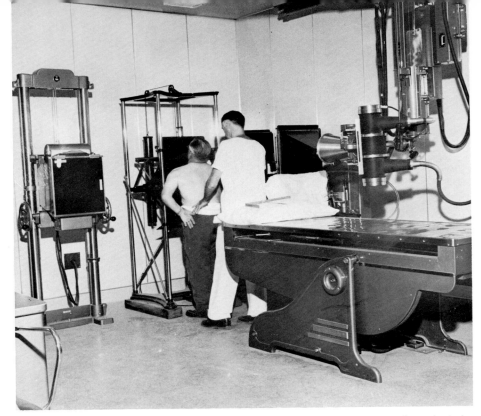

21. *Routine Chest X-rays.* Early efforts (before 1910) to stamp out tuberculosis in industry demonstrated the need for periodical physical examinations. Chest X-rays, then a rarity, are now a routine precaution. The modern equipment shown is in the medical department of the Inland Steel Company, Chicago.

22. *Medical Pioneering at McCloud, California.* Here, as chief surgeon of the McCloud River Lumber Company, Dr. R. T. Legge in 1900 introduced a community health program for employees and their families, established a model hospital staffed by graduate nurses, and combined preventive with curative medicine.

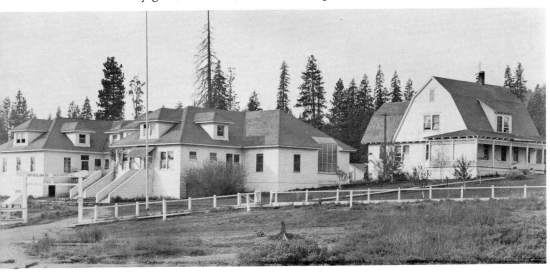

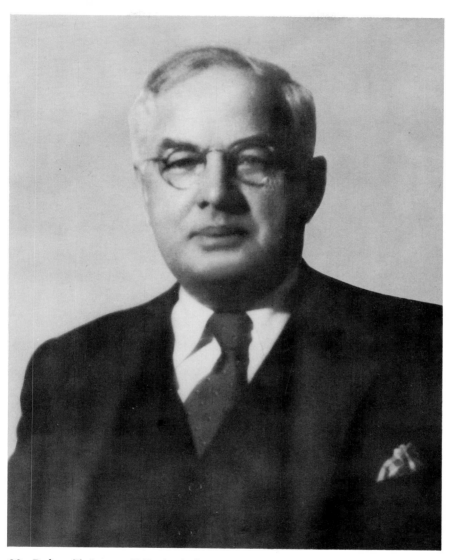

23. *Robert T. Legge, M.D.* An industrial medical pioneer. Author and teacher; a founding member of the AAIP&S, a tireless workers in the cause, and a member of the IMA History Committee.

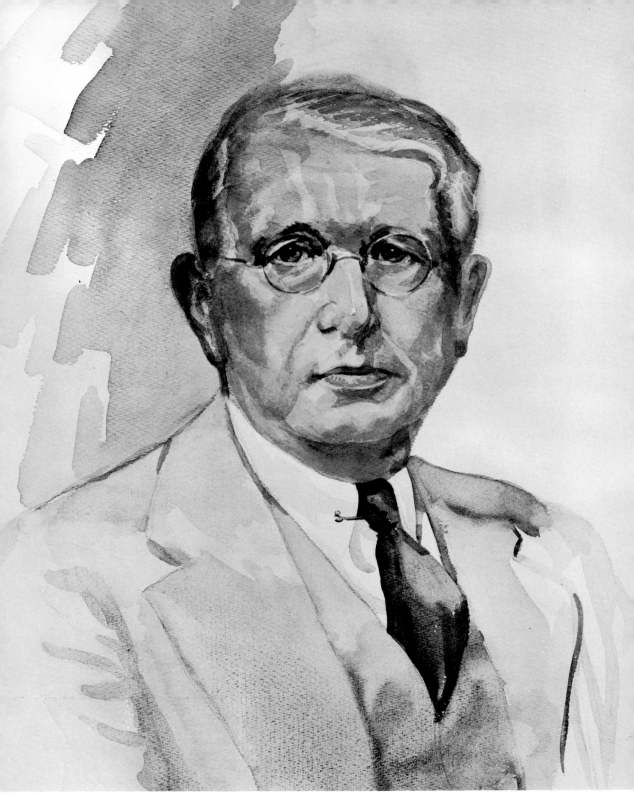

24. *Joseph W. Schereschewsky, M.D. (1873–1940). First president, AAIP&S, 1916–1918.* A man of endless energy, Schereschewsky made his mark as a surgeon in the United States Public Health Service, went on to head the federal Office of Industrial Hygiene (1915 to 1918) and later to direct the Division of Scientific Research. In him the AAIP&S found a staunch champion in high places during the transition of occupational medicine from obscurity to national importance. His talents ranged from administrative skill in upper echelons to complex mechanical hobbies at home; and he found time to write many excellent monographs on public health topics.

—All watercolor portraits in this volume were painted by G. Spurgeon Wood.

FIRST ANNUAL MEETING

of the

American Association of

Industrial Physicians and Surgeons

MONDAY, JUNE 12th, 1916

Detroit, Michigan

"The object of this Association shall be to foster the study and discussion of the problems peculiar to the practice of industrial medicine and
surgery; to develop methods adapted to the conservation of health among
workmen in the industries; to promote a more general understanding of the
purposes and results of the medical care of employees; and to unite into
one organization members of the medical profession specializing in industrial medicine and surgery for their mutual advancement in the practice of
their profession."

While the founders set their sights at the highest level with respect to the association objectives and the caliber of membership, they kept their financial program within modest bounds. A standard paragraph in committee correspondence dealt with the matter of cost in these reassuring words: "There will be some little expense connected with the organization, but this will be very slight and can easily be covered by nominal dues of one dollar per member." Actually, first-year dues were set at two dollars, but, since a maximum membership of one hundred and fifty was expected, the working budget gave no ground for charges of extravagance.

One finds a similar note of economy wisely accented in arrangements for the convention itself. Under date of May 25, R. A. Carson and C. C. Schantz, co-managers of the Cadillac Hotel, sent a banquet menu to Mock for his approval. The following exchange of letters is of passing interest as a commentary on those times:

Mock to Cadillac Hotel, May 26: "This menu is very satisfactory with the exception of cigars. Two dollars a plate should include at least one round of some good cigar."

Cadillac Hotel to Mock: "Yours of the 26th to hand with menu as selected for the American Association of Industrial Physicians & Surgeons, at $2.00 per plate—cigars extra."

Mock to Cadillac Hotel: "As we have advertised our banquet for $2.00 per plate, I wish you would kindly make some slight change in the menu so as to include one round of some good ten-cent cigar."

There was no provision for cigars.

There was, in fact, no need for either frills or festivities to whet the enthusiasm of the founding group. To a man, they realized the seriousness of the business at hand, and sensed something of the import of this new milestone in the history of American medicine.

As almost the final step in completing arrangements, Mock dispatched a night letter to Sidney M. McCurdy of Youngstown, a fellow committeeman: "Organization Committee have left it to me to choose toastmaster banquet Monday night. Have chosen one of best scouts in the bunch, namely, you. You can't refuse, for programs go to press tonight. Everything looking rosy."

There appears to have been only one advance notice of the Detroit meeting published in any periodical reaching the medical fraternity. It appeared in the *Journal of the American Medical Association*[1] under the headline:

MEETINGS OF NON-AFFILIATED ORGANIZATIONS
AMERICAN ASSOCIATION OF
INDUSTRIAL PHYSICIANS & SURGEONS

The notice stated that organization of the association was to be completed at a meeting in Detroit on June 12, 1916, and gave the essential facts about the new association, its purpose, and the character of its proposed membership—adding that the industrial doctors had been meeting during the past few years in AMA sections and with the National Safety Congress. Among the problems to be discussed at the meeting, the *Journal* listed the following:

1. Medical examinations of employees, and the results and benefits of these.
2. The surgeon as an aid in preventing accidents.
3. Emergency surgery and the standardizing of procedure in certain types of cases.
4. Standardizing of records used in this work.
5. Various forms of industrial insurance and the need of a federal health insurance law.

Through the Committee on Arrangements for the American Medical Association meeting in Detroit—with James E. Mead (Ford Motor Company) as an intermediary—reservations had been made for a "minimum of one hundred," who were expected to enroll for the session of the AAIP&S. Actually, about 125 were present when J. Chase Stubbs, as temporary chairman, called for order at 10:00 A.M.

Interest in the purpose and plans of the new organization was unquestionably much broader than actual attendance would indicate. This was evidenced by the flow of letters and telegrams Mock received from physicians and surgeons in all parts of the country, who, because of other pressing business, could not be present. Typical is this telegram from R. C. Cabot of Boston, who was prominent in organized activities of the AMA: "You are pioneers in medical service and medical organization such as the public good demands. You will meet opposition, but you should welcome it and will surely overcome it. I am heartily with you in spirit and in purpose."

Typical, too, was a message from Frank Billings of Chicago: "I congratulate you on the inauguration and first meeting of the American Association of Industrial Physicians and Surgeons because it is one of the most important subjects for the consideration of physicians and surgeons."

The Conference Board of Physicians in Industry fulfilled its promise of support, made earlier in the year by Dr. Moorhead; this organization was well represented at Detroit by leading industrial doctors from the east. The group centering around Chicago, who had engineered the incorporation and preliminary organization, were present almost to a man.

From the far West came Legge (California), Philip K. Brown (Southern Pacific Railway), Alvin Powell (Western Pacific Railroad), and William Brown (Valmora, New Mexico). Among representatives in the public health field were J. W. Schereschewsky and Anthony J. Lanza (USPHS), and F. D. Patterson (Pennsylvania). Others who were to render signal services to the association in later years included Donald B. Lowe (Akron), Clarence D. Selby (Toledo), Loyal A. Shoudy (Bethlehem, Pennsylvania), and Guy L. Kiefer (Detroit). It is unfortunate that no complete or accurate list remains today, either of those who registered at the 1916

73

meeting or of those officially qualified as founding members. Such records apparently were lost or destroyed in the years before the association established a permanent headquarters office—or lie forgotten in personal files.

The first official act of the convention was to appoint A. M. Harvey as permanent chairman of the meeting—a fitting tribute to a man whose leadership had been largely responsible for the founding of the association. Mock, as secretary, reported on the activities of the Organization Committee, then presented the proposed Constitution and Bylaws, bearing committee approval. This document, after stating the name and object of the organization, established four classes of membership: (a) Active, (b) Associate, (c) Honorary, (d) Fellowship. In essence, it provided:

> *That* only physicians who are actively engaged in the practice of industrial medicine and surgery, or who are engaged in the investigation of industrial medical problems, shall be eligible to active membership.
>
> *That* other physicians might be eligible for associate membership, though they failed to meet the requirement of active industrial practice, but provided they had the personal and professional qualifications entitling them to active membership.
>
> *That* applications for active and associate membership must be made in writing and be accompanied by the fee for annual dues; with the further provisions that the applicant be approved by a member in good standing and be certified as to ethics and good standing by the secretary of his local medical society.
>
> *That* honorary membership might be conferred upon a physician for some definite contribution toward the advancement of industrial medicine and surgery or for the performance of some special service for the association.
>
> *That* associate and honorary members should have all the privileges of active members, except the privileges of holding office and voting for officers and directors or for amendments to the Constitution and By-Laws.

Under provisions of the document the Board of Directors was empowered to elect a candidate to any class of membership by a two-thirds vote. Active members, after three or more years in the association, were permitted to apply for fellowships, to be conferred upon selected applicants who satisfactorily passed an examination by a board of examiners consisting of five members or fellows.

In essence, the original Constitution of the association does not differ greatly from the articles and regulations governing the present Industrial Medical Association, though these have been amended from time to time to meet changing conditions. That the basic provisions have stood the test of the years is a tribute to the foresight of the founders and their grasp of the fundamentals of sound organization.

The business of debate and decision proceeded swiftly, and with remarkable unanimity, at that first meeting in Detroit. The Constitution and Bylaws were adopted promptly, with a minimum of change. Records from the files of William A. Sawyer (president of the organization, 1926–1927) tell us that committees were named to deal with the matter of an association journal; standardization of forms, records, and methods in the examination of employees; and the problems of health insurance.

The chairman also appointed a nominating committee composed of R. L. Cameron, H. W. Clarke, and W. E. Post, to present the names of candidates for office in the new association. Reminiscing at the annual banquet thirty-one years later, Loyal Shoudy recalled an interesting sidelight on that first election.

"When we went up to the meeting," he commented, "the idea was that Harvey should be president and Mock, secretary. But apparently not enough people knew about the slate. There were a number who thought Harry Mock should be president, and another group that Harvey, being an older man and in the work longer, ought to be elected. When they finally got it all settled, neither one of them was president."[2]

Whatever the actual process of electioneering, the following were duly voted into office and installed at the morning meeting: president, J. W. Schereschewsky; first vice-president, R. T. Legge; second vice-president, F. D. Patterson; secretary-treasurer, Harry E. Mock.

Joseph W. Schereschewsky was born in Peking, China, and educated at Harvard and Dartmouth Medical School. He served as a private and an acting hospital steward in the Spanish-American War, then entered the United States Public Health Service, and from 1915 to 1918 was medical officer in charge of the Office of Industrial Hygiene. A hearty, dynamic man of great personal magnetism, an able administrator, and a forceful writer of medical monographs, he had worked closely with the founders of the association in the battle for recognition and was exceptionally qualified for the leadership entrusted to him. He served the association with distinction from 1916 to 1918—through two of the most trying years in its history.

The first meeting of the association in Detroit stands out in vivid contrast to meetings of the present and immediate past. All the business of complete organization—plus a program of medical talks and discussions—was crowded into a single day, concluding with an evening banquet.

The convention program, a simple four-page folder, listed only four formal addresses; and the chief participants included only about a dozen men—as compared with some three hundred scheduled for active parts at the 1954 meeting. There were no sections or sectional activities, no discussions of "specialties within the specialty," no meetings of component or affiliated groups, no scientific exhibits. The program, nevertheless, made up in quality what it lacked in length or variety. The opening address, "The Scope of Medical and Surgical Supervision," by C. G. Farnum of the Avery Company, Peoria, is remembered as an incisive definition of the doctor's place in industry. A discussion followed, with Francis D. Patterson of the Pennsylvania Department of Labor, as chairman.

Schereschewsky opened the afternoon session with an address, "The Educational Function of Industrial Physicians"; and a discussion was led by Wilbur E. Post, medical director of the Peoples Gas Light and Coke Company, Chicago.

Highlight of the session, by verdict of all who have survived to recall it, was a talk, "The Factory Doctor," by Dean S. S. Marquis, clergyman-director of Henry

Ford's famous Sociological Department. Harry Mock describes it as "a magnificent address that still further fanned the flames of enthusiasm in this young organization." The discussion was led by Dr. R. L. Cameron, of the Republic Rubber Company.

The meeting closed with an address, "Health Insurance and the Prevention of Sickness," by John B. Andrews, Ph.D., whose exposure of phosphorus poisoning in the match industry had led to sweeping reforms a few years earlier. Clarence D. Selby, Commissioner of Health in Toledo at the time, led the discussion that preceded adjournment.

Among unsung workers for the association during its entire period of organization was Miss Pauline Gunther of Chicago. "Her arduous work and cooperation," said Mock, "played no small part in the success of preconvention arrangements, and the smoothness of proceedings at the meeting." Two years later she became the first paid assistant secretary of the association.

Despite the unanimity of opinion among the founders on most matters of policy, there is record of one controversial point, which, under other circumstances, might have completely altered the future of the association, reducing it to the rank of a satellite, deprived of the independence of action that has made it a power in industrial medical affairs.

"At the meeting in Detroit," Mock wrote, "there were two factions—those who felt we must be under the American Medical Association and become a part of the preventive medicine section, and the boys who wanted to swing us to the National Conference Board. Dr. Geier, Dr. Schereschewsky, Dr. Crowder, and I fought and pushed and pleaded, and came out with an organization having a national rating."

Thus the matter of the status of industrial medicine among the specialties was settled, at least for the time being. Regrettably, the exact substance of discussions and decisions at the June 12 business meeting has become a matter of memory rather than of record. Even the texts of the principal convention addresses have vanished along the way. They do not appear to have been published either in periodicals or in reprint form. However, there survives, strangely, a letter from the public stenographer, which accompanied a transcript of proceedings under date of July 19. She explains the loss of some of this material by the fact that the speakers promised to deliver copies for the record but failed to do so.

It appears that the new association, intent upon getting its organization work done, paid little attention to publicizing its proceedings, or, seeking publicity, failed to get it. For even Detroit newspapers dismissed the event with little or no mention.

Matters of great moment were claiming the headlines in June, 1916. War was raging in Europe and going badly for the Allies. The United States was in the midst of political turmoil. Charles Evans Hughes had just announced his acceptance of the Republican nomination for the presidency—stepping down from the Supreme Court to campaign for election.

The big medical news of the day was the gathering of eight thousand delegates in Detroit for the sixty-seventh annual meeting of the American Medical Association. Its proceedings were pervaded by a sense of world crisis and the imminent need for preparedness in this country.

It was at this AMA meeting that Surgeon General Rupert Blue (USPHS) called upon the doctors of America to fight "poverty, ignorance, intemperance, cruelty, and greed."[3] The temper of the times was also reflected by the address of Charles H. Mayo, president-elect of the AMA.

"Business interests in this country," said Dr. Mayo, "get four times as much from the government for protection of hogs and cattle as the public health service gets for the care of human health. Humanity must be put above commerce. We should have skilled men at work for the public health everywhere, and each worker should receive a salary equal to the economic value of just one human life. That is only $5,000."[4]

It is not strange that in the midst of the general outcry for economic, industrial and medical preparedness, the organization of a new association of doctors should have received scant attention in the press. One paper, *The Detroit News* (June 13, 1916), gave a brief report on an inside page, which we quote for the record:

"SAFETY FIRST"
DOCTORS ORGANIZE
Work to Increase Efficiency of Employees

More than one hundred physicians and surgeons engaged in industrial branches of their profession formed the American Association of Industrial Physicians & Surgeons at a meeting at the Hotel Cadillac Monday. The organization, which has been in the process of formation for nearly a year, is composed chiefly of men attached to large industries and other corporations and others whose interests lie in the same direction. The object is the study of the problems and development of the methods of the care of employees.

In its July, 1916, issue, the *Journal of the American Medical Association* likewise stated that "more than one hundred physicians engaged in work for great corporations met at Detroit June 12, and organized the American Association of Physicians & Surgeons." The paragraph was followed by a list of officers.

Robert T. Legge and others among the founders recall an incident that occurred on the floor during that meeting. A member of the American Medical Association, seeking to discourage the formation of another medical organization, suggested that it would be unwise to start an association with such small membership. Otto Geier, pointing to the assembly, retorted: "You see that 'small group' there? Well, they represent seven million workers."

Among the banquet speakers that same evening was Dr. Joseph C. Bloodgood, of Baltimore. He was then working earnestly to promote the conservation of manpower in industry, as part of the preparedness program. He was no stranger to the philosophy, aims, and activities of the AAIP&S. He is quoted, on good authority, to have reported later to his confreres in other organizations to this effect: "I have just attended a meeting of the association which is going to become the giant of industrial medicine in the United States."

So the founding of the American Association of Industrial Physicians & Surgeons took its place in medical history. The founding, though little acclaimed, was well and thoroughly done. Within less than a year, the United States was drawn into World War I. Here was the test of a nation's strength, the test of its industry, the test of its medicine.

The question became: How would the association, fledgeling representative of the industrial aspects of health, meet its first real challenge?

WAR! INDUSTRIAL MEDICINE
WINS ITS SPURS

IN ALL human history one finds nothing to justify war, on either social or economic grounds. The ledger sheet is too tragically overbalanced on the debit side with death, suffering, and sacrifice. Yet, since wars continue—growing always in scope and destructiveness—it is the duty of medical history to weigh them and their by-products, coldly and objectively.

It is a strange anomaly that man, while devoting his entire medical skill to means of conserving life and preserving health, has used his greatest discoveries in chemistry, physics and engineering to fashion more and more deadly instruments of death. Civilization, it now appears, has a choice of erasing the institution of war or being erased by it.

Wars have progressively multiplied the hazards to life, limb, and health, not only among combatants but also among civilian populations. Yet, on the other side of the ledger, there have come from these ghastly clinics great advances in both medicine and surgery which have increased life expectancy and raised the over-all level of human health.

Medical historians have declared that America's war for independence "was the making of medicine in this country." By necessity, war injuries and war-connected disease called many young men to a profession that was backward and immature at the time, and gave them experience which could not have been obtained under ordinary circumstances.

Surgeons in the Civil War worked under the most adverse conditions, often with makeshift equipment hurriedly assembled at the fighting fronts. Anesthesia was still in its infancy; chloroform and other pain-deadening drugs were pitifully scarce. Asepsis in surgery still lay ahead, for Lister did not propose the application of his methods to military practice until 1870. Nevertheless, the war brought marked improvement in surgical techniques, and sharply increased enrollment in medical schools.

The brief Spanish-American conflict, despite its shameful record of sickness and death from noncombat causes, speeded the conquest of yellow fever and typhoid and resulted in improved sanitary safeguards in the military services.

World War I, in contrast to all preceding conflicts in human history, was a war of total resources. Its medical importance stems not alone from its greater scope and the size of the military forces engaged—not alone from the new weapons, new forms of transport, new logistical problems. It was the first of all wars in which the industries and the working populations of the combatant nations were enlisted in all-out offensive effort.

As early as December, 1915, at the behest of President Wilson, the United States committed itself to a program of preparedness, which called for mobilization of the nation's financial strength, its agricultural capacity, its material and manufacturing resources, to aid the Allies abroad and to ready the country for the eventuality of its entry into the war. Early in 1916 Congress passed an act creating the Council of National Defense. In that year at the annual conventions of banking, manufacturing, business, and medical associations, discussions centered upon the threat of war and the requirements of a wartime economy. Immediately following America's declaration of war in April, 1917, came the Selective Service Act and the creation of the sprawling, many-sided War Industries Board. In June the War Risk Insurance Act was passed. It provided a plan to rehabilitate disabled fighting men by physical reconstruction and functional re-education, under direction of the Federal Board of Vocational Education.

Suddenly, manpower assumed an importance it had never before been accorded in peace or in war. The health and usefulness of the individual American became almost overnight a critical factor, not only in the maintenance of fighting forces overseas but in the expansion of industrial and agricultural production at home. Despite months of preparation, the United States found itself on unfamiliar ground, when faced with the necessity of turning out new types of munitions in vast quantities, and of dealing with terrifying new health hazards in industry.

"Here," writes Alice Hamilton in her autobiography, "were new engineering problems, and they were being solved, not in advance of the actual production, but while it was going on."[1]

Early in the war period Dr. Hamilton was sent by the Department of Labor to investigate conditions in plants manufacturing high explosives for Britain, France, and Russia. Processing of these called for large-scale production of picric acid, dinitrotoluol, smokeless powder, military gun cotton, mixed powders and fulminate of mercury—all requiring the use of great quantities of nitric acid.

80

Shut off from German sources by the U-boat blockade, American manufacturers were forced to build coke by-product plants to catch essential gases and to work out production processes "from scratch." They were dealing, they knew, with highly poisonous substances, and they had had little or no experience even in handling the death-dealing chemicals involved.

So strict was the censorship surrounding this entire operation that Dr. Hamilton was not told where to find the industries she was investigating. But while the project was veiled in mystery, the plants themselves—scattered along the eastern seaboard —were shrouded in great clouds of orange and yellow fumes. With these as a guide, and aided by local gossip, she made her way to her goal.

Dr. Hamilton was shocked by her first sight of the "canaries" she encountered in the vicinity of these chemical works—a white man "of a leaden hue, thin and weary looking but touched into incongruous comedy by smears of orange stain on his cheekbones and deeply dyed yellow eyebrows and hair . . . black men in motley garb with great stiff aprons, colored orange, woolen shirts eaten away to rags, high boots streaked with yellow, flaps of leather hanging down against their hands."[2] Seeing these modern war workers, any student of ancient occupational diseases must have been reminded of Statius' description of miners in the first century A.D.: "Pale from the sight of Pluto, and yellow as the gold unearthed."

According to Dr. Hamilton, the landscape surrounding the nitro plants was drenched by noxious orange fumes, moving across the fields before a breeze, killing all vegetation, and driving men to safer spots until a change of wind at least partially cleared the atmosphere.

No one will ever know exactly how many deaths were caused directly by inhalation of such nitrous fumes and by their absorption through the skin or how much serious illness resulted from damage to the central nervous system, the blood, and internal organs. In some rapidly-developing, fatal cases cited, no accurate diagnosis was ever made—for "most doctors knew nothing about nitrous fumes and would pronounce such a case heart failure or heat prostration." In May, 1917, Dr. Hamilton published a report listing 2,432 cases of occupational poisoning, of which nitrous fumes accounted for 1,389 cases and 28 deaths, and TNT, for 660 cases and 13 deaths. The TNT fatalities on the list, she adds, were due to toxic jaundice or to aplastic anemia.[3]

Admittedly, these and similar accounts present a picture of occupational hazards in World War I at their very worst, and of industrial medicine at an extremely low level of efficiency. The explosives and the aniline industries, in particular, were by no means typical of industry in general. They were, nonetheless, important factors in the health of the nation's working force at a time of crisis.

Conditions in the munitions plants of 1917–1918 emphasize the inability of engineers, faced by the necessity of working with new and highly toxic material in a grave emergency, to improvise methods for their safe handling and the relative helplessness of doctors to control morbidity and mortality from exposure to chemical compounds whose very names had not yet become part of the ordinary medical vocabulary. There are no records to indicate any great improvement of conditions in the munitions industry during the first world conflict. Early in the war competent research teams were assigned to study the causes and effects of toxicological diseases traceable to the new chemicals; but time was lacking. Some employers were uncooperative. There was a natural tendency to subordinate health considerations to the production demands of the emergency.

World War I, however, taught many important medical lessons—and they were well learned. It should be noted here that the health record of the munitions industry in World War II stands in bright contrast to that of the first conflict. The difference is attributable to a quarter century of engineering experience, radically new knowledge in the fields of physics and chemistry, a more humane approach to problems of health and hygiene, and tremendous advances in industrial medicine.

Among researches developed between 1914 and 1918, and later used in industrial medicine, Dr. Legge lists the Carrell-Dakin treatment of wounds with dichloramine T, defense against poisonous gas, the geophone to detect snappers underground, aviation medicine, the investigation of trench fever, preventive inoculation against tetanus in gunshot wounds, inoculation against typhoid fever, rehabilitation for war cripples, and fatigue studies and researches in efficiency.[4]

Above all these might be placed the upsurge of social and scientific interest in industrial medicine, hygiene, and safety. It came with the recognition of manpower as the greatest of all national resources, whether in times of peace or times of war. It led to a concerted effort to conserve health and promote productivity that was unparalleled in our national life up to that time.

Within a few years prior to the war many new organizations had come into being, each devoted to specific health goals. Hitherto these had followed independent lines of effort, with little or no coordination or cooperation. Now they had a cause in common—a reason for defining areas of operation and reconciling differences of interest.

The medical profession in the United States had answered, promptly and without reservation, the call to service at home and abroad. The problem was how, where, and under what conditions the doctor could best serve both military and civilian needs.

Among health agencies the American Association of Industrial Physicians & Surgeons occupied a unique position. Newest and smallest of such national organizations, it was the only medical group dedicated exclusively to the study, treatment, and prevention of occupational trauma and disease. In one sense this was a restriction upon its area of activity; in another sense it opened up to the industrial doctor a new and specialized field in which no other medical group was equally competent to serve.

The late Dr. Geier was speaking for the association and for American industry when, in an address, "The Human Potential in Industry," in May, 1917, he declared:

82

This is a day that calls for statesmen as well as soldiers, for calmness as well as courage, for patience and patriotism, for virtue and vigor, for faith and faithfulness, for health as well as willingness to die. This day calls for social reconstruction as well as enemy destruction. Huge is the task in which all should find a place to do with all their hearts.

And what tasks has our entering the war brought to industry? Huge production? Yes! But is that all? Have not old truths as to the value of the conservation of labor taken new form, new emphasis? Has not the human potential in the nations abroad finally been the measure of their potential upon the battlefield? Has the interdependence of man ever been more fully demonstrated? Has the mutual dependence of labor and capital? Have we ever witnessed such limitless industrial energy and output?

Has it occurred to all of us Americans that Europe's industrial experience of the past three years holds not only a lesson but a warning? Militant and efficiently industrial England of war times will be succeeded by industrially militant England of peace times. Labor and capital in England, Germany, and France, having learned the mutual advantage of cooperation in war, are not likely to give up this advantage and return to the destructive internal warfare of former days.

The question that presents itself is this: Can we keep pace with them in war and will we keep pace industrially after the war? Can we stand this new type of competition unless we likewise enter upon the program of the new social order? Will not the programs of our National Association of Employers, chiefly defensive in the past, necessarily become socially constructive? Will not labor now have to seek leadership capable of best adjusting itself to these forward-looking steps?

War has lifted the discussion of the human potential in industry out of the realms of philosophy and has used it as the foundation stone of a national economic policy.[5]

This declaration was *of* its time and uttered *for* its time. Whether or not it was prophetically accurate, it may perhaps be recorded as the expression of a socioindustrial creed that is in full accord with the thinking of the industrial medical fraternity in America—now, as then.

Young though it was—with a membership of little more than 225 in 1917—the American Association of Industrial Physicians & Surgeons was a closely-knit corps of specialists who made up in determination and singleness of purpose what they lacked in numbers.

From the day of their organization, the founding members stood solidly together on controversial medical issues. They crusaded militantly for the precise objectives set forth in their charter. They opposed with equal vigor any and all programs which might vitiate the character of industrial medicine, compromise its established principles, or subordinate its activities to those of labor, governmental agencies or other health organizations.

Moreover, these pioneers had influential friends in high places. Throughout the public health services, and in other medical organizations, they found support from doctors who either were members of the association or were in sympathy with its aims. While the association, as a corporate entity, had relatively little prestige during the war period, the opinions and recommendations of its individual members were received with respectful attention wherever the health of America's working force was under discussion. A large majority of these first-year members were in active practice as plant physicians and surgeons. They had the confidence and backing of management in the industries they served. And they understood, far better than any other medical group in the country, the nature and seriousness of occupational disease hazards existing in various types of production.

In its effort to conserve manpower as a wartime measure, the federal government was confronted with the need for experience as a guide to sound planning. But experience was nowhere to be found except in plants which had established medical departments and operated them as a proving ground of policies and procedures.

Pioneer plant doctors had long since come to one unanimous conclusion: that thorough physical examinations for employees were the starting point in any effective program of preventive medicine and that physical fitness must be regarded as a determining factor in job placement. To prove this they had health records built up over a period of years in successful medical departments from coast to coast.

As always in times of national emergency, the federal government created a maze of boards, councils and committees—the interlocking machinery of a great war effort. High on the agenda of many of these agencies stood the problem of conserving manpower. It was of tremendous importance not only to the administration, but also to organized labor, to industry, to the American Medical Association, and to the American Association of Industrial Physicians & Surgeons.

Official life in Washington, in 1917 and 1918, resolved itself into an endless succession of interviews, hearings, and conferences. All the agencies involved were agreed as to the ends to be achieved, but they brought to these meetings such widely varying viewpoints, such a conflict of interests, that there seemed at times no hope of reaching a satisfactory agreement on ways and means.

The association may justly claim a large share of the credit for slicing through official red tape, overriding agencies and individuals over-mindful of their own private interests, and focusing attention on the real issue—the formulation of a program of health supervision within the plants where the nation's manpower was at work. The association had a concrete and practical plan aimed directly at this objective, while much of the thinking in governmental circles was still at an indecisive stage.

Among association members in the forefront on the fight for in-plant medical supervision were Geier and Mock. Both were left free by their enlightened employers to devote their time and effort to furtherance of the manpower program. With the full sanction of the association they acted again and again as spokesmen for the organization in a series of dramatic meetings during the early months of the war.

The first step toward cutting the Gordian knot of the manpower issue came in the spring of 1917 when a small group of founding members, headed by Geier,

84

opened up the subject of physical examinations for employees as a war measure to cut down absenteeism and increase much needed production. To speed action, they asked the influential House of Delegates of the AMA to request a meeting of the governmental medical services to discuss the problem.

The house promptly passed the required resolution, which was duly forwarded to Franklin Martin as chairman of the Medical Section of the National Defense Council. Time passed, but no word came from Washington. Geier decided to beard Martin at his office in the capital. Nearly thirty-seven years later—shortly before his death in February, 1954—Geier wrote to a friend, apropos of this meeting: "When I asked him whether he had ever called the three surgeons general[6] together, he admitted that he had done nothing. I decided to lay my last card on the table. I said: 'Well, if you don't I will, before I go home tomorrow.' The shock threw him into action. 'If I call a meeting tomorrow at 10:00 o'clock, will you meet with us?' he queried. Of course I stayed, demonstrating what a roughneck, with no standing, can do to cut red tape."

The meeting was held as scheduled, with both Geier and Mock present to plead their cause. The service chiefs listened attentively, and assented to the development of a formal program. Other conferences followed, as rapidly as they could be arranged, among them a general meeting of labor representatives, employers, and heads of the federal medical services, at which A.F. L. President Samuel Gompers and William Green were in attendance.

Scarcely had the question of physical examinations in industry been introduced when Green jumped to his feet to attack the proposal—the very heart of the program, without which, in the opinion of the industrial doctors, there could be no adequate medical supervision and no progress toward the goal of healthier, more productive manpower. In effect, Green charged that proponents of the plan were bent on "producing a human scrap heap," on which men would be discarded as a result of examinations. "Gompers," wrote Geier, "said not a word—just listened."

When Green had finished, Geier rose calmly and declared: "As for that human scrap heap, you already have it, and you are adding to it daily." Continuing, he quietly reminded his audience that workers were being put into jobs for which they were not fitted and that the unions were doing nothing about it, either by proper placement of the handicapped or by some effort to restore them to greater efficiency. "We are trying to repair these men," he concluded, "and fit them into productive jobs."

On this note the meeting ended. The issue still was far from settled, but an entering wedge had been driven into the ranks of the opposition. Each succeeding conference brought about a better understanding of the objectives of the examination program, with added support for the AAIP&S. And among the converts was Samuel Gompers, a man whose power as either friend or foe reached far and wide.

Another leaf from Otto Geier's notebook relates his experience in expediting an appropriation by Congress to carry on the government's work in industry. Even in his high place, Surgeon General Blue had been unable to get money, and the prospect for early action seemed anything but bright. Geier suggested an appeal to Gompers, whom Blue had never met; and two hours of telephoning brought an invitation to visit the labor leader at his country home the following morning—July 4, 1917. In high spirits, and in perfect holiday weather, the doctor and the surgeon general motored out to Gompers' residence.

The spirit of the occasion was apparently contagious. Introductions over, the three launched into a long discussion of patriotic music and poetry—of everything except the grim business of war. But when the visitors took their leave the mission had been accomplished.

"What a strange beginning," wrote Geier, "for a long-standing friendship between these two men! Of course Congress, thereafter, with Gompers' blessing, supplied Blue with money."

It was an equally strange chain of events that moved Harry Mock to a responsible post in wartime Washington, with the rank of lieutenant colonel and plunged him into the problems of medical supervision in industry and the rehabilitation of disabled soldiers. In his department of Sears, Roebuck, years before the war, Mock had coined the slogan: "Physical qualifications, plus occupational qualifications, equal a job." The slogan impressed Dr. J. C. Bloodgood of Baltimore, who recommended to Surgeon General William C. Gorgas of the Army that he establish a Division of Physical Reconstruction and Rehabilitation in the service. And it was his recommendation that pulled Colonel Mock from his assignment as chief surgeon of Evacuation Hospital No. 1 seven days before it sailed for France in October, 1917, and placed him in the Surgeon General's office as assistant chief of the new division.

From personal files and from memory, Mock reconstructs the story of medical supervision in industry, and of the rehabilitation program, during the remainder of the war. These projects moved ahead slowly, controversial issues were bitterly debated, but progress was made. And in the center of negotiations member-representatives of the AAIP&S worked arduously to attain the basic objectives of the association. It was a momentous period in the modern history of industrial medicine, for it marked the turning of the tide in favor of in-plant medical services, physical examinations as a criterion in job placement, and the rehabilitation of disabled and handicapped veterans.

As part of his industrial program Franklin Martin established, within his branch of the National Defense Council, a subsection on industrial medicine. Mock writes: "This group proposed elaborate plans for the supervision of the health of all workers engaged in essential war occupations. Few of those in authority were familiar with this new field in medicine, and it took weeks and weeks of patient endeavor to sell the idea."

Discussing with Martin the plan to place doctors in all strategic industries contributing to the national defense, Mock pointed out that many of these plants already had full-fledged medical staffs and that there was an organization known as the American Association of Industrial Physicians & Surgeons, which was uniquely qualified to serve in programming such an activity. He recommended that a committee representing the association be appointed to consult with him. Martin agreed, and in late October, 1917, such a group was appointed, consisting of Loyal A. Shoudy, Clarence D. Selby, and Mock—with Otto Geier as chairman. About this group, Mock wrote:

> We had an all-day meeting with Franklin Martin. It was evident that he wanted and felt that he had the power to appoint doctors to industry in the name of national defense. The committee felt that our association could appeal to members who were already in industry and were in the best position to recommend other doctors for this type of work.
>
> Dr. Geier was asked to draw up a letter to the AAIP&S, asking that it assume this duty. The next day he presented his memorandum. It was returned the following morning so changed in scope and meaning that the committee refused to accept it. Thus, the association's part in the war was never made official. However, a list of doctors assigned to industry was drawn up and given to Surgeon General Gorgas—with the result that a great many active medical men in industry were not called for army service but were left to continue in their essential positions.

Oddly, this negative decision probably constituted the greatest victory the association could have won. It was, in principle and effect, a recognition of the status of industrial medicine as a function of private enterprise; it prevented a disastrous division of authority and a duplication of activity; it forestalled the regimentation of doctors in industry under federal control—with unpredictable consequences.

The war years brought about developments of equal moment in the sphere of military medicine, broadening its scope to include a concept of physical reconstruction and rehabilitation entirely new in our national thinking. Only now, at a distance of more than four decades, are we beginning to envision the ultimate contributions to social progress and human happiness that can be made by restoring the disabled and handicapped to useful, productive occupations.

At the very beginning of hostilities the medical staff of the United States Army launched plans to rehabilitate disabled soldiers by therapeutic treatment and vocational training. In all previous wars the great majority of such men had been condemned to lives of helpless resignation in hospitals and soldiers' homes or to eking out a bare existence at the few simple tasks they could perform. The World War I program, by contrast, held out the hope of a return to normal, or nearly normal living, and the dignity of self-support.

It was to this great project that Colonel Mock, in his new Washington post, was assigned. In its first phase the problem was to work out a plan that would enable the Army to utilize, on limited duty, volunteers and draftees who had been rejected for active service because of physical handicaps. To Mock, the field of job placement was familiar ground. In his own department at Sears, Roebuck he had followed the principle of picking jobs for handicapped applicants, rather than selecting only those who were fit, and discarding the others. This principle furnished the text for a memorandum to Surgeon General Gorgas, recommending establishment of a station at which draftees rejected at their first examinations could be re-examined and re-classified for limited service. The memorandum was approved by Secretary of War Baker in May, 1918, and under the direction of general staff officers a limited service station was established in the Fair Grounds at Syracuse, New York. Orders were issued to fifty thousand rejected draftees to report there for re-examination, after which they were assigned to vocational officers who studied their fitness for limited Army occupations.

Four classifications were used in the final disposition of the previously rejected draftees:

Class A—Fit for regular army service anywhere
Class B—Fit for limited service back of the lines overseas
Class C—Fit for limited service in the United States only
Class D—Unfit for any type of army service.

Results of this re-classification were surprising. In the three months that the station functioned, between 5,000 and 8,000 Class B soldiers were sent overseas and some 32,000 Class C men were assigned to duty in the United States as stenographers, clerks, and messengers—releasing equal numbers of able-bodied soldiers for combat service. Less than five thousand of the total examined were placed in Class D.

Thus was the blueprint drawn for limited service procedures which have become a fixture in the Army and which were followed with conspicuous success, on a far larger scale, in World War II.

Along with the development of this limited service cadre in the military forces, the federal program for the reconstruction of disabled veterans was rapidly expanded, with the aid of a vigorous promotional campaign by the federal Board of Vocational Education, the American Red Cross, and several state governments. At the end of the war forty-seven large Army hospitals were carrying on the work, handling every conceivable type of physical and mental disability.

Viewing this work in retrospect, Mock commented: "The rehabilitation of disabled veterans and the introduction of limited service are two of the great contributions to the nation's fighting forces that can be regarded as outgrowths of industrial medicine."

In the second year of the war Clarence D. Selby was called to Washington by Surgeon General Blue, at Otto Geier's suggestion, to act as a consulting hygienist in the United States Public Health Service. A prominent industrial surgeon in Toledo, and a founding member of the AAIP&S, Selby had served his city brilliantly as Commissioner of Health from 1916 to 1918. During his stay in Washington (1918–1919), he was thrown into intimate contact with all phases of national medical problems. As a close observer of the wartime reconstruction program for disabled veterans, he comments: "Mock did more for the advancement of rehabilitation than any other living man."

Specifically, Selby was assigned to make a fact-finding survey of the medical services which were being rendered in industry—activities which were all grouped conveniently under the broad heading of "welfare." He recalls: "It didn't work out; it savored too much of policing the lives of American workers."

In the very failure of the project, however, lay its success. The study demonstrated the folly of government intrusion into this phase of industrial management and served as a deterrent to further paternalistic ventures, thus materially strengthening the position of organized industrial medicine in the federal scheme of things. More importantly, it enabled Selby to conduct the research from which emerged the famous *Bulletin 99*,[7] his most significant contribution to the literature of the profession. Its main findings will be discussed in later chapters.

Like its doctor members, the AAIP&S made war its official business until hostilities ended in November, 1918. Annual meetings in the war years were one-day affairs and were well attended despite the heavy schedules under which all the doctors were working. Medical problems of national importance crowded the agenda; discussions continued into the night—all with the objective of maintaining industrial health and conserving precious manpower.

The 1917 convention was held in New York on June 4, with J. W. Schereschewsky presiding. The program lists papers by J. C. Bloodgood, "The Application of Our Knowledge of Industrial Surgery to Military Surgery"; Alice Hamilton, "Health Hazards in the Munition Industries"; Wilbur E. Post, "The Need for Health Insurance as Seen by the Industrial Physician"; and John J. Moorhead, "The Operative Findings in So-called Traumatic Inguinal Hernia." Discussions at this session were led by Charles A. Lauffer (Westinghouse), John D. Ellis (Rush Medical College), John H. McClellan (Chicago Telephone Company), and C. W. Hopkins (Chicago and North Western Railway).

The 1918 meeting, held in Chicago on June 10, took on an even more warlike flavor. The program included an important address by Doctor Selby, "The Relation of the Medical Profession to Industrial Efficiency in Wartime," based on the research in which he was engaged. Discussion was led by D. B. Lowe (B. F. Goodrich Company).

It was at this meeting that Schereschewsky turned over the presidency of the association to his successor, Mock, who described the rehabilitation program of the Army in a paper, "Lessons from the Reconstruction of the War Disabled Applicable to the Industrial Army." Other speakers and topics were: Lieutenant Colonel James Cordley, Jr., "Reclaiming the Blind from War—from Industry" and Dr. Francis Patterson, "The Employment of the Rehabilitated Disabled Soldier in Industry."

No better demonstration of the value of preventive medicine—of early diagnosis and reporting of illnesses in industry—can be found than in the experience of the

Cincinnati Milling Machine Company during the influenza epidemic of 1918, which took an appalling toll of lives among the military and civilian populations and cost an untold number of productive hours. Otto Geier is authority for the statement that while Cincinnati industries as a whole reported an average of 35 percent absenteeism during the epidemic, the average was only 7½ percent for his plant, in which a progressive system of medical supervision had been in effect for several years. "This was accomplished," he wrote, "with no miracle drugs or formulae."

The contributions of the Association to the war effort have been ably summed up by both Mock and Geier. The former wrote, in 1919: "The combined efforts of this association have undoubtedly done more to raise the standards of the physician engaged in industrial practice and to increase the benefits from this work to both employees and employers, than any other one agency which has entered this field."[8]

The American Association of Industrial Physicians & Surgeons emerged from the war immeasurably strengthened and firmly established as a potent factor in the national health. But there remained another battle to be won. The gains must be consolidated by the introduction, across the nation, of medical programs that would apply wartime and rehabilitation principles to peacetime industrial manpower. How would the association meet this challenge?

IX

THE DOCTOR'S PLACE IN INDUSTRY

ORGANIZED industrial medicine, or, more specifically, the American Association of Industrial Physicians & Surgeons, found itself in a peculiar position at the close of World War I.

There was widespread and steadily growing interest in the entire subject of manpower and health. There was strong agitation for the reclamation of disabled and handicapped workers and for their employment on productive jobs. More and more employers, particularly large corporations, were organizing medical departments worthy of the name. But there were many problems, all of them difficult of solution. For every ably-manned and well-equipped department, there were many that had not progressed beyond the first aid stage. The place of the physician and surgeon in industry was not firmly established, nor was it clearly defined. There remained more than a modicum of suspicion from labor and resentment from management.

Great strides in the advancement of medical science had been matched by equal progress in industrial surgery, thanks to the work of such men as J. J. Moorhead, W. D. Clark, C. G. Farnum, R. W. Corwin, A. M. Harvey, C. A. Lauffer, Loyal A. Shoudy, J. C. Bloodgood, Edward Martin, Richard and Hugh Cabot. But the benefits of their work had been extended to only a small fraction of the nation's working force.

World War time, like all wartimes, had been a period of high wages and lush spending. At the gates of war plants, when shifts changed, taxi drivers commonly did a thriving business from the fares of tired, grimy, silk-shirted workers. Bars, restaurants, and merchants prospered. And peace, of a sort, prevailed along the labor front during the emergency. With the end of the war this uneasy truce erupted into

91

an epidemic of unrest, wage demands, and strikes—seemingly the inevitable consequence of economic inflation. In the turbulent period that followed the climate was definitely unfavorable to the orderly progress of industrial medicine.

In an article titled "The Physician and Surgeon in the Industrial Crisis," Otto Geier painted a vivid picture of labor conditions in 1919 and their relation to health services in industry. The paper was first read before the American College of Surgeons in October of that year, at the invitation of Dr. Will Mayo, and was repeated in 1920 at a meeting of the National Tool Builders Association.

With characteristic bluntness Geier analyzed developments in the labor-capital controversy and their relationship to the problems of industrial medicine. He spared none of his associates. Salient points in his address well deserve a place in the archives of the Association, to which he was so devotedly attached:

> This is not only the industrial era, but also the era of greatest industrial strife. Public disorder and strife originate almost wholly in the clash of opinion between organized money and organized labor. Strikes and lockouts and their attendant turmoil are but outward signs of a constant warfare that is going on between these groups.
>
> Thus we are uncomfortably reminded daily . . . that the individualistic viewpoint no longer holds; that we must adjust our work and our thinking to large groups and great units of society; that we must think in terms of the mass rather than the individual; that this is the time for mass treatment.
>
> Recall, if you will, the national peril of business stagnation and starvation that England has just faced. Recall also the similar situation in our own country three years ago (1916), when the railroad brotherhoods forced the nation to its knees in the passage of the Adamson law. Its recent arrogant progeny is the Plumb Bill. We have . . . just passed the crisis of the steel strike, only to be threatened by a coal famine with its almost limitless possibilities for national disaster. . . .
>
> What part is our profession playing in this post-war psychology, this industrial and social crisis? Are we making our contribution to the study of the problems of industry and labor? Have we adjusted the science of medicine to the needs of these two groups, or have we practiced our profession with individuals just as was appropriate one hundred years ago? Have we not failed to develop a consciousness of group problems?
>
> Bear with me in asking these personal questions. Is it not paradoxical that the physician, who to his patient appears as the most socially minded individual, should prove so unsocial and so inactive in his public thinking? Is it not strange that we, who have the closest view of the intimate living and thinking of the people, should play so small a part in the disposition of their individual and group lives? . . .
>
> As an illustration, were our surgeons carefully considered when workmen's compensation acts for the care of industrial accidents were established? Are we satisfied with the application of these laws? Is it not a fact, that, generally speaking, medical men, not qualified surgeons, are tinkering with the industrially injured?
>
> For the worker, this means prolongation of the case, greater loss of wage, unnecessary invalidity, with practically no scientific rehabilitation. For the employer this

means the idle machine, lowered production with higher cost. For society, it inevitably means lower standards of living and higher costs of living.

On the other hand, was the profession entitled to such consideration? Is it not a fact that for years we blindly went on repairing the injured and maimed, without public protest and without suggesting an improved program? It occurred to labor to seek compensation for time lost from accidents and payment by the state of the surgeons' fees. In the very nature of the case, labor could have no knowledge as to how to obtain the best surgical results for the injured, yet they dictated the law.

Moreover, it remained for industry, not the medical profession, to get under way that wonderful safety first movement which has reduced death and accidents by approximately 50 percent. . . .

Are we not assuming the same negative attitude toward the movement for the better organized application of group curative medicine? Are not the physicians being practically ignored by the framers of compulsory sickness insurance, another group program? And yet we shall all admit that the future of the scientific teaching of medicine as well as its economic practice or application will be absolutely determined by the enactment of such a law.

Unless the profession comes out of its social, or rather, unsocial torpor, we may be sure that such legislation will be made to fit the whims of the perniciously active reformer, whether or not it pleases us or benefits labor or capital.

These are strong words, from a strong fiery man. It must be remembered that they were spoken in 1919. Judged from a distance of more than forty years, they plot a course which is remarkably close to that which organized industrial medicine has since followed.

Geier was appealing to the profession to assume its rightful place and responsibilities in industry; to study minutely the medical and surgical needs of production workers; to institute more comprehensive programs of plant service; to apply to civilian employees the rehabilitation and placement procedures adopted for war veterans; to take a more active part in the framing of compensation codes. Tremendous progress has been made toward these goals, and far greater progress is in the offing.

In all her early research, Dr. Alice Hamilton found that without the voluntary collaboration of management the best laid plans of the industrial doctor were doomed to frustration and failure. Many employers were indignant and incredulous when she declared she was sure men were being poisoned by the materials they were handling. The manager of one white lead works retorted: "Why, that sounds as if you think that when a man gets lead poisoning in my plant I ought to be held responsible."[1]

Recalling his early experiences as an industrial surgeon, Loyal A. Shoudy once declared: "Employers steered clear of us. They said, 'We don't want it to get around that we injure anybody so badly that we have to have a doctor around to take care of him.' "

Alcoholism was commonly blamed by some employers for accidents and sickness, of whatever sort. In fact, the "boiler maker" got its name from the whiskey-and-beer bombs with which many a man fortified himself before he went on the job. But as a reason for failure to provide health safeguards in a plant, the excuse was only a convenient refuge for the indifferent and unwilling employer.

Actually, the real problems of industrial medicine in the post World War I period rose from the age-old conflict between capital and labor. Each was struggling to hold the balance of power; each was fearful that the other would gain ascendancy. Dr. Geier remarked at the time: The autocratic employer of yesterday is more than matched by the autocratic employee of today. The medical profession, along with a great mass of people, is in the arc of the swing, and must needs be on its guard.[2]

A true balance of power between these two groups is, of course, as delicate as a true balance in the nation's economy—and as impossible to maintain. Then, as now, the field of industrial medicine was one of the battlegrounds in the capital-labor conflict, and recurrent strife was one of the most serious deterrents to the establishment of adequate health programs.

At the start of the reconstruction period following the war, practicing industrial doctors were agreed on one cardinal point: that a comprehensive program of physical examinations must be established as a basis for employment and as a determining factor in job placement, if industrial medicine was to accomplish its long-term objectives. The doctor's place was in the plant, and he must have a free hand in setting up medical procedures. The groundwork for such procedures had already been laid in pioneer medical departments across the country, a majority of them under the direction of AAIP&S members. These pilot procedures had crystallized the needs and had broadly indicated the types of organization best suited to meet them.

In an address on "The Human Potential in Industry," given to the American Society of Mechanical Engineers in Cincinnati in May, 1917, Geier pleaded for the establishment of "all-day" dispensaries as the best means of winning the confidence of workers in plant medical services. He declared:

> Here, the virtues and weaknesses of the men will be most apparent. The physician will also be confessor, adviser, priest. . . . An industrial dispensary, with a dental clinic as its adjunct, will advertise itself. It will come in daily contact with 5 percent of the force, the equivalent of the whole force each month. To respond to all the possible services that grow out of these frequent contacts, it will require one full-time physician to every 750 employees.

In this address Geier cited case after case of faulty diagnosis that had come to his attention in plants that lacked well-organized medical departments—a gastric ailment treated with headache remedies, muscular pain from broken arches diagnosed as rheumatism, and infection from pyorrhea diagnosed as neuralgia. Systematic examinations and accurate records, he pointed out, would have prevented the resultant suffering and loss of working time.

In his "Physician and Surgeon in the Industrial Crisis," he wrote:

> It may surprise you to know that the average worker receives his first complete physical examination in the industrial clinic. He is too often the victim of blind, gunshot prescriptions. The industrial clinic is teaching him to seek a better type of physician for himself and his family, and in that sense the industrial physican is tending to raise the standard of private practice on the outside.[3]

Publication in 1919 of Harry Mock's *Industrial Medicine and Surgery* served further to focus attention on the organization and operation of medical departments in industry. It is an omnibus of information and practical suggestion on every phase of the subject, covering, in scrupulous detail, types of organization, requirements in the way of service, medical and surgical procedures, staff and technical personnel, questions of equipment and cost. One of the most ambitious early works of its kind, this volume served as a guide to many corporations, large and small, in the establishment of new medical departments. Beyond this, it set standards of service and of examination procedure that were accepted as criteria in the profession for many years.

Not the least important of the forty-eight chapters of this work are those dealing with the reconstruction and reclamation of handicapped and disabled workers. The success of the Army's rehabilitation program turned the spotlight on a vast, and practically unexplored, field of medical endeavor. Leaders in industrial medicine were asking: "Why, for humanity, health and productivity, can we not apply similar procedures in reclaiming the handicapped among civilian workers?"

Mock's tables show that some 200,000 soldiers were disabled annually by wounds and disease in wartime. Of these, 50,000 had to be physically reconstructed, and 20,000 others vocationally retrained. He estimated that in the industrial army at least 800,000 were disabled each year by disease and accident, of whom 200,000 needed training for new and better occupations.

Because of his work for the rehabilitation of war veterans, Mock was sent to Italy in 1919 to represent the United States at the Third Interallied Conference for the Assistance of the Disabled of the War. Here he voiced again the appeal he had made at the AAIP&S convention the year before for the extension of veteran rehabilitation methods to industrial workers. He expressed the hope that, as the work for disabled soldiers diminished in volume, it might "extend its functions to the salvaging of disabled humanity throughout the world."[4]

During the decade following passage of the first workmen's compensation laws, pressure for this type of legislation had increased steadily, and by 1920 all but six of the forty-eight states had compensation statutes of one kind or another. Workers in Hawaii, Alaska and Puerto Rico and civil employees in the District of Columbia had similar protection.

One of the first effects of such legislation on industrial practice was to promote the use of pre-employment examinations. Without medical histories there could be no records; without records industry was practically defenseless against compensation claims. Thus the trend to compensation furthered one of the primary objectives of the AAIP&S, the maintenance of accurate clinical data, on which all modern health programs are based.

C. D. Selby is authority for the statement that a further effect of compensation was to discourage the rehabilitation of disabled workers. "Many men in management," he said, "took the attitude that their responsibility ended with the payment of compensation."

Nevertheless, the concept of conserving and utilizing manpower to its full potential had found a place in the thinking of management, labor, and medicine—to remain there, ineradicably. From this concept have come the enlightened programs of today, which aim to fit the task to the capacity of the handicapped.

At its annual meeting in Atlantic City in June, 1919, the association turned its attention to postwar problems, and they were many. The association had no capital; its membership had grown, slowly, to 275 in 1918 and to 340 in 1919. The doctor's position in industry had been materially strengthened, but recognition of industrial medicine had been accorded, for the most part, to individuals rather than to the association they represented.

In the same year Mock reported: "We are able to point to approximately eight million of the workers of the nation who are receiving the benefits of this enlightened era in industrial medicine to a more or less degree." If the estimate was accurate, there remained some thirty million workers in production who were getting no health supervision. To extend protective coverage the number of industrial physicians and surgeons had to be sharply increased. What sort of practice could be assured to attract able men to industry? They would require better pay, greater responsibility, a broader field of activity. The scope and functions of industrial medicine would need to be precisely defined, and its relation to other spheres of medical practice accurately determined. Until this was done, industrial medicine could not hope to win recognition as a specialty.

PART THREE

A NEW SPECIALTY

THE SCOPE AND FUNCTIONS OF INDUSTRIAL
MEDICINE IN THE MODERN WORLD

*Industrial medicine, at its best,
is applied science in the fullest and
finest sense of the term.*

X

WHAT IS INDUSTRIAL MEDICINE?

INDUSTRIAL medicine is as difficult to define as democracy, or patriotism, or any other concept that suggests many different things to many different people, the difficulty being, of course, to arrive at a brief and understandable definition which includes all that the term does mean and excludes all that it does not.

The word *industrial* does not appear in any of the early literature on this special phase of medicine, even in translation. Ramazzini used the title *De morbis artificum* (Of the Diseases of Artificers—or Workers, as commonly translated). Writers, down to relatively modern times, referred to "occupational" rather than "industrial" diseases.

The concept of industry itself also has changed materially within our century. More often than not, in present popular usage, the word is accepted as referring to the mass production of goods by modern machine methods. In this sense the term *industrial medicine* is obviously too restrictive, since musicians, farmers, divers, barbers, painters, and hosts of other workers are subject to diseases peculiar to their callings, and hence within the province of this medical specialty. In recent years, we have seen a growing tendency to describe the field as "occupational" or "environmental" medicine. The nomenclature, perhaps, is not too important so long as the meaning is clear—and for our purposes the three terms may be used interchangeably.

Occupational medicine and occupational diseases have been variously defined by countless writers, and no doubt many more will attempt the task. From a long list we select a few of these definitions, each of which expresses a somewhat different point of view and all of which have the virtue of clarifying the everyday terminology of the profession.

Carey P. McCord, educator, writer, and authority on industrial toxicology, has interpreted occupational diseases as including "abnormal body and mental states directly resulting from extended exposure to the harmful substances or conditions directly related to work."[1]

C. O. Sappington, noted writer, and consulting industrial hygienist, states: "An occupational disease is one which occurs with characteristic frequency and regularity in occupations where there is a specific hazard as the cause which operates to produce effects in the human body recognized clinically by the medical profession as pathological changes and effects produced by the specific hazard involved."[2]

Emery R. Hayhurst, teacher and author, defines the term as follows: "An occupational disease is an affliction which is the result of exposure to an industrial health hazard, while the latter is any condition or manner of work that is unnatural to the physiology of the human being so engaged."[3]

The Michigan Department of Labor and Industry offers this definition: "The term *occupational disease* means a disease which is due to causes and conditions which are characteristic of and peculiar to a particular trade, occupation, process, or employment."[4]

The Industrial Medical Association has its own official definition of occupational medicine, adopted after careful consideration of its scope and functions. It reads as follows: "Occupational medicine deals with the restoration and conservation of health in relation to work, the working environment, and maximum efficiency. It involves prevention, recognition and treatment of occupational disabilities, and requires the application of special techniques in the fields of rehabilitation, environmental hygiene, toxicology, sanitation, and human relations."

An interesting parallel is found in the definition published by the American Medical Association, which, though it has differed strongly with the Industrial Medical Association in some areas of thinking, has consistently agreed as to the ultimate objectives to be attained, as the following statement indicates:

> Occupational medicine concerns itself with all aspects of health in relation to occupation. Industrial medicine is a component of occupational medicine applied to employed groups by an employer or other third party with a valid interest.
>
> The broad purpose of industrial medicine is promotion of the healthful well-being of employed persons through services provided at the place of employment or at another convenient facility or location. This purpose is served by: (1) prevention of disease and injury through medical supervision of workers, the work places, materials, and processes; (2) constructive measures such as medical examinations, counseling, and health education; and (3) medical and surgical care to restore health and productive capacity as promptly as possible after occupational illness or injury.[5]

On this same subject Clarence D. Selby, while a consulting hygienist with the USPHS, wrote: "Industrial medicine may be defined as the theory and practice of medicine applied to the purpose of preventing and alleviating sickness and injury among industrial workers in order that they may enjoy the benefits of continuous productive employment."[6]

The value of these and other similar definitions may be judged as much by what they exclude as by what they include. As may be seen, all reflect thoroughly modern viewpoints; all avoid controversial implications; all seek to draw clearly the thin and elusive line that separates industrial medicine from other closely related fields. There is probably little to be gained by any restatement of what industrial or occupational medicine is. The need is for more complete and specific definition of its scope—the nature and extent of its functions and responsibilities—as distinct from those of other specialties in the field of health. These questions have been a source of disagreement and contention for a generation or more.

The key to an understanding of the proper role of medicine in industry is found in the story of its evolution from small beginnings, long before the turn of the century. The first steps toward improvement in the health of workers came in the form of legislation calling for factory inspection and the observance of higher sanitary standards.

Great progress was made in this direction during the early nineteen hundreds. Industry was quick to see the economic advantage of replacing dark, insanitary workshops with clean, well lighted, and ventilated buildings. On the practical side, the change materially reduced both accident and disease hazards; idealistically, it led to further recognition, by management, of its social obligations to labor.

In 1917 Otto Geier wrote:

> It was at about this same period that many abortive attempts at so-called welfare work were started, which in most instances failed to make any real contribution to the better understanding of labor and capital.
>
> This sort of welfare work was established on purely paternalistic lines, was imposed upon the group of workers without their desire or consent, and all too frequently furnished that for which they had no real need. This type of welfare contributed to the social and superficial requirements of the man, and overlooked the fundamentals. It did not take into account the basic principle that the workman is very human, and to get the best results from any socializing effort you must first engage his cooperation. . . .
>
> Welfare work of the former kind deserved failure and did fail. It was "built upon the sands" and was all too frequently washed away by the least wave of discontent among the workers. After the first strike, the returning man found the doors of the dining rooms, libraries, and club rooms closed upon him. The whole structure was weak and crumbled at the mere sign of a storm. Is it any wonder, then, that welfare work came into such disrepute with the worker and was so continuously and effectively used by the labor agitator?[7]

Conspicuous among the welfare experiments of that era was the ill-advised sociological department established by Henry Ford in the heyday of expansion that followed introduction of the Model T. Built upon a sand foundation of paternalism, it sought to teach employees the virtues of thrift and to monitor their personal habits.

Such experiments belonged to a period in which some employers, seemingly desirous of impressing labor with their beneficence, were saying in effect: "Look at all we are doing for you!" Labor was unimpressed. The experiments failed because they did not take into account the fact that the workers' eyes were fixed not upon frills and gratuities but upon such tangibles as working conditions, hours, and wages and living standards.

The doctor played little or no part in these early "reforms," social or sanitary. He came into the industrial picture when he entered a plant in his professional capacity with the one intention of doing what he could to heal the sick and mend the injured, to prevent accidents and disease, and to improve the health of the labor force. Health was something the working man could understand. It was an absolute essential in his program of self-betterment.

In his USPHS *Bulletin No. 99* (p. 106), Dr. Selby summed up the advantages of industrial medicine to management, with commendable restraint, and in a minimum of words.

> It appears, that industrial medical service is not a gift to labor, but purely a function of good business. The reasons which induce employers to provide their workers with medical service may be summarized as follows:
> 1. It is an acknowledgment of their obligation toward the workers who sustain injuries during employment and an economical means of procuring expert attention for them.
> 2. It is deemed capable of removing or minimizing certain causes of lost time.
> 3. It is one of several activities that have been found to be of use in removing certain unstabilizing influences from employment and as such can be expected to assist in holding down the labor turnover.
> 4. It enables the workers to produce more.
> 5. It prevents litigation and reduces compensation expense.
> 6. It contributes to a sense of security among employees and promotes a feeling of good will toward the management.
> 7. Conditions make it imperative in isolated industrial establishments.

With slight elaboration, and the addition of a few items, this listing might be considered fully up-to-date even by present mid-century standards. In its time (1919), it represented a radically new viewpoint. For the reason that it merits the attention of any serious analyst of today's industrial medicine, the quotation has been lifted from the obscurity of a pamphlet long out of print.

In his study of the science of human relations, Stuart Chase observes: "The scientific method does not tell us how things *ought* to behave but how they *do* behave. Clearly there is no reason why the method should not be applied to the behavior of men as well as to the behavior of electrons."[8]

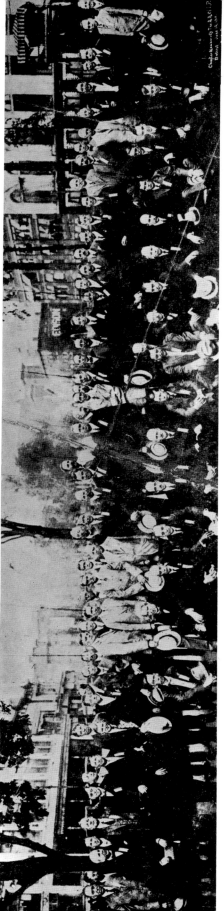

25. *Founders Meeting of AAIP&S, June 12, 1916.* These are the men who, within the space of a few decades, converted a random idea into a great coast-to-coast organization of industrial physicians and surgeons. From its very beginnings, the AAIP&S was held together by an unusual bond of comradeship. Unity of thought led to unity of action, and won the recognition and respect of older, larger agencies. No organization has done more for the safety and health of the American working force. It may be that some surviving founders who attended the 1916 Detroit meeting will be able to identify themselves in this picture—taken on Washington Boulevard on that historic occasion.

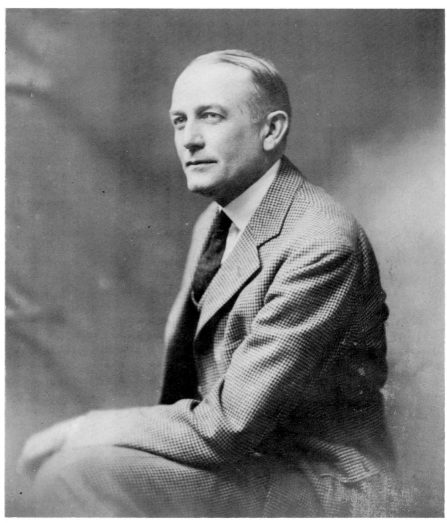

26. *Otto P. Geier, M.D., about 1920 or 1921.* By logic and persuasive oratory young Otto Geier, during World War I, won reluctant concessions from governmental health agencies and respect for the new AAIP&S. In 1925 he went to Europe as a member of the League of Nations medical committee to study living and working conditions in Europe.

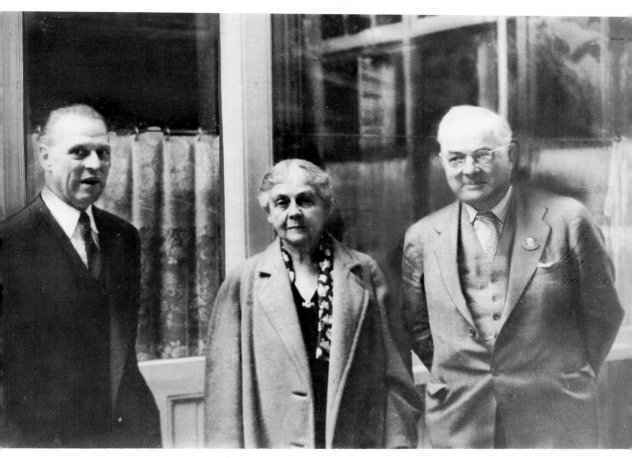

27. *Drs. Sayers, Hamilton, and Legge.* These three doctors had attended the 8th International Congress of Accidents and Diseases, held in Frankfurt am Main, Germany, from September 26 to October 1, 1938. The Munich conference between Chamberlain and Hitler was in session; war seemed imminent. The American delegates left early and crossed the border to Nijmegen, Netherlands, where the picture was taken. Dr. Hamilton, in her book *Exploring the Dangerous Trades,* gives a detailed account.

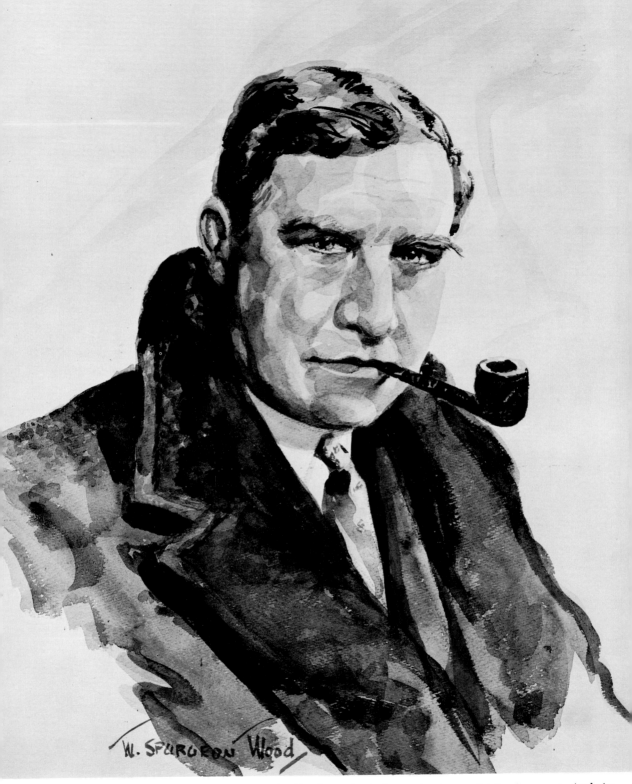

W. Spurgeon Wood

28. *Harry E. Mock, M.D. (1880–1959). President, AAIP&S, 1918–1920.* In one simple sentence, Harry Mock unwittingly summed up the guiding principle of his career: "Physical qualifications, plus occupational qualifications, equal a job." This concept led Sears, Roebuck & Company, in 1909, to give him a free hand in his program of physical examination and job placement. And the same phrase took him to Washington during World War I to establish the Division of Physical Reconstruction and Rehabilitation, in which he rendered distinguished service. Mock's literary output totaled nearly seventy publications, including three books.

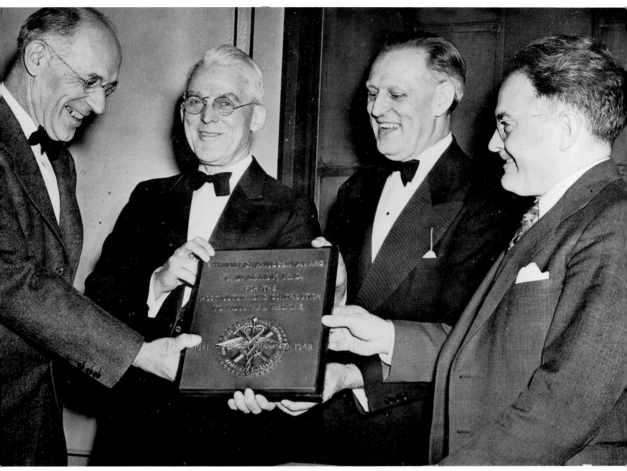

29. *Four Knudsen Award Winners.* From left to right, Drs. Leroy U. Gardner (1940), Clarence D. Selby (1942), Royd R. Sayers (1941), and Clarence O. Sappington (1939). Sayers is presenting the award to Selby. In 1941 Selby presented it to Sayers, for his studies of sickness absenteeism.

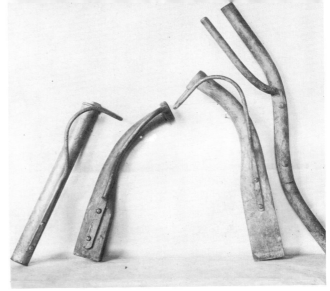

30. *Hand Guards about 1900.* Hand guards for hand operated trucks, wheelbarrows and similar vehicles. These rudimentary devices were constructed by Crane Company employees.

—Courtesy of the Crane Company

31. *Mobile Medical Unit.* This well equipped mobile unit, owned by the Humble Oil & Refining Company, Houston, Texas, takes medical service to the "front" in the oil fields.

—Courtesy of the Humble Oil & Refining Company

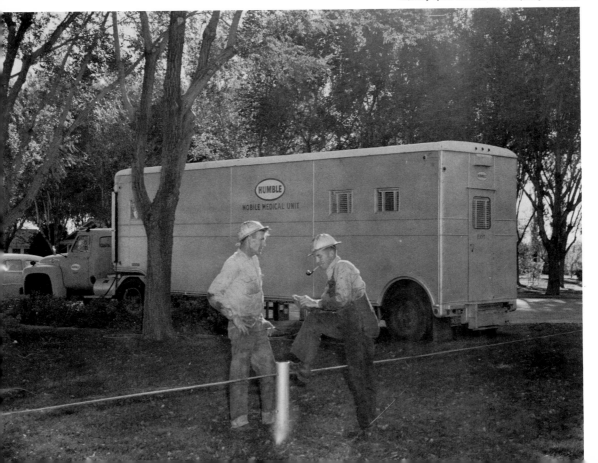

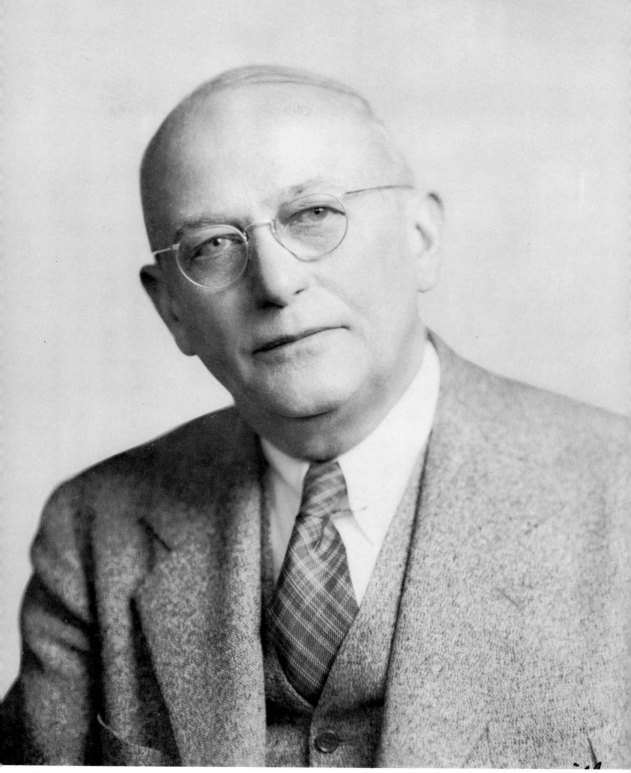

32. *Otto P. Geier, M.D. (1874–1954). President, AAIP&S, 1920–1921.* Otto Geier compressed three notable careers into one professional lifetime. A graduate of the Medical College of Ohio in 1897, he installed and directed one of the earliest complete medical departments in an industrial plant (1914), a model of its time. To the end of his life he was active in the civic health affairs of his native Cincinnati, serving as city welfare director, fighting TB, and pressing campaigns in the interests of pure milk, charities and penal institutions. He played an important role in shaping the destinies of the AAIP&S and the specialty at a national level.

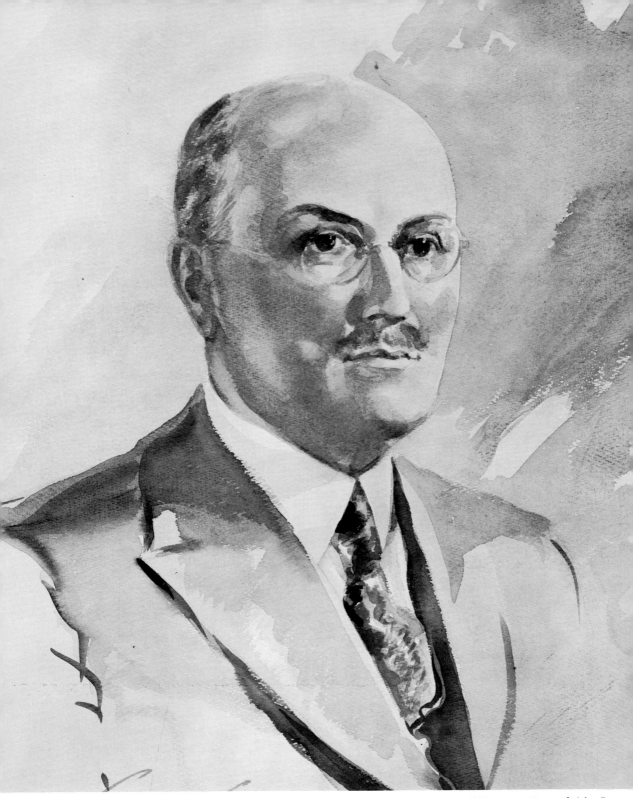

33. *Clyde E. Ford, M.D. (1874–1928). President, AAIP&S, 1921–1923.* A founding member of the AAIP&S, Dr. Ford was elected its president in 1921 and thus resolved a near-deadlock among rival factions. In the confusion of conflicting opinions and diverse plans at the founding, Ford saw the immediate need of clear thinking and a great deal of executive trail-blazing. One of his first official acts was to lay before the membership an eleven-point program defining the field of industrial practice, suggesting educational and research activities, and urging standardization of methods and records. His program established a policy trend that was followed well into the thirties.

When industrial physicians and surgeons, in appreciable numbers, went to work in American plants they were following exactly this precept. They demanded clinical evidence, rather than presumption or theory, as the basis of their health programs, and they recognized physical examinations and systematic record-keeping as the only solid foundation on which they could build.

Until examinations became an established procedure, the doctor in most plants had few regular duties and was given little or no professional recognition. Industrial medicine, in practical application, was limited for many years to first aid and emergency surgery, for which the surgeon was paid substantially less than he could have earned in a private capacity.

"With few exceptions," says Mock, "his work consisted of bandaging cuts, caring for bruises and other minor injuries, treating simple fractures, and prescribing in cases of acute illness. Major surgical cases were usually sent to outside surgeons. The job within the plant had few attractions for the well trained, alert physicians or surgeons."

It was in this period that industrial practitioners first acquired the sobriquet of "finger wrappers," a term which, unfortunately, is still used occasionally by the few medical men who remain blind to the progress of forty-odd years. The evolution of the medical director from the finger-wrapper was a slow process, attended by many difficulties and discouragements. In his *Bulletin No. 99,* Selby pointed out that examinations for employment, as usually made, were exceedingly superficial, amounting to little more than inspections for obvious defects, and, although the avowed purpose was properly to place employees, the real purpose in some places seemed to be the exclusion or the recording of defects that might subsequently complicate injuries or become involved in claims for compensation.

Some concerns, he observed, had ceased to require examinations of applicants when labor became scarce—a fact that would appear to confirm the impression that their motive had been the exclusion of defectives. In times of labor shortage, when employers were forced to bid for labor and accept all applicants regardless of their qualifications, age, or sex, the use of physical examinations as an aid to the intelligent assignment of employees and their subsequent maintenance as efficient workers would seem to be more necessary than in times when labor was abundant.

Selby also noted that in plants which he surveyed the time required for examination averaged probably ten minutes. However, time is not the only factor determining effectiveness. With today's improved instruments, today's criteria of health, and today's scientific studies of job requirements, more may be revealed in a ten-minute examination than was possible in twice that time under older methods.

Where examinations were sketchy, where physicians failed to follow up their findings, rejection of the obviously unfit was the principal, if not the only, result that could be expected. Under such conditions there could be no reclamation or intelligent placement of the handicapped. Employees simply passed from observation by the medical department until injury or illness forced them to reappear. Under such makeshift procedures, the partially disabled and unfit were thrown on the scrapheap of nonproductive labor, or they were hired, defects notwithstanding, and put to work alongside the fit with whom they could not compete on equal terms. Of such indiscriminate hiring, Mock wrote: "The placing of all comers on jobs without any effort at a physical selection for their work is responsible for a great financial waste, which cannot be shown in dollars and cents but which nevertheless is very evident."[9] He went on to cite six sources of this waste:

1. Employment of physically unfit who later must be discharged because of inability to do their work.

2. Employment of physically unfit who continue to work for a while, but with a gradual decrease of efficiency because of disease.

3. Employment of physically unfit who are subject to frequent accidents because of their condition.

4. Employment of physically unfit who suffer death or prolonged disability from accidents which would not be serious for the physically fit.

5. Employment of persons with contagious diseases, acute or chronic, who communicate them to healthy workers.

6. Employment of the mentally deficient who never could be fitted to jobs.

Such were the hazards—to management and to workers—of examination procedures so loose and nonselective as to permit applicants with serious physical or mental deficiencies to attempt work suited only to the whole and healthy. What of the other extreme—a policy which barred handicapped applicants from productive work of any kind? Here too there was waste of manpower and earning capacity.

"The selection of qualified employees," wrote Selby in his *Bulletin No. 99,* "implies the rejection of disqualified applicants." Among examples revealed in his survey as reasons for rejection he lists heart and kidney lesions, hernia, variocele, varicose veins and ulcers, deformities which impair functions, deafness, imperfect vision. It was his belief that physicians who were familiar with working conditions in their establishments could assist in the assignment of a large proportion of the physically defective, and by subsequent supervision aid them to do their work well.

Selby went on to cite the case of a worker with flat feet, whose job required him to walk among machines. Because his feet hurt he took short-cuts—a dangerous path instead of a safe one—and the inevitable accident occurred. He should, the doctor points out, have been given sedentary employment if his feet were so bad and should not have been exposed to this hazard. By contrast, it may be noted that the same survey brought to light a storage battery company in Philadelphia with a department manned by mutes; a large electric motor company in Springfield, Ohio, which had two blind men engaged in production work; an Ohio shoe factory with fifty-one crippled employees on its payroll. Such placement policies are, of course, common today, but they were decidedly exceptions to the rule at the close of the first World War. These and other examples emphasize the wide spread between the best and the worst in industrial medicine during its formative years. It is a spread that still exists today, though the gap has been narrowed by steadily rising standards within the profession and growing acceptance of social responsibilities by management.

Selby recognized the field of industrial medicine as embracing sanitation and preventive medicine, emergency and orthopedic surgery, laboratory technique and interpretation, orthodontia, dental prophylaxis, specialties of the eyes, ears, nose and throat, and other branches of practice. There were, in some plants, chiropodists, bacteriologists, pharmacists, and masseurs. And there was mention of hydrotherapy and heliotherapy.

Such coverage was, of course, far from representative of industry as a whole or even of the largest corporations. In the final analysis, the effectiveness or ineffectiveness of a medical department depended, then as now, upon management policies, labor relations, and the caliber of the physician or surgeon in charge of health activities. From harmony came success; discord spelled failure.

At the close of World War I these three factors were sadly out of balance. Management-labor-medical relations were neither clearly crystallized nor properly coordinated. Nor was the status of the physician or surgeon in the industrial scheme of things established with any degree of uniformity. Depending on the labor policy of the employer, it varied from that of an out-and-out representative of management to that of a glorified medical handyman reporting to any one of several department heads.

Of medical departments in the establishments surveyed by Selby in 1918, it was found that 42 percent were responsible to officers who had supervision over production, 21 percent to officers who handled compensation for injuries, 18 percent to administrative officers, and 15 percent to those who directed employment and labor relations. Only in the remaining 4 percent was the physician a real medical director, with the freedom, responsibility, and authority to which he was entitled.

Commenting on the situation, Selby declared: "If the purpose of the medical department is broad and includes activities that concern several or all of the functions which are necessary to manufacturing, it should be accountable to the directing head only."[10]

Under such conditions medical accomplishment lagged far behind medical thinking. Progress was discouragingly slow with respect to scientific job analysis, selective placement, evaluation of disability, preventive medicine, and many other activities which are under constant study in modern medical departments.

Despite the promising results of rehabilitation work in Army hospitals, the average disabled veteran found anything but a warm welcome in factory employment offices at the close of World War I. Progressive industrial doctors were quick to see the rewards, economic as well as social, to be reaped from therapeutic treatment and job adjustment, but management in general did not share their enthusiasm.

How different was the reception, and the treatment, accorded the disabled on their return from World War II! And the difference was due more to radical changes in management and public thinking on social questions than to advances in medical science, important though these were.

This sharp contrast provided the theme for a dramatic motion picture produced by General Motors Corporation after the second world conflict. The widespread interest in reclamation of the handicapped is indicated by the fact that this picture was shown more than ten thousand times in a ten-year period to industrial, business, and other groups, totaling nearly one and a quarter million persons.

There was nothing lacking in the way of scientific knowledge in the years between 1917 and 1920 which prohibited the operation of industrial medical departments along advanced lines. Rather, the lack was a lack of common understanding by management, labor, and medicine of the ends to be achieved and the means of achieving them. The ingredients for rapid progress were at hand, even in that early day, but they were the scattered pieces of a jigsaw puzzle which had not yet been put into place to form a complete and meaningful picture.

Scores of medical writers, in the interval between the first World War and the present, have defined the basic relationships that must exist within a plant if industrial medicine is to accomplish its ultimate objectives. These writers have spared neither their own profession, nor management, nor labor in pinpointing responsibility. A few brief comments, by qualified authorities, serve to place the intraplant relationships of these three groups in proper perspective.

Selby wrote, in *Bulletin No. 99:*

> Although fundamentally the science of medicine, the position which industrial medicine occupies is similar to that of employment, safety, and compensation. All are specialties in the science of management.
>
> Physicians who do not understand this relationship (and medical training does not necessarily contribute to this understanding) have reluctance in accepting the materialistic viewpoint of employers and, conversely, have difficulty in persuading employers to accept their professional points of view.
>
> Physicians who do not understand this relationship must realize that industrial medicine is, in a measure, a compromise between the ideals of medicine and the necessities of business. In approaching the compromise this fact should not be overlooked, that medical service in the industries, to be of the greatest possible usefulness, must benefit primarily the working people. The benefit to industry naturally follows.[11]

Nearly thirty-five years later R. B. O'Connor, in a discussion of industrial health programs at the University of Michigan, said:

> The development of rapport between the worker and the plant physician first requires an understanding of the average worker's initial reaction to the company's purchase of a plant physician.
>
> When a man goes to his family physician, he has chosen this physician himself and pays his fee out of his own pocket. There is no reason for him to feel that the

doctor has anything but the patient's own interest at heart. The plant physician, however, is chosen and paid for by management. It is wholly understandable that the worker initially wonders if the physician places management's interest above that of the employee.

Subsequently the plant physician may say to the worker, "You may not work because I do not feel you should," or "I feel that you are able to work and therefore you should." These decisions materially affect the worker's pocketbook. They are, therefore, construed by him as a prerogative of a plant supervisor, further clinching the idea that the plant doctor is a member of management and so logically places management's interest first. . . .

Most physicians in industry are primarily physicians; they have a genuine and personal concern about their patients. The workers recognize this and respond readily with complete cooperation and confidence. Unfortunately there are some physicians with the opposite approach. One such physician in industry is one too many. Labor leaders are frequently vehement in their criticism of such doctors.

All of us physicians in industry fall somewhere between the two extremes, the beloved and the despised. The farther we are away from the latter extreme, the better employee acceptance we will receive and the more effectively we will develop the cooperation of the employee in trying to assist him in maintaining and improving his health.[12]

These comments are widely separated in time, but there is no dissimilarity in viewpoint or approach. They are typical of opinions expressed again and again over the years. They ask, for the doctor, freedom from the label of "management man" or of "labor man"; for management, tolerance for labor's viewpoint and recognition of its stake in industrial health; and for the worker, realization that team play is necessary if his future well-being is to be assured.

The problems of industrial medicine start within the plant, but their scope extends far beyond the limits of management and labor relations. Of equal importance is the complex question of the industrial doctor's multiple relationships with other health agencies, public and private.

Not until the dividing lines between industrial medicine and related fields of health activity were sharply drawn, could a blueprint for future accomplishment emerge.

XI

THE BATTLE OF THE SPECIALTIES

Times of great upheaval, national and international, are invariably attended by sweeping changes in public thinking. Suddenly there appears a need for re-examination of old standards and ways of life and for wholesale readjustment to new conditions.

The period covering World War I and the immediately subsequent years was no exception. It brought global problems closer to the United States than they had ever been. With unparalleled expansion of business and industry came an explosive broadening of national interests, responsibilities, activities. This was the end of an age of simplicity, the beginning of an era in which human relations have become progressively, unendingly, more complex.

The meaning of these changes, insofar as they affected problems of health, was sketched in bold strokes by Otto Geier in 1917, when, as presiding officer of the Preventive Medicine Section of the American Medical Association, he declared:

> It is evident that we have for all time passed beyond the absolutely individual and personal relationship of family physican and patient to one where the community steps in to safeguard itself against any abuse of this circumscribed relationship and demands collective action in matters of health for the benefit of all.
>
> The concentration of population in cities has developed problems beyond the control of the private physician. In the train of density of population have come the tenement sweatshop, bad housing and living conditions, tuberculosis, alcoholism, venereal disease, poverty, delinquency, and crime.
>
> The development of industry, with its occupational hazards, has created another series of health impairments which the family physician may have the knowledge to alleviate but whose prevention is entirely beyond his control. Establishment of the public health department was a partial answer to these new social requirements.

Unemployment, seasonal employment, the physically unfit, the unemployable, the industrial hobo, the labor turnover, all loomed up as medical and social problems of such huge size as to spell defeat of their solution.

Society is realizing that problems of industry are largely its problems, that the major portion of the community is engaged in industry, that when badly administered it is therefore a menace to the peace, health, and happiness of the whole community. When properly administered it is of inestimable value socially and economically. Whatever industry does, because of its size, is impressive.[1]

Geier's listing of health hazards that trail in the wake of mass industry and mass movements to urban centers is a startling echo from a distant past. Almost to the letter it repeats the story of nineteenth-century English workers in the dawn of the Machine Age—repeats it on a gigantic scale.

In 1919, as editor of *Medicine and Industry,* Geier wrote prophetically:

The profession must either assume leadership in new medical organization and legislation, or it will have forced upon it all sorts of quack legislation, devised by unmedical minds, that will not only not secure to the public the predicted improvement of community and personal health but will still further lower the economic and social status of the physician. . . .

In self-protection, as well as to dignify his profession, every physician must become less of an individual and think more in terms of the mass and its problems as they relate themselves to medicine.[2]

Fortunately, American medicine has found the means for its own salvation. It has produced the leadership needed not only to preserve its standards but also to raise them immeasurably. It has had the wisdom to tailor its activities to the changing requirements of management, labor, and the public health. Thus it has averted disastrous domination "by unmedical minds" in matters of professional procedure.

As we have seen, the emergency of 1914–1918 brought about in America a new evaluation of health as a national asset, and a new sense of responsibility toward the disabled and handicapped. Among the earliest benefits from this trend were notable improvements in the surgery of trauma, which have profoundly affected not only the treatment of industrial accident cases but also the rehabilitation of the disabled and surgical procedures in hospitals, clinics, and other medical centers. So important are these advances that they will be discussed in detail in later chapters.

The new postwar thinking had equal impact upon industrial medicine, as distinct from surgery, and opened up opportunities for greater service in broader areas of activity. The same was true of all other agencies in related fields: general medicine, public health, safety, hygiene, and sanitation. Their scope was extended; their duties multiplied.

Each of these groups provides essential services not performed by any other group. Each functions in a field which is in itself a specialty or which includes one or more specialties. There is no conflict of purpose among these agencies; there is little or no important duplication of services. But, with a host of organizations engaged in a multitude of health activities, there is necessarily an overlapping of interests and areas of operation which can be a source of both confusion and conflict. The confusion comes in some degree from confusion in terminology. Broad, general terms are not sufficiently definitive. Exactly what do we mean by *hygiene, sanitation, preventive medicine,* even *safety?* All are worthwhile ends in themselves, legitimate goals for every person dedicated to the pursuit of human health.

Again, the need is for better definition, for coordination of effort in the various fields, in place of competitive strife. It is easier to state the problem than to solve it. The area in which any health organization operates is sacrosanct territory, jealously guarded. The tendency within any agency is to expand its activities to maximum limits. Yet boundary lines must be drawn if there is to be harmony and progress toward common objectives.

What is the place of industrial medicine in this apparent hodgepodge? What are its proper relationships with other aspects of health and welfare? Which of its functions can it alone perform; which does it rightfully share with other special groups?

Long and earnest discussion of these questions led to a few basic conclusions on which medical men are still in general agreement: that an industrial physician is simply a doctor who prefers to treat masses of people—groups from one or more types of industry—rather than individuals regardless of occupation; that he is concerned first and foremost with diseases of occupational origin; and that his work thus requires a more specialized knowledge of such hazards than it would be possible for him to acquire in any other kind of practice.

This concept is entirely compatible with the comment of Clarence Selby, who wrote many years before: "If it is true that industrial medicine has a claim to specialism, it is in its application of all the branches of practice to the needs of industry rather than in pursuit of any one branch."[3]

It would seem, then, that the industrial physician is as truly a specialist as the doctor whose major interest is diseases of the heart or of the lungs, or of urology, or gynecology. There is no other branch of medicine which limits its practice to workers in industry and at the same time provides all possible services for the detection, treatment and prevention of occupational diseases.

In this day and age, however, it is not enough to label a man a specialist or his field a specialty. Such controversy as there has been on this point has resulted largely from failure to define specifically the duties of the medical director. Where do his obligations to employers and employees begin and where do they end?

A list of services for which the medical department is primarily or exclusively responsible must certainly include:

1. Over-all supervision of the health of personnel.
2. Placement examinations which make possible the selection of employees for work which they are physically, psychically, and by training fitted to perform.

3. Periodic examinations of certain groups—at intervals determined by the nature of their work and other special considerations.

4. Medical, surgical and dental services, when such services are necessitated by conditions for which employment is responsible.

5. Protection (within the plant) against communicable disease.

6. A reasonable degree of medical and dental prophylaxis.

7. Maintenance of records giving complete histories and providing accurate data on morbidity.

There are other areas in which the industrial physician has at least a half-interest, areas which concern him because of their direct bearing on health and in which he must cooperate fully with other departments and/or agencies. No one will question the logic of his interest in, and partial responsibility for, many health factors that are largely nonmedical, such as:

1. Lighting, heating, ventilation, noise and other environmental considerations—important in their physiological effects on the working forces.

2. Safety precautions, chiefly mechanical, which reduce health and body hazards to a minimum.

3. Provisions of various kinds which minimize the element of fatigue.

4. Specific instruction on how to keep well and avoid injury on the job.

5. Provisions which assure proper nourishment at reasonable cost during the working day.

6. Help in adjusting social and financial difficulties which may seriously affect the employee's ability to do his work.

These are at best partial lists, itemizing some of the major considerations that govern the organization and operation of industrial medical departments in general. From such lists have evolved the so-called "minimum standards" established through years of study and improvement. By the degree of efficiency with which these services are performed the position of a department on the rating scale is finally determined. It is of course the duty of management to establish medical policies: to provide the environment and conditions which enable the department to function and to allocate responsibilities among supervisory personnel. It is the duty, and privilege, of labor to take full advantage of available health facilities, protecting its rights on the one hand and conforming with policies on the other. And upon the medical director rests responsibility for the quality and effectiveness of services rendered.

The duties of the physician and surgeon in industry, however, extend in several directions beyond the boundaries of in-plant service. The intricate codes of compensation laws have made him the important figure in medicolegal testimony to determine liability. Court procedures in this field have, in recent years, come under withering fire, chiefly from the medical profession in its effort to correct abuses which cast discredit upon both medicine and the law. So important is this controversy in its financial and ethical implications that the problem will be discussed more fully later in this volume. The fact remains that the industrial doctor, though not a lawyer, must possess more than a passing knowledge of compensation law if he is to discharge capably his medicolegal obligations.

The doctor goes to court in the capacity of an expert, presumptively unprejudiced and uninfluenced by either side in the dispute at issue. He is armed with clinical data, from meticulously-kept case records, to validate his evidence. His professional opinions axiomatically should carry more weight as medical testimony than those of nonprofessional witnesses, provided he is competent in his field and is ethically unimpeachable. Only by the clarification and improvement of medicolegal procedures can the ends of justice in compensation cases be more adequately served. But after years of verbal crossfire the problem still awaits satisfactory settlement through the joint efforts of the two professions.

Considerably more progress has been made in harmonizing relationships between industrial medicine and other specialized fields of health activity which touch it on all sides and overlap its boundaries at some points. At the risk of oversimplifying a complex subject we can bring some of these relationships into sharper focus by a brief comparison of objectives and procedures.

The National Safety Council, oldest of national organizations devoted to accident prevention, created a Committee on Industrial Hygiene in 1914 at the insistence of employers who saw a need for extending safety services to broader areas of health care. There was no other recognized agency to undertake the task. Prominent industrial doctors were active in promoting this committee, recognizing in it a new ally for their profession. Among them were such men as Geier, Patterson, Harvey, Farnum, W. Irving Clark, McCurdy, Lauffer, Mock, and Shoudy, all proponents of a line of thinking that led, two years later, to the organization of the AAIP&S.

Understandably, management the country over received the idea of a new industrial medical association without great enthusiasm. Why, they could well have argued, deal with two organizations when the National Safety Council has already committed itself to the job of improving hygienic conditions among their workers? Time has given us convincing answers to this question.

Looking back, in 1944, at the early years, the general secretary of the National Safety Council, W. C. Cameron, wrote as follows to Loyal Shoudy, medical director of Bethlehem Steel:

> The NSC just drifted into its health services section because in 1912–13–14 and later years its membership asked for the discussion of health problems at its congress meetings, and later for some general services such as the health practice pamphlets and other incidental services familiar to you.
>
> There are eleven thousand national organizations in the USA. Most of them were organized for one specific service. The NSC was organized as an accident prevention national association, but many times pressures have been put upon it to do something on related problems.
>
> Do you remember the pressure in 1919 to become active in industrial relations?

112

After six months this enterprise was dropped like a hot cake because it did not relate directly to accident prevention. And the policy-making Executive Committee decided that the council had its hands full with the many complicated phases of safety.

In 1925 the NSC Health Division was created. C. O. Sappington was its director for four years, but it was discontinued at the beginning of the depression because it was necessary to throw some cargo overboard, and this was considered by the Executive Committee to be the least valuable. . . .

The NSC, like other associations, has always been willing to bring its members and others together for the interchange of experience on related problems. The council has recognized the sphere of the American Association of Industrial Physicians & Surgeons, and the activities of other groups in the industrial, traffic, home, and other divisions of accident prevention. . . .

Recently I was asked to recommend a safety program for the Society for the Advancement of Management. I have told the officers not to embark on a safety service unless they have a natural interest in the problem; that if within their organization there are persons and interests who really know something about safety, and can interpret it to their group, then they might undertake a service to their particular clientele—management.

Safety, by dictionary definition, is "freedom from danger or hazard," with no distinction between dangers from accident and dangers from disease. Accident prevention, industrially, is to a large extent a matter of providing adequate mechanical safeguards for the protection of workers and thus is primarily the province of management and its engineers. The industrial physician or surgeon, however, would be remiss if he failed to take an active part in this phase of safety promotion. He can and does perform valuable safety services, even down to the suggestion of practical devices to improve mechanical protection; and his department is a potent force in safety education.

Conversely, the medical department is responsible for the treatment of both trauma and disease. Yet the safety engineer fails to meet his full obligations unless he lends his skill and experience for the elimination of disease hazards. As long ago as 1927, Otto Geier, in an address before the National Safety Council, paid tribute to that organization for its contributions to industrial medicine:

"In the case of ill-health, where losses to industry are eight to ten times as great as from accident, we have an agency like the Safety Council that has been able to command the attention of management in its propaganda to induce the habits of health and safety with its magnificent lifesaving and misery-saving results."

These comments, expressing the viewpoints of men intimately familiar with the problems of both industrial trauma and occupational disease, emphasize the clarity with which lines can be drawn between two major fields of health endeavor, to the advantage of both. Potentially controversial issues melt away when the objectives of the agencies are soundly conceived and when each recognizes the other as a member of the same team.

A further paragraph in the Cameron letter (1944) to Shoudy is of interest in this connection: "It is frequently said nowadays that after the war the industrial relations program will be adopted by practically all industries. The personnel and industrial relations leaders are claiming that accident prevention, and related problems, should come within the jurisdiction and control of the industrial relations or personnel staffs. You will hear much more about this a little later."

It is a matter of record that safety as a mainline activity is still in the hands of safety experts; medicine and surgery are still the responsibility of medical men; industrial relations and personnel problems remain under supervision of specialists in those fields. Nor is there reason to think that these vast and diverse enterprises could be successfully handled by a single administrative head except in small organizations.

These same considerations apply in the relationships of industrial medicine to the specialized fields of hygiene and public health, both of which have their own exclusive objectives but perforce rub shoulders on common ground in industries of every type and size. Hygiene, "the science of the preservation of health" or "the science of sanitation," is by dictionary definition an extremely broad term. Even in its limited application to industry it includes plant sanitation, the prevention of occupational diseases, and most of the basic procedures to assure the health of employees. In higher education it is a convenient classification covering instruction in widely varying phases of health maintenance.

"From the employer's viewpoint," wrote Doctor Mock in 1919, "industrial hygiene is now recognized as the cornerstone of maximum production. From the standpoint of the medical man it is the cornerstone of preventive medicine."[4] But what of its specific functions and responsibilities in industrial health?

As William R. Bradley, chief of the Industrial Hygiene Division of the American Cyanimid Company, explains it:

> The field of industrial hygiene is composed of those interested in the total environment of people while at work. The industrial hygienist may be a person more particularly interested in microchemical sampling and analysis, or his main interest or training may be in that distinct phase of engineering involving work-place environmental control from the standpoint of health maintenance.
>
> Likewise, he may be interested particularly in the field of toxicology or in the field of health physics. Again he may be one who embraces more knowledge and experience in the field of atmospheric pollution prevention or in the field of industrial sanitation.
>
> The industrial hygienist, then, is one who has a knowledge and appreciation of the general body of information regarding worker health preservation, although his specific interest or activity from time to time may be more closely directed towards one or more phases of the industrial hygiene field.
>
> The American Industrial Hygiene Association now [in 1952] in its fourteenth year, provides a common ground upon which these closely related and associated disciplines may properly meet to exchange information.[5]

114

Nowhere in such definitive comments does one find any basis for controversy between the industrial physician and the industrial hygienist, with respect to objectives, jurisdiction, or procedures. The hygienist's goal is an environment as free as possible of injurious materials, processes, and conditions. The physician's responsibility is the treatment and prevention of diseases resulting from injurious hazards. The work of one complements, and makes more effective, the work of the other. Again and again, at medical meetings over the years, doctors have been reminded that one of their duties is to act as "deputy health officer." So universally is this obligation recognized that is requires little comment. As a member of a community, serving the people of a community, the physician cannot divorce himself from public health activities. The relationship is reciprocal, direct, and absolute.

In a University of Michigan symposium, Adolph G. Kammer (president of the Industrial Medical Association, 1951–52) declared: "A specialist in this [industrial medicine] field may metaphorically be stated to function with one foot in each of two camps—clinical medicine and public health. He must be capable of dealing with the problems of individuals and with problems that have their expression as group findings."[6]

Industrial participation in public health affairs is not new. One of the earliest results of employee examinations was the discovery of tuberculosis, active and incipient, on a large scale. For more than forty years industry has vigorously supported the drive to eliminate this disease from the nation's mortality statistics. Examples can be multiplied indefinitely, in almost every category of communicable ailments.

Thanks to advanced medical science and alert public health services, epidemics of catastrophic proportions have become a dim memory in America. But the price of immunity is eternal vigilance. There is an ever present possibility that a health problem in a single plant may become a community health problem or that disease of outside origin may invade basic industries.

Thus, the health groups in any area, large or small, are completely interdependent. The public health agencies would be helpless without medical personnel and facilities, and the doctors would be impotent without sanitation, quarantine, inoculation and other safeguards. Government is the enforcement agency; hygienists and sanitary engineers provide the machinery of operation; the medical profession determines and administers procedures.

The American Association of Industrial Physicians & Surgeons, in its formative years, found many staunch friends in the United States Public Health Service, including such men as J. W. Schereschewky, C. F. Rucker, B. S. Warren and Anthony J. Lanza, with David Edsall, George M. Price, W. Gilman Thompson, A. S. Stengel, and C. D. Selby then serving the USPHS as consultants. This group helped greatly to win initial recognition of industrial medicine as a force for the improvement of national health. Subsequent years have seen a steady growth of governmental interest in the industrial phases of medicine and hygiene and have developed constantly closer relationships between the profession and federal, state, and local health agencies.

The expansion of government activities at every level has been fully as spectacular in the field of health as in other social and economic areas. The 1951 *Guide to Health Organization in the United States,* a USPHS publication, lists no less than twenty-five separate federal agencies, including eight departments of Cabinet status, which are "concerned with public health and medical care activities."[7] A catalog of their functions fills eight solid pages of small type. The size and scope of state and local government agencies have grown proportionately.

What are the logical limits of governmental activity in the field of health? In what direction will future trends develop? The answers to these questions have not been written. They involve social ideologies and political factors which make prediction futile. Properly mindful of their own prerogatives, organized medical groups —both specialized and general—have stood firm in their opposition to any extension of government authority that might dilute the quality of medical care or endanger the ethical codes on which the practice of medicine is based. Beyond these considerations, the profession has worked earnestly to improve and cement its operative relationships with the public health services, for the common good.

Writing editorially in the August, 1927, *Bulletin of the American Association of Industrial Physicians & Surgeons,* Guy L. Kiefer, an authority on public health and for many years head of the Detroit Board of Health, stated: "No field offers greater opportunity for preventive medicine than industry." Among the important contributions of industrial medicine in this direction he listed:

> Early detection of skin diseases and other infections to keep them from being spread among families at home
>
> Establishment of methods for the control of communicable diseases, helping local health departments in isolation and quarantine
>
> Systems of placement and periodic examinations which detect signs of incipient disease long before the family physician would be consulted
>
> Keeping of data on defective conditions at certain ages and under certain conditions, which help the public health organizations and encourage family physicians to make regular examinations.

Otto Geier also has pointed out the value of such preventive services as a means of lightening the burden laid upon taxpayers to finance public assistance.

> The clinics of the hospitals or medical colleges meet only a fraction of the problem. The work there is with those who have fallen below the poverty line, in whom it is too late to do preventive social work and often too late to do preventive medical or social work.
>
> What a wondrous waste of energy! For only about 15 percent of your clinical cases ever return for further observation. The clinic within industry prevents the un-

116

fortunate but good American workman from reaching the poverty line; it keeps him out of the charity class.[8]

Times, conditions and statistics have changed. The problem, basically, remains and grows in size and complexity. Its solution lies not in curative medicine but in prevention. And no more economical or effective means to this end has yet been devised than capable medical supervision at the point of closest contact, the worker's place of employment—while he is still productive, self-supporting, and responsive to preventive treatment.

No analysis of the relationships of industrial medicine to other health organizations is complete without some consideration of the so-called "voluntary" agencies, which have expanded enormously in number and scope within our generation.

The Federal Security Agency, an adjunct of the public health services, estimates that there are more than twenty thousand separate agencies of this type, "pioneering groups of citizens whose work is supported largely from private sources."[9] Of these, the great majority operate at the city or county level but nearly three hundred carry on state-wide activities and about thirty are national in scope.

Such agencies have, in recent years, assumed an increasing share of the nation's total health burdens. Their interests range from the study and prevention of specific diseases (tuberculosis, venereal disease, cancer, poliomyelitis, diabetes, etc.) to the safeguarding of specific organs or functions (eyes, ears, heart, muscular and skeletal defects) to the promotion of the health of special groups (including mothers and children). These organizations, by and large, are splendid examples of "man's humanity to man." Supported largely by foundations and public donations, they are carrying on notable work in scientific research and remedial and preventive treatment. They present no particular problems of relationship, except those of integration with other health facilities and regulation to eliminate racketeering, inferior medical standards, and similar abuses.

On what common grounds do the private physician and the industrial physician meet? What sort of working relationship is best calculated to serve the interest of both and infringe upon the rights of neither?

These questions have been the subject of widespread discussion for more than forty years. There have been differences of viewpoint and abuses in practice, demanding prompt attention. But rarely has any controversy reached the point of official pronouncement or action. Criticisms for the most part have been voiced by individuals, as a result of local conditions or personal experience.

C. O. Sappington took a rational attitude toward this problem when he wrote in 1943:

Medical and surgical service for nonindustrial injuries and illnesses has provided a cause for some misunderstanding between the industrial physician and the private practitioner. There need not, however, be any difficulty here. Industry should not engage in the practice of medicine. By this is meant that industry should not provide medical and surgical services for employees or employees' families for nonindustrial injuries or illnesses.

It is now recognized by competent authorities on these questions of industrial medical service that industry itself should go no farther than the actual treatment of industrial injuries and illness, except that there should be given reasonable first aid or advice for nonindustrial illnesses to those employees who are still on duty when these exigencies occur. If further diagnosis or treatment is necessary, these cases should be referred promptly to their own physicians.[10]

The American Medical Association has had a vital interest in industrial medicine since its beginnings as a specialized type of practice; yet this fact received its first recognition rather casually in 1922, when the name of the AMA Section of Preventive Medicine and Public Health was formally changed to the Section of Pretive and Industrial Medicine and Public Health.

This name, while suited to the administrative pattern of the AMA at the time, left much to be desired. It blanketed two great fields of medical effort which were closely related but differed widely in objectives and areas of operation. Both were, and are, preventive in practice as well as in theory.

When, in 1937, the AMA created its Council on Industrial Health, it eliminated much of the confusion as to purpose and functions inherent in the former section. The council has repeatedly clarified the physician's place in the industrial picture and his relations with affiliated professional groups. In 1942 it published an outline of procedure for physicians in industry, a clear, concise statement of AMA policies with respect to the conduct of industrial medical departments.[11]

Despite the harmonious relations prevailing officially among health organizations, sharp criticism of industrial medicine and physicians in industry still persists in some quarters. It stems, perhaps, from isolated violations of professional ethics; it may be an echo from the old days of so-called contract practice, a time when standards of industrial medicine were low and all conditions of employment were ruthlessly dominated by management.

Under the title "Company and Private M.D.'s—Must They Feud?" Michael Fooner reported that frictions appeared to be growing as the number of M.D.'s with a stake in industrial medicine increased. He found that the chief cause of irritation was the amount of treatment given by industrial physicians to workers who otherwise might consult their family doctors. Workers liked it, he declared, because they had a good excuse for layoffs if the doctor told them to "take it easy." On the other hand, he said, doctors replied that they were usually paid by the hour and not by the case and were generally hired for specific purposes. In short, they had nothing to gain by trespassing on the private doctor's domain, but were more likely to increase the general practitioner's case load by referrals.[12]

In this connection, Fooner quoted Robert Collier Page: "The industrial doctor, through his program of employee examinations and periodic checkups, discovers conditions that would otherwise remain unknown to the employees, and he sends them to their family doctors or physicians of their own choice. Thus he expands the "demand for outside practitioners' services, helps to develop practice for them that they wouldn't get otherwise."

Close study of literature dealing with industrial-general medical relationships provides ample evidence of the truth of Dr. Page's contention and reveals nothing to indicate that the normal procedures in industrial medicine impose any greater penalty on the private practitioner than do those of any other specialty.

In a searching analysis of these relationships Earl F. Lutz, associate medical director of General Motors Corporation, states:

> Most physicians are well aware of the fact that the average general practitioner takes care of an occasional patient whose case is an industrial medical one, but few realize that surveys have established that from 70 to 80 percent of the employed population in the United States receive their industrial medical service from general practitioners and that 94 percent of all general practitioners surveyed indicated that they carry on some industrial practice. . . .

> In spite of this, however, most general practitioners are not primarily interested in industrial medicine. They concentrate most of their attention on problems in internal medicine, acute infectious diseases, obstetrics, metabolic diseases, etc.

> Likewise, top managements of industry are not primarily interested in and do not want to practice medicine. Their primary objective is to manufacture automobiles, washing machines, locomotives, or what have you, and their chief concern is that the article they are manufacturing be of superior quality and that it be produced in an economical manner.

Dr. Lutz lists four main classifications in which workers may be placed as the result of pre-employment examinations: workers with 1) nondisqualifying ailments, 2) with ailments causing temporary disqualifications, 3) with ailments causing special placement problems, 4) with ailments causing disqualifying conditions.

> After the physical examination is completed, each applicant is informed of his physical condition. Those applicants having nondisqualifying ailments are permitted to start work immediately, with the understanding that they will consult their family physicians at the earliest opportunity and have their ailments treated. In many cases the new employee is required to bring a statement from his physician indicating that he is receiving adequate medical care.

> Those applicants having ailments causing temporary disqualifications are not permitted to begin work until their ailments are corrected. Such applicants are promptly referred to their family physicians who have the opportunity to cure or correct these neglected ailments. Upon their recovery these applicants can be reappraised for employment.

In cases involving special placement requirements or disqualifying conditions, the problem is more serious. "Here," says Lutz, "the private practitioner and the industrial physician share a responsibility that frequently can only be properly discharged when both are in complete agreement.

In cases of arrested tuberculosis, epilepsy, or serious heart disease, for example, the family physician upon request should inform the industrial physician as to his opinion of his patient's physical condition and prognosis. The industrial physician then has the responsibility of placing the applicant at a job which is in keeping with the physical abilities of the applicant and in the environment in which there can be no aggravation of his disease state.

Differences of opinion are bound to arise in some of these instances. However, if the family physician is explicit in his information and the industrial physician explains in detail just what the applicant will be required to do and describes the environment in which he expects to work, these differences in opinion rapidly disappear. In general, the private practitioner knows far more about the applicant's past medical history and physical condition, while the industrial physician knows far more about the physical requirements of the job and the working environment.[13]

That the number of annual referrals to private practitioners reaches a surprising figure in large corporations is shown by records kept for a one-year period by a division of General Motors. Lutz says "that more than twenty thousand referrals were made in one year. Or, in other words, each employee was referred on the average of once every six months to his private physician."

If these analyses of relationships between the industrial doctor and other important health groups lead to any single conclusion, it is this: that the specialized profession of industrial medicine is a business of give and take; that reciprocal obligations are many and meticulous; and that they must be faithfully discharged if society is to reap the full benefits of modern medical science.

Seen from this viewpoint the "battle of the specialties" ceases to be a battle. It remains competitive in the sense that all businesses and professions in America are traditionally competitive, but only in the sense that one member of a team seeks to excel another in performance. Beyond this, it will be apparent that modern industrial practice has come to impose upon physicians and surgeons special requirements which test to the utmost not only their professional skill, but also their knowledge of other fields, their understanding of basic social trends, and their devotion to the betterment of human health.

XII

THE MIDDLEMAN IN INDUSTRY

T HE stop watch ticks the tempo of today. Business has become a contest in which speed and timing are paramount. It is a race to design, perfect, and manufacture products that meet human needs and satisfy human desires, a race to reach profitable mass markets ahead of competition. We see this elementary principle at work every year in the introduction of new motor cars, with emphasis on advanced styling, comfort, and convenience, mechanical features that contribute to performance and economy. To be first, with most, at the right price—that is the goal of the industry.

In the battle for business, no production advantage is small enough to be unimportant. Millions of dollars in profit or loss may depend upon items of cost which are individually insignificant but which in the aggregate materially affect price as a final factor in success or failure.

Thus, quality and volume of production are related directly to the physical fitness and morale of the employees in any industry. Management's concern for the health of the working force is actuated by this cold financial fact rather than by humanitarianism.

Clarence Selby summed up this viewpoint succinctly when he wrote:

Anything that is capable of facilitating production is welcome to industry so long as its cost is not excessive. The test is its ability to increase the quantity or to reduce the cost of production without impairing the quality. . . . On the contrary, anything that retards or does not facilitate production is tolerated by industry only so long as it is unavoidable.

Accidental injuries are such. By incapacitating the worker partially or wholly, they retard production. Necessitating always surgical treatment, frequently the payment of compensation, and occasionally the substitution of untrained labor, they are sources of expense.

121

Employers generally are accustomed to provide surgical attention for their injured workers, but they do not solicit the aid of physicians for this purpose any more than they seek the accidents that cause the injuries. Exigent, humane, and economic reasons force them to accept and endure the burden of surgical service as a penalty for accidents which industry does not seem to be able wholly to prevent.[1]

At the time of this commentary, trauma was the principal hazard recognized by industry; the doctor's services were almost exclusively surgical. But the same economic conditions—lost time, labor turnover, and other production penalties—which then focused attention on accident prevention, now apply far more importantly to entire categories of occupational disease for which industry has assumed financial and moral responsibility.

We have seen in our time an infinite number of metals and alloys, chemical elements and their compounds, come into general industrial use, along with innumerable new processes. Electronics alone has written a whole new vocabulary for science and engineering. The new technology is the work of chemists, physicists, engineers, and production men in every industrial field. Their objectives are simple: to create new products for new purposes, to improve existing products, to make all available to the largest possible number of people at the lowest possible cost.

It cannot be said that the hazards inherent in either materials or processes are ignored in the engineering stages of production, but they are bound to be of secondary interest. It is not likely that the medical tragedies of the phosphorus match industry, or of munitions production in World War I, could be repeated today. But of the raw materials and compounds now in general use in industry, a high percentage are toxic in one way or another, under one set of conditions or another, and in varying degrees of severity. Their toxic effects are not always immediately apparent. Exposure may be hazardous to some workers, while others suffer no ill consequences.

Modern industry, pouring hundreds of millions of dollars into research and development, is constantly complicating the health problem. Mechanization of labor, according to a report by the United States Department of Commerce (*Detroit Free Press,* December 20, 1954), has more than doubled since the late 1920's, and production per worker has increased by about the same amount. Most of the increase in mechanization, the report adds, has taken place since 1946.

As a result we are now witnessing another never-ending race within industry. On the one side there are the engineer and technician, aiming at new production goals; on the other, is the team of doctor, hygienist, and safety expert—all alert to new disease and accident hazards and to means for their control.

Keeping pace with the unparalleled development of production techniques, medical services in industry have undergone corresponding changes in character and scope. T. Lyle Hazlett, professor of industrial hygiene at the University of Pittsburgh Medical School and president of the American Association of Industrial Physicians

& Surgeons, 1941–42, recognized three distinct cycles through which industrial medicine had passed up to 1939:

1. The cycle prior to 1910, when such services were practically unknown, when employees injured while at work were sent to the office of the nearest physician, and management gave little thought to their surgical care and rehabilitation.

2. The surgical cycle predominant from 1910 to 1926, marked by the development of the group system of production with an increased concentration of workers. Industry was the greatest source of traumatic injuries in that period which saw the enactment of early compensation laws and the remarkable growth of the organized safety movement.

3. The medical-engineering cycle, which continued through the 1930's, a period marked by increasing attention to environment in its relation to the health and well-being of the worker; the beginning of cooperative effort by physicians and engineers in preventive programs.[2]

To those three cycles Hazlett has now added a fourth, as a contemporary record for this history:

Maturity of industrial medicine might well be traced to the commencement of World War II, when the urgent need of health maintenance among our industrial groups became essential with the greatly increased production necessary for our country's needs. This might well be described as the cycle of medical relations.

With the passage of these years we have seen an important increase of interest in healthful standards of working environment, control of these standards, and the toxicity of many materials and processes; [in] health education, placement of the worker, absenteeism, and many other phases which enter into employee and community relationships.

Both management and labor have become more cognizant of the importance of good health in its relation to production. Our professional schools have gone far in promoting industrial medicine in their curricula. Our own Industrial Medical Association, together with the American Medical Association, has brought to all physicians the importance of this particular branch of medicine.

This is new thinking emerging from old. We had primitive science in the primitive world, and it was adequate for its time. But at no stage in the history of civilized people has more than a fraction of human knowledge been applied for the betterment of society. Physical science, particularly in modern times, has far outstripped the social or humane sciences in its application to practical needs. Stuart Chase attributes many of the most perplexing problems of the present to this "cultural lag," a term he attributes to the sociologist W. F. Ogburn.[3]

In an address to the graduating class of Brown University in 1953, Alexander Meiklejohn, philosopher, educator, and author, made a penetrating analysis of inventive and technical progress in its relation to what he called "the present desperate crisis in human thinking." He said, in part:

Inventions destroy a social order as well as share in its creation. The inquiring, discovering mind has given to man the use of earth and water, fire and air. It has fashioned the wheel, the road, the boat, the clock, money, the bank and credit, the multifarious uses of power, and, most powerful of all, new methods of mind by which still other inventions may be made. But each of these devices, in turn, displaces older devices, and thus shatters and renders obsolete some earlier mode of life, the customs and beliefs, the habits and values, which the earlier devices had kept alive. . . .

As inventions thus lead the way, the forces of wisdom lag along behind. Theirs is the task of reconstruction. They must, by reasoned creative, imaginative thinking, bring into being new beliefs and plans, make out of chaos a new order of individual and social action. The inventions have widened out the range of human choices. And now, a new philosophy, informed by knowledge but not directed by it, must make a plan of life to fit the novel situation. In our present time of troubles, disaster has come upon our planning because inventions are being devised so fast that wisdom cannot keep the pace. Philosophy, the tortoise, is far outdistanced by science, the hare. And for that reason, our civilization is becoming more externalized, more mechanized in mind, more fascinated by gadgets and techniques, more avid for power, more barren of clearness of purpose, than any other the world has seen. . . .

If you and your friends can, by rigorous thinking, understand and master the process of invention, there can be established a human community in which no woman or man or child will lack for proper food, or proper housing, or proper care of health, or proper education to fit him for friendship and human understanding with his fellow man.[4]

Seen from this viewpoint, advances in the materialistic sciences can hinder, rather than help, the progress of civilization. If invention and technology draw further and further ahead of their integration into the practical procedures of daily life, the end can be confusion, instability, chaos.

We are faced today, in almost every American community, with the tragic effects of this "cultural lag." They are inherent in the patterns of cities that have grown enormously without central planning; in the jamming of traffic and other facilities; in disgracefully inadequate housing; in the growing need for more and better highways; in the shortage of schools and hospitals.

Labor, like every other segment of society, has had to cope with these inadequacies in adjusting itself to modern life. Mechanization of industry has made specialists of millions of workers in the various "handicraft" trades. The American worker has learned thousands of new skills which have given him mastery of the machine, multiplied his productivity, and raised his standard of living to an enviable level. But there is urgent need for a better understanding, on his part, of the basic relationships—economic, social and political—on which his continued well-being depends.

In no other area is there a more critical need for harmony of thought and action than in the "proper care of health" mentioned by Alexander Meiklejohn. Herein lies the opportunity of, and the challenge to, the industrial physician or surgeon. The new technology has broadened immensely the scope of his duties and by the addition of important responsibilities has dignified his profession beyond the dreams of even a generation ago.

* * *

What sort of man is the doctor in industry? What are the requirements for his success in matters of training, viewpoint and procedure?

Definitely he is not the man to whom Mock referred in 1919, when he wrote: "It is less than ten years since the majority of leaders in our profession could see naught but a questionable future, a sort of lowering of the prescribed method and standards, for those physicians who entered the field of the plant doctor."[5]

Nor does the status of today's industrial practitioner resemble that of his early prototypes, of whom Selby wrote in his war time study: "Physicians are drawn definitely into the accident problem after the damages have been done, and their relations are apt to be, in the eyes of the management, on a parity with those of a wrecking crew, necessary but not desirable."[6]

Listing specific conclusions from the same study, Selby declared:

> Knowledge of the theory and practice of medicine, such as is possessed by the ordinary physician in general practice, does not necessarily mean that the possessor of that knowledge is able to apply it to industrial needs. Physicians who intend going into industrial service should seek special training in that direction which will enable them to adapt their knowledge to the requirements of industrial work.[7]

Many other doctors prominent in the industrial field have pointed to this need for a thorough understanding of all environmental, economic and social factors that affect the health and well-being of workers. Their comments are in no way disparaging to the general practitioner, but they serve to draw a needed line of distinction between the two fields.

In the *Bulletin of the American Association of Industrial Physicians & Surgeons*, 1929, C.F.N. Schram, president in that year, made the general observation that the field of medicine had become "too broad for any one mind to grasp it all or even a large part of it." In this fact, he declared, lay the justification of all medical specialties; they required not only a more intimate knowledge of some phase or phases of medicine but knowledge of the relationship of the specialty to the great body of medicine.

Many employers of that time, said Schram, made the mistake of thinking that any man with an M.D. after his name was qualified to run a medical department—to be a chemical, electrical, mechanical, and efficiency engineer, all in one—even though he was a "third-rate man from a Class C school."

"There are physicians," he continued, "who are still putting greases, ointments, and medicated mud packs on infections, who feel that the immediate care of fractures is unimportant and that a good surgical result is more important than a good functional one."

Nearly twenty-five years later Earl F. Lutz asked an assembly of the American Academy of General Practice:

> Have you ever wondered just how the general practitioner differs from the average full-time industrial physician? After all, all of us went to the same colleges, studied under the same professors, interned at the same hospitals, took the same board examinations, belong to the same medical societies and hospital staffs. We treat a laceration or a fracture occurring on the highway, in the home, or in the factory in the same manner; nevertheless, there is one point on which most general practitioners differ from full-time industrial physicians. Almost invariably the general practitioners lack familiarity with the working environment of the employees they are treating.
>
> It is my sincere belief that every physician doing industrial medicine, whether he be a full-time industrial physician or a general practitioner, should be thoroughly familiar with every process occurring in those plants to which he gives attention if he expects to render the best service possible.[8]

The relative status and duties of the full-time and the part-time physicians in industry have been the subject of much discussion over the years. C. O. Sappington groups them into four commonly recognized classifications: those who devote their entire time to industrial practice; those who give only part-time service; those called in emergencies only; and those who serve as consultants. He adds that emergency practice "may be called obsolete."[9]

Of the three other classifications Selby writes:

> The full-time group, as the name indicates, gives its whole attention to industrial practice, and always in one establishment. These are the only true industrial physicians, who, as a group, apply the principles of preventive medicine to the maintenance of employee health.
>
> Of these three groups it is difficult to understand how any except the full-time physicians are in a position to assume appreciable responsibility in industrial hygiene. The extent to which they do or can largely depends upon their knowledge, vision, professional ability, and capacity to organize or fit into the organization that employs them.
>
> Physicians of the other two groups, the part-time and on-call, should frankly admit their dependence upon the industrial hygienist; but, though admitting dependence, they should be sufficiently informed of the principles of industrial hygiene to interpret and use the information obtained by engineering methods.[10]

Elsewhere, Selby has made this further pertinent comment on the two types of practice: "The essential argument favoring the part-time physician seems to be that he remains in intimate contact with the practice of medicine and is thereby likely to be a broader-minded medical man. The essential argument against the part-time doctor is that so long as he remains a part-time man, he is not wholly an industrial physician."[11]

It may be noted that these differences in training and experience have been largely offset in recent years by a joint approach to common problems. At the annual Industrial Health Conferences, as now programmed, the Industrial Medical Association meets with the American Industrial Hygiene Association, the American Conference of Governmental Industrial Hygienists, the American Association of Industrial Nurses, and the American Association of Industrial Dentists. The free exchange of information and ideas by these related groups has resulted in a harmony of viewpoint and procedure that could be accomplished in no other way. The sessions are invaluable as refresher courses. They crystallize the benefits of co-operative action and emphasize again and again the need for further extension of education in the basic problems and principles of industrial health by the nation's colleges and medical schools.

Industrial medicine, as a professional specialty, has gained immeasurably by these and other similar cooperative policies. Through the close association of the industrial practitioner, the hygienist and the sanitary engineer, the public health official and the safety expert, there has developed a rapport that recognizes the essential functions of each, along with the limitations of their various jurisdictions.

Moreover, the industrial doctor has become highly skilled in the diagnosis and prognosis of occupational diseases characteristic of the industries he serves and ingenious in suggesting measures for their prevention. By a well-rounded system of physical examination, the modern industrial medical department separates the fit from the unfit and brings under control medical supervision of the sick, the handicapped, the mentally disturbed, the accident-prone. It discovers who can work and in what kind of work he can productively engage. It prescribes medical and surgical treatment and undertakes the rehabilitation of the disabled and the handi-capped.

Beyond these purely medical and surgical responsibilities the doctor in industry, as we have seen, discharges other important obligations to his chosen profession. He must have more than a cursory knowledge of compensation law, as well as a basic understanding of the broad social and economic aspects of industry.

How can we best sum up these numerous and onerous responsibilities? The answer, perhaps, is found in a phase of the problem that has been relatively little discussed. Actually, the physician in industry has become, or is in the process of becoming, an essential middleman between management and labor, representative of both, biased toward neither. It is a role for which he is ideally fitted by the training and discipline of a profession that places health above all partisan considera-tion.

The machine was largely responsible for creating the gulf between capital and labor. Modern health care, as envisioned by all agencies dedicated to it, may well be the means of narrowing, if not closing, the gulf. Otto Geier, more than thirty-five years ago, wrote pointedly of this aspect of industrial medicine:

In the old days master and man worked elbow to elbow. The master largely molded the thought and living of the man. Often the man graduated from his ap-

127

prenticeship to set up a business of his own. Now industrial concentration practically hinders the establishment of new small units. Now the employee's work is more and more repetitive and limited to a single part of some machine. Now the employer and employee not only work apart but live farther apart. Industrial discontent is easily bred, and both employers and employees organize themselves to meet strife.[12]

On a later occasion, he wrote: "We can narrow the gulf (between labor and capital) by humanizing industry. This approachment will come not by the fact that the physicians will act as mediators in any active struggle, but by daily furnishing human contacts on which better understanding and greater tolerance are created. In actual practice the physician acts as the liaison between employer and employee."[13]

And, in an address to the AAIP & S in 1920, he made this further comment:

> Industry and society need today an ever increasing group of seriously minded, well trained physicians and surgeons who realize the great social and economic contributions that they may make to industry and society by special studies of their opportunities to serve both employer and employee.
>
> In conserving the body and mind of the worker, the industrial physician is able frequently not only to add to the earning capacity of the man, but also to change the worker's attitude toward his job. Incidentally, he educates the employer to the dollar-and-cents value of individual and community health.[14]

Since these words were written, in the early years of organized industrial medicine, industry and its labor relations have undergone changes of tremendous importance. Yet Geier's observations retain their force as a commentary on modern conditions. There are signs today that management and labor may yet find, in effective programs of health care, a common meeting ground on which an enduring peace may be established.

If we discuss the question of professional responsibilities with an experienced industrial physician or surgeon, we find him acutely aware of his obligation to promote better labor-management relations, and both ready and able to discharge that obligation. His purpose, however, is altruistic. He has no wish to pre-empt administrative duties in this field—to engage in labor negotiations or to extend the functions of his department beyond those which affect the health and fitness of workers.

Even when reduced to its simplest essentials, the task of the industrial medical practitioner is many-sided and complex, demanding of time, skill, understanding, stamina. Aside from professional routine he participates actively in the affairs of his Industrial Medical Association as well as in those of local, state and national organizations in general medicine and the various specialties.

Yet the industrial physician has still another duty to perform: a duty to the history of his profession, to young men studying in this field, to industry seeking a better grasp of the medical problems inherent in modern business. In a personal letter, Edward C. Holmblad, managing director of the IMA, commented with deep insight upon this obligation:

> I have frequently been impressed by a feeling of tragedy while paying respects to the survivors of recently deceased friends or professional allies. I then realize the vast amount of knowledge, information, facts, judgments, and valuable opinions they [industrial physicians] have accumulated during their lifetimes. If they have not been prolific writers, there is real tragedy as we realize that all of this knowledge and ability is being buried and forever lost to posterity.

Ideally, then, the medical specialist is also a writer: a recorder of clinical developments in medicine as they occur; an authority on the etiology, treatment and prevention of disease; a commentator on the ethics and standards of his profession, its goals, and the means of reaching them.

PART FOUR

TRENDS

AN "ENTR'ACTE" IN THE DRAMA
OF INDUSTRIAL MEDICINE

From never ending societal evolution comes an ever changing picture of occupational health.

XIII

TRENDS IN THE LITERATURE
OF ENVIRONMENTAL MEDICINE

Tʜᴇʀᴇ are two simple reasons for the insertion here of the three following chapters in the story of occupational medicine in America: First, although industrial health care of a sort was practiced in scattered areas late in the nineteenth century—and although the beginnings of mass production after 1900 created an urgent need for expanded medical programs—long-term trends in the growth and development of this specialty did not become apparent until the 1920's. Second, major trends in thought and practice offer the only reliable index by which the progress of occupational medicine and surgery can be measured in any single period. A knowledge of such factors is essential if we are to understand the full significance of health activities in the remarkable era of industrial expansion during and after World War I.

"That which is important," said the great Thomas Huxley, "is that which is persistent." The series of graphs with descriptive text (Figure 2), on the following pages, covers a cycle extending from the earliest years of the American Association of Industrial Physicians & Surgeons to a point well into the 1950's. It reveals trends that are not only persistent but in some cases spectacular. Some of these graphs reflect the progress made in the development of medical departments and the improvement of departmental procedures. Others visualize trends of interest in persistent occupational health hazards, some of them recognized for centuries (such as tuberculosis, silicosis and other respiratory diseases, and a few forms of metal poisoning) and some of relatively recent origin (notably dermatoses and other ailments ascribed to new toxic metals and chemical compounds.

133

In its twenty-first anniversary issue *Industrial Medicine and Surgery* refers to the diagnostic problems presented by "the near 3,000 forms in which occupational diseases have appeared."[1] In the aggregate, all of these health hazards are of professional interest to the industrial specialist, at least in the degree that he encounters them in medical departments for which he is responsible.

Indicating the size and complexity of this field, the association's journal printed in its first few issues (in the early 1930's) a list of some two hundred specific topics which it considered pertinent to the specialty and within the scope of its editorial policy. As a basis for the graphs presented here, we have selected from this wealth of subject matter twenty-seven main categories, all thoroughly representative of the continuing problems of occupational medicine, and, hence, of importance to business management and labor as well as to medical department personnel.

Statistically, these graphs are scaled to visualize fluctuations in the number of significant professional papers read at clinics and medical meetings and/or published, in each of the subject categories over a period of thirty-five years. The total number of such papers and articles is not impressively large, for the media devoted, wholly or principally, to the field of occupational health have always been relatively few. The sample used in this study is, however, large enough and selective enough to produce dependable data and lead to valid conclusions.

The material selected for these graphs was produced originally because of its professional importance; it interested publishers because of its scientific and news value; it attracted readers for the same reasons. The topics covered have been discussed year after year in conventions, debated perennially at medical board meetings, and studied constantly by special committees.

It is safe to say that this picture story of trends, during the most momentous period in the history of occupational medicine, accurately reflects the thinking, research and accomplishment of men most familiar with problems in this field and most eager to help in their solution.*

Pre-employment, periodic and placement examinations: One of the important requirements for certification of medical departments is a program of examinations before employment, at the time of transfer to a different job or department, and periodically during employment. Note that as early as 1921 increasing recognition of the desirability of this program, important to both employer and employee, was evident in medical literature and in papers delivered at medical meetings. Improved employment brought a further increase in interest after the depression of the early 1930's and again during World War II. Sustained emphasis continued until 1955, when the requirement for these examinations had become an established custom.

Health insurance: Although there was some consideration of health insurance as early as 1916 (when the AAIP&S was founded), there was no widespread interest on the part of

* These graphs are based on statistical material from publications of the AAIP&S—IMA (including *The Bulletin, Convention Programs,* and *Industrial Medicine and Surgery*) and from goverment bulletins and selected books bearing on various phases of occupational medicine.

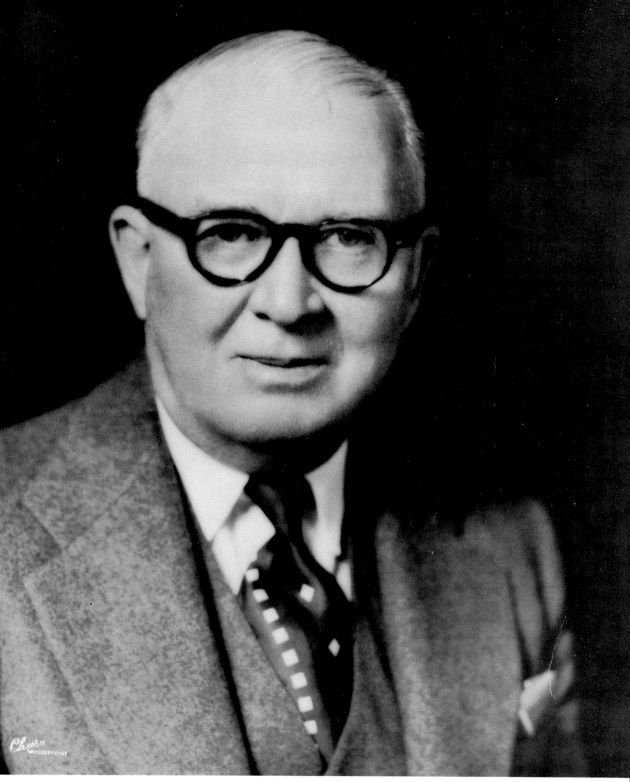

34. *Loyal A. Shoudy, M.D. (1880–1950). President, AAIP&S, 1923–1925, 1946–1947.* Loyal Shoudy was one of an active compact group at the organization of the AAIP&S in 1916. From that year until his last illness he remained an association leader in both thought and action. In 1917 he was a member of a committee, with Geier, Mock and Selby, opposing national defense plans to regiment the doctors in industry. A graduate of the University of Pennsylvania School of Medicine in 1909, he joined the Bethlehem Steel staff in 1914; became chief of medical service in 1918 and medical director in 1945. There he did his research on salt as a preventive of heat sickness.

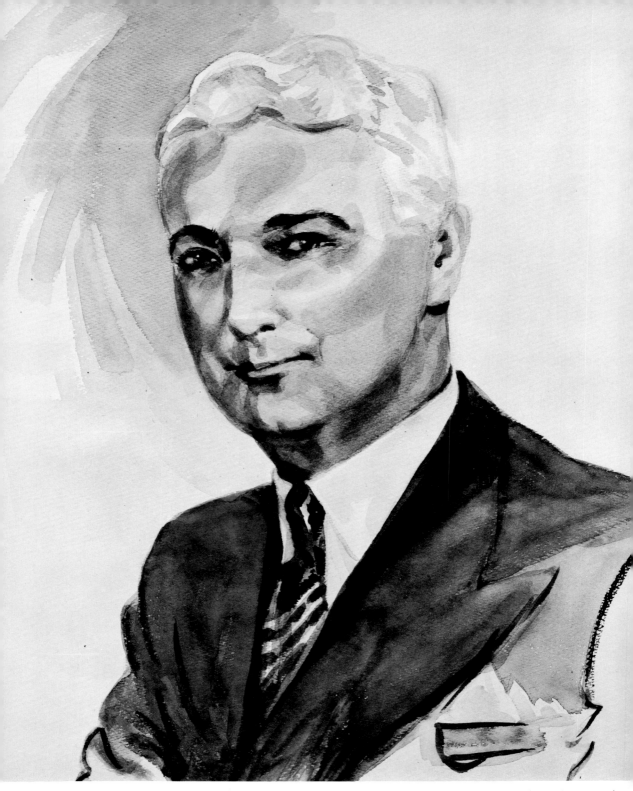

35. *William B. Fisk, M.D. (1871–1941). President, AAIP&S, 1925–1926.* Dr. Fisk was one of the six who formed the nucleus of the founding group. About 1900 he became chief surgeon of the International Harvester Company and later took over direction of its Industrial Relations Department. He worked quietly, efficiently. Incessantly he expounded the value of physical examinations in industry. As AAIP&S president, one of his first acts was to push through the directorate a vote against a proposed merger with the AMA. His final act was a move to establish permanent headquarters for the association's staff.

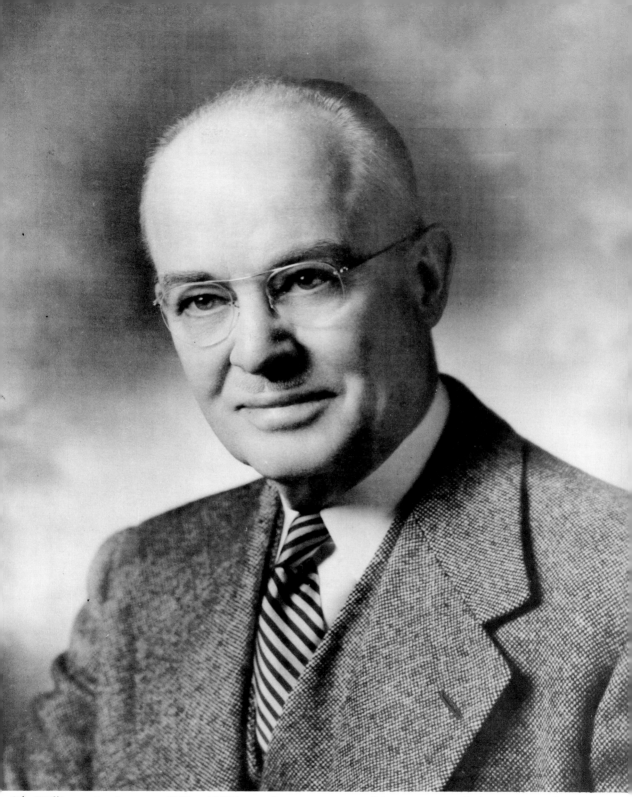

36. *William A. Sawyer, M.D.* (1884–   ). *President, AAIP&S, 1926–1927.* A graduate of the University of Pennsylvania School of Medicine, Sawyer started a long association with the Eastman Kodak Company in 1919, as medical director. In 1921, while secretary of the AAIP&S, he was involved in controversial issues by his strong opposition to merger "with any organization" and by a notable paper entitled "Nurses in the Guise of Industrial Physicians." As incoming AAIP&S president in 1926 he handled problems of membership and finance boldly, decisively. He was noted for his work on nutrition and his use of serial X-rays for early diagnosis of TB.

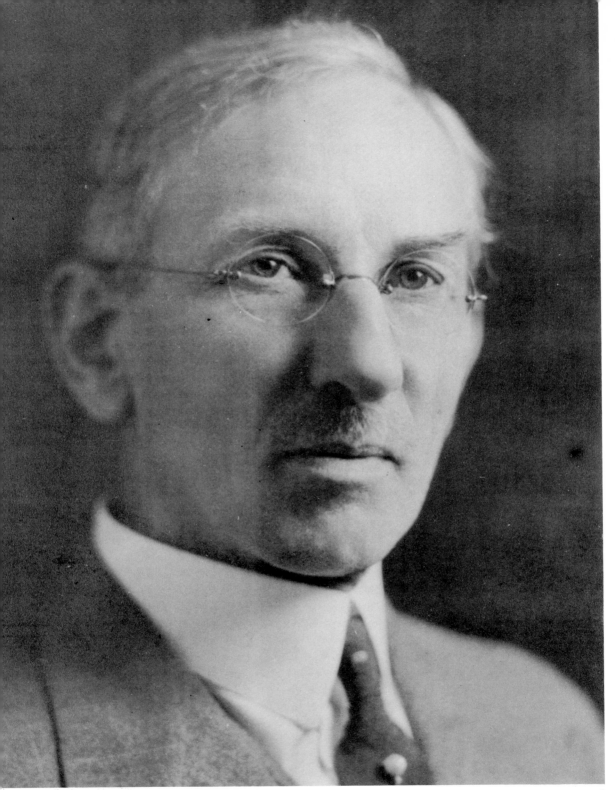

37. *Thomas R. Crowder, M.D. (1872–1942). President, AAIP&S, 1927–1928.* Educated at De-Pauw, at Rush Medical College, and in Vienna, Crowder built up a special practice in genito-urinary diseases. In 1905, he became medical direc-tor of the Pullman Company, in charge of sanitary matters. He wrote with authority on various as-pects of tuberculosis, and published a score of studies on railway sanitation, car ventilation and the diseases of travel. Crowder was one of the founders of the AAIP&S. As association president he devoted himself to furthering a steady and normal growth, and he remained active in associa-tion affairs until his death.

Year 1917–18

June 4, 1917.   Receipts   Dues.   Misc.   Year 1917–18   Disbursements   Cr.

	Dues	Misc	1917		
Bro't forward	44 00	1662	June 13	Prize to M. Shie	100 00
Ralph Walker 1917 X	2 00		20	Watson – 250 Regis. cards	2 00
422 Chestnut St. Lebanon, Pa. ✓			29	S. S. Corpin – stenographic report (2nd annual meeting)	76 75
Dr. M. Holtz – 1917 X	2 00			Stamps	5 00
Randall Zimmerman – new X	2 00		6	Check set for endorsement – V. A. Paul	2 00
J. B. Hileman – 1917 X	2 00		July 11	Banquet – 2nd annual	225 00
Jean S. Millard – new 1917 X	2 00			39 sold. 75 reserved X 3.00	
C. E. Ford – 1917 X	2 00			Badges – 2nd meeting	11 25
W. A. Lucas X	2 00			Menu cards – " "	5 00
J. W. Ellenberger ✓	2 00			Signs	4 00
Myers S. Bloom X	2 00			Incidentals – Dr. Ford, chairman arrangements 2nd meeting	4 00
Theodore Joepel – new X	2 00				
Herbert J. Cronin X	2 00				

38. AAIP&S Ledger Pages, 1917–18. These fading pages record some of the first business transactions of the AAIP&S, when dues were $2.00 per year and costs proportionate. It has survived where other, more important, papers have not.

39. Detroit Public Library Exhibit, 1958. Display cabinets in the main library have helped create public understanding of the nature and purpose of United States social and labor legislation.

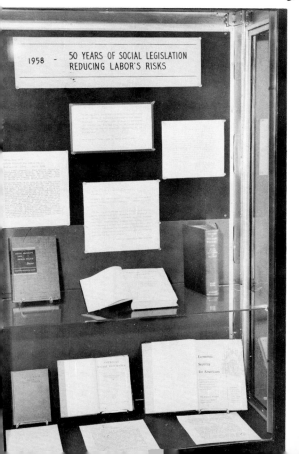

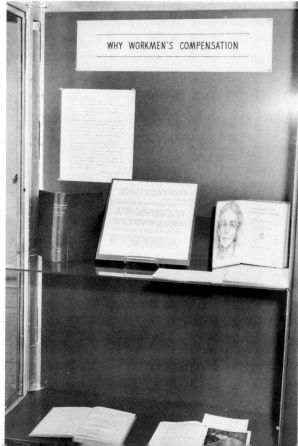

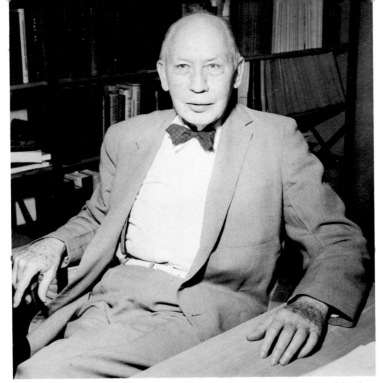

40. *Carey P. McCord, M.D.* A distinguished research physiologist, teacher and medical director; consultant to industries, associations and governmental bureaus; editor of *Industrial Medicine and Surgery* since 1951.

41. *Robert A. Kehoe, M.D.* Famous for research in the toxicology of lead absorption; research professor in Cincinnati University College of Medicine; widely sought as consultant. Named vice-chairman of the new AMA Board of Preventive Medicine, 1955.

—Photo, Chase News Photo, Washington, D.C.

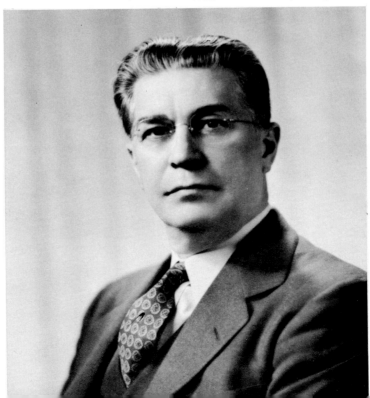

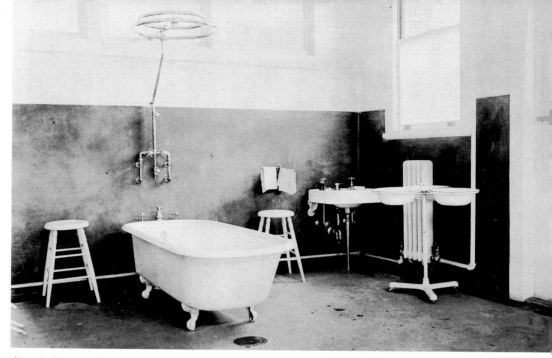

42. *A Corner of Dr. Harvey's Operating Room at the Crane Company, Late 1890's.*

43. *A Mid-Twentieth Century Operating Room, Arabian-American Oil Company.*

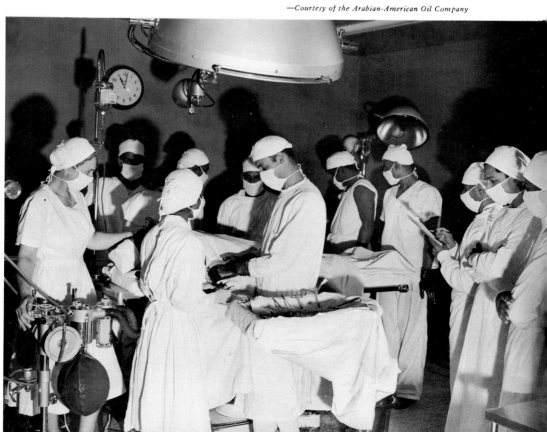

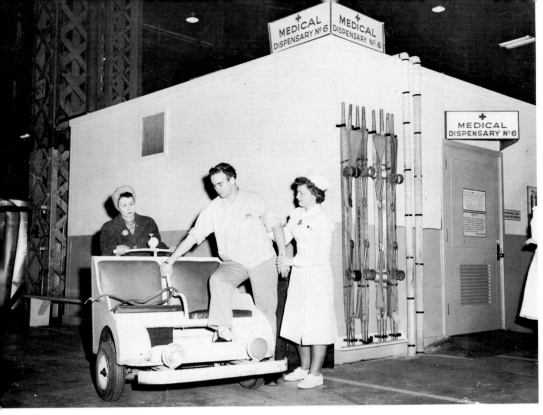

44. *Factory Medical Dispensary, Boeing Aircraft Company.*

—*Courtesy of the Boeing Medical Department*

45. *The Original Central Medical Clinic of Boeing Aircraft Company.*

—*Courtesy of the Boeing Medical Department*

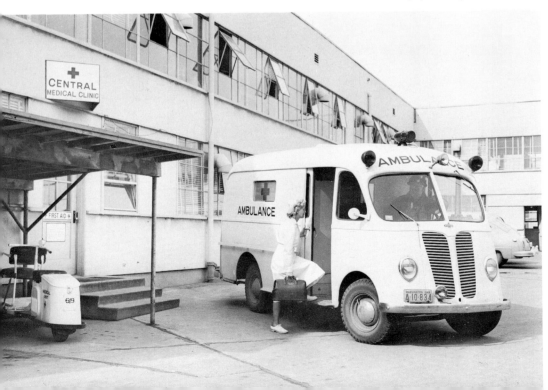

the public, employers, or the labor unions until 1932, when the severe economic conditions created a desire for greater social security. In the labor movement and in Congress and the national administration during the "New Deal" increasing attention was given to health protection, but there was very little discussion of the problem by physicians in industry. This situation persisted until 1955, with the result that many plans were established which lacked expert medical guidance.

The Specialty: Almost from the establishment of industrial medicine as a formal branch of medicine (in 1916), there was expressed in literature and at meetings a wish to place the practice on such a high plane that it could be regarded and designated as a specialty. This interest increased steadily, until 1945 found industrial physicians insistent that educational facilities be made available at the undergraduate level and that hospital opportuni-

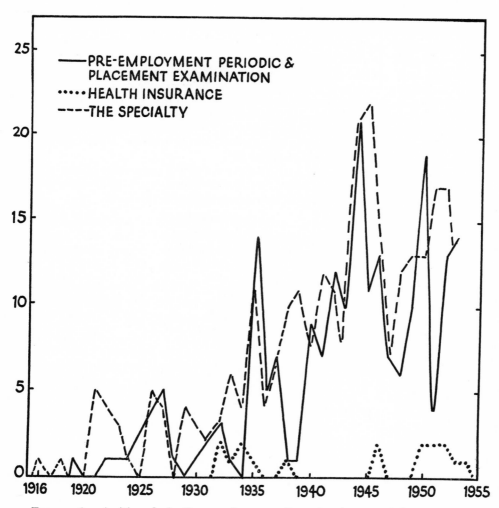

FIGURE 2. A. *Trends in Pre-employment Examination, Health Insurance and the Specialty*

135

ties be opened for graduates, thus paving the way to establishment of a specialty board in occupational medicine. Rapidly growing emphasis on health conservation, and the complexity of special problems which set industrial practice apart from surgery and general medical practice, resulted in 1955 in the designation of a Division of Occupational Health under the American Board of Preventive Medicine, followed by creation of the American Academy of Preventive Medicine. (See Chapter XXXII)

Medical Departments: A review of the literature and programs of meetings of industrial physicians reveals that in the early 1920's the importance of medical department records was recognized. In 1942 a special committee, of which Dr. Stuart F. Meek of Detroit was chairman, presented a report to the AAIP&S prepared by Dr. Carey Pratt McCord emphasizing the importance of records. In 1943 Dr. William J. Fulton, of the medical department of General Motors Corporation, presented a paper before the Industrial Nursing Session of the Thirty-Second National Safety Congress titled "Records—the 'Seeing Eye' of Industrial Medicine." He stated:

> The present is the sum total of the past. Had man left no records, the present sum total would be infinitely less. We are what we are, largely because of records, and the future sum total is moulded by what we, in turn, add.

> Of necessity, such records must be of a simplicity capable of accumulating the maximum information concerning each individual with the least cost of time, effort and space. They should be records of a high degree of efficiency in their practical application; readily accessible records that, day by day, can be consistently applied toward bettering and studying the safety, health and environment of each and every individual; *records to use—not simply to file.*

The graph of the records curve continues to reflect the importance of this phase of medical are. A requirement for AMA Certification is that records meet an established proficiency and that they be available only to the medical department.

Environment: Industrial medical literature reflects a constant recognition of the importance to the employee and the employer of the working environment. This recognition has developed along with the broad acceptance of health conservation in contrast to the mere treatment of accidental injury.

War: World War I created an increased interest in industrial medical problems. The mechanization of combat and the need for the utmost production in World War II caused a skyrocketing of interest in all phases of employee health and safety, which continued through the Korean War and into the cold war period.

Industrial Dentistry: Industrial Dentistry has received increasing recognition. Starting in the early thirties, physical examinations revealed the effect of the economic depression and a resulting neglect of teeth. The American Dental Association gave important consideration to the dental problems of the employee, some industries established dental departments in their medical divisions, and the American Association of Industrial Dentists, meeting annually with the industrial physicians, stimulated an increased interest in the improvement of dental care of the employee.

Trauma: As pioneers in occupational medicine will recall, trauma was the main problem of industrial health in and around 1916, and practically all medical discussions had to do with the treatment and prevention of injuries. In later years, when health conservation began to occupy an ever larger part of the physician's attention, it was assumed that this shift in industrial health was due to a decreased interest in surgery. Figures, however, do not justify this assumption. The graph reveals a greatly increased interest in trauma and the surgery of trauma, a fact borne out by the large attendance at the surgical sections of medical sessions. In the fifties—although surgery, percentage-wise, occupied a relatively small part—the increase in interest and the emphasis on improved surgical care were striking indeed.

Nutrition: World War II created potentially dangerous nutritional deficiencies among industrial workers, because many of them, under food rationing, did not buy food that gave them a balanced diet. Many employers in that period introduced carefully studied nutri-

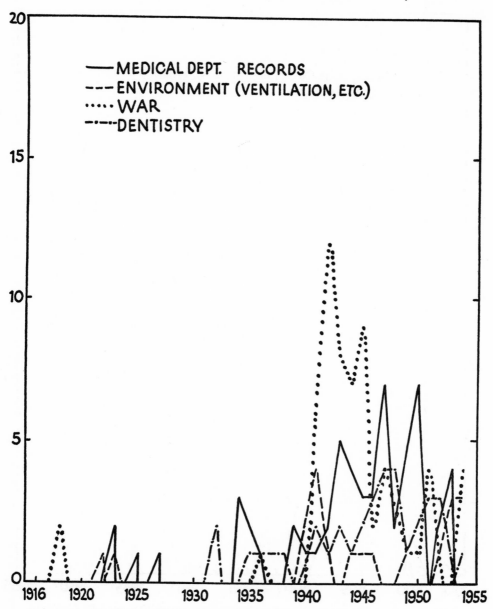

FIGURE 2. B. *Trends in Medical Department Records, Environment, War, and Dentistry*

tional programs into their plants, feeling that to do so would go far to maintain a healthy working force and hoping that employees would follow the example and carry better dietary habits into their homes.

Disability: The graph reflects the need for a comprehensive survey and program dealing with the problems of disability in industry. Although interest in this subject received early

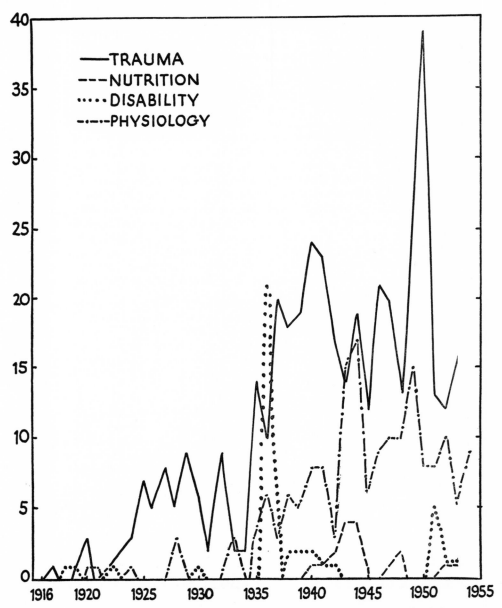

FIGURE 2. C. *Trends in Trauma, Nutrition, Disability, and Physiology*

138

impetus from workmen's compensation legislation, and later from laws affecting war veterans, interest remained sporadic over the years, partly because physicians as a whole did not thoroughly understand the psychological, sociological and ideological factors involved, and partly because medical societies were reluctant to get involved in highly controversial matters.

Physiology: As could be expected, both medicine and surgery have benefited by the application of great advances in physiological knowledge to preventive as well as curative procedures in industry. The graph reflects the steadily increasing inclusion of physiological principles in the development of occupational medicine. Indirectly, it also reflects the interest of the many highly trained chemists in industry and the ability of medical personnel to call upon their specialized knowledge.

Workmen's Compensation and Medicolegal Problems: As the graph indicates, medical literature has faithfully reflected the steady growth of American interest in workmen's compensation, a growth that reached its climax during and immediately after World War II. The national movement toward legislation in that field received strong impetus in 1907 when the Illinois Commission on Workmen's Insurance reported. This report attracted attention of both employers and employees, particularly after its findings had been presented and discussed at the First National Conference on Industrial Diseases in June 1910 at Chicago. Unions requested brief, plain, practicable directions for workingmen in various trades to help them avoid disease. Employers asked for information and advice as to better methods of guarding the health of employees. It soon became apparent that a new social concept was finding acceptance in industry. Despite some points of conflict, there developed a profound harmony of interest, based on recognition that health among workers was an asset to the employer and sickness a liability; that money wisely and carefully spent was not a burden upon capital but a profitable investment.

Maryland, in 1902, was the first state in the Union to provide legislation for certain benefits payable without suit. This, however, was limited to certain occupations and was declared unconstitutional, as were the early laws of Montana (1909), New York (1910) and Kentucky (1914). Wisconsin on May 3, 1911, was the first state whose compensation laws became effective. Along with Illinois, nine other states enacted compensation legislation in that same year. Steadily, state after state followed suit until by 1940, forty-seven of the forty-eight states had passed similar laws.

While this activity indicates fairly rapid progress, once the trend started, it does not explain the long period of inactivity in the nineteenth century. Thirty years before the first effective American laws, Switzerland had boldly established compensation for accidents in certain types of employment without proof of fault on the employer's part. And protection of one kind or another was in force in Europe a century before the Swiss declaration.

Germany remained far ahead in this field in the 1800's. The German plan had its roots in the medieval guilds, whose welfare organizations were officially recognized by the Prussian *Landrecht* in 1784 and developed in the next fifty years into a complete system of socialized medicine. Indeed, up to 1913, when the United States was still taking its first steps in industrial compensation, forty-one foreign countries had introduced some form of compensation for accidental injuries in industry.

Preventive Medicine and Safety, closely allied with the problems of workmen's compensation, attracted serious attention as early as 1920, gradually replacing in importance the surgical and reparative services in industry and reaching their greatest emphasis in the early 1940's. This emphasis was marked in 1955 by the creation of a Division of Occupational Medicine under the American Board of Preventive Medicine.

Sociology in Industry likewise received steadily growing emphasis because of its importance in general planning during the period of the New Deal. With government, unions,

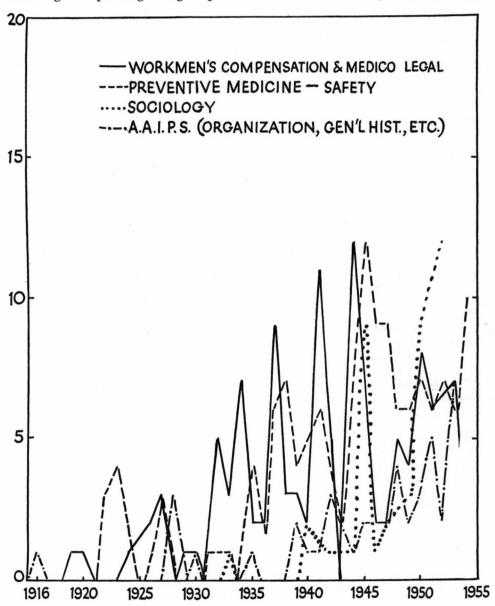

FIGURE 2. D. *Trends in Workmen's Compensation, Preventive Medicine, Sociology and the AAIP&S*

140

and doctors pressing for more consideration of employees, the term *Health Conservation* appeared in medical literature, and fringe benefits were written into union contracts. Under this new concept social progress in health care has since assumed major importance.

American Association of Industrial Physicians & Surgeons (Industrial Medical Association): This association has had a constantly growing influence in guiding the evaluation

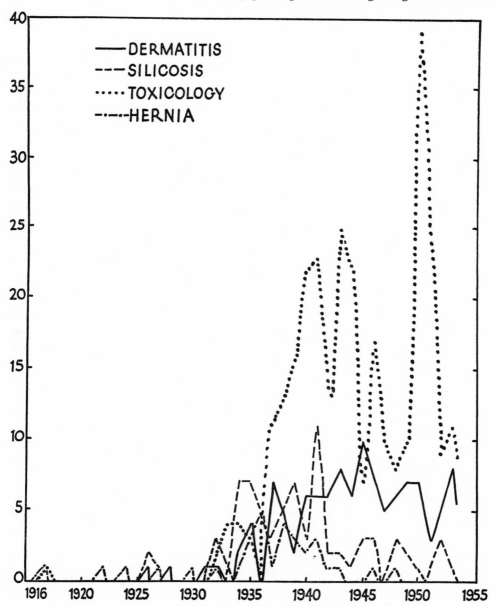

FIGURE 2. E. *Trends in Dermatitis, Silicosis, Toxicology, and Hernia*

141

of factors entering into the health, safety and welfare of the American industrial employee. This influence has continued at a high level.

Dermatitis: By 1925 the skin problems of industrial workers were receiving serious attention. They have steadily increased as more and more chemical compounds of greater complexity have come into use in production, until in the mid-century dermatologists actively participated in industrial medical meetings and contributed to industrial medical journals.

Silicosis: Although the effect of the dust of mines upon human lungs had been recognized by the ancients—and Isbrand de Diemerbroeck had described the pathological changes found at autopsy—it was not until the 1930's that physicians both in and out of industry, as well as radiologists, gave serious consideration to silicosis. So immediate was acceptance of the importance of the disease, and so efficient the communication, that workers in the dusty trades—helped by legislation—were given the protection needed. Then, and only then, did medical interest, as reflected in the literature, return to routine discussion.

Toxicology: In the study of the advance in occupational medicine during the present century, there is no more important development than the recognition of the necessity for a full understanding, by specialists in occupational medicine, of the toxicological aspects of health in industry. Starting in the 1930's and continuing into the 1960's, the literature and the programs of meetings reflect this development.

Hernia: The problems of herniae among industrial workers were discussed at the founding of the AAIP&S. For a time labor legislation and interpretation by workmen's compensation boards accented emphasis on this health hazard, which continues today to be a subject of minor interest.

Human Back: The graph indicates that the human back (including the cervical region to the coccyx and referred symptoms into the extremities) has been a problem from the time that industrial medical literature appeared and industrial medical meetings were arranged. Interest continues to mount in spite of automation, for the biological inadequacy of the back cannot meet the requirements of industry, especially of heavy industry.

Psychology and Psychiatry: By 1920 mental illness and emotional instability received careful consideration by physicians in industry, and as knowledge increased they received more and more emphasis. With recognition of the fact that the stresses of employment directly affect the emotional and behavioral tendencies of employees, both industrial medical departments and management have been obtaining personnel capable of coping with the problems involved.

Nursing: While the industrial nurse since 1920 has played a broadening role in environmental health, it was not until a large group became available and nursing organizations were formed that medicine finally recognized the true stature of the position occupied by the nurse. Still handicapped by the refusal of training schools in nursing to provide special training for the industrial nurse, she has become, by in-plant experience, a full partner in the health conservation programs of industry.

Geriatrics: The most recent concern of medical departments and of medicine in general is the great new field of opportunity in preparing the aging employee for retirement and in counseling him in his post-retirement plan. This concern is greatest in industry because of retirement requirements and the increasing number of employees living to a more advanced age. The graph reflects the recent emphasis on geriatric programs.

Education and Research: The graph depicts one of the most important problems of environmental medicine, the lack of a sustained increase in educational resources. Educators, as well as industrial management, which depends for its existence today upon health su-

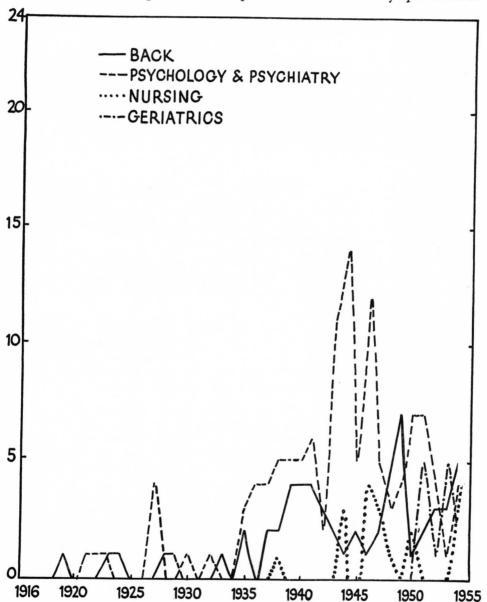

FIGURE 2. F. *Trends in Human Back, Psychology and Psychiatry, Nursing, Geriatrics*

pervision, have failed to realize fully the importance of training facilities and to support their development.

Even as environmental medicine receives recognition as a specialty by the creation of an accrediting board, and although a few universities have added departments and facilities, the opportunities for training are woefully inadequate and are almost entirely de-

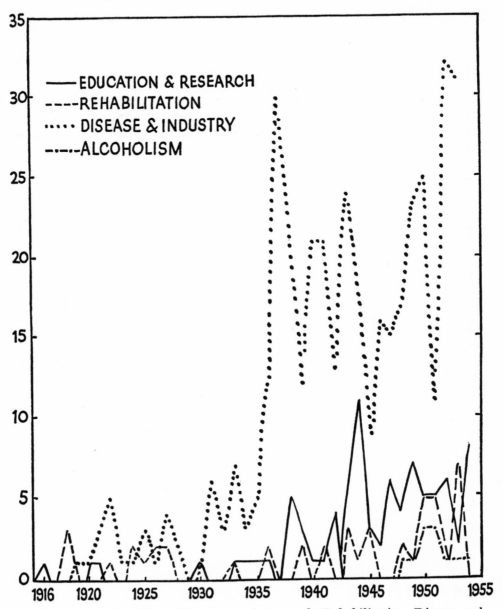

FIGURE 2. G. *Trends in Education and Research, Rehabilitation, Disease and Industry, and Alcoholism*

pendent on graduate instruction. Residencies are nonexistent, and the undergraduate is afforded little contact with the discipline which determines the opportunities for service and success in industrial medicine.

Rehabilitation: After each war we see the passage of liberal legislation to make rehabilitation less expensive than neglect of the handicapped. Accompanying this we see a rapid creation of rehabilitation institutes, headed by specially trained directors and personnel. Naturally, the literature of a post-war era is large and important—devoted as it is to the introduction of new techniques and social viewpoints and to a program that aims at "the return of the disabled workman to the highest possible skill consistent with his physical or mental capacity."

Disease and Industry: From a modest beginning at the turn of the century there has been a gradual but steady increase in recognition of the problem presented by disease in industry. The lessening of illness is one program in which success benefits the employee, who profits directly by health and the employer, whose greatest asset is a healthy work force. The dramatic lines in the graph reflect the programs of meetings and the content of medical journals devoted in large part to this problem.

Alcoholism: Although alcoholism has always been a serious problem in industry—and although rapid strides have been made in recognizing it as a disease that can be cured—medical departments in industry have been slow to apply advanced methods to meet its threat. Thanks to the directors of several centers of research and the efforts of a few dedicated workers,* industrial medical society meetings since the late 1940's have included the problem in their deliberations. Presented in dramatic form to well attended conferences, the literature has reflected increased interest, and the attitude of physicians as well as employers is undergoing rapid change.

* For example, the work of R. G. Bell, M.D., of the University of Toronto, and J. K. W. Ferguson, M.D., of the Shadowbrook Foundation, Toronto; and the studies by Yale University.

XIV

INDUSTRIAL SURGERY *

I T IS A remarkable fact that the transition of industrial surgery from the period of cigar-box first-aid kit limitations[1] to the present mid-century medical department, scientifically planned, efficient in physical arrangement, and presenting the highest skills available in modern surgery, has taken place within the work-span of many living surgeons.

The great mystery is why at the beginning of the present century, when great advances already were being made in surgical procedures and when the United States was already passing other countries as an industrial nation,[2] the workman should have been considered entitled to only the barest necessities of medical care administered by a fellow worker or by a plant doctor of dubious skill and state of sobriety.

Several wars had produced a knowledge of the special problems encountered in the surgery of trauma. Friedrich Esmarch[3] in the Franco-Prussian War developed methods helpful in emergency and definitive stages of treatment of war injuries. Larrey,[4] as surgeon to Napoleon in all his campaigns, not only was a brilliant surgical technician, but had made his experience and his methods available through his writings.

* We have not attempted to draw a clear line between the functions of the physician and the surgeon in occupational practice. Although the early work of doctors in scattered American industries was predominantly surgical, new concepts of health, along with phenomenal advances in medical science, have attracted a rapidly growing proportion of physicians to this field and have increased the emphasis on the medical aspects of occupational health. Industrial surgery has undergone an equally dramatic transformation in recent decades. And it is to place this transformation in its proper perspective that this chapter, which covers the historic evolution of surgery, is included.

146

The surgical experiences of our own war between the states had been well documented[5] and pictorially recorded by Matthew Brady[6] and Surgeon-General Joseph K. Barnes.[7] Lister,[8] using the research of Louis Pasteur,[9] had demonstrated the principles of antisepsis and cleanliness, and James T. Whittaker[10] had demonstrated the importance of physiological changes and the part played by parasites and bacteria.

The year 1900 found the industrial plants of America, with a few exceptions, totally without facilities to provide even the most primitive first aid other than a meager supply of unsterile bandages, kept in a cigar box on a shelf and supplemented by the proverbial chew of tobacco to be applied to a wound.

The exceptions included the first major prepayment program of record, started in 1868[11] by the Southern Pacific Railroad in Sacramento, California, where a hospital was opened in 1869. This project, financed jointly by employer and employees, provided service by a medical staff through arrangements with surgeons along the railway.

In 1882 the first major employee-sponsored mutual benefit association was formed: as the Northern Pacific Railway Beneficial Association. This organization developed a program of complete medical care and other benefits financed by employer-employee payments. Medical services were provided through group practice in the Northern Pacific Hospital in St. Paul, Minnesota, and through arrangements with surgeons along the line.

Through the years following those humble beginnings, the railroads continued their support of progressive health programs, with the close cooperation of the American Association of Railway Surgeons. It is interesting to note that at the 41st annual banquet of the Industrial Medical Association held in Philadelphia, April 25, 1956, the Health Achievement in Industry Award was presented to the Pennsylvania Railroad for the excellence of its modern facilities in Philadelphia, which developed from one of the earliest medical departments.

Nineteenth-century efforts to safeguard the health of workers were not, however, limited entirely to the railroads. In 1887 the Homestead Mining Company[12] of Lead, South Dakota, established a company-financed medical department, with a full-time staff providing complete medical service to employees and their families. Other mines and kindred establishments in remote areas followed suit with programs of one kind or another.

Andrew Magee Harvey's introduction of protective goggles for workers[13] in 1897 heralded a similar trend in large industrial centers. As medical director of the Crane Company in Chicago, he set an example which profoundly affected the development of truly modern industrial medicine.

Another pioneer of that period was Dr. Robert T. Legge, who in 1899 joined the McCloud Lumber Company of California as chief surgeon.[14] Though traumatic injuries were of first importance among the hazards in this isolated community, Legge soon discovered the need for more basic planning. With company cooperation he built a modern hospital, launched a general welfare measure and introduced a successful program of preventive medicine.

Industrial medicine in the United States is generally considered to have its roots in the surgery of trauma, as these early activities indicate. If this is so, then the steel industry was the place of its beginning. Steel history for more than a hundred years has been an unbroken record of efforts to reduce occupational hazards, and the industry has always been in the forefront in developing improved methods of surgical care.

In 1836, Joseph Whitaker purchased the Principio Iron Works in Maryland, and he and his descendants were leaders in this field for many generations, distinguished by their thoughtfulness for their employees. Moving west with the industry they finally settled in Wheeling on the Ohio River, where they developed larger and larger mills. The story of early years in the expanding industry is well told by Earl Chapin May, who writes: "Danger stalked in the steel mills, but steel men were unafraid—tough men in a tough business." He adds: "Traditionally the smelters, rollers, roughers, heaters and catchers resented any attempts to 'nurse-maid' them. . . . Death might come in the afternoon or evening, yet fatalistic steel workers seldom if ever dodged it."[15]

For a dozen years prior to 1907, the various steelworking plants which later merged into the Wheeling Steel Corporation employed local physicians "on call" to attend any employee hurt in line of duty. It was in one of those units, the Wheeling Corrugating Company, that an effort at in-plant care was made in 1907. It was a modest experiment but nonetheless it proved to be, in effect, the beginning of American industry's safety first movement. Among the office employees of the company was Lewis McC. Steenrod, member of an old Wheeling family. He had a degree in medicine, but like many young men in Wheeling he had taken a job in the rapidly expanding corrugating works. While holding this job, Dr. Steenrod moved his operating chair and surgical bag into a small vacant storeroom of the company's warehouse, and there, from time to time, he rendered first aid to any worker who had suffered an accident.

During that same period, James Farrington of the Steubenville plant of LaBelle Iron Works was outlining to fellow superintendents his plan for a national association of iron and steel engineers, an organization designed to promote plant safety.

While that plan was under consideration, Corrugating's safety program was progressing steadily. Because of the cost as well as the suffering entailed in accidents, instructions were soon issued to all employees that even the most minor injuries had to be reported in person to the company's so-called hospital. There, wounds were dressed and infection was prevented; if necessary, patients were sent or taken to one of Wheeling's hospitals.

These precautions promptly proved their value. Quick action in the improvised plant hospital radically reduced cases of infection, and patients treated there were required to report daily until redressing was no longer necessary.

Similar programs were independently adopted by the Wheeling Steel and Iron company, LaBelle Iron Works, and Whitaker-Glessner Company plants, as well as in Corrugating's Martins Ferry and Wheeling plants. By 1908 top management and superintendents and foremen of these plants were working together to install protecting machine guards.

While humanitarian activities were getting under way in widely separated Wheeling district plants, James Farrington's idea had become a fact. During the 1912 convention of the Association of Iron and Steel Engineers the Farrington plan developed into the first cooperative alignment of industrial leaders with federal and state officials to protect workers during working hours. And that alignment, in turn, developed into the National Safety Council.

When the Wheeling Steel Corporation was organized in 1920, E. A. Ellis, director of the safety program at the Steubenville plant, became director of the corporation's Safety First Department. The chief source of injuries was removed by discarding the customary foot-pedal controlled presses and replacing them with hand operated presses. Experience readily poved that when a worker's hands were busy operating a machine, they were less likely to get caught in the machinery than when foot presses were used and hands could be under the dies.

As the corporation's safety program progressed, top management furnished its mill workers, over a long period, with seven thousand pairs of goggles and specially ground prescription glasses. Employees were also supplied with 240,000 pairs of canvas, leather-palm, rubber-dipped, riggers' steel-studded, acid rubber or asbestos gloves where use of gloves was advisable to secure safety in certain operations. Later, the company distributed through its Safety First Department hand pads, aprons, skull guards, ear defenders, helmets, masks and respirators.

One phase of this protective program required salesmanship by management, superintendents, foremen, and the state Department of Labor. Because of a feeling that there is a point beyond which American workmen do not wish to have things done for them *gratis,* safety shoes were sold to them at cost, and more than 5,000 pairs were distributed on that basis in one year.

It was not easy, in that early period, to induce workers to use safety equipment or to follow safe procedures. So, warning signs were posted where employees could not avoid reading them. And campaigns of education—publicity, motion pictures, safety posters, interdepartmental and interplant safety contests—became an important part of the program.

Obviously, there can be no permanent solution of the safety problem as long as it concerns human beings. Gradually, however, taking care of themselves became a habit among mill hands, and statistics began to prove that employees of a steel mill were much safer than they were on the streets and public highways and even safer than they were in their own homes.

Safety education has, of course, continued, growing in scope and in success, until, today, it may be said that employees in all industries are convinced that accidents are preventable and that employees are sincere in their efforts to prevent them.

For many years after the founding of the American Association of Industrial Physicians & Surgeons (1916), the surgery of trauma still held its pre-eminent place in industrial medicine. The program for the fourteenth annual meeting of the association (Detroit, May 10–11, 1929) emphasized the importance the organization itself placed on surgical care of injured employees, in contrast to the programs of today, which emphasize medical and toxicological aspects of health care.

The 1929 program listed a total of fourteen professional papers and addresses, of which four dealt with the treatment of various types of fractures, one, with statistics on accidental deaths, one, with spinal anesthesia, one, with industrial surgery of the eye, one, with lame backs, one, with the debridement of wounds, and one with the treatment of burns. None of the remaining four talks was on a specific *medical* subject.

In the 1929 issue of the *Bulletin of the American Association of Industrial Physicians & Surgeons,* Frederick A. Besley, speaking as chairman of the Committee on Industrial Medicine and Traumatic Surgery, described the program of the American College of Surgeons to improve the surgical standards in industry. "Admittedly," he said, "the industrial surgeons and medical men, both as individuals and through their associations, have succeeded in bringing about many important reforms in the treatment of the sick and the injured workers."[16]

For more than ten years prior to that time the College had been working on the standardization of hospitals and had spent $750,000 in the undertaking. As a result, it was able to point to an average saving of three to five days' stay in the standardized hospitals as compared to those not standardized. Now the College hoped to raise the standard of treatment throughout industry by creating a similar procedure for the standardization of medical departments—using a system of inspection by agents of the College.

Dr. Besley referred specifically to the pioneering work of Drs. Hart E. Fisher, C. H. Watson, Loyal A. Shoudy, William O. Sherman, Andrew Harvey, and Volney S. Cheney, and stated that the College hoped to make more nearly universal the high standards established by those surgeons. Expressing the highest regard for the splendid work done by those and other individual surgeons, he declared that the College would endeavor to win the cooperation of willing and competent men who were interested in industrial surgery.

The College proposed to further its program chiefly through educational channels, with a particular effort to enlist the interest of the deans of all medical schools in arranging the surgical instruction of students in the principles of the surgery of trauma and by demanding a high standard of efficiency for men desiring to practice it. It was also proposed that educational propaganda be developed for the public, which should enable the laymen to discriminate intelligently between trained and untrained surgeons. These objectives were to be accomplished (with the help of the

College's Committee on Fractures and Other Traumas) by promoting standards of care that would ensure proper attention to adequate equipment, methods of transporting the injured, emergency rooms, X-ray facilities, trained technicians, all varieties of splints, and controlled physical therapy departments.

Citing the compensation laws involved, the College recognized that a prolonged disability was a great economic loss. It pointed out that all surveys and reports emphasized the importance of providing the best possible surgical care for the injured employee, to the end that the immediate and permanent disability be reduced to a minimum.

These activities of the ACS were responsible for the start of a program providing for certification of approved medical departments in industry and business. This program, described in detail in a later chapter, was to become a prime factor in elevating the standards of surgical care in industry. It was administered by the ACS until 1950, when, because of the increased importance of health conservation in occupational medicine and the radical reduction of injuries through safety measures, it was taken over by the American Association of Industrial Physicians & Surgeons.

Even a very brief chronology of industrial medicine in this country is sufficient to indicate the emphasis placed on surgery (from the earliest crude attempts at in-plant health care down to the present time) and the notable part played by the steel industry in its evolution.

The first so-called "plant surgeon" of record was William J. Middleton, who was appointed surgeon for the Pennyslvania Steel Company, Steelton, Pennsylvania, in 1884. He was succeeded in 1888 by J. F. Culp.

W. B. Lowman became chief surgeon for the Cambria Iron Company at Johnstown in 1886 and continued until 1904. In that year A. W. Colcord was appointed chief surgeon at the Clairton plant of the Carnegie Steel Company. At Johnstown, in that period, Cambria Steel Company opened the oldest industrial hospital, and Lackawanna Steel completed a thirty-bed hospital at Lackawanna.

The Bethlehem Steel Company established a hospital at its San Francisco shipyards in 1907. Two years later William O'Neil Sherman was appointed chief surgeon at Carnegie Steel.

It was at Bethlehem that Loyal Shoudy wrote a brilliant chapter in the history of occupational medicine. Shoudy, a Fellow of the American College of Surgeons and trained at the Lankenau Hospital in Philadelphia under Doctor Deaver, spent a short time at the Bethlehem Steel Company in 1913. He became medical director and spent the remainder of his life developing the medical service of that company. Thanks to his friendship with Eugene Grace he was able to provide the finest of facilities throughout the countrywide divisions, and as one of the leaders in the activities of the Industrial Medical Association he imparted his enthusiasm and his standards to other doctors from coast to coast.

While these activities were going on, interest in occupational medicine was spreading, slowly but steadily, beyond the scope of the mining, railroad and steel industries. We have mentioned the work of Harvey and of Legge. In 1908 Harry E. Mock (trained in surgery) came to an agreement with Julius Rosenwald, president of Sears, Roebuck & Company, to develop medical service for its employees. Mock's experiences constitute one of the amazing chapters in the evolution of occupational health in this country. Out of this effort and the extensive surgical experience that followed, he wrote the first book dealing with surgery in industry, as well as health supervision, compensation, insurance, and the medico-legal phase of industrial practice.[17]

Back in 1901, George M. Kober, professor of hygiene at Georgetown University, addressed the 52nd annual meeting of the American Medical Association, discussing industrial hygiene.[18] In 1908 he published a lengthy report of studies dealing with the health of American workmen.[19]

In 1914 W. Gilman Thompson, professor of medicine at Cornell Medical College, published the first comprehensive American book on industrial medicine,[20] and the trend away from surgery and toward emphasis on the health and occupation-connected diseases of the workman was under way.

In 1915 Dr. Hayhurst, professor of industrial hygiene at Ohio State University, reported the findings of a study of working conditions in the industries of Ohio.[21] He was later to collaborate with Kober[22] as co-editor of an exhaustive contribution by thirty-three writers in the industrial health field and conducted a course in industrial hygiene for the junior class in medicine.

At the same time Dr. W. J. Means, dean of the Medical College at Ohio State, accepted an invitation from the Jeffrys Manufacturing Company in Columbus to develop a medical department. In this work he was helped by Alfred H. Whittaker. Not only was a surgical service organized, but preplacement examinations were made, preventive medicine was introduced in the form of inoculation of all employees against contagious diseases, and safety education was stressed. John W. Means, son of W. J. Means and professor of surgery at Ohio State, continues as the Jeffrys medical director.

In Toledo, Ohio, Clarence D. Selby, also a surgeon, became health commissioner, and he and his associates, Paul and Howard Holmes, developed an industrial medical service. Selby's contributions to early awareness of the importance of highly competent surgical care are recorded elsewhere in this history. His accomplishments were later recognized by his appointment as medical director of General Motors Corporation.

By 1918, in New York City, the accident room of Roosevelt Hospital had gradually assumed responsibility for the surgery of the many industrial plants in northern Manhattan, the surgical staff alternating in this service.

Before 1920, at the New York Postgraduate Medical School and Hospital, John J. Moorhead, ably assisted by Henry Ritter, was conducting courses in the surgery of trauma. Many industrial surgeons benefited from this training, and the standards of surgical care were improved.

The same period was marked by a rapidly growing interest in industrial health on the part of large insurance organizations. In Boston the American Mutual Liability Insurance Company, under the direction of Henry Marble and with the consulting help of Frederick Cotton, developed a medical clinic in which all problem cases of the many industries insured by that company across the country were reviewed. It also held conferences in many cities from year to year to bring to surgeons in industry the newest developments in the surgery of trauma, in physical medicine, and in the problems created by changes in the workmen's compensation laws.

The Liberty Mutual Insurance, also of Boston, established rehabilitation clinics and arranged for local consultants throughout the country to aid in the more difficult problems of injured employees.

In Wausau, Winsconsin, the Employers Mutual Liability Insurance Company conducted a department of rehabilitation. By inviting surgeons who were associated with the company to Wausau, interest in the rehabilitation and reconditioning of injured employees was greatly stimulated.

Almost exactly twenty years after Mock's remarkable volume on industrial medicine appeared, a second book dealing with industrial surgery was published, written by Willis W. Lasher.[23] This, too, was a helpful contribution to the steadily improving quality of surgery as practiced in the field of trauma.

In Chicago, in 1937, the Inland Steel Company selected a young orthopaedic surgeon as medical director, Edward H. Carleton, who developed a fine medical department. Later (as president of the Industrial Medical Association and one of the most important trustees of the Occupational Health Foundation) he emphasized eduction in the field of occupational health, thus making a lasting contribution to this branch of medicine, which was by then becoming highly specialized.

Also in Chicago, Edward C. Holmblad and Frederick W. Slobe had established surgical clinics which provided competent care for the employees of many small plants and companies. In Cleveland Richard P. Bell rendered a similar service.

Detroit, with its many large industries and with management which from the time of the early expansion of the automotive industry had been interested in the health of the employee, rapidly developed medical departments with large staffs. Parts for these industries are supplied by thousands of small plants, and several clinics were established in the early 1920's which still fulfill a need and which carry on an unremitting program to influence the small plants to adopt the methods of the large industries, in safety programs, control of environmental hazards, and particularly, prompt and skilled care for industrial accidents.

An industrial city such as Detroit has been likened to a battle area. If all structures could be eliminated except the medical facilities of industry, there would remain an arrangement which resembles the forward first aid stations, the collecting stations which are the medical departments in industry, and the ambulance centers and base hospitals, which are the city's well arranged hospital centers. This set-up provides full-time personnel to render immediate emergency care and prompt transportation to the central hospital. On arrival there a specially trained surgeon is available, or an internist, if the emergency is medical in nature. All the special facilities such as radiology, shock team, and operating rooms are ready for instant use.

The efficiency with which industrial employees are cared for sets a standard which the physicians responsible for care in highway accidents and home emergencies have not been able to approach.

Early in the development of industrial medicine in Detroit, the late Dr. Thomas Mullen was active, as were Grover C. Penberthy and Glenn Carpenter. In 1922 Alfred Whittaker established a surgical clinic, which over the years has rendered a service to the smaller industries of the city, and with associated internists and specialists in other fields such as ophthalmology, dermatology and physical medicine, has provided, as far as possible, the kind of services that are available to large industries. Other clinics, such as the Detroit Industrial Clinic, of which Theodore Roth is director, also have provided service in the field of industrial trauma.

In other localities, clinics like that of the late Richard E. Newberry in the South, whose work has been carried on by Allen M. Collingsworth, and that of the late Fenn E. Poole in California have provided efficient surgical care for the industries there.

Before we pass on to the later, advanced scientific concept of the physiological and mechanical problems presented by severely injured employees, it will be helpful to consider briefly the social and economic stresses involved in the life of our age and day.

The modern complex problem[24] presented by exposure to industrial hazards is the result of an ancient evolution. Man progressed slowly by changes in biological differentiation—the physical structure of the chromosomes being zealously guarded, permitting improvement but resisting retrogression. Man has improved rapidly, however, by education and by increased stature in human dignity. Attempting to lessen his physical burden and fatigue, he has fashioned tools more and more complex in nature, which increase the danger of accidents.

Beginning with the eleventh century, and especially in the twelfth and thirteenth, the social structure changed in a manner to affect industry. Cities began to free themselves. Serfs left their native villages to go to the cities. Merchants and artisans freed themselves from their lords or bishops. "The air of cities sets you free," the peasants thought, for they legally became so after "one year and one day" if no one reclaimed them. Thus, cities increased in size. Commerce thrived, great international merchants appeared, and trade achieved such proportions that we speak of "the world economy of the Middle Ages." This commercial progress stimulated industry.

Improvement in transportation and increase in commerce resulted in increased production. The labor force grew proportionately, and larger and larger groups of workers became subject to the authority of one man. Workmen could be replaced without difficulty, so there was no incentive to develop safeguards or to improve environmental conditions. The great mass of employees led a precarious existence, subject to injuries, undesirable working conditions, economic crises and unemployment.

During the Renaissance great scientific and geographic discoveries opened new fields of conquest and added impetus to commercial development. With the concentration of capital as well as production, great cities sprang up, with subsequent crowding and exposure of workers not only to increased accident hazards due to more complicated processes but to disease resulting from lack of sanitation and light. Noise and fatigue also influenced the accident rate adversely.

Factories of a later date, in the dawn of the Machine Age, were run by steam and lighted by gas, so that they could produce by day and night. At that time the work day was sixteen hours. Entire cities became factories, with little regard for working or living conditions. Increased production was the goal, and only immediate profits counted. The deplorable state of workers in that era brought about a clamor for protective laws; and such laws appeared in England, protecting children in industry and controlling the length of the work day, as well as restricting the physical hazards in places of employment.

In Germany, a plan for compensation for industrial accidents first appeared in 1883. In France, Leon Losseau in 1897 published a 376-page volume, listing books, treatises, articles and laws dealing with the compensation of work accidents.[25] In England an Employers' Liability Bill was considered, and in 1897 the Workman's Compensation Act was passed, providing for compensation to be paid to an injured employee or to his dependents in case of death.

Although the United States was changing rapidly from an agrarian to an industrial economy, the social advances made in England and on the Continent unfortunately were ignored for many years, the safety of workers being regarded as secondary in importance to production. Keen competition resulted in wages which did not permit the employee to establish a financial reserve. In case of accident he had to sue under the common law, which required a great deal of time and expense. And although such action at times resulted in loss to the employer, he was relieved of responsibility if he could prove negligence on the part of a fellow employee.

Despite strong pressure, protective legislation was long delayed on this side of the Atlantic in comparison to other countries. Maryland, in 1902, enacted a law (of limited scope) substituting compensation for liability. New York passed the first comprehensive act in 1910, but it was declared unconstitutional, as was a Montana law of 1909. Other states and other legislation followed slowly, however, until the national work force was protected in a way to make it advantageous for employers to observe safety codes and to supply surgical care, at first very inadequate but later providing the highest skilled services available. This development had an important effect in creating the specialty of Occupational Medicine.

In spite of the preponderance of *medicine* in occupational health care, the *surgeon* is more affected by the compensation and compulsory disability laws, and it was recognized that he should be thoroughly conversant with the mass pressures at work on industrial employees, so that, as changes occurred, surgical skill could still be made available to them at its highest possible level.

While states have changed from agricultural areas to industrial communities, laws too have been adjusted to meet the problems of a growing industrial economy. Fortunately, most corporations have come to a clear awareness of their public responsibility and have developed a philosophy rooted in a sense of service to the people. Management today is acutely aware of its social obligations, apart from its obligation to make money for stockholders.

But while society was working on measures to solve the problems presented by big business, there was developing the problem of big labor. Men and women brought together in our huge industrial establishments not only organized themselves but turned to a sympathetic government for help. Their fight for recognition of those fundamental rights which they regarded as essential placed them in a position to deal with such matters on equal terms with management. Labor organizations, numbering about fifteen million members in the United States to-day, represent a force to be reckoned with when plans are being made to provide medical services. As a result of the revolution in power and influence, organized labor no longer can be designated as the under-dog in our society. Thus, the surgeon in industry is working in a labor economy.

It is important to recognize this force, which is seeking a form of protection that legislative bodies of our various states are interpreting as a request and a demand for a *disability* type of protection above that afforded by workmen's compensation laws—a type, in short, that will protect the citizen against disabilities arising outside of employment. Already, four states have such legislation, and since disability basically requires medical evaluation, another great responsibility is rapidly developing for the industrial surgeon.

It is well to remember that since the adoption of workmen's compensation laws, the estimation of disability has been within the surgeon's province. At first, a mechanical determination of degrees of limited motion in a local area of the human body was thought to be adequate—an approach unfortunately perpetuated by recent publications in this field,[26] but now the experienced surgeon learns to approach the problem of evaluation from the standpoint of the whole patient, taking into consideration not only the immediate region of the body injured, but the psychological, economic and social factors that influence recovery.

The use here of two terms should be understood, because of frequent confusion. Webster defines "evaluation" as "accurate appraisal of value" and "rating" as "classification according to a standard; grade; rank." To the administrator in the

156

field of workmen's compensation, "evaluation" usually means: how much money the commission is going to pay, while "rating" generally means the percentage of anatomical and functional use.

Since today's surgeon is functioning in an era of social security,[27] in which some states already have compulsory disability laws and in which all states have workmen's compensation laws, every unemployed person claiming disability presents a potential problem to the medical profession. A large percentage of the people of this country are insured under voluntary plans of hospital and medical care, and this care is granted only upon a doctor's certificate of temporary or permanent disability.

Pre-employment and periodic examinations (now a requirement of many industries), placement studies, pension plans, advancement by seniority, forced retirement, early requests for retirement, and requests for employment beyond the retirement age—all shift a great responsibility to the physician. These are evaluations in addition to those required by life insurance applicants, candidates for military service induction, and Veterans Administration claims.

In appraising its accomplishments, on its tenth anniversary, the United Nations pointed out the emphasis being placed on human rights. These rights are inseparably linked with the health and physical condition of the people of fifty-eight nations, and only the doctor can interpret the disability involved.

Medical officers in the overseas forces must pass upon the physical condition of applicants for marriage, and under a ruling of the commissioner of baseball, no ball player can be placed on the inactive list without a doctor's certificate. In the courtroom doctors play an important part in judicial proceedings, the extent of damages awarded depending, in many cases, directly upon medical testimony, which is a disability evaluation.

Unfortunately, disability evaluation is not an exact science resting on exact rules inevitably resulting in the same conclusion irrespective of the person operating the formula. As Chester C. Schneider has pointed out, the conclusions vary with the evidence and concomitant significance, the experience of the physician, and the condition and reaction of the patient.[28] Appraisal of injuries, including the disability potential, is a complicated and important subject. It requires extensive knowledge of all diagnostic procedures, in order to evaluate the nature of the injury and the probable consequences in terms of healing and degenerative changes.

It has been remarked that a speedy evaluation of injury insures elimination of uncertainty on the part of the patient, a more rapid recovery, and an earlier return to work. It is axiomatic that the earlier the injury is competently handled, the better the chance of orienting the patient for future capacity. It is difficult to understand the surgical neglect of injured employees by physicians at the beginning of our century, as there were available excellent reference books and reports from the medical centers of the world—dating back to the work of Ambroise Paré[29] in the 1500's.

To the list of master teachers already mentioned, we should add the contributions of less well known surgeons in a much later period. Examples would include the careful comparisons of methods of amputation by Teale[30] in 1858; and in 1893, the Carpenter Lectureship address on "Surgery of the Hand" before the New York Academy of Medicine by Robert Abbee. Reprints of this were widely circulated. The problem of hand surgery, important then, proved to be of such interest that during the two world wars special teams were selected and special centers designated (such as the Valley Forge Military Hospital) for clinical demonstrations. Later, a hand trauma society was organized, and stories appeared in the lay press emphasizing the value of the human hand.[31]

In 1868 Edwin Morris published a book on shock "with special reference to shock caused by railway accidents,"[32] which was followed in 1890 by a book titled *Railway Surgery* by C. B. Stemen.[33] A year later, Herbert W. Page presented a book discussing railway injuries of the back and nervous system, in their medico-legal and clinical aspects.[34] In 1898 came a paper by Eskridge, also dealing with railroad surgery.[35]

Over the same period of roughly fifty years, fractures likewise received a great deal of attention from American surgeons, who added substantially to the literature of the surgery of trauma. When, in 1917, Royal Whitman developed the treatment of fractures of the hip,[36] he was carrying on the work of Sayre,[37] who established and occupied the first chair of bone and joint surgery in America at Bellevue Medical College in 1861.

As early as 1896 Helferich, professor at the University of Greifswald, presented an *Atlas of Traumatic Fractures and Luxations*,[38] well illustrated, with many of the reproductions in color, which was available to the surgeon in industry.

The year 1900 was particularly productive of literature on this subject. It was then that Estes wrote his book, stating in the preface that he would "discuss the treatment of fractures and only consider the supposed mechanics."[39] Bigelow's work on fractures of the hip appeared in the same year, as did the first edition of Scudder's[40] text book. Scudder was assisted by Frederick J. Cotton, who in 1910 developed his own text book.[41] Both of these surgeons, by their enthusiasm and frequent visits and talks to surgeons in industry, made important contributions to the surgical treatment of accidents.

During the first seventeen years of this century there were developments in surgery which set the stage for the rapid advances which were to come with World War II. In general, the larger medical centers were making the greater contributions to the surgery of trauma, but by the time of the first World War clinics were being formed to provide surgical service to small industries, clinics such as that of Meyer Wolf on the lower East Side of New York City and the hospital of the Michigan Mutual Liability Company in Detroit, where H. N. Torrey was chief surgeon, assisted by Pemberthy and A. H. Whittaker shortly after the war.

By 1918, interest had reached a new peak. In the early stages of the war the mortality had been high, especially in open fractures. In 1914 injuries involving the femur had resulted in a mortality of 80 percent. But the rate dropped to 15 percent, as the result of four developments: the Thomas splint, which provided traction to immobilize the fractures[42]; the administration of morphine at the time of first aid; heated ambulances; small teams formed of young surgeons specially trained in the surgery of trauma and highly mobile in action, who could be made promptly available at the point of most urgent need.

Naturally, injuries occurring in industry varied from those of the battlefield because of differences in environment, such as freedom from the bacterial content of field manure and the fatigue and filth of trench warfare. Yet many industrial injuries equaled in severity those of warfare, and with modifications the industrial surgeon quickly applied the knowledge gained by war experience.

It had been demonstrated in 1875 that infusion of physiologic saline solution was beneficial in combating shock, and on November 14, 1914, the first transfusion of human citrated blood was administered. The blood being incoagulable during transfusion, the procedure was simple, safe and practical.

Lives were being saved by untiring and brilliant surgery, but too many patients had to live what must have seemed to them endless periods of treatment until their wounds were soundly healed. With the occurrence of a great number of severely injured men in a war which for the first time used missiles of high velocity and great explosive force and of injuries in war industries which created serious trauma due to the handling of materials under need for speed, it became apparent that the carefully developed aseptic surgical ritual that had brought rich reward in all branches of surgery was inadequate. The annoying discovery was made that a perfect antiseptic did not exist. The problem was taken to the bacteriologists. One of them, the famous Sir Almroth Wright, stated that he never expected anything too much of antiseptics and pointed out that surgeons must place less reliance on the antibacterial powers of antiseptics when applied to wounds. He suggested that the surgeon regard the wound as a natural experiment. The physiological processes of its walls must be studied and so far as possible be better understood; its exudates and natural processes of repair must be encouraged.[43]

The surgeons of the period felt that chemical solutions would kill or inhibit the growth of microbes, but it became apparent that while the solutions would sterilize instruments they would not sterilize wounds. Lister had eradicated the septic infections which had devastated the wards of hospitals, but his was a prophylactic method. We know now that, although contaminating organisms may be killed and new ones prevented from entering, infecting bacteria cannot be reached by external application. Once infection has occurred, once an active invasion of the tissues has commenced, antiseptics are of little value.

Experiments during 1914–1917 showed that wound discharges and tissue fluids reduced the powers of antiseptics, and it was learned that drugs like lysol, creosote and guaiacol would have to be administered in lethal doses before they would come into operation in the blood, and it was recognized that the only really potent antibacterial agent was one which would circulate in the blood. In spite of this knowledge the techniques in that period called for the constant application of chemicals which were thought able to destroy the organisms without injuring the tissues, such as hypochlorite solutions and the flavine compounds, the Carrell-Dakin treatment so brilliantly carried out by Alexis Carrell[44] at his hospital at Compiègne, and the B.I.P.P. of Rutherford Morison.

Also used were techniques based on the insertion of gauze saturated with a 5 percent solution of salt or continuous introduction of salt solution, the object of the hypertonic salt solution being to promote the normal transudation of tissue fluids.

Toward the end of World War I, however, the major conclusion reached was that the right and only way of treating wounds was by very early excision, by the immediate elimination of contaminants before contamination could turn into infection, and by the so-called delayed primary suture of wounds.[45]

The time requirement was met, as mentioned, by making available highly trained surgeons, who were moved to areas near the scenes of battle, that is, at the advanced casualty clearing stations. The easy availability of highly trained men is now an integral part of the care of industrial trauma. Recognition of the importance of specialized nursing also was helpful, and since that war the major centers of acute trauma have been placed in charge of accident ward nurses specially trained in the care of injuries.

At the close of the war, Doctor Alexander Fleming (1919) said: "All the great successes of primary wound treatment have been due to efficient surgery, and it seems a pity that the surgeon should wish to share his glory with a chemical antiseptic of more than doubtful utility."[46]

Complications developed, however, as a result of wounds being left open. Yet the danger of infection was so great that they could not be tightly closed, and it was realized that a closed wound could be contaminated even if a small tube or sliver of rubber was introduced for drainage.

Then came the sulfa drugs, and through their use improvement in wound care. In 1935, Gerhardt Domagk recommended prontosil in the treatment of streptococcal infections.[47] Numerous other clinical reports shortly made it obvious that a new form of chemotherapy with surprising effectiveness against bacterial infections had been discovered. Sulphanilamide had been first prepared by Gelmo in 1908.[48] Its first trial with certain results was made by Kinser in 1936. The next great advance was the introduction of sulphapyridine, synthesized by Evans and Phillips in 1937. Then the method of controlling treatment by estimation of the level of the drug in the blood and the use of sulfathiozole soon followed.

Years before (in 1922) Fleming, in the small, old-fashioned laboratory of St. Mary's Hospital at the University of London, where he was hospital pathologist, had found that human tears and saliva contained a peculiar substance capable of destroying germs. Fleming's report attracted the attention of Jules Bordet, director of the Pasteur Institute in Brussels. André Gratia and Sara Dath, while working on pus-producing *staphylococcus aureus,* found that some plates filled with agar culture media became contaminated with molds. One day they observed a whitish mold around which germs had been killed. This was reported to Bordet. They then identified a mold-contaminated ampoule of vaccine as a mold of the penicillin family which had the same power. Four years later, Fleming observed the same phenomenon. He preserved the culture, and from it are descended most of the cultures used today in the production of penicillin in the United States.

The importance of penicillin was first discovered and described in September, 1928. Howard W. Florey, professor of pathology in the Sir William Dunn School of Pathology at Oxford and formerly a Rockefeller Fellow, foresaw the possibilities of penicillin and decided to recultivate the mold discovered by Fleming. Assisted by a group of twenty scientists, pathologists, biochemists, bacteriologists and physicians, working together as a perfect team, in a little over a year he laid the foundation for penicillin therapy, established the potentialities of the drug, and pointed out its limitations.

Years later the Oxford doctors were still working on penicillin, while only fifty-five miles away from their laboratory and clinics, war was making a hell of once-peaceful London. Florey and his assistant, Dr. Heatley, accepted an invitation from the Rockefeller Foundation to come to the United States to continue their research. Late in June, 1941, penicillin was enthusiastically received by American scientists. Clinical investigation was begun on a large scale, and manufacture carried out in the American way—the way of mass production—with two dozen large pharmaceutical companies starting manufacture at the same time.[49]

Penicillin immediately proved its value to the military in treating diseases and injuries. And its benefits were promptly implemented in industry by the industrial surgeons, who were putting forth every effort to maintain America's working force to further the war effort.

Standards of surgical care throughout the country were greatly improved during that entire period of discovery and research, particularly in the field of industrial surgery. Fine industrial surgeons, serving on the American College of Surgeons Committee on Fractures and Other Traumas, played an active part in its proceedings. The American Association of the Surgery of Trauma, formed in 1942, took over an important role in establishing the prestige of this specialized type of surgery. And, over the years, authoritative programs presented by the Industrial Medical Association have been a major factor in bringing the rapid advances in surgical knowledge directly to the surgeon in industry.

The broad movement to upgrade industrial surgical standards attained world significance in 1947 with the appointment, by the International College of Surgeons, of a committee now known as the Committee on the Surgery of Trauma.

XV

THE EVOLUTION OF SHOCK CONTROL
IN INDUSTRY

As industrialization in America proceeded at a faster and faster pace during and after World War I, trauma became as important on the home front as it had been on the battlefield. A major portion of the literature dealing with surgery was already devoted to consideration of the specific physical changes resulting from disease or trauma. Gradually, there developed an appreciation of the importance of physiological changes, and, with it, a realization that to secure the best end results, or to assure recovery, attention must be focused on the response of an injured employee to the stresses involved. And since this response or lack of response is based upon the degree of shock produced by the trauma, there followed an upsurge of both medical and surgical research into the nature, the effects, and the treatment of shock.

It goes without saying that the literature on this subject is immense. It is also growing rapidly. Volumes are required for thorough discussion of any of the many phases of traumatic shock; and obviously all of its clinical and pathological aspects cannot be covered here. We can, however, profitably mention a few important milestones marking the progress, and list reference works that may be of interest and value to readers.

In 1940, Blalock classified shock, in terms of origin and characteristics, as follows: hematogenic (characterized by a reduction in blood volume), neurogenic (reduction in blood pressure but not in volume), vasogenic (including histamine shock), and cardiogenic (reduction in blood pressure due to cardiac failure).[1]

162

A later classification, based on a descriptive terminology which relates circulatory failure to the clinical condition, has come into wide use. It recognizes these seven types of shock: traumatic, hemorrhagic, burn, obstetric, medical, anesthetic, and operative.

If we go from the multiplicity of causes of shock to the behavior of the organism itself, we find that certain patterns of response to stress constantly recur.[2] To understand this fact we must turn to a basic concept in biology first introduced by Claude Bernard in his book, *Experimental Medicine:* All vital mechanisms, however varied they may be, have only one object, that of preserving constant conditions of life in the internal environment. The importance of this concept lies in the fact that it provides the foundation for our understanding of the response of living organisms to various types of stress, for it is logical to assume that since the character of the internal environment is relatively constant, the pattern of response to stress must also be uniform. Cannon in 1923 extended Bernard's work by analyzing the mechanism by which the body maintains the constancy of the internal environment, or fluid matrix. He pointed out that this state of equilibrium was preserved by the integrated cooperative function of many organs, including the nervous system, heart, lungs, kidneys, spleen and liver.[3]

If we analyze such forms of stress as trauma and hemorrhage, it becomes apparent that when they are mild they will cause little or no disturbance of the internal environment, but when sufficiently severe they will cause injury to the organism. This damage may extend to the point of impairment of cellular nutrition, particularly in relation to oxygen, and the final result of all forms of stress, if severe enough, will be anoxia of varying degree. This concept, known as the triphasic response to stress, recognizes three phases in the reaction to such disturbances: the phase of anoxic injury to the cells, the catabolic phase, during which there is a breakdown of the cells of the organism, the anabolic phase, during which the reparative processes are active.

The anoxic phase extends from the time of the injury for a variable period, usually not exceeding twenty-four to seventy-two hours, during which there is a decreased supply of oxygen to the tissues. This is associated with a diminished flow of oxygen through the tissues, a fall in blood pressure, a decrease in the oxygen consumption rate, a fall in body temperature, and decreased function in various organs, particularly the kidneys, liver and central nervous system, the brain being most affected. Histologic studies demonstrate, for example, that the earliest necrotic changes in the liver occur some twenty-four hours after injury, the necrosis being due to hepatic anoxia.

The catabolic phase begins *during* the anoxic phase, and may last as long as two to five weeks. It is characterized by a breakdown of body constituents, shown by a rise in creatine and urea nitrogen levels in the blood. There is a rise, of variable degree, in the blood potassium level. The urine shows an increased nitrogen output, and the post-shock metabolic response may show a loss of body nitrogen of over

220 grams. Frequently there is hemolysis and even hemoglobenuria. Fever develops, there is a loss of fluids from the tissues, and there may be an increased volume of vitamin C in the urine.

The anabolic phase begins after the catabolic phase has started, and not infrequently before completion of the anoxic phase. It may last as long as ten weeks. During this phase regeneration of tissues takes place, the plasma proteins are restored, and there is formation of new red blood cells. Visceral function, particularly that of the kidneys and liver, is restored, as are the water and electrolyte balance and the blood volume. A positive nitrogen balance also replaces the negative balance.

The symptom complex we call "shock" may have many origins leading to a fundamental circulatory failure characterized by a disparity between the circulating blood volume and the capacity of the vascular bed.[4] While it was formerly thought that vaso-constriction in the early stages of shock tended to compensate for decrease in blood volume and cardiac output, it was found that total peripheral resistance was increased only moderately in early shock and was never maximal.[5] It was probable that generalized arteriolar vaso-constriction had only a negligible effect in sustaining arterial pressure and that the constriction was a net *unfavorable* influence because it decreased blood flow to vital organs.

Other studies[6] of the vascular reactions of exteriorized omentum during hemorrhagic hypotension demonstrated that the capillary bed was not a passive structure, but contained structural units which are pre-capillary sphincters having contractile properties. Observation of the behavior of these structural units revealed two phases of the development of shock: an initial *compensatory* phase characterized by the shunting of blood away from the capillary bed back into the venous system by the pre-capillary sphincters and a *decompensatory* phase characterized by progressive hyporeactivity of the terminal vascular bed, with pooling of blood in the capillaries. This latter stage is identified with irreversible shock.

These same studies develop a new concept of hemodynamic mechanisms involved in shock, based upon the demonstration of specific humoral principles which control the reactivity of the terminal vascular bed. It was found that in the initial compensatory stages of shock reaction there appears in the blood stream a vasoexcitatory material (VEM), while during the decompensatory stage the blood contains a vasodepressor material (VDM). The production of these substances is related to hypoxia of specific tissues, VEM being released by the kidneys and VDM chiefly by the liver but also by the spleen and skeletal muscles. VEM is thought to be largely responsible for the action of the pre-capillary sphincters during the compensatory stage. The liver has the ability to inactivate VDM accumulation in the blood stream, but the loss of this ability through liver damage is responsible for the phenomena associated with the hyporeactive stage and ultimately with irreversibility.

In his investigations of the effect of bacterial infections in the development and aggravation of shock, Fine also works on the premise that traumatic shock is a state of acute and persistent deficiency of blood flow through the peripheral circulation, which, if sufficiently severe and untreated, grows progressively worse and is rapidly fatal.[7]

The complete syndrome of circulatory disturbances in shock reveals a chain of reactions that are not only very extensive but of the utmost importance. All of these clinical data deserve minute study. The findings cannot be detailed here, but they are available in the reference literature cited. Briefly described, stagnation in the peripheral circulation reduces the rate of return flow from the veins to the heart, with a consequent decrease in the cardiac output per minute and a decrease in oxygen consumption and in the basal metabolic rate.

The most common cause of the disorder is a critical loss of blood volume (35 percent or more) whether from external or internal hemorrhage, soft tissue trauma, burns, etc. Thus, replacement of *volume* deficit is a primary requirement in most cases, and if this requirement is met by volume therapy without loss of time, a normal circulation is promptly restored. This replacement should be supplied in less than fourteen hours. If the anoxia is allowed to persist, whole blood given by transfusion ceases to provide any correction, and the shock continues to an irreversible stage. In septic shock, irreversibility to transfusion is present from the onset, whereas irreversibility to transfusion does not develop for many hours in hemorrhagic shock.

Shorr and his co-workers with the liver extracts in hemorrhagic shock found that the amount of VDM appears to be a function of *time,* that is, the degree and duration of hypoxia.[8] While these investigators believe that the vasodepressor action of extracts is derived from a change in the structure of normal liver protein, it is possible that minute quantities of compounds, derived not from liver proteins but from normally resident bacteria which become activated by prolonged hypoxia, are responsible for this action.

In the experimental work it was demonstrated that there are many bacterial toxins capable of producing shock which will not yield to fluid volume therapy. Since prolonged hemorrhagic shock can invite the added burden of shock due to bacterial action, it may be that the same thing can happen in severe and prolonged shock produced by any agent. Therefore, in the treatment of peripheral vascular collapse which persists in spite of restored fluid balance, one should consider employing whatever therapy might possibly contribute to the elimination of bacterial action. This experimental work also suggests that the prophylactic administration of an adequate dose of antibiotic is far more effective than the administration of an equal dose after shock has developed.

Since the bacteria that are resident in the liver tissue may become activated by a decrease in oxygen, the bacteria resident in the intestinal tract may also be at fault. There is some evidence that the use of aureomycin by mouth may be helpful in combating the bacterial invasion, and other measures to combat the flare-up of infection are indicated.

It should be added that of all the organs which suffer during shock, the one likely to be of the most clinical concern is the kidney. In this organ there is often a more severe deficit with respect to blood flow than in the total body economy, resulting in profound changes in this organ. The most important changes are those which have been described by France as lower nephron nephrosis.[9]

It can be seen from the preceding discussion that the treatment of acutely injured persons is closely interwoven with the problem of shock. The treatment to be carried out depends upon an interpretation of the phase of deterioration or improvement which the patient presents at the time of first examination, and the treatment necessarily must be given according to the changing picture of his condition.

There are many cases in which surgical intervention is necessary immediately. Such cases as rapid hemorrhage occurring from a rupture of the spleen or liver, cardiac tamponade, rapid bleeding from the gastro-intestinal tract, a sucking wound from a chest injury, or rapidly developing intra-cranial hemorrhage, may require attention before a full program of overcoming shock is possible. If the patient's condition permits, immediate debridement of devitalized and contaminated tissue is advisable, and in burn cases the lesion should be excised and the defect covered with skin grafts on the day of injury.

Since the great majority of cases of shock as seen in surgical patients are the result of hemorrhage, burns, trauma or dehydration, and are characterized by reduction of blood volume, the first procedure to be carried out is replacement by whole blood. There are, however, occasional cases in which cross-matching and other laboratory procedures are too time consuming, and plasma, which does not require the pre-administration studies, should be available for immediate use. There are also cases in which the severely injured patient presents so much interference with circulatory function that the circulation is unable to carry added blood to the areas in which it is oxygenated for distribution through the body. In these cases intra-arterial transfusion may be helpful in averting disaster.

Particularly in severely burned patients, replacement of fluid and electrolytic loss may be essential, and severe dehydration may occur in injuries which have resulted in intestinal obstruction, ileus or fistula. In severely injured patients, the replacement of choice is whole blood. As just mentioned, where immediate treatment is required the use of plasma is indicated, but it should be remembered that though the danger of hepatitis has been largely overcome, plasma likewise is not inexhaustible; especially in major disasters where large amounts of intravenous fluids are required, plasma expanders should be available.

In spite of the increased number of plasma substitutes that have been developed, their use should be restricted to the treatment of nonhemorrhagic shock and then only while waiting for sufficient blood to be provided. A suitable plasma substitute should be non-viscous, stable, sterilizable, non-antigenic, non-toxic, and have a colloid osmotic pressure similar to plasma. There are several such substitutes which appear to have some value, among them gelatin manufactured from hydrolyzed

166

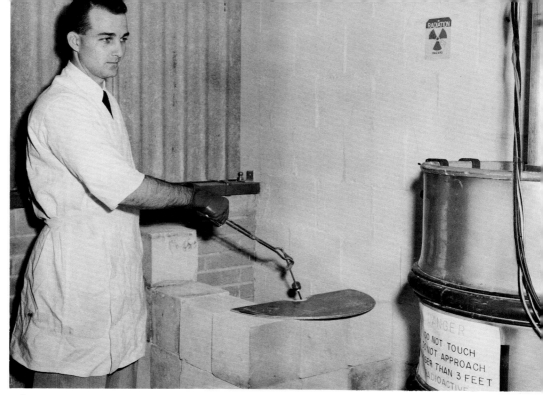

46. *The Handling of Radioactive Materials*. Since radioactive materials have become a health hazard in certain types of industry, rigid precautions are taken in many plants to prevent dangerous exposure of workers to the rays.

47. *Conference on Radiographs*. Swift advances in the science of radiology have greatly broadened the usefulness of X-ray in diagnosis and cure—and radiographs often call for close study at medical department conferences in industry.

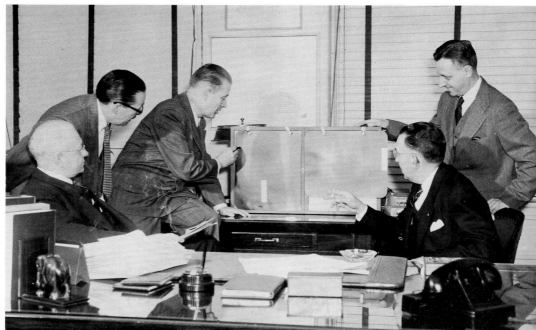

PROGRAM

University of Detroit Band

Rev. Fr. John McNichols, Presiding
Pres. University of Detroit

Mercantile Health
Dr. Arthur B. Emmons
Director, Study of Industrial Hygiene,
Howard College, Boston

Industrial Medicine and Surgery
Dr. Ralph W. Elliot, Cleveland, Ohio

Industrial Hygiene from the Standpoint
of the employer
Dr. W. Louis Hartman, Chief Surgeon,
Michigan Central Railroad

Hudson Quartette

Play—"Suppressed Desires"
Dramatic Club, U. of D.

University of Detroit Band

Owners, Managers, Employees, Foremen, Welfare, Fir
Aid Men, Surgeons, Officials of all Insurance Compani
associated with the Medical and Compensation work
the Workmen's Compensation Act of Michigan, are i
vited to attend the

Program of Industrial Hygiene at the Michigan Health Exposition on Monday Evening, June 11th, at 8 o'clock, Auditorium General Motors Building. *1923.*

It is hoped that all employers and employees in Detr
will make an effort to hear these interesting speakers
that the production and earning power, health and saf
ty of all industrial and retail employees will be improve

Respectfully,

Alfred H. Whittaker, M.
Chairman Committee of Industrial Surge

Sponsored by the Michigan Association of Industrial Physicians and Surgeons.

48. *Invitation to Michigan Health Exposition, 1923.* Factory bulletin boards carried this come-one-come-all invitation to the exposition for discussion of the then little-understood Workmen's Compensation Act of Michigan.

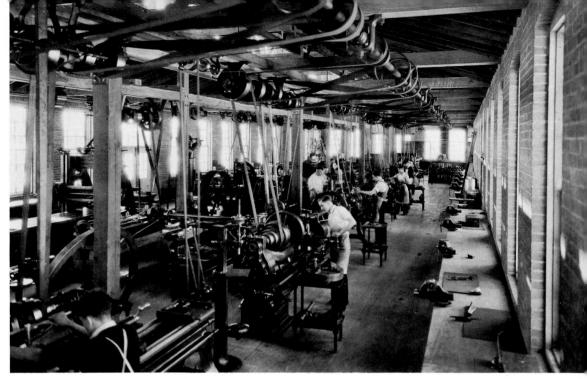

49. *Pre-electric Power Belts and Shafts.* Gone are the belts and shafts that once made jungles of our factories. The Ford Museum restoration of the Armington-Sims Machine Shop, Providence, R.I., as it was in the late 1870's.

—Courtesy of The Henry Ford Museum, Dearborn, Michigan

50. *American Production Automation of the Twentieth Century.* An electrolytic tinning line at Jones & Laughlin Aliquippa Works. Nearly 500 feet long, it is able to apply different coating weights on each side of a steel strip.

—Courtesy of the Jones & Laughlin Steel Corporation

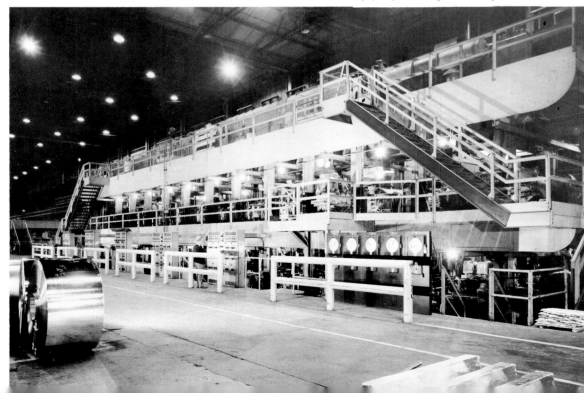

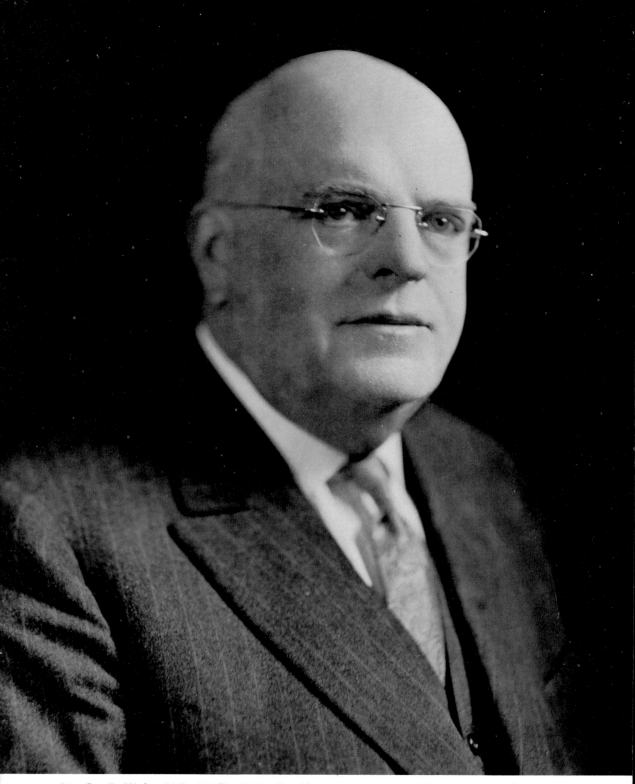

51. *Guy L. Kiefer, M.D. (1867–1930). President, AAIP&S, 1928–1929.* In his acceptance speech Kiefer said: "I know of no group of men . . . to whom you can go and talk over problems of industrial medicine as we can in this particular group." Kiefer had a brilliant career as health commissioner of Detroit (1901–1913); as a member, State Board of Health (1916–1920) and president, State Advisory Council of Health; as medical director of Michigan Bell Telephone (1921–1927); and as health director of Michigan (1927). He gave the AAIP&S a "medical administration" notable for sound research and a significant literary output.

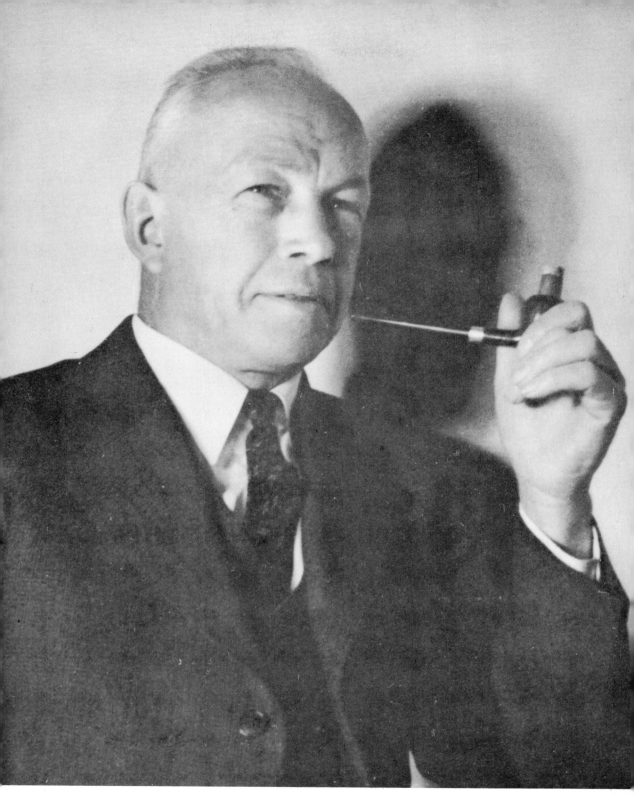

52. *C. F. N. Schram, M.D. (1884–1945). President, AAIP&S, 1928–1929.* On the eve of a great depression, with membership declining and finances in a precarious state, the association in 1928 looked about for strong leadership. C. F. N. Schram met the need. He blasted the belief that any M.D. was qualified to run a medical depart-ment, and urged doctors to "learn the business they serve." He was chief surgeon of Fairbanks, Morse & Company, 1917–1934, and then joined the Tennessee Eastman Corporation as medical director. In 1940 the *Saturday Evening Post* published his "Unmined Gold," one of the earliest articles on industrial medicine written for a mass audience.

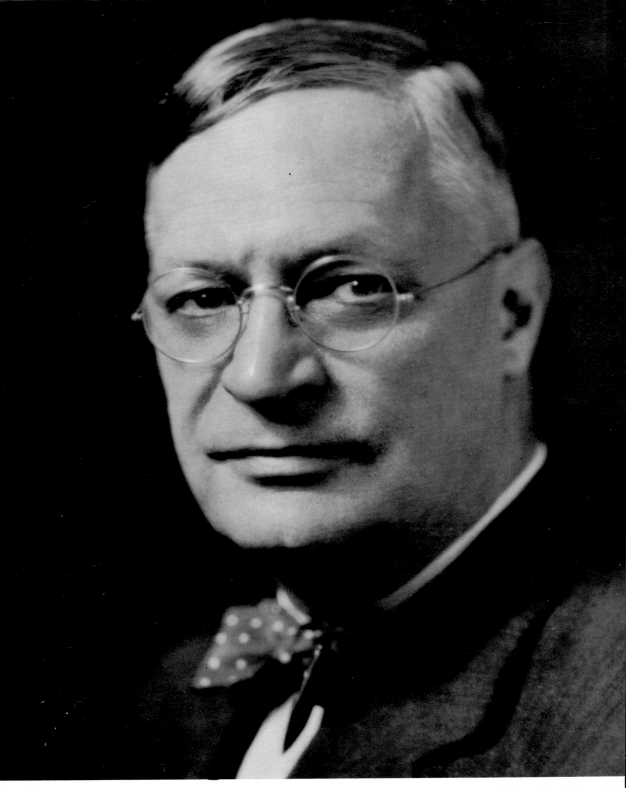

53. *Cassius H. Watson, M.D.* (1878–   ). *President, AAIP&S, 1930–1931.* For thirty years Dr. Watson served the New York Telephone Company and American Telephone & Telegraph. On his retirement in 1943 to direct the Vanderbilt Clinic of Presbyterian Hospital, New York, the AAIP&S Board wished him well in these words: "We all know you will do a fine job, and will enjoy the thrill that comes with accomplishment in a new undertaking." During his long active career Watson won distinction for development of diagnostic work in industrial medicine and surgery. To the association he gave a businesslike administration on a high professional level.

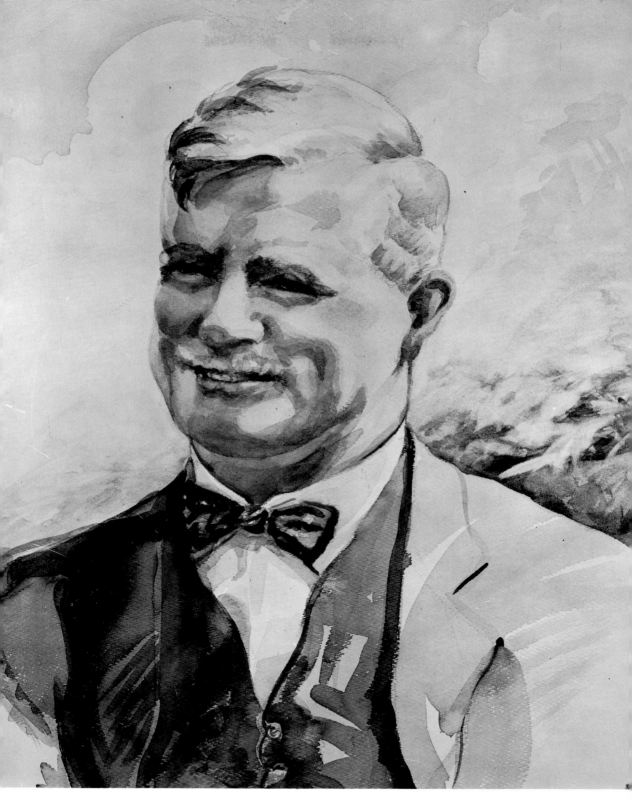

54. *Donald B. Lowe, M.D. (1883–1946). President, AAIP&S, 1931–1934.* When the association elected Lowe president in June, 1931, none could know that this was to be the last annual meeting for three years and that because of the economic situation Lowe's term was to extend, by executive order, until the spring of 1934. His was the diffi-cult task of transacting organization business—maintaining services and standards—without even adequate means of communication with the membership as a whole. At that time, he was at the height of his career with the B. F. Goodrich Company, manifesting the talents that led Dr. Legge to describe him as "a real humanitarian."

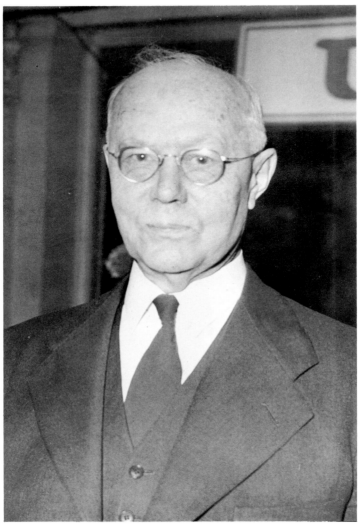

55. *Volney S. Cheney, M.D.* Secretary and treasurer of the AAIP&S from the late 1920's into the 1940's; helped shape editorial and publication policies in that period. At 76, retired, he found a new career in medicine.

bone, which was recommended for use by the committee for blood and blood substitutes during World War II. The material from which it is made is not, however, inexhaustible. Certainly a large supply of blood substitutes should be on hand, perhaps held by Civil Defense authorities to be available for distribution where required, if a large-scale disaster should occur.

The treatment of severely injured patients can be carried out efficiently only if the nature of the reaction of the human organism to the trauma can be carefully evaluated by clinical and laboratory studies and the requirements of treatment determined. Upon such definitive data depends the decision whether to institute immediate treatment or to delay it until after recovery from shock.

The speed with which circulatory adjustments take place under shock conditions and their far-reaching effects on vital organs, emphasize the great importance of immediate or emergency treatment in severe cases, to prevent rapid deterioration of the organism involved. Also important in preventing further damage are the method of transportation of the patient and prompt care on admission to hospital.

Evans has reported that in civilian injuries there is a direct correlation between the degree of shock and the reduction in blood volume as measured by the T. 1824 dye method.[10] Signs of shock do not appear until the blood loss is 15 percent. The average loss in severe shock he found was 38 percent.

To meet such needs whole blood, of course, is available in most communities, as are various intravenous solutions with special reparative properties, all of which have a useful place in various stages of treatment. Antibiotics, also available in a wide range, should be administered early; and where tetanus or gas infection is a factor, immunizing or protective injections should be used.

Important in shock, however, is the fact that reparative processes vary in individuals. Under stress some patients are more prone to failure of the circulation. These may be termed "circulatory weaklings," who should always be looked for. It is interesting to note that circulatory weakness may be corrected by training in some people; athletes participating in body contact games, for example, may be conditioned to meet great stress.

Shock cases should be analyzed on admission to determine whether the surgeon is dealing with a circulatory cripple, which the physical examination will reveal. In fact, a survey to locate all evidence of trauma should be made, since the stresses may be multiple in nature. The examination will provide a blood sample for cross-matching, a determination of the blood sugar level, the blood urea nitrogen, blood volume and general cellular morphology, as well as the Kline reaction.

Obviously, where immediate surgical intervention is necessary it should be carried out rapidly by a specially trained team, with importance placed upon the anesthesia involved, the laboratory workers to provide the studies that are so essential, and provision for constant expert nursing. If immediate surgical intervention is not indicated, the patient should be placed in an oxygen tent and a procedure

167

outlined to have various symptoms and signs observed and recorded to permit of treatment designed to fit the needs of the severely injured patient and, at the proper time, the repair of tissue damage caused by the injury.

Just as complex toxicological problems constantly confront the physician in industry, so the physiological aspects of trauma challenge the industrial surgeon in mid-twentieth century practice. Because the pattern of trauma cases aptly illustrates the complexity of the problems facing the surgeon in industry, we are justified in discussing in some detail the nature and effects of occupational traumatic injury.

The parallel between the treatment of war-produced trauma and the care of employees injured in industry has already been noted. It has been said that the greatest similarity of non-military wounds to military wounds is found in those types of injury occurring on the mass production line which starts in Detroit and runs across the nation.[11] Severe injuries encountered on the assembly line and in the operations of suppliers—injuries to young people who have the responsibility of families to support and community obligations to fulfill—led the surgeon in industry to his goal of "a return to gainful employment at the highest attainable skill"—and at the earliest possible moment.

Crile in 1913 pointed out the serious effects of trauma upon the human organism and advocated the blocking off of the traumatized area by local anesthetic to prevent the transmission of the harmful impulses to the central nervous system.[12] We now know that these reflexes produce acute biochemical, endocrine and metabolic changes which prevent a dynamic convalescence.[13]

In military combat the "tuning up" of environmental and psychological factors that might stimulate bodily changes occurs for many hours. If it exists at all in industrial accidents it is only of momentary duration.

Conduction of nerve impulses proximally from the injury, their sorting out in the brain, the stimulus of pituitary output of ACTH and the increase of adrenal steroid production, all take place so rapidly that no matter how soon we reach the patient these changes will have already occurred. Alterations in the function of the adrenal medulla, as indicated by tachycardia and vaso-constriction, may take place very early. There is an alteration of renal excretion of water and salt, probably traceable to the posterior pituitary and the adrenal.

With free-blood 17-hydroxycorticoids at four to six times their normal level, adrenal medullary activity intense, maximal sodium resorption from the renal tubular fluid and strong conservation of body water, the injured employee is lying on the floor or ground—conscious, frightened, in pain, perhaps bleeding—awaiting his first help. Where there is efficient planning, this help is prompt. The patient is transported to the plant medical department, and if the injury is severe, he is immediately given temporary wound care and medication for pain. Splints are applied and clothing is adjusted. All bleeding is controlled and, accompanied by a trained attendant, he is taken by ambulance to a hospital where required emergency care is given, to be followed by the definitive treatment when his condition permits.

We now know that hormones are not the only chemical messengers which alter the metabolism of the body after injury. Although, in recent years, there has been a good deal of study of the endocrine changes after trauma, they have been overshadowed in importance by the tissue factors that arise from the injury and affect the organism as a whole. These tissue factors are the product of the anatomic injury itself and occur quite independently of any endocrine changes. Moore has called them the "wound cycle."[14] Briefly, the specific systemic results of such local tissue injury are as follows:

Injury to the central nervous system—alteration in its function, resulting from direct trauma to the brain and spinal cord, with respiratory paralysis and deficient ventilation or inability to achieve vaso-constriction.

Ventilatory inadequacy—often due to anoxia and respiratory acidosis from injury to the air way. Wounds of the face, neck, nose, throat, thorax or diaphragm are fatal primarily because of this inadequacy. Experience in trauma has emphasized the importance of prompt intubation, tracheotomy, thoracentesis or traction on the chest wall.

Prolonged deficiency of blood flow due to hemorrhage or shock—resulting in loss of effective blood volume and lack of blood to vital organs.

Cross-sectional tissue disruption—necrosis or crushing of tissue which releases intra-cellular substances into the extra-cellular fluid, resulting in metabolic acidosis.

Contamination leading to infection—often a deciding factor. This results from a break in the ectoderm or the entoderm, permitting bacteria to enter sterile tissues which may be deficient in blood supply as a result of the trauma. Perforation of the esophagus, stomach, intestine, liver, bile ducts, pancreas, bladder or ureters may produce breaks in the internal mucosal barrier.

Absence of nutritional intake—or lack of assimilation of any taken early in a severe injury. Care should be used not to be overzealous in correcting this deficiency; surgeons of trauma have learned that starvation does not occur early, though it can become important after 72 hours.

It has been customary, in clean surgical wounds, to expect that endocrine alterations due to the surgical insult will subside quickly. By contrast, in the severe trauma described above, the systemic changes persist as does the disordered biochemistry of the wound, maintaining endocrine activity at a high rate and continuing to threaten the injured by deficient neurological function, blood flow and oxygenation, or by development of acidosis or sepsis.

The object of modern emergency care at the plant level is to initiate battle with these factors. Attention is given first to recognition of hemorrhage and respiratory obstruction, then to the temporary immobilization of fractures, prompt transportation, carefully controlled to minimize the severity of the continuing injury, and the management of pain and fear.

Here, the person giving first aid can be of great help by assuring the injured that he is under the care of a fine surgeon, that he will be in a hospital specially equipped and organized to provide the best of care, and that there is no need for financial worries, thanks to arrangements made by his employer.

However, the first aid room in a small factory may be an illusory trap for the unwary. It should give the required emergency treatment with as little delay as possible, and when that is done there should be no stop until the patient is in the hospital. On admission there, immediate evaluation takes place—by history, by physical examination and, at the right time, by x-ray.

In the first twelve hours there are two ways in which the injured man dies—by injury to the brain and to the circulatory system. When brain and circulatory functions are lost the patient is lost, even though cellular activity may continue in other parts of the body. The things that stop the heart and brain, other than direct trauma, are anoxia and acidosis. These two, between them, can produce complete cessation of nervous or circulatory activity within minutes—anoxia (circulatory or respiratory) by stopping the metabolism of the brain cells, and acidosis (usually respiratory) by ventricular fibrillation.

One of the most important factors in the present-day evaluation of trauma is an understanding of the part played by metabolic changes in the early post-trauma stages. Metabolic changes (necessarily limited to cursory discussion here) are many and of vital importance. They are characterized by a lysis of tissues, with consequent involvement of vital organs to one degree or another. As a whole, this process represents the reactions of the body in its effort to preserve a state of equilibrium in the internal environment.

The surgeon now recognizes that there also occurs a utilization of body tissue for energy. Body carbohydrate is small and quickly consumed. One kilogram of lean tissue contributes less than twelve hundred calories as the protein is burned, whereas one kilogram of fat contributes about nine thousand calories, fatty tissue being rapidly oxidized after severe injury.

Many of the endocrine changes in soft tissue injury, burns and skeletal trauma resemble one another closely, while the metabolic patterns vary widely. The nature of the wound seems to influence the metabolic pattern. It is evident that alterations in the adrenal cortical function are not the only stimuli to post-traumatic metabolism. Probably the wound affects metabolism directly, the hormones being necessarily present for metabolic change, but not as an initiating stimulus. In this function the hormones may be permissive in character, acting to permit tissue changes to occur.

The disordered biochemistry of the wound (exemplified by the six systemic effects of local trauma previously listed) could be a stimulus to body change. However, on occasion when these effects are minimal, marked metabolic alterations still occur. This suggests that some substance elaborated from damaged tissue acts diffusely to alter the pattern of tissue metabolism, and that this in turn acts in concert or synergistically with the neuroendocrine product of the pituitary and adrenals to produce the clinical picture as we see it.[15]

170

There has been frequent reference in these pages to the contributions that war has made to the improvement of industrial surgery by the adaptation of battlefront techniques to civilian life. The *indirect* effects of war have been almost as important as the direct changes in occupational practice. First, war inevitably creates a shortage of surgeons; and because programs of deferment of medical personnel have never received the emphasis that a successful conclusion of the war effort warrants, the result has been the introduction of many new surgeons to the industrial field. Second, increased production under forced draft creates a greater volume of trauma, which in turn results in a quest for improved methods of surgical care.

The importance of today's industrial surgeon is reflected in studies by such men as Gaylord R. Hess, an administrative staff member in the Industrial Division of the American College of Surgeons. In an article titled "Influences of War on Medical Service in Industry," published by the College in June, 1944, Hess cited figures showing that accidental injuries, on an average, accounted for 61 percent of all permanent physical disabilities, with 33 percent due to disease and 6 percent, to physical defects.[16] The challenge implied in statistics of this sort greatly stimulated organized activities to protect the safety and health of workers. In succeeding years accidents have come to be regarded with abhorrence as human and social evils to be prevented by the use of the best engineering skills and to be treated by highly trained surgical personnel once they have occurred. As a sequel to such efforts, Dwight H. Murray, while president of the American Medical Association, was able to announce at the Seventeenth Annual Congress on Industrial Health a 30 percent reduction in accidental deaths in industry, through the expansion of industrial programs between 1940 and 1955.[17]

Although engaged by the employer or an insurance company, the surgeon in industry continues to be motivated by a set of principles which have been summed up in the phrase "the amazing new science of love."[18] For science, finally, has discovered love—the biblical loving kindness, not the kind depicted in motion pictures but the love of humanity. Moreover, doctors are learning to prescribe it. For example, at the Menninger Clinic in Topeka, Kansas, a standard prescription used on the order sheets is "love unsolicited." And the most effective industrial surgeon is one who, knowingly or unknowingly, uses this type of prescription along with the mechanical skills at his command.

We have devoted much space in this volume to America's crusade for safety, with reference to the leadership of the American College of Surgeons in the field of trauma and to the work of the American Medical Association and various councils and committees. Credit is also due to such organizations as the Council on Scientific Assembly for arranging panel discussions and papers dealing with the management of the severely injured. Additional information has become available as the result of such studies as those of Schulzinger, who again emphasizes the accident syndrome,[19] and studies of the accident-prone employee by A. F. Lecklider, formerly medical director of the Fisher Body Corporation.

During the past thirty years the techniques of physiological study of the parts of animals, the organs and the cells, have been supplemented by a newer approach—that of biochemistry. Instead of starting with large objects and working downward, biochemistry attacks the problem from the opposite end, starting with simple, naturally occurring chemical substances and working upward to progressively larger units and more complex chemical systems.

Like the other biologies, biochemistry has had its two stages, the purely descriptive study of structure preceding that of function. In its first, or structural, stage it was in effect a highly specialized branch of organized chemistry, requiring all the skills of classical chemistry for the solution of its problems. The question to be answered was: "What is living stuff made of?" But recently, while still necessarily concerned with questions of structure, biochemistry has become interested in functional or dynamic problems, and the question is: "How does it work?"

Such a question starts with a realization that no matter where we look in the world of living things, we find that chemical reactions are taking place, that all biological processes—digestion, locomotion, fermentation, putrefaction—are essentially chemical changes; and all chemical changes are associated with exchanges of energy. From these beginnings biochemistry has gone on to explore the mysteries of photosynthesis, the process by which green plants and certain bacteria trap solar energy and use it to build up complex substances of high energy content. While animal organisms are barred from full utilization of solar radiation at first hand, they have access to it at second hand by consuming and decomposing these complex plant products, the intrinsic energy of which they can use for their own purposes: growth, locomotion, reproduction, etc.

The trail, in turn, leads to studies of that complicated and extensive network of chemical changes collectively called metabolism. It is significant that nearly all of these chemical changes, in the absence of living matter, take place very slowly but, in order to support the life and activities of living cells, are enormously accelerated by the actions of a large number of biological catalysts called enzymes.

Still more significant is the fact that the energy made available by these changes is not liberated all at once, with explosive violence, but is captured and chemically stored in the living organism, much as a battery stores up energy fed into it by a dynamo, and can subsequently be transformed into the mechanical work done by the muscles. There are various ways in which this chemical energy can be used, for example, in the synthesis of complex chemical substances. The starch of plants, in its animal counterpart, is glycogen, which serves as a store of energy-rich carbohydrate material. The other main constituents of food, the fats and proteins, are also digestively dismantled before being absorbed, each animal having its own characteristic way of carrying out a reassembly. If it can be said that any one of these groups of substances is more characteristic of life than any other, that distinction must go to the proteins. They play a large part not only in the structure of the cells but in their metabolism, for the enzymes which control and direct the metabolic processes are themselves proteins.

In recent years a great deal of interest has centered on one particular group of these conjugated proteins, the nucleoproteins. These are fascinating substances. Viruses are nucleoproteins, and chromosones (which are the material basis of heredity) are perhaps composed entirely of nucleoprotein.

Thus the chain of physiological research has irrevocably linked man—his health, his hazards, and his productivity—to chemical processes within him. And so we come to recognize how important is the application of biochemistry to clinical medicine and how essential this biochemical knowledge is to an understanding of the problems presented by seriously injured employees.[20]

Although Callander[21] and others have frequently referred to the problem of the industrial surgeon as that of the relationship between employer, employee and insurance carrier, we now see that the complex clinical problem is the really challenging aspect of industrial surgery.

The importance of readjusting the injured to their work is more appreciated in this era than ever before.[22] In fact, that readjustment is the goal to be attained throughout the course of treatment of complicated metabolic and physiological disturbances. And it is obvious that medical department personnel must be thoroughly familiar with possible exposures, methods of clinical examination, chemical and other laboratory techniques, and emergency measures.

Great progress has already been made in the recognition of the problem presented by the unconscious or comatose employee admitted to the medical department or hospital. The complexity of that problem is indicated by the fact that nearly a score of possible pathological factors are recognized in charts provided by industrial medical departments, to be memorized or consulted in such emergencies.

Over a period of twenty years, exhaustive studies in several university centers[23] have demonstrated the importance of prompt determination of water loss and existing proportion to body weight, the acid base balance in the presence of shock, and methods of treatment aimed to restore equilibrium in the internal environment.

Long since, the use of oral salt has practically eliminated heat cramps by replacement of electrolyte loss due to excessive sweating. The identification of normal and diseased tissues by histological configuration of biopsied specimens also has been long recognized in establishing diagnoses.

In recent years there has been further concentration of research on the problems of fluid loss and replacement, such as the work done by the Abbott Laboratories[24] and many other organizations interested in furthering the development of biochemical knowledge.

From intensive studies in this field it began to appear that various diseases may result in enzymatic tissue alterations as profound as the morphological changes identified with inflammatory, neoplastic and degenerative states. The disease of an organ may at times be inferred from the examination of accessible body fluids.

Just as localized inflammation in an organ may be reflected peripherally by a morphologic change such as an increase in the circulating leukocytes, so tissue insults may result in equally impressive enzymatic alterations in the blood stream and other body fluids. Thus it is evident that a tissue may be characterized by its enzymatic as well as its cellular composition, and correlation of clinical facts with quantitative and serial enzyme changes in body fluids contributes to the differential diagnosis of disease-states.[25]

Here again there developed a challenge to the industrial surgeon to improve his diagnostic approach by working closely with the biochemist and the laboratory.

Among the most significant achievements of biochemical research in the twentieth century, one must rank the study and classification of the vitamins and recognition of their value in aiding recovery from disease and the prevention of deficiency diseases which affect a large part of the industrial population. Today, of course, vitamin therapy is a major field in itself, and the enormous literature on the subject demands detailed study by all students of occupational health.

Long before these later developments, the value of vitamins in the anemias and in wound healing had been recognized. It was this understanding, decades ago, which roused the interest of employers in providing eating facilities in their plants and promoting programs of dietary education. And to minimize vitamin deficiency due to faulty dietary habits, many placed bowls of balanced vitamin preparations in their cafeterias.

The present scope of vitamin therapy in the treatment of previously uncontrolled diseases is indicated (in brief summary) by the influence of vitamins C and B12 upon the degenerative diseases with accompanying osteoarthrosis and osteoporosis; by the part played by vitamin C in controlling diabetes; and by vitamin C bioflavonoid therapy, which has permitted the use of coagulant drugs in coronary thrombosis, all resulting in a return to work by many employees who otherwise would be permanently disabled.

Pain intensity, being a subjective symptom, until recent years has been considered incapable of measurement. The development of a new technique—"dolorimetry"—now makes it possible to measure the intensity of pain and to record it accurately on a scale based upon the ability of a patient to distinguish differences in the intensity, an advance of considerable value to the industrial surgeon in accident cases presented to courts of law. ("Dol" is the name given to the unit of painfulness, its value being about one-tenth of the intensity of maximal pain.)[26]

By mid-century, physiologists and pharmacologists had produced drugs which gave the surgeon a commanding control of shock. So great is their number, so broad their field of utility, that it is obviously impossible to present here even a fractional list. They range from drugs administered to assist in bringing about specific corrections of body metabolism, whether in the emergency treatment of trauma or as an aid in surgery, to multi-purpose drugs (such as ACTH), which find a place in the treatment of shock and burns, as well as in rheumatoid arthritis, gout, lupus erithematosis and other diseases which are allergies or are related to the so-called "collogen" diseases.

Clinical research brought about a greater appreciation of the value of oxygen, and various forms of apparatus were developed to provide emergency administration, as well as tents in which cooled oxygen could be supplied in carefully measured quantities.

Notable, too, was recognition of the importance of the Rh factor; and in preparing injured patients for transfusion not only was the blood grouping determined, but cross matching between donor and recipient was also universally carried out.

Again, war experience was to benefit the work of the industrial surgeon, by throwing needed light upon what came to be called the "crush" syndrome. During the blitz in 1940, patients were treated who had been buried for several hours. Despite severely crushed extremities, with swelling and shock, the local condition presented a good clinical response, but urinary output progressively decreased to a daily output as low as 25–50 cc. Only about one-third of the patients recovered; the remainder died of uremia.

Acute renal failure after trauma without direct injury to the kidneys had been noted in World War I, but in the intervening years much had been learned about kidney function, and further microscopic study traced the trouble to severe and prolonged reduction in renal blood flow, which caused anoxia of the kidney, leading, in turn, to disrupting lesions in the renal tubules. Realizing, from these findings, the early damage that occurs to the kidneys in shock, the industrial surgeon planned his strategy accordingly.

Critically crushed chests are not unusual and may well be fatal. Adequate ventilation alone can break the vicious cycle of reduced pulmonary capacity, hypoxia, pulmonary edema, pneumonitis and exhaustion. Significant among the technical advances of the mid-century was the development of apparatus for use in cases requiring cardiorespiratory resuscitation, such as the Morch piston respirator and the Morris defibrillator-pacemaker.[27]

Modern warfare, with the rapid development of high powered explosives, likewise resulted in a sharp increase in "blast" injuries, producing mechanism and cellular changes which were described by Dr. George M. Curtis.[28] An understanding of these traumatic factors also fell within the province of the industrial surgeon.

It soon became apparent that the surgical facilities of industry would play an all-important role in case of disaster and that the entire subject was of major concern to the industrial surgeon. The federal Civil Defense Administration issued instructions in 1950 that special provisions for the care of casualties be made in hospitals operated by industrial plants and prepared complete plans of procedure, accompanied by illustrative charts.[29] America's industrial surgeons not only cooperated closely in C.D.A. activities but followed with care the plans for disaster control developed at numerous conferences, both national[30] and local.[31]

There ensued a great deal of discussion and many important contributions to the literature of *serendipity,* the finding of valuable or useful things by chance encounter.[32] In the field of industrial surgery, progress was made by carefully planned programs based on a large clinical experience, but accidental discoveries were also put to good use, penicillin being a good example.

So numerous, and so broad in scope, are the modern advances made in occupa-

175

tional health that a detailed description is impossible here. The accomplishments of the past half-century constitute an evolution from inadequate first aid measures to mastery of the stresses produced upon the physiological and metabolic mechanisms of the worker by exposure to conditions in space and in ocean depths, by low- and high-degree thermal agents, by complicated chemical substances, by the mechanical effects of the atomic age, and by social and economic pressures affecting accident proneness.

A skeleton listing of major advances, however, serves to indicate both their direction and their importance:

Entirely new techniques in the care of soft tissue wounds—large or small, clean or contaminated—resulting in better healing, almost total absence of infection, less disfigurement and loss of function.[33]

Successful treatment (with newly developed drugs) *of "static" ulcers* caused by capillary blocking and previously considered incapable of healing.[34]

Effective treatment of frostbite—developed from Korean War experience, which demonstrated the value of rapid thawing by immersion in warm water, the use of antibiotics and anticoagulants, and prompt physical therapy to stimulate circulation and minimize muscle atrophy.

Professional recognition of rapidly increasing athletic activities as a source of trauma (particularly in contact sports), and formation of a national association of surgeons interested in athletic trauma, which added an important group to the field of occupational surgery.

Concentrated attack upon the various forms of arthritis, marked by great strides in knowledge and control of rheumatoid arthritis and the development of effective drugs to combat joint-disabling inflammation. The importance of this problem to industry was highlighted by the Conference on Rheumatic Disorders in Industry in 1953, of which A. J. Lanza was the chairman.[35]

Introduction of new drugs effective in reducing the painful symptoms of involuntary spasms of skeletal muscles,[36] a problem frequently confronting the industrial surgeon.

Surgical attack upon back injuries (which often presented an element of collogen disease); stabilization or surgical reconstruction of joints sometimes indicated in addition to local physical medical measures.

Successful operation for removal of nerve root pressure in a small group (about 3 percent) of patients suffering from back pain due to herniated intervertebral disc.

A new (1955) *method of artificial respiration* introduced by the American Red Cross, known as the Holger Nielsen Arm Lift, an advance so important that it produced a mass movement in first aid training among industrial safety and medical personnel, exemplified in Detroit by the development of a manual[37] and courses of instruction available to industrial employees throughout the area.

Studies of x-radiation problems created by the development of atomic energy plants and the great number of workers in this and the expanding missile industry; important findings on use of transfusions in case of mass irradiation.[38]

New methods in rehabilitation and reconditioning of injured employees under

176

supervision until their return to work; growth of rehabilitation centers with trained staffs and development of self-help devices by the New York University-Bellevue Medical Center.

The use of equipment designed for community facilities by manufacturers of physical fitness and play equipment,[39] development by the National Recreation Association of a large group sponsoring techniques of rehabiliation.

New techniques of cineplastic operations on the upper extremity,[40] steady improvement in prosthesis manufacture (helped by the use of lighter materials), and progress in developing electrically operated and air pressure prosthesis to eliminate the use of straps.[41]

Increased emphasis by medical colleges upon physical medicine, that the younger surgeons coming into industry may be better trained in the use of prostheses, braces and rehabilitation procedures.

Notable improvement in surgical techniques to insure the preservation of function in hand injuries, one of the great accomplishments of industrial surgery in an area that accounts for an important percentage of occupational trauma; problems created by amputations, fractures (including mallet finger), tendon injuries and contractures solved since World War II to an incredible degree, occasionally helped by muscle and tendon transplants, nerve suture and substitution of a finger for a thumb,[42] and replacement of an injured thumb web (at least in part) by a skin graft.[43]

Increasingly successful surgical repair of inguinal hernia, rarely traumatic, as pointed out by Coley in 1922,[44] but a responsibility of the surgeon inasmuch as compensation boards have regarded nearly all hernias as the result of occupational strain.[45]

Growing concern, on the part of the industrial surgeon, *with malignancies,* benign growths about the hip which require amputation through the pelvic bones, that is, interinnomino-abdominal or hind quarter amputation.[46]

Improved techniques in the operative care of fractures; replacement, for the most part, of metal plates (introduced by an industrial surgeon, William Sherman) by pins, and the more recent replacement of the Kuencher pin by the Rush pin, which permits better approximation of bone ends and requires less tissue damage.[47]

Replacement of the head of the radius (when removed in treatment of a comminuted fracture), by a vitallium head—providing a much more stable elbow joint and permitting a return to fairly heavy work.

Reduction of a two-year disability to three months, through new operative procedures in the treatment of comminuted fractures of the *os calcis.* Surgeons, formerly reluctant to operate on the *os calcis,* fearing necrosis,[48] now use open reduction and internal fixation by screws, which permit excellent anatomical restoration and retention of the reduction.[49]

Important improvements in the treatment of brain and spinal cord injuries, by the development of specially staffed and equipped neurosurgical centers, permitting many injured employees to return to work who formerly would have been permanently disabled. Reduced mortality in severe head injuries also promised by the use of hypothermia.[50]

Corresponding improvement in blood vessel surgery,[51] which now permits replacement of injured arteries and the excision of diseased vessels (even the aorta), with substitution carried out by the use of an aortic bifurcation graft of chemically treated nylon.[52]

So goes the parade of progress, a seemingly endless list of advances in medical knowledge, techniques and procedures. If a single example were to be selected as exemplifying the nature and importance of such innovations, it might well be the dramatic evolution of the treatment of burns, always a critical problem in foundries and certain other industries.

In the 1920's, the tannic acid method of Davison had replaced Doctor William Sherman's paraffin treatment. When the use of tannic acid, in turn, was discredited because of hepatic damage, the use of compression dressings after thorough cleansing was instituted, with some surgeons preferring the open method of treatment. The disability was so prolonged, however, and the morbidity so severe, that in an effort to avoid the toxic "after-48-hours" phase and the serious shock and electrolyte imbalance that developed, the procedure of immediate excision with split-thickness skin grafting on the day of injury was instituted.[53] At first only localized deep burns, such as electrical burns and those caused by hot metal, were excised. Then followed the immediate grafting of an extremity. Under these procedures the local grafts healed so well (with joints protected from contractures), and the systemic reaction was so improved, that extensive burns were excised and immediately grafted. Where the burns were too extensive to be covered by available skin, homografts were used in alternal strips with the patient's split-thickness grafts. It was found that as the homografts were absorbed, the adjacent grafts spread to cover the defects so that no additional grafting was necessary. Great saving in length of hospital stay was accomplished, function was preserved, and loss of time from work was greatly reduced.[54]

These contemporary advances of science are part of the heritage of modern occupational medicine from its colorful beginnings early in this century. They are a common denominator in any practice of the specialty but are of vital interest to the surgeon because they are so closely linked with the treatment and prevention of trauma.

Industry provides a challenging field in this specialized surgery, one in which great satisfaction can be experienced in returning the men who actually produce the wealth of the world to gainful employment at the highest attainable skill and in the shortest possible time.

PART FIVE

THE TURBULENT TWENTIES

INDUSTRIAL MEDICINE IN THE ERA OF BOOM AND BUST

An association, like an individual, succeeds only as it serves.

XVI

GROWING UP:

MEN, MONEY, AND MEMBERSHIP

Born in a period of grave world crisis, the young American Association of Industrial Physicians & Surgeons cut its teeth on knotty problems involving the nation's war potential. Its members performed distinguished services to industry and to the country. Industrial medicine gained widespread recognition, and some prestige, as a professional specialty.

At the end of the war the association faced another immediate crisis—this time in its own internal affairs. Its membership was small. It had no money, no permanent headquarters-office, no source of revenue other than dues, amounting at best to some $600 a year.

From 1916 to 1919, association activities had been dictated almost wholly by government needs: the conservation of health for maximum industrial production, the utmost utilization of available manpower, and the rehabilitation of sick and disabled veterans. Now the association was on its own, beset with administrative and policy problems which at times threatened its very existence.

No organization can thrive forever on the zeal and enthusiasm of its founders. This new association had set up sound and well-defined objectives, but it had formulated no practical program for attainment of its goals. Momentum was lacking in the crusade for anything approaching uniform procedures in industrial medical departments. There was need for new blood, young blood, to meet the challenge of the times.

John J. McCloy, former High Commissioner for Germany, has written nostalgically of "that simple, untaxed, untelevised, uninvolved life which was the pattern of these United States in the early part of this century."[1] One thing was apparent

181

even before the signing of the Treaty of Versailles which officially ended World War I—the day of leisurely progress and national self-sufficiency in America was gone, never to return. The United States had emerged from the conflict as a dominant power in world politics. It had assumed international and domestic responsibilities that could not be relinquished. Industry, trade, and commerce entered on a new and higher plateau of activity. And tremendous social upheavals were already in the making.

Such was the national atmosphere when the association opened its fifth annual meeting in New Orleans on April 26, 1920. No record of registration has survived, but reports indicate that attendance was small, not for lack of interest, but because the press of business at home kept members in many sections of the country from making the long trip. At this meeting Harry E. Mock gave his farewell address as president, yielding the gavel after two years of faithful and efficient service as head of the association, in whose interests he had labored unceasingly since 1912.

On his return from military service after the war, Mock had decided against resuming his work at Sears, Roebuck. He also declined an opportunity to join the International Health Board of the Rockefeller Foundation in a mission to Australia to organize a Department of Industrial Health for the Australian government. The association, however, was well represented on this project. Anthony J. Lanza, prominently identified with the USPHS and active in the work of the association from its earliest years, accompanied the group overseas in 1921, serving as a special staff member until the spring of 1924.

Mock writes in a letter to Alfred Whittaker: "I considered this recognition as another example of the influence of our association. As for myself, I decided to continue my surgical practice in Chicago, applying to it many of the ideas I had learned in industry and especially using my experience to promote the physical reconstruction and rehabilitation of the handicapped."

At its two-day session in New Orleans in 1920, the association chose Otto Geier to succeed Mock as president. During the war, Geier had served as an assistant surgeon in the USPHS, in charge of health matters in the powder works at Anchor, Ohio, but he had returned to take up his full-time duties as medical director at the Cincinnati Milling Machine Company. Unfortunately, he was unable even to attend the convention that elected him to its highest office, being detained in Cincinnati by labor troubles.

A shrewd observer of the current scene, and thoroughly steeped in association affairs, Geier wasted no time in taking the helm and setting up a program for his administration. He recognized the need for long-range planning and for a nationwide program of activity. With characteristic modesty he wrote, on May 15, 1920, to Francis D. Patterson, association secretary-treasurer since 1918:

> In my sane moments I appreciate that great honor has been done me. I almost regret, however, that any of us of the old guard were put back in official positions. I have a fear that the feeling is getting about through the membership that some of

us seem to believe that we have squatters' claim on all the jobs loose in the organization.

It shall be my purpose, therefore, when I get out of the present fog, to try to plan with you some communications that will tend to dispel this idea and secure, if possible, the cooperation of the membership in our plans for the next meeting.

I assume that we will meet in Boston with the AMA. I would thank you to advise me very promptly as to who the other officers of the association are, with their addresses. I suppose you are going to have some stationery printed at once, and that you will let me have some for my correspondence.

With his usual candor and forthrightness, Geier likewise struck, in the same letter, at the heart of association problems which he believed most urgently called for action:

It has occurred to me that it might be advisable for us to plan a mid-season meeting of the association in the Middle West, perhaps at Chicago, some time during the late fall or winter. We might want to work that up in connection with some other association meeting. I should like to have your reaction on this. It would certainly help to bring up our membership in this thickly-populated industrial section.

I wish you would also have your secretary give me a complete comparative review, by years, of the membership and income, as well as the expenditures. Add to this your estimate of the income on the basis of the new dues, as well as a complete statement of our budgetary requirements.

Most important of all right now, it seems to me, my dear Dr. Patterson, is a complete reversal of form in the matter of our proceedings. Coming out as they did this year, after the men had gone to the convention, makes the subject matter so stale that I really believe the money invested in printing was wasted.

We should either adopt an official journal which would agree to carry the papers within a reasonable period of time or edit and print them at once. This may be impossible, due to the cost of printing and your inability to take time to edit same. We might consider, on the other hand, giving our main papers to some official journal to be printed in due time, and have all of the papers abstracted for immediate distribution.

I am of course at a disadvantage in discussing these subjects because I was not present at the New Orleans meeting and do not know what conclusions the Board of Directors reached in these matters. I want to repeat, however, that I think it is highly important that we reach a conclusion at once as to which method is to be followed. The vitality of our association depends upon following some vigorous policy at this time and continuing to follow it throughout the year.

The letter is printed almost in its entirety because it dealt with the principal problems of the association in the twenties, and sparked the programs undertaken during those eventful years. Men, money, and membership, year-round activity and some channel through which the text of important papers could be placed in the hands of members! These were the subjects marked for immediate action.

Patterson replied in a letter dated May 18:

Everyone agreed that you were the one and only man to head our association as president, and you were unanimously elected, so cheer up.

I send you enclosed a comparative review of the income and disbursements, and I feel that with the new dues of $5.00 per year as agreed to at our New Orleans meeting, it will give us enough to run on.

I absolutely agree with you about the proceedings. It is a crime and a shame that they did not come out for a year. . . . I intend to have the proceedings out by the first of July at the latest.

As I have written you, we are trying to agree upon an official journal and my choice is in favor of *Modern Medicine,* about which I have written you. The journal would devote an entire number to the proceedings of our annual meeting, and then we could print enough copies from that type to have for distribution.

This correspondence contains the earliest available references to selection of a publication to represent the association and to print its proceedings and papers in any detail. Also on record is mention of a committee headed by Dr. W. Irving Clark, of Worcester, Massachusetts, which was studying the problem. The issue aroused a surprising degree of partisanship for and against the few periodicals in the field at the time. It was not settled to everyone's satisfaction until the appearance of *Industrial Medicine* in 1932.[2]

Some sort of arrangement with *Modern Medicine* was made in 1920, and the treasurer's report for the year ending April 30, 1921, lists a disbursement of $368.61 for copies of the magazine and/or reprints. The contractual relationship, however, was tenuous. In 1921 *Modern Medicine* was absorbed as a department of *The Nation's Health,* which remained the official journal of the association through 1922. The subscription cost, $1.50 per year, was paid from dues.

The fiscal affairs of the association, in the years immediately following its founding, presented a picture that was anything but encouraging. Lack of money, obviously, was the root of most evils during that difficult period. One may doubt that any organization of equal size has ever operated on a smaller budget, or stretched so little so far.

Fortunately for historical verity, the original ledger of the association has survived its travels from treasurer to treasurer to treasurer and has come to rest in the archives of the Industrial Medical Association. Entries, carefully inked in a round, schoolgirl hand, reveal the nakedness of the exchequer and hint at a perpetual struggle to make ends meet. Ends, in fact, did *not* always meet. Ledger pages covering the period to June 16, 1916 (immediately following the first annual meeting), list a total of 176 dues-paying members, with a $2.00 credit opposite each name. The balance for fiscal 1916–1917 shows that the association was solvent, by a margin of $16.62. Total disbursements of that period were $737.38, for scores of items of every description.

During the next four years, membership grew slowly but steadily—to 220 to 275 to 340 and, in 1920, to the 400 mark. But finances did not follow the membership pattern. For the fiscal year, 1917–1918, there was a deficit of $24.98; in 1918–1919 the deficit was $264.71. For 1919–1920, by some financial magic, the books showed a credit balance of $26.09.

In his May, 1920, report to President Geier, Secretary-Treasurer Patterson wrote: "I furthermore am sending out a circular letter to every industrial physician, some 2,000 in number, who has not yet joined our association, and hope to secure the membership of at least the majority of them."

The forecast was optimistic, to say the least. Still, there was a net gain of 99 members in the following year, bringing the total to 499. This was the largest number on record during the entire 1920's, except for brief peaks between annual reports. From that point on, membership followed an irregular downward trend, reaching a low of 252 in 1929. Not until 1937 did enrollment again pass the 400 level.[3]

By 1921 it had become apparent to officers and directors that something had to be done to improve the condition of the treasury, the obvious remedy being an increase in dues to $10 per year. There also was a strong feeling on the part of many members that administrative responsibility should be distributed on a broader geographical basis, introducing new names, new faces, fresh thinking. It was a viewpoint to which most of the wheel horses among the founders, who had shouldered the bulk of the burden, heartily subscribed.

These and other policy problems were vigorously debated, in intra-association correspondence, during 1921. The annual meeting at Boston in June did not solve them all, but it did produce one of the few heated political campaigns in the association's history, in which a faction representing the public health services was aligned against a ticket supported by Geier and Sawyer. The result—a victory for C. E. Ford, medical director of the General Chemical Company, of New York, who won by a wide margin over Clarence C. Burlingame to succeed Geier as president. Burlingame, medical director of Chaney Brothers, South Manchester, Connecticut, held several responsible posts in the Army medical service during his long and active career.

Ford, a founding member of the association, had served as a director in 1920–1921. He was a clear thinker, a man of decision and action, who plotted a sound course for the organization during his first year and in a second term, which carried over to October, 1923.

The remainder of the successful ticket in the 1921 election consisted of C. F. N. Schram, of Fairbanks, Morse & Company, Beloit, Wisconsin, as first vice-president; Loyal A. Shoudy, of Bethlehem Steel, as second vice-president; and William A. Sawyer, of the Eastman Kodak Company, Rochester, as secretary-treasurer. Their names recur again and again in industrial medical literature as outstanding contributors to the progress of the profession and of the association.

Sawyer, a close friend and ardent admirer of Otto Geier, makes this comment on his early impressions:

Dr. Geier was a great inspiration to me, especially since he was president at a time when we felt that the association was undergoing a reorganization. He stood for the finest of ideals in industrial medicine. I remember an article he wrote for one of the trade journals, in which he likened the industrial physician to the parish priest, someone who was interested not only in their [his parishioners'] ills but also in their social and environmental and mental problems.

There was very much more of a spirit of service and concern for the general welfare of workers in those early days than there has been latterly. I think it was upon that note that industrial medicine made its first impression upon me, and I still believe, after all these years of experience, that it is upon that note of service and of interest in the whole man that its greatest usefulness is attained.

I do not believe that in any of the specialties of medicine do you find the close association or the intimate understanding of problems involved that you do in industrial medicine. It is very much a part of real living and has in it all the real attributes of humane and social advancement.

My only regret is that it has not advanced rapidly enough, it is not applied to enough workers, and I always see in it the great possibilities for improvement which would mean so much to the betterment of mankind and to the economic advantage of all concerned.

A few weeks after his election President Ford suggested, in a letter to Sawyer, closer cooperation with the Conference Board of Physicians in Industry, which would make possible wide distribution of "great masses of statistics" gathered by the Board, thus performing a needed service to the association and offsetting to some extent its lack of funds for such purposes.

Ford proposed an eleven-point program "that the association attempt to further during the term of our administration." It is outlined here, in substance, as indicating the broad policy followed during the twenties and into the succeeding decade:

1. Definition of the proper limitations of the industrial physician in relation to general community health activities, and to the work of the private practitioner.

2. Coordination and standardization of first aid methods to be applied in industry.

3. Collection of mortality statistics and standardization of record keeping in cases of illness, accident, and absenteeism from other causes.

4. Education of management, with the aim of raising the status of the heads of plant medical departments to such a plane as will command respect and make for responsibility directly to executives.

5. A practical scheme for supplying health service in small plants.

6. Making available to the medical profession at large, special methods of treatment and technique which have been used to advantage by individuals or by a group in more or less restricted territory.

7. Efforts to produce high types of papers for publication in the journal, featuring problems dealing with industrial hygiene and medicine.

8. Production of scientific data.

9. Stimulation of active interest among members in national and state legislation having to do with medical economics.

10. Printing of monthly abstracts of industrial literature for distribution through the Conference Board.

11. Closer cooperation with associated industries of different states and with chambers of commerce. We need plenty of contact with the sources of our existence.

Sawyer tackled the job of secretary-treasurer with great enthusiasm. His correspondence was voluminous, and, in the absence of a full-time paid assistant, he was obliged to call on his office help to carry on the program. "Getting the dues paid was a problem," he writes. "I remember rather clearly that the work consumed so much time of the medical department staff that there was finally a complaint from some of the people in the Kodak Company, and I then began to realize what a burden I had taken over."

Money and membership problems continued to plague the association, not only during Sawyer's tenure (1921–1923) but for the next decade and more. Oddly, membership drives did not produce the response that was to be expected in a time of prosperity and expansion. Interest in industrial medicine was spreading rapidly, more and larger medical departments were being established, but Association enrollment remained in the doldrums. It seems probable that the association was undergoing a natural readjustment in which many of the original joiners dropped out because of waning interest, death, or retirement. Late in 1921 Sawyer launched a vigorous letter campaign to a selected list of desirable men, aimed at the goal of "a thousand members by May 1." Returns were gratifying, but losses more than offset gains in the next few years. Dues-delinquency was commonly 30 percent or more.

Ford and Sawyer enlisted the help of influential members from every section of the country in their campaign. Typical of the appeal is a letter from Sawyer to Geier in January, 1922: "As the past-perfect president of the association, won't you please do a little something for the expanding organization? I would appreciate it greatly if you would stir up a few members down your way, and I would also greatly thank you for a letter to be addressed to the present membership to be published in an early issue of *The Nation's Health*."

Geier and others of the old guard did their best. They succeeded in winning the interest and support of many men prominent in industrial medicine and allied fields, who immeasurably strengthened the prestige of the association. Their addition to the membership rolls, however, did not materially improve the financial picture. The annual report in May, 1922, showed another deficit, the largest in the association's history.

There was the question of quality as well as quantity to be considered. Sawyer hoped for quantity but insisted on quality. It undoubtedly was a wise policy, for the association gained in vigor and purposeful activity despite its slow numerical growth. Adherence to the same policy over the years has since brought the organization to a membership of more than 4,000, representative, across the country, of the highest standards and most progressive procedures in industrial medicine.

The fiscal situation in 1922 brought to a head the perennial debate on an increase of dues. On the surface, an item of $5.00 per year seemed unimportant, but many believed it might mean the difference between survival and death by attrition.

Thomas R. Crowder, medical director of the Pullman Company and first vice-president of the association in 1920–1922, militantly opposed any increase. He urged rigorous retrenchment regardless of the membership trend, even to the extent of eliminating the annual hundred-dollar prize essay contest and the free banquet at conventions.

The question of a virile and influential journal to represent the organization was closely linked with the problem of revenue. Nearly one-third of every $5.00 of income from dues had been earmarked for subscriptions to *The Nation's Health,* published by the Modern Hospital Publishing Company and edited by Frank L. Rector. This arrangement was under fire as early as October, 1921. Correspondence indicates that the magazine was losing money, and there was some doubt that it could continue publication. From this fact stemmed a proposal to substitute the *Journal of Industrial Hygiene,* issued by the Medical School of Harvard University under the direction of Cecil K. Drinker, a strong and active worker in the cause of industrial health.

Settlement of this question hinged largely on cold fiscal facts. An annual levy of $5.00 obviously could not provide a publication costing $4.00 per year. No decision was made until the end of 1922, when a contract was signed giving *Industrial Hygiene* the exclusive right to publish papers presented at meetings of the AAIP&S. The journal (said to have been the first professional periodical in its field) agreed, in turn, to print membership data and other association news each month.

Dr. Rector's allegiance to the profession extended far deeper than his interest in an editorial connection with *The Nation's Health.* He remained active in the association for many years, until his retirement from professional service. As secretary-treasurer, 1925–1927, he devoted much time and energy to upgrading the literature of industrial medicine. He was largely responsible for the founding of the association's *Bulletin,* which he edited through 1927.

The *Bulletin* represented an important forward step in the relations between the association and its members. First issued in August, 1926, it continued as the official organ until 1932, when the establishment of *Industrial Medicine* at long last brought the publication policies of the association to full maturity.

The Bulletin was a modest, inexpensive little sheet of four to eight pages, published with some irregularity at intervals varying from once a month to four times a year. But it was the members' own magazine; it brought them the Association's intimate news and reprints or abstracts of important papers. They took a vast, and justifiable, pride in it.

The debate over an increase of annual dues for association membership dragged on through 1922 and well into 1923. On September 27, 1923, V. S. Cheney, president of the Chicago Society of Industrial Medicine & Surgery, wrote to Sawyer to protest against the proposed increase to $10.00 a year:

There is a strong feeling in the west that the American Association of Industrial Physicians & Surgeons has developed into an eastern-controlled association, which is gradually being dominated by theorists and teachers of the Harvard Medical School; men with no practical experience in industrial work. This sentiment was strongly in evidence at our meeting in St. Louis two years ago at which quite a few western men were present, and instead of growing less, it has steadily increased.

There has been organized recently in Illinois a State Society of Industrial Surgeons, and at the time of organization the question came up of affiliation with the American Association of Industrial Physicians & Surgeons, and it was decided that it was not a thing to be desired.

We have a very strong local society which contains many members of the American Association of Industrial Physicians & Surgeons, and as president of that society I am in close touch with them and know just how they feel toward the national association.

I am confident that any raise in dues will cause the withdrawal from membership of practically all the western members, especially those in Illinois and surrounding states. I am almost sure that many western men will withdraw at the end of the present year unless the policy of the association is changed and a western man (by western, I mean west of Cleveland, Ohio) is put in as president or secretary of the organization.

There is no doubt that the feeling expressed by Cheney did exist. It may have been fairly widespread, and it had been aggravated by the selection of a Harvard Medical School publication as the association's official journal, despite the high quality of its service and the fine cooperation of its staff.

Proof that this apprehension was not universal came at the 1923 annual meeting in Buffalo, which for some unexplained reason was postponed until the first of October. The Board of Directors promptly approved a constitutional amendment raising dues to $10.00 per year. In the following December Sawyer wrote to Cheney:

"The dues were increased, and it was done without the slightest opposition. I expect that a goodly number will withdraw from the association, but it seems impossible to conduct affairs on anything less."

Geographical peace also reigned at Buffalo. Nor did the heavens fall. The delegates elected a ticket headed by Loyal A. Shoudy, Pennsylvania, as president, with D. B. Lowe, of the B. F. Goodrich Company, Akron, as first vice-president; Sawyer, Rochester, New York, as second vice-president; and A. G. Cranch, of the National Carbon Company, Cleveland, as secretary-treasurer. And in his letter to Cheney, Sawyer had this comment to make: "I think if you had been at Buffalo, you would have realized that the offices went to those men who have given considerable thought and time to the interests of the association. No one seems to care what part of the country the officers come from."

The new president was well named Loyal Shoudy. As a vice-president in the two preceding administrations he had endeared himself to the entire membership by his magnetic personality and dedication to association interests. He served two consecutive terms (1923 to 1925) as its administrative head and was one of its most valued counselors until his death in August, 1950.

Retiring at the end of an unprecedented third term as president in 1947, Shoudy reviewed the early years, and early struggles, of the association in a memorable fare-well address. Fortunately, a verbatim transcript of the entire banquet meeting was made. It was discovered, years later, among his papers, and thus it remains in the archives. Among other things, he said:

> When we were small we all knew each other better, and the friendships formed over the years are something you can't wipe out. Boys, I ask you when you are carry-ing on, please, please, please, keep it that way.
>
> In those [Directors'] meetings where the twelve or fifteen got together and started in at four o'clock in the afternoon and ended at two o'clock in the morning, something sprang up between us that you cannot take away. Keep our friendships. Keep our association known as the friendly association.

Of such stuff are vital and successful organizations made. It is a monument to Loyal Shoudy and others of his quality that the association has "kept it that way."

Speaking of conditions in the latter half of the twenties, he said:

> In 1927 we were at Johns Hopkins. The going was a little bit tough. Our mem-bership was around 250, if that many. Our meetings were small. We had good times. And I am proud to say that we didn't have much money, and as Patterson may have done with the Commonwealth of Pennsylvania, I went down into the pockets of Bethlehem Steel and dug up what money was necessary to keep this association to-gether. We are happy that we could do that. I am happy I work for a company that didn't say "No."

It was at the close of Shoudy's second term that the most fateful of all crises in association affairs came to a head. The issue was whether the AAIP&S could continue to exist as an independent entity. The question had been raised, more or less casually, as early as 1921.

In his first report to President Ford in June of that year, Secretary Sawyer wrote: "I also am interested in the suggestion of Dr. Geier regarding the affiliation with the AMA. I talked the matter over with a number of people in Boston last week, and the consensus seemed to be that it might be undesirable right now to merge our society with any organization, that we would have a great deal to lose and very little to gain by such action."

The idea was given only passing attention at the time, but it was kept alive by a coterie of men who were discouraged by the continuing lack of funds and the difficulty of gaining new members. In March, 1922, Sawyer wrote to Ford: "I notice on going over the files that you, Dr. Geier and I are on the committee to consider union with the AMA. Can we do anything further before the annual meeting in May?"

No action was taken at that time, or during the following two years. By 1925 the issue was recognized for what it really was, a question of whether the association should remain the big toad in a then little puddle, or should surrender its freedom of action and direction, and become at best an adjunct of the American Medical Association. The issue demanded immediate decision. The answer would be final and irrevocable; there could be no compromise. In a directors' meeting at the Atlantic City convention in May, President Shoudy appointed another committee to study the question. It was one of his last official acts at the close of his second term.

As a result of the Atlantic City election William B. Fisk, director of the Industrial Relations Department of International Harvester, succeeded to the presidency; Sawyer moved up to the first vice-presidency; C. W. Hopkins, of the Chicago and North Western Railway, Chicago, became second vice-president; and Frank L. Rector, who was still affiliated with *The Nation's Health,* took over as secretary-treasurer.

Fisk had joined the association in June, 1919, serving as a director, 1921–1923, and as first vice-president, 1924–1925. He was an able administrator, highly regarded professionally, and continuously active in organization affairs. As president, he pressed for prompt action on the proposed merger with the AMA, and four months later, at a meeting in Cleveland, the new Board voted without dissent that the association retain its identity and its full functions as an independent organization. Truly, September 28, 1925, was a day of "great decision."

This administration was marked by another notable milestone, a move to establish permanent association headquarters and to provide adequate secretarial help for the conduct of official business. Need for these facilities had been long apparent, but they could not be financed with red ink. By May, 1926, the financial picture had improved materially; at their annual meeting in Philadelphia the directors recommended the opening of a central office and employment of a full-time assistant secretary at $2,000 per year.

It was in Philadelphia that Sawyer took over the presidency of the association, with C. F. N. Schram, of the Fairbanks-Morse Company, as first vice-president, and Robert S. Quinby, of the Hood Rubber Company, Watertown, Massachusetts, as second vice-president. Rector continued as secretary and was already busy with plans for the forthcoming *Bulletin.*

The headquarters plan was officially approved by the Board of Directors at their meeting in Detroit on October 26, 1926. In its February, 1927, issue the *Bulletin* announced the opening of a permanent office at 22 E. Ontario Street, Chicago, under supervision of the secretary-treasurer, with Miss Louise Ragan, of Lafayette, Indiana, in charge as full-time assistant. "For the first time in its history," the notice declared, "the association is now able to carry on continuous work for the members."

To increase the value of the organization to its members and others, President Sawyer appointed a standing committee to which problems that the secretary's office could not handle were to be referred. It consisted of A. W. George, A. Girard Cranch, T. Lyle Hazlett, V. S. Cheney, Louis G. Harney, A. W. Colcord, R. J. DeMotte, Lloyd Noland, J. M. Wainwright, D. B. Lowe, Robert P. Knapp, and Wade Wright. A star-studded team, it functioned well.

"It is expected," said the *Bulletin,* "that this committee will serve in an advisory capacity; so that from out of the experience of our own organization we will be able to supply the desired information to inquirers. . . . Out of this small beginning it is hoped that a wide field of usefulness may be developed which will do much to stimulate an appreciation of industrial health problems and place the work of the physician in industry upon the high plane where it properly belongs."

The salutary effects of these simple steps are not to be underestimated. They smoothed immeasurably the path of succeeding administrations, lifted a growing burden of detail from the shoulders of overworked officers and directors, and gave them time to concentrate upon the larger aspects of association activity, which were medical, not fiscal or political.

Professional interests were uppermost in the minds of the association's members. They were keenly aware that the future of the organization would be determined by the value of its services to industry, to the worker, and to the membership. But such services—the *raison d'être* of the association—were bound to suffer if they were allowed to become secondary to a battle for solvency and the treadmill performance of administrative routine.

Now, in the latter half of the twenties, industrial medicine in America had emerged from what Lyle Hazlett has called the "surgical cycle" and had entered what he describes as the "medical-engineering cycle." It was an era in which the *total environment* of workers assumed its rightful place as the prime factor in the conservation of health.

The accent on problems of membership and finance in the early twenties was justified by circumstances that were difficult to control. Until the association had achieved stability, coherence, and orderly operational procedure, it could not concentrate on the achievement of its medical goals.

Medical men, on the whole, are not noted for financial wizardry, nor for devotion to the humdrum of correspondence and clerical detail. Largely for lack of centralized operation and adequate help, administrative procedures left much to be desired in those formative years. Directors' meetings were held irregularly—if, when, and where expediency dictated. Dates were juggled. There was little long-range planning. Records were a sort of traveling library, which too often failed to travel as administrations changed. Books were audited by committees of doctors, who more than once described the financial situation as "a hell of a mess."

When Loyal Shoudy took over the presidency in 1923 he wrote, rather plaintively, to Sawyer on December 7: "To date I have not heard from Dr. Cranch or anybody concerning anything about the association. Will you please give me Dr. Cranch's address and any other information I should have?" It seems to have been a reasonable request, since Shoudy had already been in office for more than three months. Secretary Sawyer replied on December 17: "I have not turned over the affairs of the association to Dr. Cranch [his successor] as yet, partly because of my inability to get affairs in such shape that they could be turned over."

The annual election at Baltimore in May, 1927, was a vote of confidence in the new turn of affairs under the administrations immediately preceding. T. R. (Tom) Crowder, beloved among the founding pioneers, became president after five consecutive years as a director. Schram, Quinby and Rector were re-elected to the other three top offices. Late in that year Rector was forced by outside commitments to relinquish his duties. For more than five years they were discharged with distinction by his successor, V. S. Cheney.

In the June, 1927, issue of the *Bulletin*—under the title "Growing Up," President Crowder wrote:

> I have no revolutionary policies to propose. Our twelve-year-old association has ceased to be an infant and has become a sturdy youngster. Having successfully passed through the perils of childhood it is beginning now to give service to those who reared it.
>
> Delicate still, perhaps, and not as well nourished as we would like, but growing and full of the promise of progress, challenging our affection and the world's respect.
>
> As the temporary chief of its guardians it is my duty to see that definite growth and increased usefulness are registered during the year.

Reminiscing about Tom Crowder and his services to medicine, Selby comments: "He was seriously handicapped by deafness, but he could always hear the voice of a patient in distress."

There was ample evidence during the remainder of the twenties that the association was indeed growing up and entering a period of rapidly expanding service and increasing prestige.

At the annual meeting in June, 1928, at Minneapolis and at the Mayo Clinic in Rochester, Minnesota, Guy L. Kiefer was elected to the presidency. Climaxing a brilliant career in the Detroit public health service and as medical director of the Michigan Bell Telephone Company, he had been appointed Health Director of the State of Michigan in the preceding year. At the Detroit meeting in May, 1929, C. F. N. Schram succeeded him as president.

Both Kiefer's and Schram's administrations were truly "medical" in purpose and activity. Internal affairs were progressing more smoothly than in any previous period in association history. Years of solid accomplishment in the steady march of industrial medicine lay just ahead, despite the calamitous effects of the 1929 crash and the ensuing depression.

The progress of those years is most clearly understood if considered in terms of the medical "business" discussed at the annual meetings of the twenties, a topic reserved for the following chapter.

XVII

THE SPRINGTIME OF INDUSTRIAL
MEDICINE

THERE is a good deal of mystery, but no magic, in medicine, although popular faith in sundry potions and lotions still survives. An inheritance from darker ages, it will persist as long as there is human credulity in the world. The remaining mysteries of medicine, for the most part, are found in fields that are now being subjected to concentrated study by endowed foundations and by scores of professional and volunteer groups. In our relatively enlightened age they are being resolved, one by one, under the fierce light of research.

Progress in the preservation of human health has been compounded of rapidly growing scientific knowledge, specialized education, "shared" experience, constant trial and some inevitable error, and *organization* geared to sustaining a relentless attack on the multiple conditions that result in ill-health. The pace of progress has been roughly in proportion to recognition of and attention to these factors.

The pioneers of modern industrial medicine in America had few reliable beacons to guide them in their trail-blazing. In the twenties they could only follow a course of action that appeared promising for the attainment of goals that seemed desirable.

The American Association of Industrial Physicians & Surgeons faced many problems never before encountered on a large scale either in general practice or in the field of public health. There was an entirely new relationship to be established between the industries and their medical departments. Management wanted proof that investment in medical facilities was a means to greater productivity and increased earnings. Labor was yet to be convinced that health supervision was neither a paternal gesture nor a conspiracy to ally the doctor on the side of his employer against the workers' interests. It was necessary to make clear to both groups that the area of medical services was a neutral zone in which plant politics had no place.

195

Associations, like individuals, are known by the company they keep. Very early in its history the AAIP&S demonstrated the truth that "names make news." The recognition and respect won by industrial medicine during the first World War were largely due to the professional stature and integrity of the men who espoused its cause and preached its gospel.

While still wrestling with organizational problems in the Twenties, the association began to reach out across the country to attract to its meetings the ablest authorities on industrial medical problems, who could do most to inspire and stimulate the membership, and at the same time extend the influence of the new specialty as a force in the promotion of national health.

There are few, if any, important "trade secrets" in medicine. Life still withholds from the doctor the keys to many of its mysteries, but the doctor shares his knowledge and experience with his fellows to a degree that is almost unique in American business and professional practice. This principle has remained an outstanding characteristic of industrial health activities.

In programming its annual meetings in the twenties the association followed a pattern familiar to millions in the most convention-minded nation on earth. Here was a forum for discussion of all phases of all problems, a place for the free exchange of ideas, the development of plans to improve industrial medical education, the clinical demonstration of medical and surgical techniques. Programs, as often as not, were hurriedly prepared; always they were subject to last-minute revisions and substitutions. More than once the cost of printing the simple four-page leaflets was defrayed by some generous corporation, as an alternative to deficit financing.

Despite small membership, lack of funds, and the difficulty of obtaining men of national reputation to deliver papers on currently significant topics, the AAIP&S displayed an extraordinary vitality during the turbulent twenties. Topics were never trivial. Subject matter was steadily broadened to cover more areas of medical activity. Papers were incisively written and well documented, and they bore directly on mainline problems. Important names began to appear with greater frequency on meeting programs as the years passed.

Compared with today's elaborate joint conferences of the IMA and related organizations, the early conventions were small affairs. Hard-working committees usually managed to obtain from ten to twenty papers dealing authoritatively with problems of current significance and common interest. The total membership of the association in the middle twenties could not have produced enough speakers to meet the program needs of a modern annual meeting.

The importance of any single period in medical history may be measured by two distinct and different yardsticks: first, its contributions to the scientific knowledge available to the profession; and, second, progress made in the practical application of that knowledge for the good of the people. These have been valid indices from the dawn of medicine down to the present; they apply equally to health care in its entirety and to industrial medicine as a special field.

How, from this viewpoint, shall we evaluate industrial medicine in America during the decade of 1920 to 1930? It is safe to say that, by either or both of the above criteria, greater practical progress was made than in any similar preceding period; yet these gains were to be overshadowed by the spectacular advances of succeeding decades.

The twenties will go down in history as an era of notable research in the medically important sciences. The discovery of insulin (1921) was among the monumental milestones of the period. Surgery flourished, too, extending the frontiers of operative treatment, sharpening old skills, developing new techniques, and attracting a host of brilliant young students to the profession. Still, there lay ahead revolutionary advances which, by mid-century, were to raise the curtain on a wholly new world of chemistry, physics, biochemistry, and medicine.

Emerging from the brief postwar depression of 1921, American industry moved steadily forward toward record-breaking totals of production and sales and profits, as mass manufacture and mass distribution methods were applied to an ever lengthening list of commodities. Yet this expansion, fantastic though it seemed at the time, was to be dwarfed in turn by the scale of production prevailing two decades later.

The increasing mechanization of manufacturing processes inevitably brought with it a greater concentration of the working population, larger and larger plants, more and more standardization of processes. Health problems, stemming from the growth of the labor force and the changing conditions under which men worked, assumed new importance. Industrial medicine had outgrown its old status as a first aid expedient available for emergencies; but there were many barriers to be broken through before it could win its rightful place among health agencies.

Experienced physicians and surgeons engaged in active industrial practice were acutely aware of the need for preventive medicine, for environmental safeguards to health above and beyond the safety devices installed to protect machine operators from injury. For years they had crusaded for thorough physical examinations as a condition of employment and a guide in job placement.

Many progressive employers recognized broad-scale medical service as an earmark of good management, an essential factor in profitable production, and a valuable asset in labor relations. Results of their recognition quickly proved the wisdom of their policy. Thousands of corporations, however, were slow to accept the new concepts of industrial medicine and management responsibility. Their medical departments remained little more than glorified first aid stations, headed by men who were medical directors in name only.

Adressing the memorable annual metting of the AAIP&S in Boston in 1921, Dr. William A. Sawyer succinctly summed up the wide differences of viewpoint among industrial executives in these words:

> For our present consideration employers may be grouped into two different classes: (1) Those who are doing the least possible to protect themselves under the law. The large majority of these are those hard-headed men of finance who are "pro-

ducers," not for the sake of the "game," which of course includes the "score," but whose mental processes have but one track—profits. Of course this results in a medical department conducted on a "half-a-loaf" idea. (2) The class which, in spite of the present depression, is growing steadily—those big men of vision and broad mind who maintain maximum standards because the best is such a little way ahead and because they find zest in the chase.[1]

Labor as a whole, in that period, looked at industrial health programs with little interest, a good deal of distrust, and practically no understanding of their economic and social importance.

Workmen's compensation laws, effective in all but four of the forty-eight states by 1921, were far from uniform, full of ambiguities, and open to varying interpretations. Written by non-medical men, they reflected the divergent opinions of politicians and special interests. Disability due to occupational disease was, by and large, noncompensible; and liability in claims involving injury was too often determined by the persuasiveness of attorneys and the whims of juries.

Although compensation laws have been liberally amended and substantially improved in the past thirty years, there are evils still crying for correction, a striking commentary on man's stubborn resistance to major reforms, even in the face of palpable evidence that they are urgently needed.

Judged by such statistics as were then available, the general health of the American people was steadily improving in the early twenties. The editor commented in the January, 1921, issue of *The Nation's Health* that "the year just closed will probably be recorded as the healthiest year in history." Final figures had not yet been released, but the indicated death rate for 1920 was lower than that of 1919 when only 12.87 per thousand of population died, "the lowest death rate ever known for the United States or for any large country in the world."

Over-all mortality statistics, of course, have their values and their uses. In a broad sense they reflect the advances made in medical science, striking a net balance between its successes and its failures in the battle to prolong human life. At best, however, they represent an averaging of aggregate figures on all deaths from all causes. They point to no panaceas and indicate no course of action. They bring little comfort to the physician and certainly lead to no complacency.

Organized industrial medicine, from its beginnings, has sought only one goal—maximum on-the-job protection against accident and disease for all workers in all fields. It has recognized only one way to that goal—unremitting study of industrial health hazards and direct supervision of in-plant medical care and preventive measures. By these means the doctor in industry can make his greatest contribution to that shadowy something we call "the national health."

In every decade of the present century enlightened medical directors have voiced their firm faith in physical examinations as an irreplaceable element in any effective industrial program. As we know, industry-at-large gave ground slowly—and often grudgingly—on this issue in the early years. And long after pre-employ-

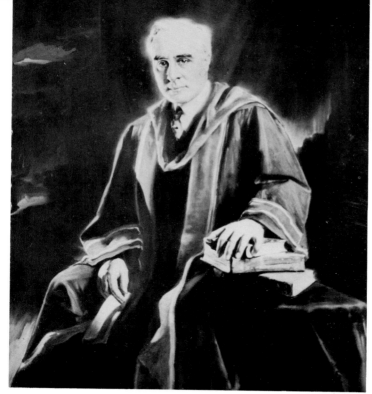

56. *Frederic A. Besley, M.D. (1868–1944).* A guiding force in the broad program launched by the American College of Surgeons in 1926 to raise the standards of surgical and medical service in industry; headed an ACS board which, between 1931 and 1951, surveyed and evaluated 2293 medical departments and certified 1459.

57. *Knudsen and Sloan in a G.M. Plant.* William S. Knudsen (left) and Alfred P. Sloan, Jr. (center) photographed on an inspection tour (circa 1937). Knudsen, then president of General Motors, was the original sponsor of the annual IMA Knudsen Award; Sloan was chairman of the board and a former GM president. Both officials had a great interest in medical service and its values in industry.

—*Courtesy of the General Motors Corporation*

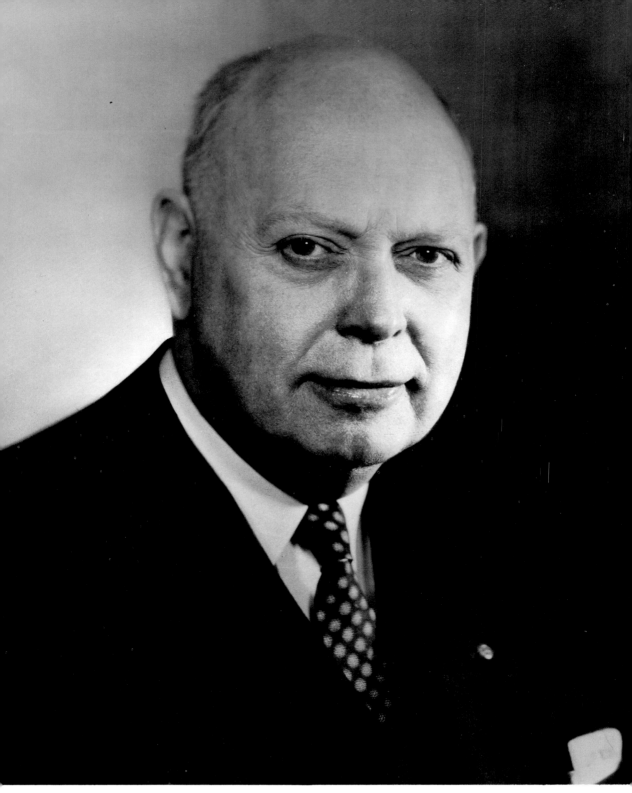

58. *Edward C. Holmblad, M.D.* (1894–). *President, AAIP&S, 1934–1935.* There are few honors within the power of the IMA to bestow that have not been accorded Dr. Holmblad. And it is likely that few members, in any period, have equalled his record in tenure of elective offices within the organization. He has served as vice-president, president, secretary, secretary-treasurer, and member of the History Committee. In 1941 he was elected managing director—on a full-time basis from 1945. Professionally, he conducted a special surgical practice in Chicago, serving the Railway Express Agency and several railroads. He is the author of many technical papers.

—Photo by Fabian Bachrach

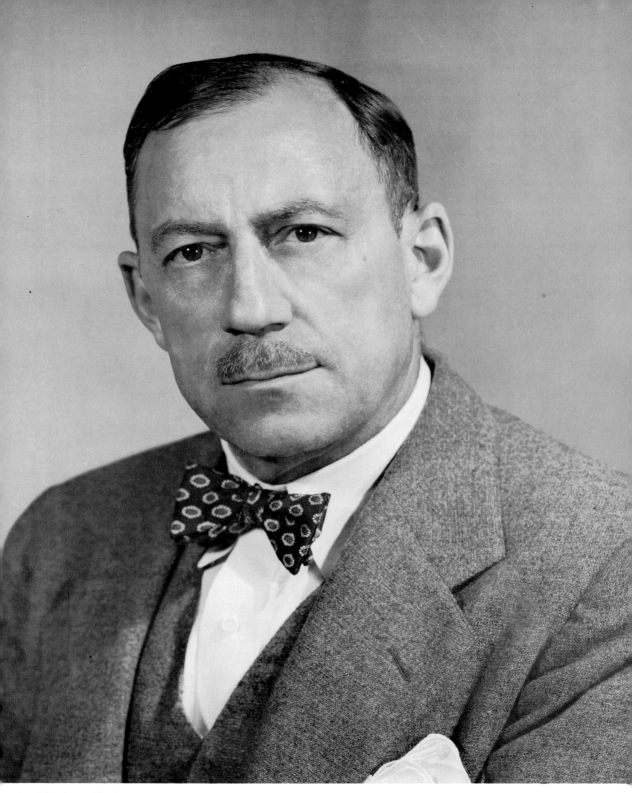

59. *Floyd E. Shaffer, M.D.* (1889–   ). *President, AAIP&S, 1935–1936.* With a medical degree from Johns Hopkins, Shaffer joined the staff of the Bethlehem Steel Company in 1917, serving at both Sparrows Point, Md., and Baltimore, as surgeon in charge of a medical department for 50,000 employees This post he held until the late forties, when he succeeded Loyal Shoudy at the Bethlehem plant. Shaffer's ingrained love of people and close contacts with employees wherever he met them stood him in good stead. His presidential year was a year of rebuilding, and his basic thinking later found expression in the expanding programs of the IMA.

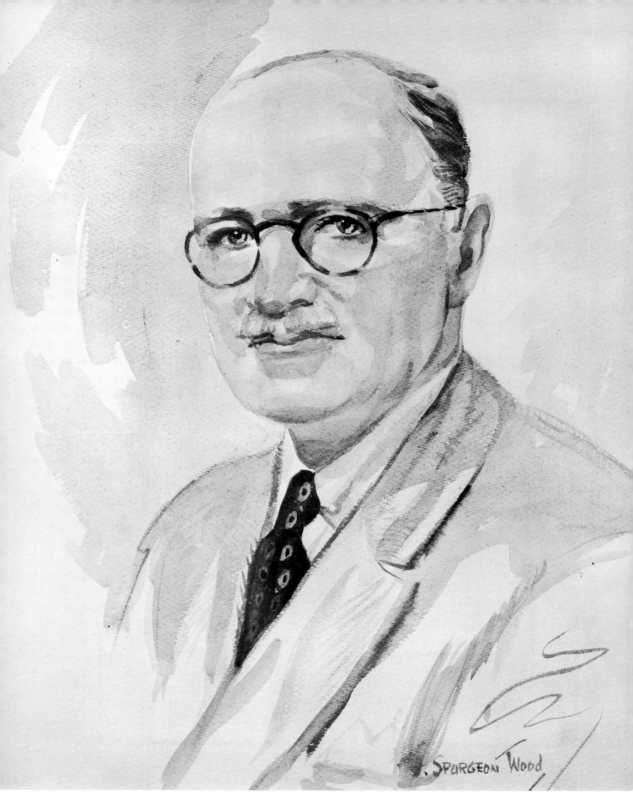

60. *Robert P. Knapp, M.D. (1885–1954). President, AAIP&S, 1936–1937.* Educated at Syracuse University and Columbia University College of Physicians & Surgeons, Knapp conducted a general practice until the United States entered World War I. As a captain in the Medical Corps he spent fifteen months in France and nine months later in the states. In 1920 he started a special practice in industrial medicine and traumatic surgery and launched a long association with Cheney Brothers (Manchester, Connecticut) as medical director. In office, Knapp did much to speed AAIP&S postdepression recovery. His writings include papers on health problems of the textile industry.

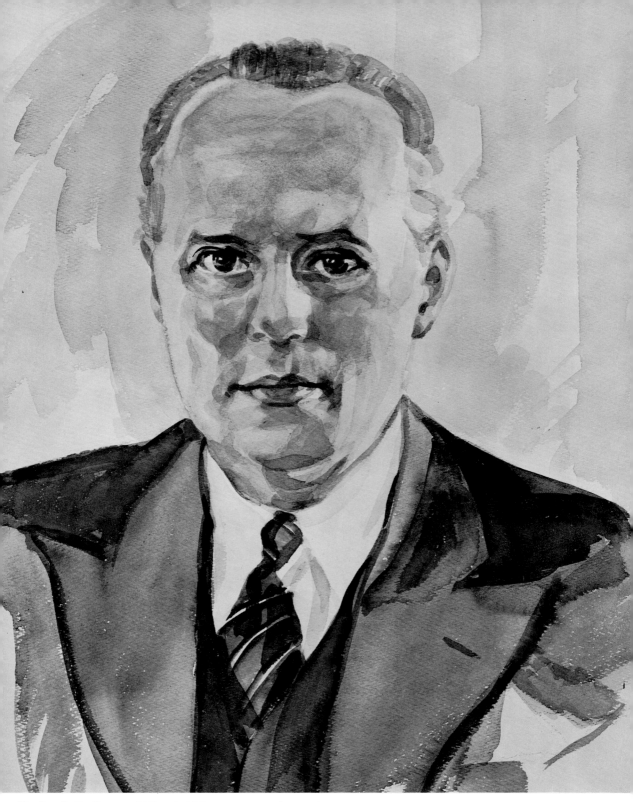

61. *Royd R. Sayers, M.D. (1885–   ). President, AAIP&S, 1937–1938.* Royd Sayers has been a man of many careers in the broad area embracing public and industrial health. From his first post in the United States Bureau of Mines (1920) he rose to become its director in 1940. He is a medical director (retired) of the United States Public Health Service and in late years served Baltimore as senior supervisor of occupational diseases. His committee assignments have been many, including several at high government level. As AAIP&S president, he was largely concerned with expansion and financing. The scope of his interests is reflected in some 200 published papers.

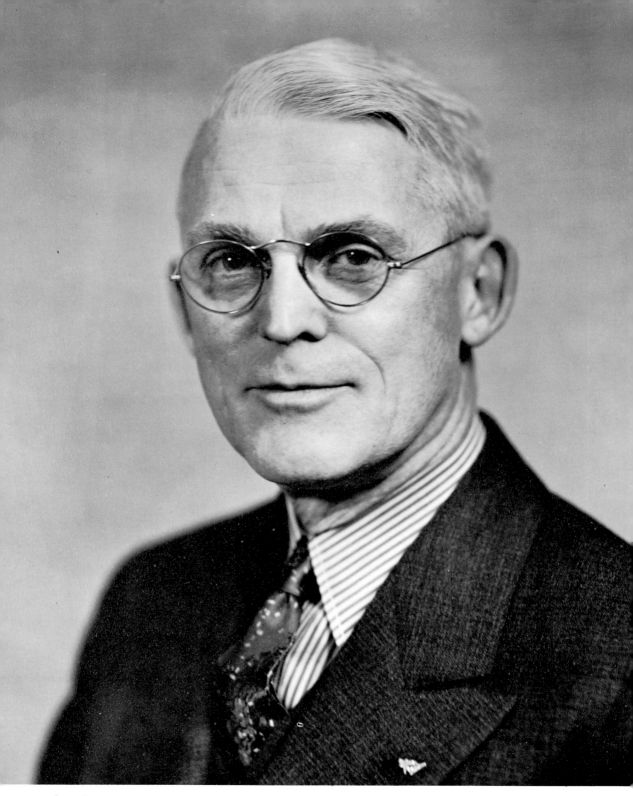

62. *Clarence D. Selby, M.D.* (1878–   ). *President, AAIP&S, 1938–1939.* Completing a hospital residency in Cleveland, Selby studied thyroid pathology as an assistant to Dr. G. W. Crile; then, in 1905, he moved to Toledo to establish an industrial medical practice. This was the first step in a career that culminated in his appointment as medical consultant to the General Motors Corporation. In 1917 he was called to Washington for special work on wartime industrial health programs, reported in his famous *USPHS Bulletin No. 99.* Manpower problems occupied him in World War II. As AAIP&S president he worked unceasingly for certification of the specialty.

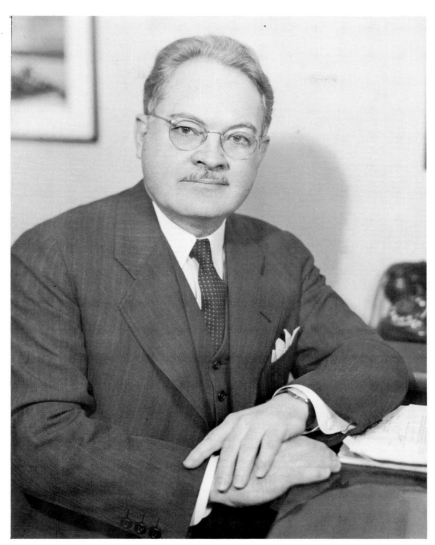

63. *Clarence O. Sappington, M.D.* A noted consultant in occupational diseases and industrial medicine, he contributed much to the literature of the specialty, and served as editor of *Industrial Medicine and Surgery* until his death.

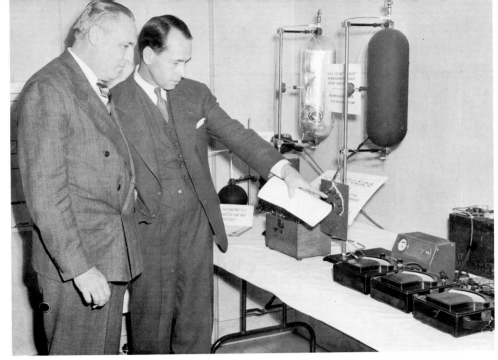

64. *Heat Study Apparatus.* Modern occupational medicine is concerned with the total environment of workers and focuses attention on all physiological factors. Here Drs. L. E. Hamlin, American Brakeshoe Company, and Dudley A. Irwin, Aluminum Company of America, examine apparatus used in heat studies.

65. *Testing Eyesight.* Visual evaluation in the eye examination room of a modern plant, the Boeing Aircraft Company.

—Courtesy of the Boeing Medical Department

66. *Mass Audiometry.* A quiet room for screening in mass audiometry at the Boeing Aircraft Company.

—Courtesy of the Boeing Medical Department

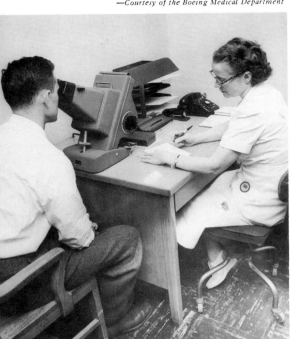

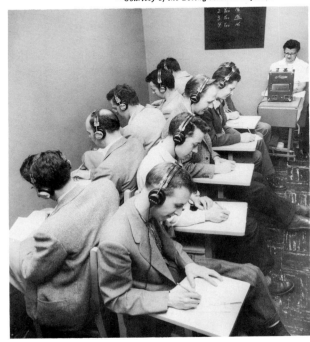

ment examinations had become routine procedure in the larger concerns, a growing demand for periodic examination of all workers in major industries met with similar resistance. Public and private discussion of this topic was at its height during the 1920's.

It was not difficult to demonstrate the need for more thorough and more frequent health inspections, particularly among employees handling metallic alloys and chemical compounds known to be, or suspected of being, toxic agents. Each year, in one industry or another, reliable surveys added new evidence to support the stand taken by medical men. Examinations of large groups of workers invariably disclosed an alarmingly high incidence of serious ailments, in acute or incipient stages, which had gone undetected and unreported. Nor was there any lack of proof that systematic re-examination at regular intervals paid off handsomely in practical benefits to management, to labor, and to the public health services. Case histories, maintained over long periods, were a source of valuable statistics for insurance companies, boards of health, and civilian and military agencies at the federal level. They were vitally necessary to the effective control of communicable diseases. Management frequently found the absence of such records a crippling disadvantage in defending compensation cases. It was apparent, finally, that without periodic examinations on a country-wide scale the practice of true preventive medicine could never become a reality.

Writing in *The Nation's Health* in 1921, Eugene L. Fisk, medical director of the Life Insurance Institute, New York City, declared that fully 50 percent of the working population of the country were in need of important medical or physical attention. His estimate probably erred, if at all, on the side of conservatism.[2]

In an illuminating paper read at the annual meeting of the AAIP&S two years later, George M. Price, director of the Union Health Center, New York City, stressed the high percentage of defects discovered in the examination of fifty thousand garment workers, and emphasized the need of constructive educational work.[3] The Center, founded twenty years previously, was a pioneer project in the field of union-sponsored health plans; its accumulated experience was probably unmatched at the time by any other organization. Price declared that, of all the service measures adopted during that period, the medical and dental dispensaries alone remained.

At this same meeting Daniel C. O'Neil, representing the medical department of the Endicott-Johnson Company, Binghampton, New York, discussed in detail the experience of that organization. Endicott-Johnson was one of the first employers in the country to provide a medical staff and full medical care for workers and their families. Its sixteen thousand employees, in 1922, produced thirty-two million pairs of shoes. The $400,000 cost of the medical program, said Dr. O'Neil, was charged not against wages, but against production. Here was further recognition of the fact that industrial medical services paid their own way in increased production per man-hour.[4]

Philadelphia, steeped in medical tradition and rich in prominent medical figures, was host to the association in 1926. Featured on the three-day program were important clinics at the University Hospital, conducted by Charles Frazier and staff of the Department of Surgery, and Alfred Stengel and staff of the Department of Medicine.

In that setting, at the mid-point of the decade, George M. Piersol, eminent Philadelphia physician and medical director of the Bell Telephone Company of Pennsylvania, delivered the address of welcome, the meat of which was a powerful plea for *compulsory* periodic examinations. His line of argument is one familiar to all present-day industrial specialists, but it deserves some quotation if only to record a revealing commentary on the status of industrial medicine at the time.

> By periodic examinations disease in its incipiency can be recognized and proper steps instituted to cure or control it before it has been allowed to go on to the point where the worker is incapacitated and becomes a charge on the employer or the community. Latent infections, notably pulmonary tuberculosis, are discovered. Sources of focal infection are unearthed and can be removed before they have caused serious damage. Numerous remedial defects can be corrected. When the health of a worker is being broken down because he or she is laboring at unsuitable work, the fact is brought to light, and a readjustment of the work can be brought about before serious impairment of efficiency has occurred. Those who are physically or morally dangerous to their fellow workmen can be removed.
>
> The existence of many factors of industrial origin that are detrimental to the health of the workers is discovered, and steps can be taken for their control. In short, the plan offers the most effective method of conserving health and of preventing disease among our workers. Yet, in how few industries has it been adopted?
>
> It is not too much to say that industrial physicians generally favor more or less compulsory periodic health examinations. Up to this time, however, we have failed to impress sufficiently the directors of industry with their importance. This is a piece of missionary work with which we should charge ourselves.
>
> The objections to these periodic examinations are based upon several reasons, the most important of which are: the time they require and the consequent interference with the routine of work; the danger of focusing the attention of susceptible employees upon their health, thereby creating in them troublesome psychoneuroses; and, the most important, the cost of such examinations to industry.[5]

Piersol's appeal was addressed alike to management, to labor, and to industrial medical specialists on the ground that an agreement on basic policies, and concerted action to effect more enlightened examination procedures, would serve *self-interests* common to all three groups while imposing unfair penalties on none.

As late as 1929 C. F. N. Schram, in his acceptance speech as incoming president of the AAIP&S, commented on the improvement in the national health as indicated by the continued decline of mortality rates but deplored the slow progress of industrial medicine.[6] His talk was, in effect, a warning to the complacent few that actual health conditions in industry can be ascertained only through close-range, *in-plant* study by qualified doctors and are not to be inferred from over-all morbidity or mortality rates.

Frequently heard in the twenties were statements that some six to eight million workers were currently covered by medical supervision and care *of one sort or another*. The figures may or may not have been accurate; the catch, of course, was in the last five words. Judged by such an elastic measuring stick, a department consisting of one part-time physician or surgeon and a nurse or two found itself under the same blanket as a fully staffed, well-equipped department operating at peak efficiency.

Such inequalities were to be expected. There was no certification of medical departments based on scope and quality of services, no honor roll reserved as a mark of distinction for plants meeting or surpassing standardized official requirements. Certification of approved departments was to come in the 1930's. It was an outgrowth of monumental studies by the American College of Surgeons, and it has probably done more to upgrade the quality of industrial practice than any other single factor.

Lest it appear that the physical examination of workers and the standards of practice in medical departments were stressed beyond their importance by the association during the twenties, it must be remembered that the growth and influence of industrial medicine in America depended very largely upon these two factors. Without thorough physical examinations at reasonable intervals, the major medical discoveries of that decade could not have borne fruit at the shop level for the treatment and prevention of many industrial diseases. Without proper staffing and organization at the administrative level, the supervision of medical service in industry might well have passed into other hands.

Tracing the progress of industrial medicine since 1900, Robert T. Legge singles out research on lead poisoning, one of the oldest of recognized occupational diseases, as an outstanding medical achievement of the twenties. "Prior to the twentieth century," he points out, "the published works of Tanquerel, the great French investigator, contained all that was known about the subject before him and in the nineteenth century as well."[7]

Legge pays high tribute to Alice Hamilton, America's first distinguished woman physician, toxicologist, and investigator of occupational diseases. "Through her devoted and tireless surveys and researches in the principal lead industries," he writes, "she laid down the principles of preventive medicine as applied to industry. . . .

"It was through her efforts that a manufacturer of white lead was induced to endow a research project at Harvard University on the action of lead in the human body. This made possible the distinguished studies of lead poisoning by Dr. Jacob Aub and his colleagues."

As the first woman professor on the Harvard faculty, Alice Hamilton in the

1920's followed up her early pioneer work in industrial toxicology with further investigations of lead ether, and trinitrotoluol and benzol poisoning, and published penetrating studies of the hazards of the fur and felt, storage battery, and enamelware industries.

On the heels of the Harvard project came new and revolutionary findings by Robert A. Kehoe, of the University of Cincinnati, famous for his painstaking laboratory researches in the physiology and toxicology of lead absorption and lead poisoning.

In the same period Carey P. McCord won national prominence as an authority on many phases of industrial medicine and hygiene. A graduate of the University of Michigan Medical School and a colonel in the Army Medical Reserve Corps, he served in responsible posts throughout the first World War, returning to private practice in 1919. Research scientist, teacher, author and editor, he has served over the years as a consultant for industries, state and federal health agencies, and industrial and labor organizations. His contributions to the profession include major laboratory investigations in industrial toxicology, and the discovery of several occupational diseases previously unrecognized. Attesting his versatility and the breadth of his medical interests are numerous books and hundreds of articles on subjects ranging from skin diseases and various types of organic poisoning to industrial fatigue and medical economics. Throughout his career his work has been inseparably linked to the activities and progress of the Industrial Medical Association.

Among others cited by Legge for significant research in the field of plumbism during the 1920's were Emery R. Hayhurst, eminent Ohio educator, scientist and author, and May R. Mayers, an assistant in industrial medicine in the Harvard School of Public Health and a member of the Committee on Lead Poisoning of the American Public Health Association, which contributed importantly to contemporary knowledge of that hazard.

Lead had been under medical observation for centuries, a persistent menace to the health of all who worked with it. Lead poisoning had produced a more extensive literature, in all probability, than any other comparable toxic agent. But for all this prodigal expenditure of time, study, and words, little real progress toward complete control of the disease had been made prior to the 1920's.

The renaissance of interest in lead poisoning was spurred by an abnormal incidence of cases in the automobile industry. With the improvement of mass production methods and the rocketing upswing of motor-car manufacture, great quantities of de-greasing compounds came into use for the cleaning of machined parts. The resulting outbreak of tetraethyl lead poisoning, widely publicized at the time, underscored the lack of adequate safeguards. Thus does the evolution of the Machine Age constantly create new hazards for workers and pose new problems for medicine.

This sudden recurrence of lead cases offers a perfect example of the tenuous connection between a given industrial health hazard and the resulting national mortality statistics. A complete analysis by Frederick L. Hoffman, consulting statistician of the Prudential Life Insurance Company, showed that the death rate from chronic lead poisoning in the United States had gradually declined "from 2.5 percent (of total cases in the report) to 1.4 percent in 1924, with slight rises in 1913, 1916, 1919, and 1921."[8] Hoffman credited this improvement to efforts in the direction of "improving factory and workshop hygiene on the one hand and the personal hygiene of the worker on the other." Commenting on these figures, the *AAIP&S Bulletin* stated: "Important to note is the considerable proportion of deaths that were non-industrial or not connected directly with lead-using industries."

Just how many deaths ultimately resulted from tetraethyl poisoning contracted in the twenties will never be known. In any event they would be spread over a period of many years and could cause only slight variations in mortality rates in that category. Nevertheless, the outbreak was of major concern to workers involved and to the employers and physicians responsible for their health. And, beyond doubt, the new outbreak was a further spur to research on lead and other toxic substances used in industry.

In the same period the spotlight of science was focused on another ancient enemy —dust. More than two centuries earlier, Ramazzini had detailed his observations on the hazard encountered by stonecutters, quarrymen, miners and other workers in the dusty trades. He reported the finding of "piles of sand" in the lungs of "asthma" victims and warned stonecutters "to be as careful as possible not to breathe in those minute fragments by mouth."[9]

The causes of the dust diseases have long been understood and their clinical symptoms generally recognized. Yet the widespread use of pneumatic rock drills, plus greatly increased employment in mining and rock-tunnel projects, brought about a sharp rise in the incidence of silicosis, which made new preventive measures imperative. The word "silicosis" itself became part of the vocabulary of the average laymen, as manufacturers advertised improved ventilating systems to replace outmoded equipment.

It was in 1924 that newspaper headlines blared the tragic story of radium poisoning among the watch dial painters. The victims were relatively few, and in a comparatively small industry, but this was one of the earliest warnings that nature had in store for mankind a menace which could threaten the very existence of life on our planet.

Thirty years later, in the summer of 1954, alert news editors in many a large city raised the ghost of this industrial-medical tragedy which had slumbered in fading memories and undisturbed newspaper files. The specter paraded in feature stories dramatized from a brief telegraph dispatch announcing the death of one Ruth Mary Williams, aged forty-eight, in an Illinois hospital. The story, in *The Detroit News,* bore this headline:

LAST SURVIVOR OF HORROR GONE
Agonizing Deaths of "Radium Girls"[10]

Mrs. Williams could not have been much over eighteen years old when the story began. She was one of many girls and young women employed, in the mid-twenties, to paint the luminous numbers on watch and clock dials in Ottawa, Illinois, and East Orange, New Jersey, plants. It was pleasant but exacting work. They dipped their delicate brushes in zinc sulphide, and "pointed" them with their lips before painting in the figures. There seems to be no record showing exactly how many of these workers died of radium necrosis and accompanying complications as a result of this practice. The victims probably numbered several score. How many escaped with light infections, or none at all, will never be known.

Radium poisoning, in these cases, destroyed oral tissue, teeth, and bones and attacked the entire skeletal structure. The initial necrosis came to be known as "radium jaw"; the sufferers dubbed themselves "The Society of the Living Dead." Most of the victims, according to *The News,* died before they were thirty, though some hung on until they were forty.

The facts, widely publicized by the press in 1924, shocked the nation. The victims were relatively few, but the manner of their death and the terrible implications of the hazard created a storm of indignation. The term "radium jaw" recalled "phossy jaw" and the outbreak of phosphorus poisoning in the match industry many years before. The watch dial tragedy was another commentary on the perverse nature of man, who so often ignores known hazards until he is aroused to action by public clamor.

The Curies may have realized that radium, the friend of medicine, was also a potential killer. Yet they handled radioactive substances as casually as they would have handled lumps of inert ore. Pierre, until his death in a street accident in 1906, suffered "attacks of pain, of intolerable violence, in the legs."[11] Mme. Curie breathed noisome fumes from her retorts for thirty-five years. Her arms and hands were frequently burned by exposures. Marie died on July 4, 1934, of aplastic pernicious anemia, but the diagnosis was made postmortem. "Mme. Curie," wrote the examiner, "can be counted among the eventual victims of the radioactive bodies which she and her husband discovered."[12] Her ailment, up to that time, had been diagnosed as *la grippe* or bronchitis. Irène Joliot-Curie, elder daughter of Marie, and herself a Nobel Prize winner, died in March, 1956, reportedly of leukemia from handling radioactive materials, a tragic repetition of her mother's fate.

The medical press of the twenties carried surprisingly little comment on the tragedy of the dial painters. An article on radium necrosis, in the *Journal of the American Medical Association* in 1925 described the cases and declared radio-active zinc sulphide to be the "probably" causative element.[13] Another paper appeared later in the same year, dealing with the unrecognized dangers of handling radio-active materials.[14]

Science, however, was spurred to immediate activity in this field of research. Private and governmental agencies united in surveys to discover the safe limits of exposure in mines, laboratories, and manufacturing plants. Protective measures were promptly devised.

Unlike phosphorous, radioactivity reappeared on the scene, as a world-wide menace, after Hiroshima and Nagasaki. In this atomic age it is "fall-out" and other forms of contamination that haunt the dreams of physicists and physiologists. Will mankind, this time, heed the warnings?

The grim statistics on silicosis and lead and radium poisoning in the twenties were medical signs of the times, incidents in the onward march of the Machine Age, heralding an even greater concentration of industrial population and proclaiming the need for a re-examination of some of the basic tenets of what may conveniently be called "mass medicine."

Before the 1920's the recognition of occupational hazards in most industrial medical departments was based on the actual occurrence of disease; the number and severity of cases determined the course of action. In other words, a health hazard did not officially exist until it had taken an appreciable toll in sickness and lost time among workers.

This concept was no longer adequate. The need was for a new approach, its goal the control and eventual prevention of disease resulting directly from the conditions of employment. The elimination of phosphorus poisoning in the match industry, some fifteen years earlier, was the classic example of what could be accomplished in that direction.

Physiology, as a science, developed rapidly in the 1920's. Its progress had been held up for hundreds of years, awaiting improvements in microscopy, the use of colors in staining bacterial organisms, and the revolutionary research of Ehrlich, Koch, Pasteur and other "greats" in the latter half of the nineteenth century.

In 1893 a book which drew heavily upon the then new findings of those pioneers was published by a prominent American physician, James T. Whittaker, a lecturer on clinical medicine and professor of the theory and practice of medicine in the Medical College of Ohio.[15] He was the first American to study under Koch, and his work was dedicated, by permission, to the master. He was also one of the first to bring to this country cultures of tubercle bacilli from the Koch laboratories. The preface to his book, a weighty tome prepared for medical students and practitioners, contains this challenging statement: "The practitioner who looks up from the signs and lesions to the cause will entertain more hope of treatment; for the practice of medicine is now not so empirical as the symptomatologists claim, or so barren as the pathologists deplore."

205

Whittaker's text strongly reflects the influence of Koch's thinking. Pathogenic microorganisms, he declares, act in two ways: by intoxication and by infection. His discussion of bacteria, and his handling of lead poisoning and other forms of toxicology, represented concepts of physiology that were new in his period.

The time was ripe for further research designed to trace the reactions and changes produced in human bodies by the absorption of toxic substances. Lead poisoning was an ideal guinea pig for use in these studies, because of the wealth of historical and clinical data available on the subject.

Armed with modern techniques and improved laboratory equipment, the pioneering physiologists of the period were able to chart the behavior of lead ingested through the respiratory and gastrointestinal tracts, to measure accurately the degree of harmful absorption, to check the effects on normal bodily functions, and thus establish the *safe limits of exposure*. Once those limits were known, it was possible to detect the weak links in the chain of defense against the toxic hazard. Studies of the working environment and manufacturing processes indicated the points at which dangerous exposure was most likely to occur. There remained, then, the practical problem of devising safeguards that would keep exposure below a normal and safe level, the final step leading to control, and prevention.

The full importance of the work of Aub, Kehoe, and their contemporaries was not immediately apparent. Their specific target was lead poisoning, but the new and improved methodology developed in their research was equally well adapted to the study of a large group of kindred hazards created by metals and compounds commonly used in industry.

Herein, it would seem, lies the chief significance of the 1920's as a chapter in the history of American industrial medicine. From the research of that period emerged a new scientific approach not only to toxic hazards but to the entire problem of industrial health. By the middle of the decade industrial medicine was passing from the so-called *surgical* cycle, and entering the *medical engineering* cycle.[16]

Physicians, hygienists, and safety engineers were beginning to look at the whole man and his total working environment in their attack on occupational disease. With this look came the first real recognition of industrial hygiene as a specialty in itself, a prelude to its spectacular progress in the next two decades.

The lead investigations were, for the most part, carried out in university laboratories and by university personnel. Their findings were promptly incorporated in medical school curricula, and were thus integrated in the training of successive classes of medical students.

The results of this and other collateral research proved to be of incalculable value in later periods, when hundreds of thousands of new alloys and chemical compounds, a large proportion of them toxic to some degree, made their appearance in basic manufacturing industries. Years of evaluation and education were to elapse, however, before the fruits of these studies could be passed on to industry, another example of the inevitable lag between scientific discoveries and their application in medical practice.

Some of the most conspicuous trends in twentieth century industrial medicine were not even foreseeable in the twenties. Many industrial health hazards, of great importance today, did not exist in that period. Others were not recognized or had not yet come within the scope of preventive planning. The strictly medical problems of the time were simple, indeed, compared with those that now confront the physician in industry.

Trends, however, were in the making, and could be read by shrewd observers. Early in 1921 Louis I. Dublin, noted medical statistician and consultant on health and welfare, discussing his work on occupational hazards and diagnostic signs, was able to declare confidently: "A great need of development along the lines of industrial toxicology is anticipated in this compilation,"[17] i.e., his article.

It is not disparagement of the profession to say that the rank and file of industrial physicians at that time had little specialized knowledge of metal poisoning, silicosis, or the multiple forms of dermatitis in the manufacturing trades. Relatively few medical directors had had the opportunity of studying these diseases at close range among large groups of workers. Periodic physical examinations were the exception rather than the rule; nor were procedures uniform. Morbidity statistics were meager and not altogether trustworthy.

Beginning in 1921, procedures at annual meetings of the AAIP&S wore a new look. In that year, at Harvard Medical School, more than a score of speakers, prominent in medicine and industry, were on the program. Papers and discussions covered a far wider range than ever before. It is interesting to note that policies and activities of the association through the remainder of the decade followed closely the plan outlined by C. E. Ford soon after his election to the presidency at that convention.[18]

Aside from committee reports, nearly 150 speakers are listed on annual meeting programs from 1920 to 1930. Of subjects covered, well over half dealt with special techniques that had proved successful in the day-to-day course of industrial practice. Of the papers and discussions in this category, fully 40 percent were devoted to trauma and related topics, including safety and first aid. By contrast, only two addresses were on silicosis and other dust diseases, only two on dermatoses, and one on toxicology—a treatise on carbon-monoxide poisoning. This is not surprising. The emphasis in industrial health care was still upon accident prevention. The new physiological doctrines had not emerged from the research stage. Existing laws provided little or no compensation for disabilities due to disease. The practice of medical directors was predominantly surgical in most industrial plants.

If the topics discussed at annual meetings may be taken as a criterion, fractures, sprains, dislocations and other injuries to joints ranked high on the list of traumatic cases in the twenties. Also, nationally known authorities discussed the more general aspects of industrial surgery. Association literature in this decade, moreover, covers a varied miscellany of medical and non-medical subjects, fully representative of the interests of its members. It must be remembered that the AAIP&S, like industrial medicine itself, was in a period of transition. The twenties were a bridge between an old and a new era.

In an effort to define accurately the status and scope of the specialty, its responsibilities and its limitations, the association at its annual meetings debated vigorously such matters as its proper relation to public health, safety engineering, hygiene and sanitation, the old problem of contract versus private practice, the education and training of industrial physicians and surgeons.

For the first time, nutrition and the diet of workers, industrial dentistry and nursing were accorded some prominence in convention proceedings. The progress of preventive medicine, group insurance, compensation, and medicolegal procedures received due attention. Electro- and physiotherapy, moot questions in the twenties, were in the limelight from time to time. Branded as quackery by some and stoutly espoused by others, these forms of treatment were frankly discussed without prejudice. However, the content of many significant addresses is left to us only in the form of titles that are not overly descriptive.

XVIII

MEDICAL PIONEERS OF THE
TWENTIES

Browsing through the medical records and literature of a bygone day is a rewarding experience, even for those whose interest in medicine is nonprofessional. Personal and official correspondence, yellowed by the years, is rich in human interest. Published papers reflect the scientific and medical thinking of their period; they yield sidelights on notable personalities and references well worth preserving, which otherwise would be buried forever in dusty files. Particularly is this true of industrial medicine in the 1920's. Its exponents—practitioners, teachers, administrators—had little time or thought to spend for the edification of future generations. Their task was to make a place for industrial medicine in history rather than to record the making for posterity.

Though its membership was at low ebb in the twenties, the American Association of Industrial Physicians & Surgeons was the only organization *fully* representative of the new specialty. Its voice was the official voice of industrial medicine in America. Its history is the history of industrial medicine, and *vice versa.*

Wisely, the association devoted the major share of its public pronouncements and papers to the instruction of physicians in the industrial aspects of medicine and surgery, which throughout the twenties were still in the early stages of definition. Even more wisely, it consistently called upon medical educators of the foremost rank to address its annual meetings, a fact which bespoke the interest of the medical schools in industrial problems and strengthened the prestige and influence of the association.

At the annual meeting in St. Louis, in 1922, a thirty-six-year-old specialist from Boston delivered a paper dealing with the problem of heart disease in industry, in

209

which he stressed the statement that heart infections, rather than occupations, were the cause of cardiac symptoms. The speaker, though not widely known outside the profession, was chief of the Outpatient Department and in charge of the Cardiac Clinic at Massachusetts General Hospital. He was recognized later as an outstanding authority on cardiology, and made notable contributions to the study of surgery in connection with hypertension. His talk aroused so much interest that the text was printed in the September, 1922, issue of *The Nation's Health,* then the official publication of the association.

In September, 1955, this specialist became, overnight, an international celebrity, his name headlined on front pages around the world. He was Dr. Paul Dudley White, who was flown from his teaching post at Harvard Medical School to the bedside of President Eisenhower to take charge of the most newsworthy medical case in contemporary history.[1]

Among red-letter dates in this calendar of the twenties were the frequent occasions when important medical centers graciously played host to the association at its annual meetings. Then, as now, staff physicians and surgeons teamed up to give their visitors the full benefit of their skill and experience, with the latest and finest facilities available for a memorable series of clinics, symposiums, and roundtable discussions. This was medical education and demonstration at their best.

Representative of the caliber of medical school personnel appearing on the programs of that period are the following: at New Orleans (1920), J. A. Watkins, from the staff of the University of Cincinnati; at Harvard Medical School (1921), Cecil K. Drinker, of the Department of Industrial Hygiene, managing editor of the *Journal of Industrial Hygiene;* at Washington University Medical School, St. Louis (1922), George W. Crile, famed Cleveland surgeon, then professor of surgery at Western Reserve Medical School, and R. Tunstall Taylor, professor of orthopedics at Johns Hopkins; in Chicago (1924), N. C. Gilbert, assistant professor of medicine at Northwestern University; at Atlantic City (1925), John J. Moorhead, professor of surgery, Postgraduate Medical School and Hospital, New York; at University of Pennsylvania Hospital (1926), Charles Frazier, Alfred Stengel, and other staff members; at Johns Hopkins (1927), staff members representing all major departments of the school; at the Mayo Clinic, Rochester, Minnesota (1928), William J. Mayo, W. H. Meyerding, associate chief of orthopedic surgery, Mayo Foundation, and other staff members.

How shall we describe that fantastic decade between 1920 and 1930? It was an era of anomaly and contradiction, like no other in the nation's history. It opened with a sharp, but brief, depression, closed with a market crash and financial collapse without equals in their impact on world events. "Back to normalcy" was the political slogan of those years, but there was no normalcy. It was the era that spawned the Charleston and sent a wave of jazz music rolling across the continent. It was the era of prohibition; but millions, having helped to vote the Twentieth Amendment into law, promptly sought to circumvent its provisions, and opened the door to bootlegging and gangsterism. The mad, exciting, unpredictable, wonderful twenties! Like the Gay Nineties they are remembered, by many who worked through them and lived at their pace, with nostalgia and affection, and some dismay.

Economically, the period is memorable for the boom in national production that built up steadily from an initial depression and reached a level never before achieved in this or any other land. Writing in his *Economic History of the United States,* Edward F. Humphrey, professor of history and political science at Trinity College, calls attention to the continuing rise in prices after World War I, and comments: "Home consumption soared, since the end of the war brought a riot of extravagance."[2] The symptom is familiar to all who recognize inflationary signs. In this instance, spending was attended by uncontrolled speculation—a sign of more tragic things to come.

Under the surface froth and apparent heedlessness of life then, one sees another picture, the picture of a people striving soberly to lift their productivity to a permanently higher level, a step closer to a destiny that is unknown because it has no prototype in history.

This colorful period may be judged, in part, by its mistakes and its excesses; but it surely is entitled to be measured in terms of the tremendous contributions it made to science and research, to the techniques of production and distribution, to medicine in general and to the consolidation of gains in the special field of industrial medicine.

*   *   *

Relatively little has ween written about the place of the professional nurse in industrial medicine during the formative years of the AAIP&S, not because she was unimportant but because her duties had not yet been clearly defined and because plant practices were far from uniform. The subject was brought into sharp focus by William A. Sawyer, of the Eastman Kodak Company, in a challenging address at the 1921 annual meeting. The title and subtitle are descriptive: "Nurses in the Guise of Industrial Physicians—The Nurse's Whole Authority Is the Physician's Order; Nursing Care Is Not Medical Service." Sawyer handled the problem with customary candor, sparing neither management nor medicine in his criticism. His paper evoked widespread discussion. Its importance lies in the fact that, by restating basic truths, it may have been the means of averting a condition which might have permanently compromised the position of organized medicine in industry. Prominently displayed beneath the title in the *Nation's Health* version are these paragraphs, quoted here because they are as applicable today as they were when written:

> Laws did not create the need of medical service to industry. Neither does obeying the letter of the law meet its requirements. Its limitations are set, not by penny-wise and pound-foolish employers, but by industrial physicians themselves.
>
> Here as elsewhere failure follows a low estimate of the problem. No specialist is confronted by greater complexities of a medical nature than those of the industrial

physician. The science of industrial medicine is yet to evolve, but it is in process, and the future is to the honest-to-goodness worker who neglects none of his tasks and delegates none of his responsibilities.

Sawyer summed up the problem in these words:

> About a month ago I received from a physician, unknown to me, the following letter—"I see that you are to read a paper before the American Association of Industrial Physicians & Surgeons in Boston, on 'Nurses in the Guise of Industrial Physicians.' As I have been visiting many plants and stores, perhaps I can give you some information on the subject.
>
> "Recently I have visited places where formerly a physician had charge of the medical work and now a trained nurse is in charge. In a certain city there is a doctor who trains nurses to do industrial work, even teaching them how to give a physical examination. At the factory where I formerly had charge of all the medical work, the superintendent hired a trained nurse to do the work when I left. The reason given was that nurses can be hired much cheaper than any doctor.
>
> "If physicians do not watch out, nurses will supersede them in medical work in industrial plants, for more and more concerns are getting rid of their doctors. What can be done about it?"
>
> There is a real dilemma apparent in this phase of the industrial crisis. Fearful for the status of industrial medicine, one group of critics tells us of nurses disguised as physicians who are about to occupy the field, while a "rosier spectacle" contingent offers equally extravagant praise for achievements made and for work projected. While all this discussion pro and con is going on, some of us are more than dubious as to the future of industrial medicine.

In his own observation of medical practices in departments of varying sizes and types, Sawyer found many instances in which nurses were performing certain functions not ordinarily allotted to a nurse. "This," he declared, "may be justified up to a certain limit. If a medical department in industry is to care for all emergency illnesses, it is necessary in the present stage of evolution that a nurse care for such proportion of these cases as standing orders and constant supervision will justify."

But he continued: "We are obviously shortsighted if in turning over the superfluity of cases to the nurse we feel satisfied that this local, or at best superficial, alleviation is getting industrial medicine very far along the road to its maximum usefulness. . . . We cannot afford to forget that we are identified *as a class,* whether we wish it or not. What industrial medicine is to become depends upon our efforts and collective personality as industrial physicians."

Speaking of the dispensing of medicine by nurses for certain superficial ailments, Sawyer commented: "Please note that I said 'dispensing,' not 'prescribing.' I consider that if the doctor in charge prepared signed orders regarding such emergencies as a nurse may safely care for, he has done the prescribing in blanket form and all the nurse does is to carry out his orders. That is all any nurse is qualified to do—*carry out the orders* of the physician in charge, thereby safeguarding herself and the department, as well as the employee."

Elementary and axiomatic? Yes. But at the time the line was seldom clearly drawn, and when drawn was often ignored. From continued emphasis on first principles, from insistence on strictly ethical procedures, the codes that now govern nursing in industry have evolved, and the present position of dignity and responsibility enjoyed by industrial nurses has emerged.

* * *

It was in the twenties, too, that dentistry received its first real recognition as an industrial specialty. The importance of oral hygiene as a factor in general health was, of course, thoroughly understood, as was the need for dental prophylaxis. There was far less agreement as to industry's responsibility for dental health and the extent to which oral examination and treatment should be included in plant medical service. Many employers had experimented in many ways with dental programs, but there had been little open discussion of the problem, and few clear-cut conclusions had been reached.

That industry had a special stake in oral health was an accepted fact, since many infections of occupational origin had direct and disastrous effects on teeth and adjacent bones and tissues. The position of the dentist in industry was analogous to that of the industrial physician, in that both faced the delicate problem of performing needed services for industry without infringement on the province of private practitioners.

A paper read at a joint meeting of the AAIP&S and the Health Service Section of the National Safety Council, in 1923, produced a spirited debate on dental problems and procedures. R. W. Elliott, of Cleveland, discussing "The Value to Industry of a Dental Clinic," declared his belief that plants should provide reparative as well as prophylactic treatment, basing his argument on his experience with the National Lamp Works.

George M. Price, director of Union Health Center, New York, cited the success of the dental clinic started by the Garment Workers Union, which employed ten dentists and made the project self-supporting by a minimum charge to employees. Louis I. Dublin pointed out that the Metropolitan Life Insurance Company had substituted dental hygienists for dentists, a compromise that had proved highly satisfactory. D. B. Lowe, of the Goodrich Rubber Company, stated his conviction that industry should do no more than provide first aid, prophylaxis, thorough examination, and education. This opinion appeared to be the consensus of those present at the meeting.

Dentistry, like medicine, continued through the twenties to strengthen its position in industry and to grow steadily in importance. The December, 1926, issue of the

AAIP&S Bulletin published a list of industrial dentists compiled by the National Association of Industrial Dental Surgeons. It contained more than a hundred names of members and their employers, who included many of the largest corporations in the country.

Time has tempered the rivalry between industrial dentistry and private dental practice. And the harmony of interests and activities in industrial practice is exemplified by the fact that the American Association of Industrial Dentists (organized in 1943) has, since 1946, sat in joint sessions with its confreres in industrial medicine at the annual meetings of the two bodies.

* * *

Never for a moment, during the twenties, did the AAIP&S relax in its efforts to improve public relations with the older medical groups and with other related health agencies. It met criticism in the open, aired its own shortcomings freely, and urged members to take corrective measures.

The stigma of "contract doctor" was resurrected and used from time to time to sting the medical man in industry, but it had lost much of its old venom. The association *Bulletin* of December, 1926, contained the following editorial comment, typifying the way in which such shafts were met and turned aside:

> There has long been opposition on the part of organized medicine to what is termed contract practice, and the Judicial Council of the American Medical Association at this time is actively considering and investigating this problem. While those who have informed themselves know that there is no relation whatever between the old-fashioned "contract" doctor and the present-day physician in industry, there are still those who persist in confusing the work of the two.
>
> Our members owe it to themselves and their colleagues in general to dispel this erroneous conception and to see that no action is taken by a committee or other group that would tend to prejudice their work.

Late in 1927 the *Journal of the American Medical Association* vigorously attacked a proprietary nostrum called "Seequit," which was being introduced into women's colleges and industries employing large numbers of women. Extolling its virtues, its manufacturers boasted: "Seequit, a swallow of water, and the worker goes right on with her duties." Analysis by AMA laboratories showed that the essential ingredient in this preparation was three and three-quarter grains of amidopyrene per tablet; yet Seequit retailed at $4.50 for a hundred tablets. The AMA concluded: "One can buy five-grain tablets of amidopyrene U.S.P. for less than $1.50 a hundred. Certainly Seequit will produce no effect that cannot be produced equally well by a plain tablet of amidopyrene U.S.P."[3]

In a subsequent bulletin the AMA listed ten well-known proprietaries, accompanied by the wholesale druggist's prices in one column and the comparative prices of nonproprietary equivalents in another. "The total cost of an ounce of each of these substances under a protected name is $16.15. The total cost of an ounce of each of these substances under an unprotected name is $4.10."

The AAIP&S was concerned because the letterhead of the manufacturers of Seequit listed eighty-eight industries, large and small, that were using the preparation, among which were several whose medical departments were supervised by members of the industrial association.

Commenting, the AMA declared: "The spectacle of physicians in charge of the health of large industrial concerns dispensing patent medicines at an exorbitant price, when the same drugs under their official names can be purchased at one-third the price, is edifying neither from the viewpoint of scientific medicine nor from that of economics." The *Journal* pointedly asked: "Why 'medical directors' if 'patent medicines' are to be prescribed?"

Why, indeed? The AAIP&S quickly repeated the question. In its own *Bulletin* of January, 1928, it republished the charges in detail, and went on to say:

> Is it any wonder that industrial medicine is so frequently discredited; that the epithet of "contract surgeon" is still applied to us? Are we under contract to the manufacturers of proprietaries or are we employed to *serve* (not exploit) our employers and their employees? It is bad enough when the physician in private practice allows himself to be inveigled into prescribing such nostrums as Seequit, but it is more reprehensible when an industrial physician, whose duty is to guard his employer and his fellow employees against all medical exploitation, lends the prestige of his position to push the sales of any nostrum.

This unsavory incident itself was not of great moment in a day when many a fraudulent panacea managed to stay on the market despite legal restrictions and the whiplash of AMA condemnation. It exemplifies, however, the unwillingness of the AAIP&A, even in those early years, to condone any hint of unethical practice; and its readiness to join the AMA in exposing violators among its own membership.

Problems involving workmen's compensation became steadily more acute as the twenties rolled on. Medicolegal questions were of as much concern to medicine as they were to law; then, as now, no case could be decided justly without reliable medical testimony. Such testimony, in turn, could be based only on opinion, unless detailed case histories were available as evidence. Thus the dilemma hinged on physical examinations and the resultant medical records.

Hernia in industry offers a good example of certain issues which have been a constant source of both medical and legal controversy over the years. This hardy perennial was the subject of an exhaustive report, in 1922, by a special committee of the Medical and Surgical Section of the American Railway Association.[4] At its annual meeting in October of the following year the AAIP&S passed the following resolution endorsing the railway committee report:

> 1. We unqualifiedly approve the definition of "traumatic and industrial hernia" together with all of the supporting data set forth in the report.

2. We especially commend that part of the report which reads, "The only thing needed to bring about greater harmony in the procedures of industrial commissions is to spread a clearer knowledge of the known medical and surgical facts relating to the etiology of hernia."

3. In endorsing the report, this association feels that it is not within its province to attempt to determine whether, for social or economic reasons, *occupational hernia* or *hernia of effort,* as these terms are used in the report, should or should not be compensated. However, the American Association of Industrial Physicians & Surgeons is prepared to cooperate with such bodies as may be called upon to determine this question.

Resolutions, however well intended and fervidly worded they may be, do not necessarily produce action. The problem of industrial hernia, with respect to compensability, has remained at a practical stalemate over the years, not for lack of medical agreement as to its etiology or treatment, but because of the difficulty of establishing in the courts its direct connection or lack of connection with an individual claimant's daily occupation. Hernia is also one of many common industrial ailments which are cited by those who urge an immediate and thorough overhaul of court procedures in cases involving compensation, particularly with reference to medical testimony. A large and vocal group, among Industrial Medical Association members today, regard such reforms as one of the most pressing needs of the profession.

Vigorous discussion of these topics in the twenties did serve one very worthwhile purpose; it focused more and more attention on physical examinations as an indispensable ingredient in the just settlement of compensation claims and the practice of true preventive medicine. The decade was one of great activity in the way of health surveys in various industrial fields; it produced many projects designed to yield valuable statistical data and to improve medical procedure.

In March, 1923, a committee on industrial medical records completed an ambitious study aimed at standardizing, at least partially, the record-keeping systems used by AAIP&S members. The committee report, signed by R. S. Quinby (chairman), D. B. Lowe, Wade Wright, Edgar Sydenstricker, and F. L. Rector (secretary), was accompanied by simple forms designed to include all vital information, exclude nonessential data, and reduce clerical work to a minimum. This early project was the forerunner of continuing studies that have progressively simplified departmental procedures and greatly increased the medical and legal value of industrial health records.

From 1919 to 1926 Dr. Arthur B. Emmons, II, as director of The Harvard Mercantile Health Work, was engaged in a then unique survey of conditions among employees of twenty-five department stores in a half-dozen large cities. His study, financed by the employers, revealed a wealth of new information on the health hazards of retail store workers. The findings were published in book form.[5] "The only book of its kind I know of," wrote Emmons some twenty years later.

216

In the summer of 1927 Edward C. Holmblad, of Chicago, was appointed chairman of the Public Utilities Group of the AAIP&S to head a survey of health and accident hazards in that field of industry. Leaving a general practice in Aurora, Illinois, six years before, he had served as local and regional surgeon for several railroads and as surgical consultant for numerous insurance companies. His activities in the twenties were the prelude to a career of continuous service to the association which led him to its presidency, and ultimately to the post of managing director of the Industrial Medical Association. The utilities study was limited in scope—confined largely to railroad employees. Its findings were significant, however, in that they again emphasized a lack of physical examination and re-examination of workers, lack of proper medical supervision, inadequate instruction and equipment for the prevention of accidents.

The complex problems of workmen's compensation and the rapid growth of group insurance were perhaps the chief factors that led large American insurance companies, in the 1920's, to more active participation in industrial medical affairs. The two groups had a common interest, social as well as economic, in accident prevention, preventive medicine, and health education for workers. Both had cogent reasons for the promotion of physical examinations and the maintenance of morbidity records.

Dr. Louis I. Dublin was one of the first insurance experts to speak formally at a meeting of the AAIP&S. At the 1923 convention he discussed the findings from annual examinations of a group of six thousand Metropolitan Life Insurance Company policyholders, covering a period of five years. The report showed that mortality was only 72 percent of what was expected, according to American experience tables. Dublin attributed the saving of lives to the knowledge gained by individuals concerning their own physical condition.

As for group insurance, its growth was phenomenal between 1911, when the first group policy was written, and 1927. In the latter year the Industrial Conference Board and the Federal Bureau of Labor Statistics reported 186 industrial concerns writing this form of insurance, with policies totaling more than $5.5-billion in force, covering 4.7 million employees.[6]

Time has broadened greatly the area of cooperation between the insurance companies and organized industrial medicine and has brought about a thorough understanding of common problems and purposes. The reciprocal benefits of this close association have been many and important. It would be difficult to find a single professional group, outside the fields of safety, hygiene, and medicine itself, that has contributed so much to public education in matters of health and health care as have the Life Insurance Institute and the individual insurance companies.

Twice in the course of the momentous twenties, signal recognition from high places was extended to prominent members of the AAIP&S, indicative perhaps of the growing stature of industrial medicine and the association. In 1925 the League of Nations appointed a medical committee to study living and working conditions in foreign countries. Among the specialists chosen for this international project was Otto Geier, whose long experience in the industrial field eminently qualified him to appraise health care and preventive practices in Europe as compared with standards in America. The Fifth International Medical Congress for Industrial Accidents and Occupational Diseases was held in Budapest during September, 1928. The list of delegates comprising the National Committee reads like a partial roster of AAIP&S membership: Emery R. Hayhurst, Columbus, Ohio (chairman); Volney S. Cheney, Chicago; R. W. Corwin, Pueblo, Colorado; Eugene L. Fisk, New York; Otto P. Geier, Cincinnati; Leonard Greenburg, New Haven; George M. Kober, Washington; W. J. McConnell, Philadelphia; George M. Price, New York; Frank L. Rector, Chicago; William A. Sawyer, Rochester, New York; Henry F. Smyth, Philadelphia; C. E. A. Winslow, New Haven.

* * *

How may we sum up, briefly, the progress of industrial medicine in the 1920's? The *Monthly Labor Review* for January, 1927, struck an optimistic note in reporting a study by the United States Bureau of Labor Statistics, citing the following points as gains made in the preceding ten years: (1) a decided extension in the medical service maintained for workers in both the hazardous and the nonhazardous industries; (2) special attention for undernourished employees; (3) means taken to guard against the dangers of old age; (4) periodic examinations required of workers urged to report for them; (5) special research brought to bear on problems of industrial health, especially upon the handling of poisonous substances; (6) a marked increase in employment of full- and part-time doctors; (7) greater employment of specialists, including dentists, oculists, and ear, nose and throat specialists.[7]

Such observations, while they winnow wheat from chaff, take no account of the *caliber* of medical men in industrial practice. Extent of facilities, amount of equipment, numbers of personnel mean little in themselves. But given men of ability, vision and determination, industrial practice will have services to match.

Dr. Guy L. Kiefer may well have had some such thought in mind when, accepting the presidency of the association in 1928, he said: "This is not a large association in point of membership. That matter has been discussed in Board meetings for several years, and I think it is the consensus of your present Board of Directors (it certainly has been all the time that I have been a member) that we do not care for an overwhelmingly large number.

"It isn't quantity that this association is looking for, it is quality; and it is quality which, in my opinion, we have."[8]

XIX

PROGRESS VIA HORSEPOWER

IT IS production, as every student knows, that lays the golden eggs of American prosperity. Any serious interruption of the flow of products of farm, mine, and factory is a debit against national wealth, and eventually affects standards of living to some degree. Along with management and workers, industrial medicine suffers in times of depression, unemployment, and strife. It cannot function at its best in a dislocated economy. This being true, major trends, up and down, in the nation's production deserve more than passing attention in any discussion of health care in industry.

The sudden reversal of business trends in 1920 has been called an "inventory" depression. There was no financial panic, but the postwar readjustment brought about a crisis in agriculture and exacted heavy toll from mining and manufacture. All commodity wholesale prices were cut by nearly half; steel and iron production dropped sharply. In the first eight months of 1921, according to Department of Labor figures, the number of unemployed increased from about 3.5 million to nearly 5 million—the highest point reached in the twenties.

"Labor unions," writes Edward F. Humphrey, "had gained much strength during the war and stood ready to test their new power, the rising cost of living determining them to resist any wage reduction."[1] The test came in the form of a wave of strikes— widespread and prolonged.

The year 1918 saw more than 4 million workers on strike in a dozen sections of the country. Employees of the United States Steel Corporation, led by a radical group in the unions, walked out in September, 1919, and returned to their jobs in the following January when the corporation substituted three eight-hour for two twelve-hour shifts. The bituminous and anthracite coal strikes in 1922, lasting five months and involving nearly 600,000 miners, came close to wrecking the industrial prosperity of the country.

Despite these setbacks, the depression ended almost as abruptly as it had begun. Unemployment proved to be an effective damper on strikes. Spurred by confidence in the basic soundness of the national economy and the demand for consumption goods, industrial production rocketed to new highs in 1923. Professor Humphrey comments: "American labor, which was militant, radical, intransigent in 1920, had become cooperative and even complacent by 1928."[2]

Commodity prices, after their plunge in 1921, stiffened and held firm for eight consecutive years. Stock prices started their spectacular climb toward a new peak, reached in 1929. Taxes settled at a moderate level. The American dollar, in point of purchasing power, was a "good dollar" during the period now known as the era of Coolidge prosperity.

Production figures mark the twenties as one of the truly great periods in our industrial history. The value of manufactured goods (for factory industries only) increased from $20.6 billion in 1909 to $62 billion in 1919. It mounted from that level to $70 billion in 1929, in a peacetime economy.[3]

The business climate in the latter decade was distinctly favorable to the growth and stabilization of industrial medicine. Many manufacturers, who had proceeded with caution during the years of postwar adjustment, now examined with new interest the problems of occupational health and began to expand their medical services along with the development of their production facilities. More and more physicians and surgeons were awakened to the opportunities in industrial practice, a trend that was to be vividly reflected in the growth of AAIP&S membership during the thirties.

The automobile industry accounted for the greater share of the production increase in the twenties. The industry, which built only 8.5 million passenger cars between 1910 and 1920, shipped 31.3 million cars in the next ten years. Their wholesale value reached a staggering total in excess of $21 billion. And production of trucks and buses more than kept pace in proportionate growth.[4]

There were, however, other developments of transcendent importance which set the twenties apart from any other era in history. These developments not only have revolutionized production procedures but have also altered the basic architecture and layout of industrial plants. They have profoundly affected the family economy of the nation and the whole mode of life in America. They have had a direct bearing, too, on the programs of sanitation, health, and hygiene in our factories. And from them has sprung another great new industry, creating national wealth and widespread employment.

For nearly a century and a half after Watt's first crude engines went to work in British mills, steam ruled the world of power. *Horsepower* was *steam* power—in shipping, in rail transportation, and in the great majority of industrial plants. America had followed the example of Europe in building its factories around central powerhouses which supplied the power to drive the machinery of production. But America led the world in nurturing the young giant—*electric* power—which soon was to challenge the supremacy of steam in industry.

"The speed age of American industry," says Professor Humphrey, "could not have been achieved by steam and gas alone; industry is being accelerated more and more by the use of electric power." This comment was made in 1931, and Humphrey goes on to observe: "The use of electric power is still in its infancy, even in the United States. . . . The whole character of American industry may be transformed in the future by the application of electric power."[5]

When it was made, this prophecy was already in the process of fulfillment. Public utility companies, by their rapid extension of light and power lines, had pointed the way to an Electrical Age. By 1929 perhaps half of the power used in industry was electric. The manufacture of electrical machinery had moved into the class of billion-dollar industries, with production values of nearly $2.3 billion in that year.

Instead of the mazes of shafts, belts, and pulleys that made dark jungles of the factories of the Steam Age in industry, are compact conduits leading from main power lines, delivering unit power direct to individual machines. Also, "plug-in" power put electricity at work on countless tasks, indoors and out, that once had been performed by brawn. It placed in the hands of workmen portable tools, limited, in range of operation, only by the length of cord required to reach a power outlet. It lightened labor, multiplied production, put a premium on skill instead of muscle.

The manufacturer whose plant was electrified made important savings in the cost of transmitting power to his machinery. No longer dependent on a nearby powerhouse, he could decentralize production. Small towns tapped the same convenient power lines that served great industrial centers. Elimination of overhead shafts and belts greatly increased flexibility of operation, particularly in machine layout for "straight-line" production and progressive assembly.

Another consequence of the shift to electric power is the change in architecture of the factory building. The modern industrial plant is a thing of beauty by comparison with its prototypes. The architect-engineer of today enjoys far greater freedom in the matter of design than in the Steam Age. He employs lighter, stronger structural materials and utilizes space to much better advantage. Problems of lighting, ventilation, and sanitation have been greatly simplified. The new concept of factory design and construction has been a real boon to the safety expert, the hygienist, and the physician in industry. The banishment of overhead shafts and belts removed a major source of accidents. Cleaner surroundings, better lighting, ventilation, have served the ends of health as well as those of efficiency and economy.

Evidence of improvement in the working environment surrounds us today for all to see. The facts are cited here not for their information value, but because there has been a tendency to underemphasize the influence of this changeover upon the health and well-being of Man: the Worker.

The transformation in industrial production was not, of course, accomplished overnight; it was spread over many years. But the Electrical Age received its first great impetus in the twenties. Wires were strung in every corner of America, extending electrical service to some 70 percent of the country's population. The United States, in 1929, generated approximately 125 billion kilowatt hours, about 41 percent of the world's total.[6] Electrification brought with it a tremendous boom in the manufacture of small electric motors, a large percentage of them for use in power tools and scores of other commercial applications. And it introduced horsepower into the home, an introduction perhaps comparable to that of the internal combustion engine.

It is a generally accepted fact that new products go through three stages before they come into universal use: experimentation, exploitation, stabilization. Automobile production and marketing followed that pattern. The industry reached the third of these stages in the twenties—shipped four-million motor vehicles of all types for the first time in 1923, passed the five-million mark in 1929.[7]

If we date the Age of Steam back to Watt's invention, surely Thomas A. Edison may be considered the father of the Electrical Age. The electric light alone was enough to assure him of historical immortality. His genius spurred experimental work on electric products of every sort in the late nineteenth and early twentieth centuries. His basic patents were involved in practically every electrical appliance produced in volume during the twenties. The list is imposing: the phonograph, vacuum cleaner, washing machine, radio, electric refrigerator, oil burner, and scores of other electrical servants now in everyday use in homes, stores, and industrial and commerical establishments. Most of these were power appliances driven by fractional horsepower motors, marvels of precision, incredibly compact, surprisingly durable and reliable.

The stage of experimentation was practically over in this field; the stage of exploitation followed. Manufacturers coupled mass production with mass distribution and skimmed the cream from virgin markets. Door-to-door selling had its heyday in the twenties. Millions will remember the advertising, which promoted "the new electrical way" by discrediting older methods. It was washing machine versus scrub-board, vacuum cleaner versus broom, oil versus coal, electric refrigeration versus ice.

At least one of these modern appliances, electric refrigeration, had a tangible relation to health problems. Adequate means of preserving foods had been long in coming to a civilized and scientific world. In old Rome, slaves carried snow from distant mountains to cool the wine for royal banquets. There was a French caterer who canned food for Napoleon's armies and won the favor of his emperor. In England Sir Francis Bacon is said to have stuffed a chicken with snow on a winter night to learn how long it would "keep," and, legend tells, died as a result of the exposure. Lord Kelvin, who discovered that the evaporation of liquids produces cold, declared: "I have found a better way." Early America had the root cellar and the spring house and ice.

With heavier concentrations of population in industrial centers, the problems of food storage and food transportation over long distances became progressively more acute. But science was learning more about the relation of nutrition to health and the need for certain vitamins and other elements in everyday diet. Electric refrigeration has come to the aid of medicine in solving most of the practical problems of food preservation; and it has been the means of introducing needed variety in the diet of the people, wherever they may live.

There can be no doubt that the combination of physiological research and electrical invention in the 1920's was largely responsible for the growing interest in nutrition as a factor in industrial health. The subject was discussed in detail at AAIP&S meetings and in the medical press. More and more corporations undertook the education of employees in matters of diet, following the lead of such pioneers as Eastman Kodak and the Metropolitan Life Insurance Company.

* * *

Every era of radical change in industrial products and processes calls for a reappraisal of the status of labor with respect to compensation, conditions of employment, and standards of living. In late years union leaders have declared that "take home" pay is the big issue in which workers are interested, the key to labor peace or labor strife. The problem is not so simple as that. The bitter strikes of the early twenties came at a time when wages were at a peak and industrial employees were prospering as never before.

Medical services and benefits have repeatedly demonstrated their value in the promotion of good labor relations. New York's clean-up of intolerable conditions in the sweatshop trades did not, in itself, materially improve the health of the garment workers; nor did it resolve all their grievances. On the other hand the harmonious relations prevailing in later years were largely credited to the benefits provided by Union Health Center, established in 1919.

In England, rioting and sabotage followed the introduction of steam power in the textile mills. Idled workers clamored that the machine was "stealing the bread from the mouths of the poor." That cry has echoed and re-echoed in successive generations, with the expansion of machine production to its present awesome dimensions. The protests, on the whole, have been less violent, but they have voiced the same fear, that technical progress, by reducing manpower, will eventually reduce man, the worker, to idleness and misery.

Who, in Watt's time, could have foreseen the material blessings that the textile industry would bestow not only on labor but on all humanity? And who, during the resurgence of industry in the latter part of the nineteenth century, could have known that the age of the motor car was just around the corner, creating thousands of jobs for every one it eliminated? Carroll Wright, in his *Industrial Evolution of the United States* (1895), comments quaintly but pointedly on this aspect of the labor problem:

> No one can claim that labor-saving machinery, so-called, but which more properly should be called labor-making or labor-assisting machinery, does not displace labor so far as men individually are concerned, yet all men of sound minds admit the permanent good effects of the application of machinery to industrial development.
>
> The permanent good effects, however, do not prevent the temporary displacement, which, so far as the particular labor displaced is concerned, assists in crippling the consuming power of the community in which it takes place.[8]

Humphrey, in his economic history of the United States, quotes national statistics to indicate the startling increase in American productivity as a result of improved manufacturing techniques. Between 1880 and 1930, he states, labor production per man per day increased "from 500 to 5,000 pounds of iron, 100 to 750 feet of lumber, 5 to 500 pounds of nails, ¼ pair to 10 pairs of shoes, ½ to 10 tons of coal, 20 to 200 square feet of paper."[9]

The conclusion is obvious. The over-all increase in national production was offset by the growing need for consumer goods. Increasing activity in manufacture added tremendously to the national income and created far more employment than it destroyed. The worker, producing more per day with less effort, received more for his work. He was, in short, in the process of becoming a manager of machines rather than their slave.

As the Age of Electricity gained momentum in the twenties, the man-versus-machine controversy again came to life. A new term, "technological unemployment," became part of the American vocabulary. Such unemployment existed, of course, and to a serious extent, as it always will exist, since the new always replaces the old, and dislocations and readjustments are among the penalties of progress. But who, at that time, could have foreseen that the manufacture of electric power and electrical machinery was soon to become one of the giants among American industries, again creating hundreds of thousands of jobs that had never before existed?

The two most spectacular production booms of the period between 1910 and 1930—in the automotive and electrical industries—differed in one important respect from any prior manufacturing development in world history. For the first time, the rank and file of industrial workers became purchasers, on a large scale, of commodities which even today are considered luxury items in most other countries.

Because of mass production and distribution, because volume manufacture has cut costs, because of high wages and high purchasing power, industrial labor has been able to buy the commodities it builds; and automobiles, along with scores of labor-saving appliances, are standard equipment in every remote corner of the land. These facts offer the best possible vindication of the machine, and of the American enterprise system.

224

Apropos of employment and standards of living in the twenties, the Industrial Relations Section of Princeton University found that 21 percent of the owners of stock in twenty large corporations in 1926 were employees of those corporations.[10] And employment statistics show that in October, 1929 (when the United States had a population of 122 million), 47.6 million people were gainfully employed, as compared with 46 million at work in 1940 (when the population stood at 131 million).[11]

Industrial medicine must ever work closely, and in harmony, with both management and labor, sharing their fortunes and misfortunes. Therein lies the revelancy of this business chronicle to the activities of the physician in industry. Prosperity built new plants in the twenties, added new thousands of workers to payrolls. New processes created new health hazards. Small medical departments were expanded. The industrial medical profession, like industry itself, set its sights higher for the future.

But a dark chapter in history, for America and the world, lay just ahead. As the twenties moved into their closing years there appeared to be a popular belief that the horn of plenty could never be emptied. "This is the millenium," said many. Even the wisest financiers seemed oblivious to pitfalls and dangers. Rich and poor alike snapped up stock offerings at fantastic prices—on perilously thin margins. Commodities of every sort were absorbed in a wave of buying—on installment terms. Manufacturers, in the flush of prosperity, overextended production—stretching credit to the breaking point. Then came Black Thursday, October 24, 1929, "the day," as one reporter put it, "that the roof fell in on our national economy, and the glorious boom of the Roaring Twenties came to an end with a sickening thud. . . ."

PART SIX

TRIAL BY DEPRESSION

INDUSTRIAL MEDICINE AND THE ASSOCIATION
IN THE TROUBLED THIRTIES

Always, on the heels of advancing science and technology, comes the problem of distributing their benefits among the people.

XX

THE GAULEY BRIDGE EPISODE

THERE was no lack of warning that a major economic disaster was in the offing as the nineteen-twenties drew to a close. The signs were clear to all who understood the dangers inherent in unbridled stock speculation, installment buying on a huge scale, and the continued outpouring of factory products to increase already swollen retail inventories.

American complacency was perhaps at an all-time peak in those free and easy days. Industrial workers happily carried full dinner pails to jobs that seemed secure forever. Their pay was good, and it was practically all "take home" pay. Corporations set their sights on higher and higher sales volume. Amateur stock speculators, busily pyramiding small cash investments into tidy profits, *on paper,* were in no mood to quit that fascinating game. What an easy way to quick riches! Why had no one thought of it before?

The current stock market, indeed, seemed to recognize only one direction, *up.* Bankers, brokers, and many others who should have known better were blind to the flash of danger signals and deaf to the voice of prudence. It was not many months before the crash of 1929 that a nationally respected investment counselor solemnly announced: "Stock values in this country have reached a new and permanently higher level."

It is odd that events of world-wide importance are so often remembered for dramatic but superficial incidents, after deeper and more significant aspects are forgotten. To many millions, mention of the big depression recalls the much-publicized apple vendors on street corners; migratory workers rioting in Western states; the "bonus army" on its futile trek to Washington; rows of vacant shops, their shelves gathering dust; juke boxes playing "Brother, Can You Spare a Dime?"; a popular cartoon picturing silk-hatted college alumni "thumbing" their way to a class reunion.

Such phenomena were among the symbols or symptoms of the economic illness from which the country suffered. Behind them lay a sobering mass of facts and figures. The depression struck hard and marched fast. Three weeks after the market collapse, quoted values of listed stocks had dropped $20 billion, and this was only the beginning. Retail sales dwindled to a trickle; wholesale and manufacturing volume followed suit. Foreclosures and repossessions were the order of the day. Failures and layoffs brought the total of unemployed to some fifteen million. Welfare agencies were swamped by applicants for relief.

Discussion of the causes or control of business ups-and-downs has no place in this narrative. The consequences of this particular depression, however, were of the utmost importance to medicine at large and to industrial medicine in particular. It may, indeed, be argued that no single sequence of events in the scientific age has so profoundly affected the progress of organized industrial health care.

The early nineteen-thirties found the familiar American production-consumption-employment formula badly out of balance. The upward spiral of prosperity had halted, then reversed itself in a tailspin. Stagnation spread like a creeping paralysis that attacked business of every type and individuals in every income bracket.

The economic dislocation, as a matter of course, struck its most crippling blow directly at the beneficiaries of industrial medical service—industrial and commercial employers and their employees—the two groups which together provide the real reasons for the existence of occupational medicine as a specialty.

It is safe to say that a very substantial percentage of the fifteen million workers idled by the depression had been employed in plants that provided medical and surgical care of some sort. It was to be expected that the withdrawal of so large a group from the nation's active labor force should result in the widespread curtailment of medical department activities, and that the need for in-plant medical personnel should be correspondingly reduced.[1]

At worst, however, this interruption could be regarded as only a temporary setback in the progress of the American Association of Industrial Physicians & Surgeons and the specialty it represented. In the ordinary course of events, economic recovery would balance the books and industry would resume something like normal operation. The pinch of hard times was keenly felt in the field of medicine, as it was in every field of endeavor; but the plight of the professional few was certainly of less over-all importance than that of millions in other walks of life.

This is to say that the depression years could be dismissed in this volume as a period of relative inactivity, of little significance in the history of industrial medicine, were it not for a few unrelated happenings of far-reaching importance to the profession and the association. Most dramatic of these was an explosive development that focused the nation's attention on the entire problem of occupational diseases and the disability resulting from them.

230

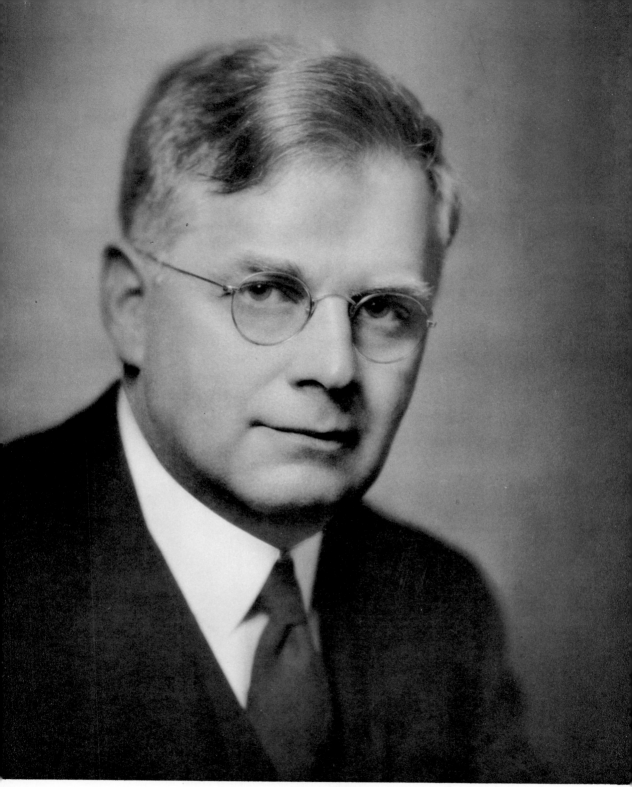

67. *McIver Woody, M.D. (1886–   ). President, AAIP&S, 1939–1940.* As secretary of the faculty of medicine at Harvard in 1917 and 1918, McIver Woody launched a professional career that has led to army service in the Office of the Surgeon General (1918–1919), to the University of Tennessee College of Medicine and Baylor University as dean and professor of surgery, and, in 1922, to Standard Oil of New Jersey, culminating in his appointment as medical director of Esso Standard Oil in 1944. Woody's recognized talent for organization found expression during his presidential term in expansion of AAIP&S and the development of component societies.

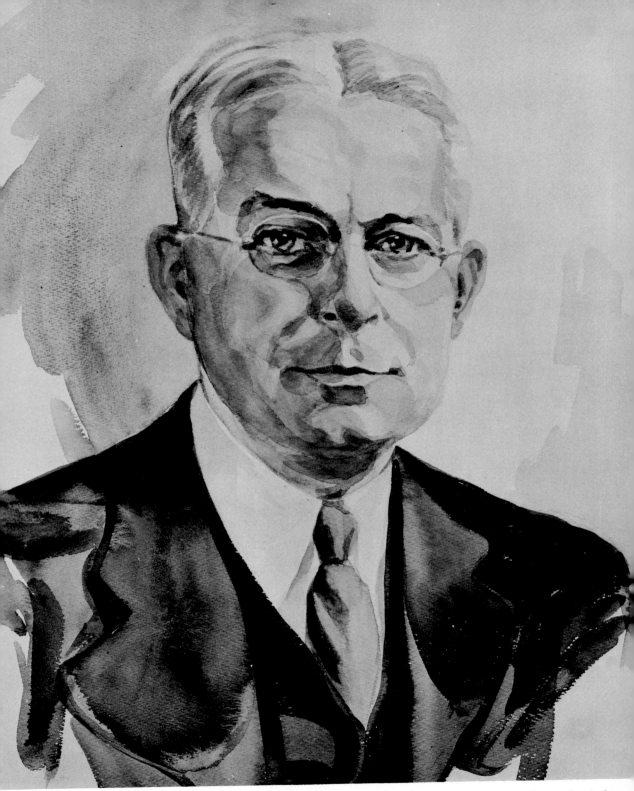

68. *Daniel L. Lynch, M.D. (1883–1956). President, AAIP&S, 1940–1941.* While still engaged in general practice Lynch became affiliated with the New England Bell Telephone Company, serving as its medical director from 1918 to 1948, and was largely instrumental in building its medical department into a model of efficiency. He proclaimed the need of special education for industrial doctors, who, he pointed out, "should have had training quite beyond the field of private practice." In the 1930's his influence brought the New England Conference of Industrial Physicians into the AAIP&S as a component, and as president he did much to strengthen such affiliations.

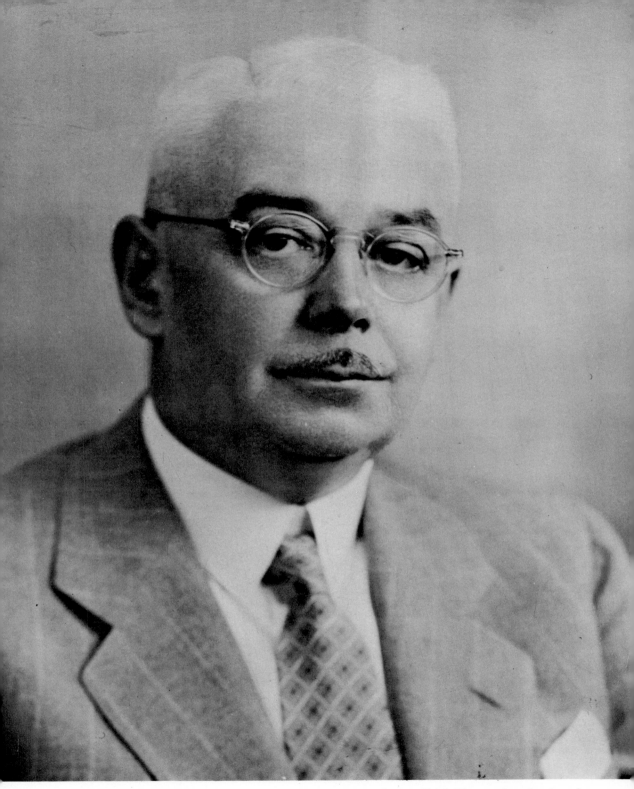

69. *T. Lyle Hazlett, M.D. (1885–   ). President, AAIP&S, 1941–1942.* Twice, after Lyle Hazlett received his medical degree from the University of Pittsburgh (1912), war intruded upon his private professional career. From 1914 to 1916 he served with the Red Cross in Russia and from 1917 to 1919 as an officer in the USMC. At the time of Pearl Harbor he was president of the AAIP&S, and his official life was largely shaped by the exigencies of World War II. Hazlett made his most important industrial affiliation in 1920, with Westinghouse. In a long association with the University of Pittsburgh school of medicine, he also set a pattern for the development of special industrial education in medical schools.

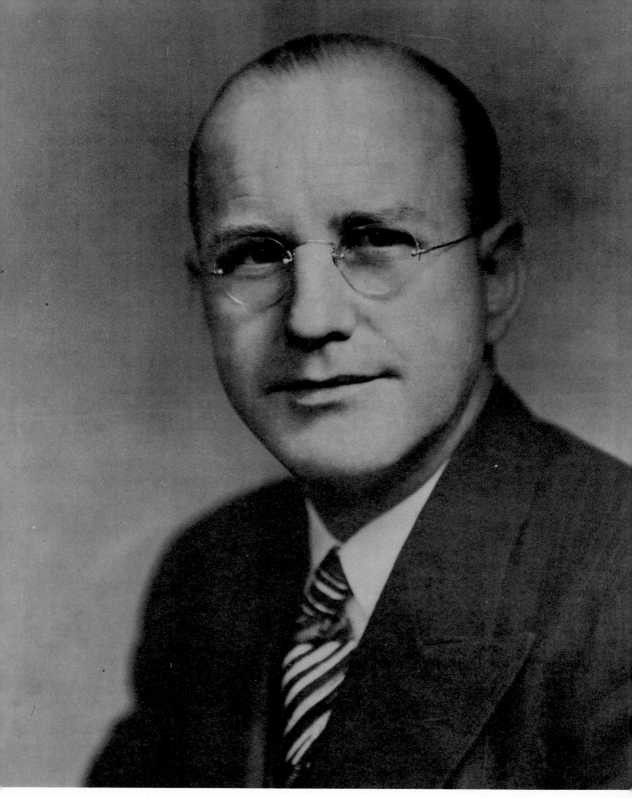

70. *John J. Wittmer, M.D.* (1895–1951). *President, AAIP&S, 1942–1943.* In Wittmer's presidential term America was facing the discouragements of its first full year of war. A critical shortage of manpower in industry was complicated by a similar dearth of medical manpower. The AAIP&S found itself immersed in problems of civil defense and first aid procedure, coupled with vital new problems in war industries. With the support of seasoned officers and a strong Board, and despite serious illness, Dr. Wittmer gave the association the adept leadership demanded at a time when the health and productivity of the nation's working force were all-important.

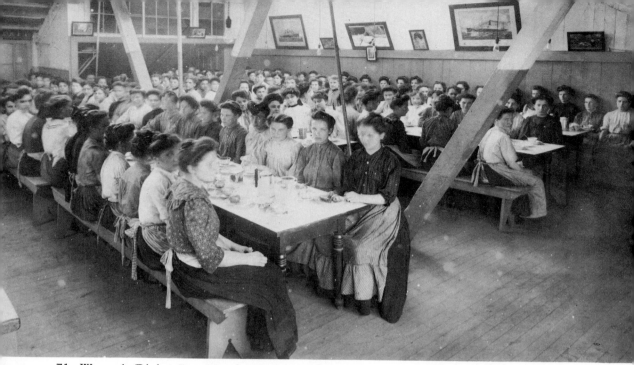

71. *Women's Dining Room at the Crane Malleable Iron Foundry.* Such facilities were typical of ordinary working conditions around 1900.

—Courtesy of the Crane Company

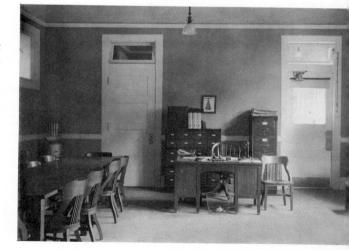

72. *Dr. Harvey's Waiting Room.* A neat, but plain, waiting room in the late 1890's at the Crane Company.

—Courtesy of the Crane Company

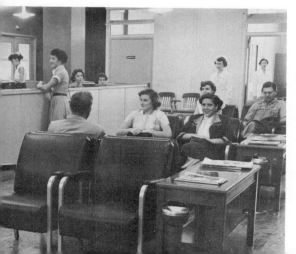

73. *A Modern Reception Room.* Clinical files are in the background.

—Courtesy of the Prudential Insurance Company

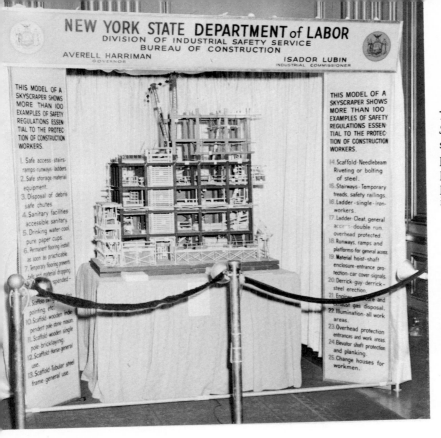

74. *Model of Skyscraper to Show Safety Regulations.* This exhibit, sponsored by the New York Department of Labor, emphasizes important safety regulations for the protection of construction workers in an age of skyscrapers.

75. *The Ramazzini Society.* The society was established in 1942, with Carey P. McCord and C. D. Selby as moving spirits, to sponsor an annual Ramazzini lecture to honor the memory and achievement of the patron saint of occupational medicine. In August 1946 Dr. Robert Legge delivered the first lecture. Members, seldom more than a score, are specialists in Ramazzini as well as in medicine. Pictured at the Muskoka Beach Inn (Ontario) in 1949 are Elston L. Belknap, J. G. Cunningham, Rutherford T. Johnstone, Robert A. Kehoe, Anthony J. Lanza, Robert T. Legge, Christopher Leggo, William J. McConnell, Carey P. McCord, Carl M. Peterson, Andrew R. Riddell, Oscar A. Sander, Clarence O. Sappington, Clarence D. Selby, Henry F. Smyth, James H. Sterner, Harley L. Krieger, L. E. Hamlin, F. J. Tourangeau, James M. Carlisle, F. S. Parney, Lemuel C. McGee.

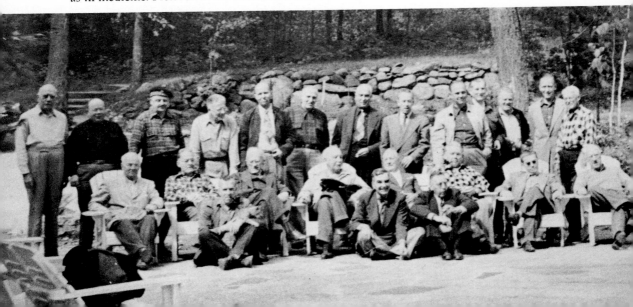

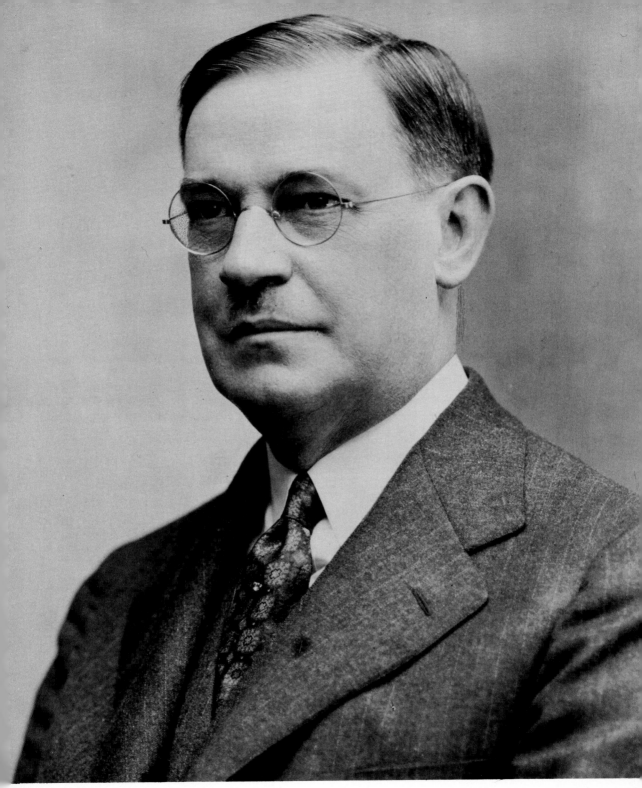

76. *Harvey Bartle, M.D.* (1874–   ). *President, AAIP&S, 1943–1944.* Looking back on fifty years of activity in the field of occupational health, Harvey Bartle has summed up the accomplishments of the AAIP&S in these words: "We have purposely, persistently and practically developed and brought into existence a fellowship of kindred profes-sionals and glorified a task which in the past was not too highly commended." A respected member of the AMA Council on Industrial Health for ten years (1937–1947), he has been equally influen-tial in the AAIP&S. As president he concentrated on the settlement of disputes that were barring a joint approach to certification problems.

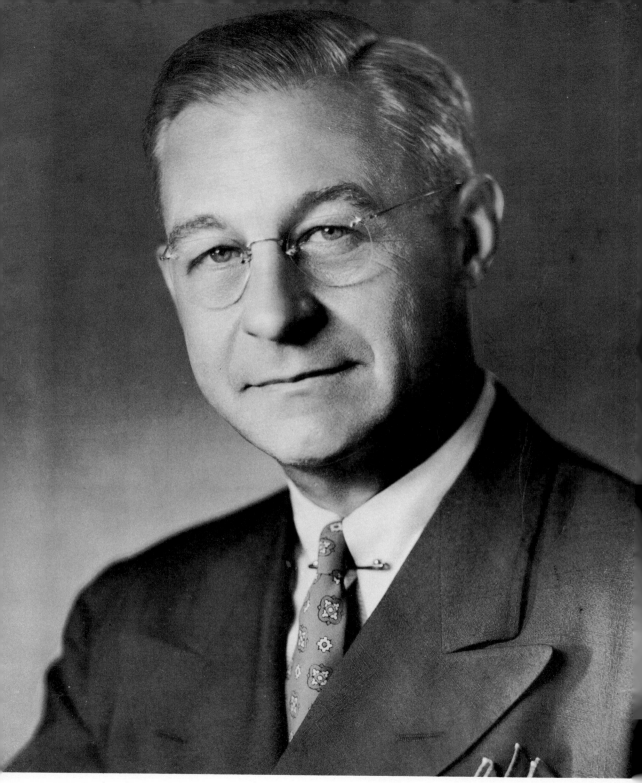

77. *Frederick W. Slobe, M.D.* (1893–   ). *President, AAIP&S, 1944–1945.* Dr. Slobe was a surgeon in the Army Medical Corps, 1918–1919, and a diplomat of the National Board of Medical Examiners. Entering the industrial field in 1921, he practiced until 1949, when he became medical director of the Illinois Blue Cross and Blue Shield.

His activities have been many and varied—author of many medical and surgical papers, founder of the Occupational Health Institute, crusader for industrial medical education, and ardent worker for certification. His presidential term ended in the famous "proxy" year, in which members balloted by mail for elective officers.

Like a bolt out of nowhere, at the very bottom of the depression, came the fantastic Gauley Bridge tunnel episode, an industrial tragedy involving the deaths of nearly five hundred tunnel workers from silicosis and kindred lung-dust diseases, under circumstances that led to highly sensational and unfavorable publicity.

So much has been written over the years about Gauley Bridge that it is difficult today to separate simple fact from unreliable rumor and to arrive at an account uncolored by controversial opinions. In 1936, nearly four years after the tunneling operation was completed, *Time Magazine* reviewed the episode in a straightforward and apparently well substantiated story. Following are excerpts from the *Time* account:

> In 1929 a water power tunnel was begun at Gauley Bridge along the forest-fringed New River in southern West Virginia, with cheap transient labor, black and white, from mountain districts as far away as Georgia. The tunnel went through white sandstone and quartz which were 99 percent pure silica. Every blast of dynamite puffed deadly silica dust down the throats of sappers who wore no protective masks over their mouths and noses. Rapidly men began to die of silicosis, pneumonia, and tuberculosis.
>
> When workmen refused to go into the tunnel heads, foremen, according to subsequent court testimoney, often clubbed them on. But the foremen dutifully followed their gangs into the dust, and many of them died too. . . .
>
> Digging of the Gauley Bridge tunnel ended in 1932. By that time about five hundred silicosis deaths had spread terror throughout the territory. A smart Kentucky lawyer went over the mountains, instigated damage suits (against the tunnel contractors). Some relicts won. Some derelicts won. Many lost or sued too late to accomplish anything for themselves. But as a result West Virginia passed its silicosis compensation law, which in turn prompted the radical press to dig up the Gauley Bridge skeleton and rattle its bones.[2]

It is interesting to note the long lapse of time between the actual construction of the Gauley tunnel and the peak of the public outcry over its medical and legal aftermath. Some of the most sensational and unsavory publicity flared up at least three years after the job itself was done and many of Gauley's dead lay in forgotten graves. Investigation, remedial legislation, and court action progressed even more slowly.

There was no lag, however, in the response of industrial medical men to the silicosis challenge. As if sensing the oncoming storm, authorities on the dust diseases, from the membership of the AAIP&S and allied organizations, were busy with important research and writing. It was in the December, 1932, issue of the association's than-new journal, *Industrial Medicine,* that C. O. Sappington published his "Silicosis and Other Dust Diseases." Carey P. McCord's "Silicosis in the Foundry," also appeared in 1932, as did "Inhalation of Quartz Dust," by Leroy U. Gardner, director of the Saranac Lake Laboratory.[3]

As the *Time* report states, the sickness and mortality at the Gauley tunnel site had become a scandal by 1932. But the same article points out that the West Virginia legislature did not pass its silicosis compensation law until March, 1935, and that in the following December "the radical U.S. press . . . was belatedly trying to distill national bitterness" from the episode.

In their intensive investigation of pneumoconiosis for the John B. Pierce Foundation several years later, Drs. Lewis G. and William G. Cole (father and son) emphasized the same point with this statement: "Popular interest in silicosis, stimulating social and legislative activities and affecting judicial decisions, was notably accentuated by the newspaper notoriety of the Gauley Bridge episode in 1935. The relation of dust and disease has been brought into the limelight, and the work of its investigators emerged for wide study and appraisal."[4]

One highly important consequence of the delayed airing of the Gauley tragedy is stressed in a report, "Silicosis and Allied Disorders," made by a medical committee of the Air Hygiene Foundation in 1937. It states:

> The tunnel was completed in two years, but a great many of the workers had died. Reports were highly colored as to the conditions under which they were living and working in the tunnel, and a committee appointed to investigate came to the conclusion that "acute" silicosis had been a contributing factor in these men's deaths.
>
> There seems to be no doubt that they worked under very severe dust conditions; but no facts are available [in 1937] as to the dust counts, previous exposures, or physical condition of the men when they started this work. Subsequent inquiries, which resulted in a congressional investigation, found the job completed and workmen scattered all over the country.[5]

Under these deplorable circumstances, thorough medical investigation was virtually impossible. Medical testimony, in court actions, often became a battle of opinions. Much of the evidence, from whatever source, was of questionable validity. Judges were even more seriously handicapped by the absence of laws and the dearth of legal precedent adequate to the silicosis situation. Organized industrial medicine (represented by the AAIP&S) gave liberally of time and talent for discussion of the medical aspects of the controversy. In fact, years before the report by the Coles was finished, the association's *Industrial Medicine* had used its columns as an open forum for the "wider study and appraisal" suggested by them.

An analysis of a dozen typical issues of *Industrial Medicine* between late 1932 and early 1935, show that no less than twenty-five major addresses and papers dealing with medical and legal phases of the silicosis problem appeared in its pages, along with at least seventy reprints, abstracts, and editorials on the same subjects. These were of profound importance to a select audience consisting mainly of doctors responsible for health care in American industrial plants.

George G. Davis, Chicago industrial surgeon, teacher, and editor of the "Silicosis Literature and Laws" series, reported in his 1934 edition, "No states have as yet enacted silicosis compensation laws," and pointed out that only six of them (Missouri, California, Connecticut, Massachusetts, North Dakota, and Wisconsin) had occupational disease legislation "worded broadly to permit its coverage."[6]

The very fact that the entire subject of compensation for occupational diseases lay in a legal twilight zone may well have enouraged, rather than retarded, the filing of claims in such cases. At least, while lawmakers investigated, pondered, and maneuvered, a torrent of civil suits poured into courts in every section of the country, seeking damages on behalf of industrial workers and former workers on the grounds of death or illness in the course of their employment.

As early as 1934, Davis reported the conclusion that "$300 million in silicosis claims have originated in the last few years."[7] During a symposium on silicosis, held by the American Institute of Mining and Metallurgical Engineering in the same year, a speaker declared that in one state alone there were claims pending for more than $58 million, and that a single suit might cost an operator $50,000.[8] An article in the *Engineering & Mining Journal,* citing the high cost of silicosis compensation, told of suits brought for $100,000 per individual affected.[9]

Also in 1934 Dr. Sappington, then consultant editor of *Industrial Medicine,* warned AAIP&S members that "the relationship of pneumoconiosis and silicosis does not seem to be very well understood by persons who file claims, by their physicians, and by their attorneys. In many instances silicosis is claimed on clinical evidence which in no way differs from that of normal persons who are symptomless and without disability."[10]

A wave of industrial compensation claims was to be expected in the early thirties as a normal by-product of the depression, compounded of unemployment, deprivation, hardship, desperation, and in many cases a certain amount of cupidity and disregard of legal niceties. In a very real sense, however, the Gauley episode triggered the chain of events that made silicosis front-page news across the land.

The tunnel tragedy, at the outset, created only local publicity and local indignation, but the story could not long be hidden among the West Virginia hills. Because of the working conditions and number of deaths involved, compensation cases emanating from the project were highly sensational; they set a pattern that was widely followed. The silicosis scandal soon became a national issue, which some segments of the press did their best to build into a *cause célèbre.*

Thus, Gauley Bridge became a symbol of the disease hazards and consequent suffering risked by the industrial worker, just as the apple vendor and the breadline came to symbolize his economic plight during the big depression. In the silicosis cases of the thirties medical history was being repeated. Like the "phossy jaw" scandal early in the century and like the tragedy of the radium dial painters in the twenties, the Gauley Bridge episode shocked the nation, and an outraged public opinion pointed attention to deficiencies in the protection of industrial workers from occupation-connected disease hazards, and to the over-all inadequacy of the medicolegal system in dealing with resultant claims. Therein lies its great significance.

On this point in 1936, James W. Ferguson, industrial physician, surgeon, and roentgenologist, wrote:

> The importance of this subject is emphasized by the number of commissions lately formed to study the conditions dealing with dust and health and by the num-

ber of articles dealing with pneumoconiosis, silicosis, asbestosis, etc., that have appeared recently in medical literature.

It is also interesting to note that in cases concerning dust ills brought before the courts of several states, industry has received a verdict of adverse character. All this affects the trend of social thought, and, in turn, points out that disease due to the inhalation of dust at one's occupation concerns not only the employee and his dependents but also the industry and society.[11]

The so-called "dusty-lung" diseases were an inviting legal target because of their frequent incidence and wide distribution, their severity, and the long duration of many chronic cases. The "duration" of a disease is of special interest as an illustration of how far-reaching the effects of such a factor can be. In its 1936 article on the silicosis cases, *Time Magazine* noted:

Because silicosis may terminate fatally as long as forty years after silica inhalations, the California Supreme Court last year [1935] declared that there is no time limit to bar a silicotic employee from bringing a damage suit against an employer. Industrial insurance companies immediately wanted to increase their rates.

Operators of deep California gold mines, which are difficult to ventilate, would be obliged to pay $22.25 instead of the current $11 premium for every $100 they pay their men. Some mines of low-profit margin have already shut down. Others threaten to do so. Mine owners and miners who face loss of employment were last week beseeching California's insurance commissioner to forbid any such rate upping on account of silicosis hazards.[12]

From scores of articles dealing with one or another phase of the pneumoconiosis problem, gathered from widely scattered sources and covering the first half of the thirties, one can put together a fairly adequate account of what went on in that period. We find some oddities, some absurdities, many detailed records of court action, all freely punctuated by loud charges of "racket" and "fraud."

For today's specialist in, or student of, industrial medicine, the chief interest of these sidelights lies in the fact that they give us a realistic picture of the legal confusion produced by the compensation claims, the dilemma in which many employers found themselves, and the tremendous impetus given to scientific research in the field of industrial lung diseases by specialists both in and outside the AAIP&S.

As early as 1932 Andrew J. Farrell, a Chicago insurance lawyer, writing in the first issue of *Industrial Medicine* (now *Industrial Medicine and Surgery*), charged that the instigation of silicosis damage suits had become an organized racket. Pointing out that approximately 200 silicosis cases were already pending in the common law courts of Illinois, he commented: "Because of the unemployment situation and the activity of ambulance chasers there probably will be many more, with the resultant closing of industrial plants and a vast economic loss." "In those states where silicosis and kindred sicknesses are controlled by the workmen's compensation act there is not so much activity in stirring up claims, as the amount to be recovered is limited by the statutes." Elsewhere, however, sharp practices apparently flourished, according to Farrell's account of the recruiting method followed:

As the fees of ambulance chasers range from one-third to one-half of the sums recovered, it can readily be seen that it is a racket which appeals to chasers, unscrupulous lawyers, and doctors who put the dollar ahead of the ethics of their profession.

In various industrial centers the chief ambulance chaser has a representative. The latter might be a local storekeeper or a small business man who has connections with the workers in the various plants. The steady, consistent worker is not ordinarily prey for the chaser; it is usually the worker who has been discharged for inefficiency who is ready to sign a contract.

Lawyer Farrell's description went on to tell of staged "examinations" at so-called "clinics," of faked silicosis symptoms, and of impressive webs of testimony skillfully concocted for use before juries. Regarding actual trials in such cases, he had this to say:

> There is rarely a defense in a court of law to a well-prepared silicosis case regardless of whether the plaintiff has silicosis or not. This statement may be astounding to the reader, but a little explanation will be conclusive of its truth.
>
> It is always a question of fact for a jury as to whether or not the plaintiff has silicosis and whether or not it resulted from conditions in the plant or factory in which he was working. Where does the jury get the facts? From the witnesses. And where do the witnesses come from? The plaintiff produces witnesses to prove his contentions and theories and the defendant produces witnesses to negative the testimony of the plaintiff's witnesses or to establish the contrary facts.
>
> Included in the witnesses for the plaintiff will be a doctor or doctors who will testify that from a clinical and x-ray examination they are of the opinion that the plaintiff has silicosis and further that it resulted from working conditions in the defendant's plant or factory. The working conditions are described by the plaintiff and four or five of his fellow workers. If it isn't tuberculosis, it is tuberculosis superinduced by silicosis, or tuberculosis aggravated by silicosis. Exhibit "A," the plaintiff himself, if he has a sickly appearance, has more influence on the sympathetic jurors than have all the medical experts from here to the North Pole. . . .

This, described by an experienced attorney, was the kind of fraud that could be, and was, practiced on an extensive scale when the occasional unscrupulous lawyer and conscienceless doctor got together to betray their professions.

Farrell's observations led him to these conclusions: First, that silicosis and kindred sicknesses be taken out of the common law and made a part of the workmen's compensation acts of the various states; and, second, that later legislation "should have the benefit of thorough study and research by capable and skilled medical men as well as the attention of lawyers fully cognizant of the needs and with original ideas as to the proper remedy."[13]

This was in 1932. The gist of these recommendations have been many, many times repeated by both doctors and lawyers in intervening years, but the goals still remain only fractionally realized.

Two years later Farrell gave readers a follow-up report on the silicosis situation, at a time when many of the early suits were in the process of trial or decision. "Nothing has been done in a legislative way," he commented, "to ameliorate what might well be termed another 'racket' " and, continuing:

> It is not the contention of the writer that all silicosis claims are fraudulent. There are many cases coming up for trial at this time that are meritorious. But there are many more that have no intrinsic merit whatsoever but are built up to a degree by those interested, but settled because of high verdicts in meritorious cases.
>
> Within the last month or two in the state of Illinois there have been several verdicts in silicosis cases ranging from $12,000 to $20,000 in each case. It is not long before such verdicts become common knowledge, especially among the co-employees of the plaintiffs, and in the remaining cases, whether meritorious or not, the companies involved are forced to expend a large sum of money in defending the claims or to pay a rather large nuisance value. . . .
>
> There are a large number of executives of plants in industries in which the hazard exists who are under the impression that they can go into a court of law and defeat all these suits by putting up a strong defense. With this in mind quite a number of companies have declined liability on practically all silicosis claims and are going to await the results of some of their cases in court before taking action toward making amicable settlements.
>
> This is a very shortsighted policy because there is no question but that the lawyers having a large number of such claims will try their more effective and meritorious cases first, knowing that high verdicts in individual cases will boost the market value of the other cases.[14]

The Farrell articles appeared at a time when AAIP&S members, individually and collectively, were extremely active in seeking solutions to dust disease problems. In 1934, Sappington was urging legal and medical groups to bridge the gap between them, and to work out together a sound medicolegal code. The 1934 AAIP&S meeting in Cleveland could truthfully be dubbed a "silicosis" convention. There were also publications of importance by Drs. McCord, Gardner, Hayburst, and others in this special field.

What can happen in the legal testing of silicosis claims, or, at least, what could happen in those depression years, is succinctly described in *Pneumoconiosis (Silicosis) Literature and Laws of 1934* under the headline, "Cement Plants Fight Silicosis Racket." Abstracting printed reports of the first case of the kind filed against a Portland cement manufacturer in Illinois, the article notes that the Circuit Court at Chicago instructed a verdict holding that the plaintiff failed to make a *prima facie* case. In fact, the case collapsed before the defendant had submitted any evidence. Herewith, the facts as reported: "The so-called experts testifying for the plaintiff were confounded. One of them testified in substance that he had examined and diagnosed from 300 to 400 cases of pneumoconiosis, but admitted under cross-examination that all but one had come to him through the plaintiff's lawyers.[15]

In the same material we find a revealing abstract of two cases against a Missouri cement company, heard in a St. Louis court. One of the plaintiffs won a $25,000 judgment, the other, $15,000. Both verdicts were appealed. The abstract goes on to comment:

> Missouri is a paradise for this type of racketeering. Under its law, nine jurors out of twelve may decide a case. . . . Plaintiffs' attorneys have employed runners or solicitors to comb the state, paying particular attention to the unemployed. As much as $25 a case is paid to solicitors for every signed contract brought in. Cases are taken on a 50 percent contingent basis, and notices under the attorney's lien law are promptly served on the employer. At first the solicitors confined themselves to cases where some disability existed. More lately solicitation has been carried on among workers still engaged in active work, who have no more outward appearance of disability than dust on their clothes and some outward appearance of age.[16]

Among the interesting dust-disease cases of the period is a suit decided in 1935 by the Supreme Court of Illinois. The plaintiff, a woman, claimed damages under the state occupational disease act on the ground that she had been "exposed to irritating and injurious dust" while employed in pouring pepper and other ground spices into cans. A lower court had found for the defendant, and the case went to the Supreme bench on appeal.

In its decision the Supreme Court upheld the ruling of the lower court, declaring Section I of the Illinois act unconstitutional. The section in question dealt with precautions required of industrial employers to protect their employees from diseases incident to the kind of work in which they were engaged. "Section I," the court held, "does not include employees engaged in extra-hazardous occupations especially dangerous to the employees but only those employees engaged in nonhazardous occupations." The opinion terms the section "vague and indefinite," declaring it in violation not only of the Illinois Constitution but of the Fourteenth Amendment to the federal Constitution, in that it did not provide due process of law.[17]

The Illinois Occupational Disease Act was passed in 1911, but, oddly, the provisions of this section had never been seriously questioned before 1935. "There has never," the court reported, "been a judicial pronouncement here upon the constitutionality of Section I." The inference is that the framers of this old law had in mind the provision of reasonable and effective safeguards to protect workers from ordinary occupational disease hazards in industry, but had no intention of producing a clear, complete code covering the intricacies of disease compensation in the modern sense. This inference gains weight from the following comment on the 1911 Illinois statute, taken from the decision:

"This type of legislation was a complete stranger to the common law, and Section I under consideration here has no common law origin or history. The section has no generally accepted body of precedents, no established standards of conduct and no common knowledge or understanding on which it is bottomed."

Judged from present perspective, the foregoing abstract of the Illinois decision emphasizes one historically important fact, that even in the latter thirties, years after the onset of the silicosis suits, neither American legislatures nor American industries were at all prepared to deal adequately with the problem of compensation for disability from occupational diseases. Obviously, there was immediate and desperate need for remedial action by those groups, with technical cooperation and counsel from the bar associations and the industrial medical profession.

From many quarters, in that period, came proposals for legislation setting up specific provisions dealing with silica diseases. The New York legislature, in fact, passed such an amendment to the Workmen's Compensation Law in 1935. But it was vetoed by the governor, with the approval of the very industrialists and insurance companies that had originally supported its passage. Mature thought had shown up the disadvantages of "one-disease" legislation, as compared with a broadening of existing compensation law to bring all occupational diseases within its scope. Incidentally, it was estimated that the proposed amendment, had it not been vetoed, would have exposed industry to some $10 million cost in the form of extra compensation insurance premiums.[18]

Evidence of increasing legal confusion in the mid-thirties on the subject of compensation for pneumoconiosis also appears in a widely discussed Wisconsin case. A well-known foundry company, finding it necessary to reinsure all its employees, chose the expendient of discharging the entire working force, then rehiring after a health survey. Some of those affected, however, were not re-employed, and filed suits against the company. The Wisconsin Supreme Court ruled that the controversy was a matter for legislation and not for the courts; it further ruled that the cases were not compensable, inasmuch as no employees had suffered disability within the meaning of the law during their term of employment.

Dr. James W. Ferguson, in discussing this decision, commented: "The last occupation is not always the one actually responsible for all of the trouble. The person may have had pneumoconiosis when he was hired. He may have contracted it during some occupation of short duration, and on account of frequent changes of occupation the one that caused the exposure was forgotten. But if the industry does not know the condition that existed when it hired him, it may be required to assume responsibility for all the existing conditions."[19]

Addressing a joint meeting of the Chicago Medical Society and the Central States Society of Medicine and Surgery, in January, 1936, George G. Davis, then an associate clinical professor at the University of Chicago, brushed away some of the fog obscuring the medicolegal aspects of compensation for pneumoconiosis; damned with no praise "certain fast-thinking members of the legal profession" and "certain colleagues of our medical profession appearing in the role of expert witness"; and gave his audience some startling facts drawn from his personal experience, backed by detailed x-ray reports.

In preparing his paper, Dr. Davis stated, he had gathered data from the study of 182 suits filed against one company during the period from 1932 to 1936, asking total damages of more than $9 million. An exhaustive analysis of more than a dozen typical cases, accompanied by the x-ray readings of experts, led to his findings:

I have been closely associated with attorneys representing defendants in the examination and the medical preparation for defense in some 200 to 300 cases in which the claim was silicosis, pneumoconiosis, tuberculosis, and a general dragnet of any occupational disease which the plaintiff's attorney conceived could be remediable under the old and antiquated occupational disease act of Illinois. I venture to say that in an examination by the x-ray, and in some cases followed up by work history and physical examination, less than 1 percent of these two hundred or more suits disclosed any basis for a claim for silicosis or other pneumoconiosis as the result of exposure to harmful dusts. . . .

It is . . . the duty of the Bar of this state to eliminate as far as possible the ambulance-chasing and quack lawyer. It is the corresponding duty of the medical profession of this state to eliminate the ambulance-chasing and quack doctor. If both the Bar and the medical profession of Illinois will perform these duties, I submit the problem of the pneumoconioses in the industry of Illinois . . . can and will be solved to the benefit of all.[20]

So the inconclusive battle raged, back and forth, with lawmakers making little progress; with courts feeling their way through a practically uncharted area of law; with employers defending themselves against multiple compensation claims, ranging from the justifiable to the fraudulent. Organized industrial medicine was placed in a peculiar position. Its function was to serve the best interests of both employer and employee and the interests of justice as well. Though the doctors had absolutely no official powers of decision in any phase of the controversy, they were far from "sitting it out" as sideline spectators. They were the medical interpreters in cases involved. They spiced discussions and stimulated action by every possible means.

Early 1936 found the Air Hygiene Foundation of Pittsburgh at work to furnish scientific information for state lawmakers who were planning safety measures to prevent silicosis in industries within their jurisdiction. An excerpt from a news story of this study declared: "Dust diseases and fatalities alleged in connection with the Gauley Bridge tunnel have aroused legislatures to consider silicosis problems."[21] The program of the Foundation was centered on preventive measures (as was right and proper), but it did not contemplate legislation clearly defining liability in the field of occupational illness (which was also needed).

In the same year a resolution was introduced in the national House of Representatives calling for an investigation of deaths "reported to have occurred" in connection with the Gauley project. The preamble informed the House that 476 tunnel workers "have from time to time died from silicosis contracted while digging out a tunnel at Gauley Bridge, West Virginia."[22]

This nearly four years after the tunneling operation was completed! Truly, the mills of the legislative gods grind slowly in matters that call for new thinking and forehanded action, even though they vitally concern the public good.

Why, one may ask, this formidable recital of court proceedings and decisions, these references to compensation laws and lawsuits, since they involved only a single group of industrial diseases? It is a fair question. Pneumoconiosis (in the generic sense of the term) has been a dangerous enemy of man since the beginning of re-corded time. It was a serious hazard, in the thirties, to the health of an estimated half-million workers in many trades.[23]

Nevertheless, it is neither the incidence nor the severity of silicosis and related ailments that commands such extended discussion in a history of modern indus-trial medicine. As noted earlier in this chapter, the consequences of the silicosis cases that stemmed from Gauley Bridge greatly magnify their historical importance. The public furor created by these suits, their impact on industry, the medical and legal issues they involved, all conspired to center more and more attention upon compensa-tion for occupational disease and less attention, relatively, upon trauma.

Actually, the disease aspect of compensation had not been either thoroughly or systematically explored up to that time. State laws then in effect had been framed to provide compensation for injury only. Manufacturers recognized that obligation, and industrial doctors everywhere were mainly interested in that type of practice.

As Dr. Sappington pointed out in 1935: "No such incentive . . . has been pro-vided in the case of occupational diseases. Because of the relatively few men spe-cializing in this kind of work, many cases of occupational diseases have gone un-recognized where reporting was required."[24] There was then, he declared, no adequate measure of the occurrence of such diseases, and their frequency and financial cost were considered of little importance.

It was fortunate for the progress of industrial medicine that problems of com-pensation for work-connected sickness began to receive serious study when they did, for America was nearing an era in which that emphasis was to become predominant. Just ahead, the great scientific boom of the 1940's was to bring forth a flood of new metals, chemicals and compounds, multiplying the number of potential health hazards to be kept under control by industrial physicians, hygienists, and safety experts. Medical research in the intervening years was of inestimable value in preparing in-dustrial practitioners for the bigger and broader responsibilities soon to be laid upon them.

Effects of the publicity given to the silicosis cases became almost immediately ap-parent in the legal field. Speaking of pneumoconiosis in its November, 1936, issue, the *Columbia Law Review* said:

> This menace has for some time been universally recognized by experts in public health and labor legislation, has become increasingly a familiar problem to employers during the depression, and has resulted in a resurgence of legislative interest within the last two years. But the problem was not brought forcefully to popular attention until, in the present year, a concentrated outburst of deaths from silicosis aroused indignant comment and a congressional investigation.
>
> Despite this growing notoriety, insufficient effort has been expended to prevent the disease, and clear provision is today made for its victims in the workmen's com-pensation acts of only twelve states. . . . Ordinarily in the vast majority of states whose statutes do not clearly compensate for dust diseases, the remedy for the worker afflicted with pneumoconiosis lies only in the common law.[25]

If reports like the foregoing do not seem to spell out progress in industrial disease legislation, it must be remembered that the twelve states referred to included practically all the large and important industrial states in the northeast and Middle West, as well as in California. One should also bear in mind that state law specifically providing compensation for industrial diseases was virtually nonexistent only a few years before.

The *Columbia Law Review* article carried with it nearly five solid magazine pages of bibliography, including references to books and reports, legal decisions and opinions. Articles in *Industrial Medicine* were repeatedly cited in the bibliography; Hayhurst received frequent mention, along with material supplied by Doctors G. G. Davis, L. U. Gardner, and other contemporary researchers. Almost all of the reference works were published in the thirties, further indicating the tremendous interest in the legal aspects of industrial medicine at the time.

This interest was nationwide. It is quite likely that, in the same period, every state and territory in the Union was studying or writing or amending industrial compensation legislation. Some states passed "blanket" acts broad enough to include occupational diseases; some states specifically excluded them; still others listed compensable ailments, with little or no mention of silicosis. Because of wide differences in state laws and their constant amendment, it is impossible to describe in a general statement, the exact status of compensation legislation nationally at any particular time.

In spite of this activity, the controversy about compensation for job-connected illness was far from settlement when the decade drew to a close. There was wide disagreement over the principle of employer liability, the kind and extent of statutory regulation best suited to the needs of the various states, and the medicolegal procedures, particularly with reference to medical testimony.

These and other issues remained for study and debate in the forties and beyond. There have been continued discussion and continued progress toward solution of those issues down to the present. It was the agitation, the public clamor, in the thirties, however, that brought the subject of occupational disease and compensation into the open and kept it there, heralding a new approach by society to an ancient and ever present problem and marking a definite turning point in the history of industrial medicine.

The impact of common-law suits after Gauley Bridge set many a corporation back on its heels. Employers realized, of course, that a good proportion of the claims would not stand up in court and that judgments assessed would be only a fraction of damages asked. Nevertheless, defense was costly in time and money; publicity was often unfairly partisan; the suits were another burden on already heavily burdened businesses.

It is obviously impossible to sum up, in specific terms, the effects of this legal landslide on industrial medical practices and procedures as a whole. Plants differ too widely in products, processes, disease hazards, and other conditions of employment.

Medical departments vary too greatly in size, problems, character, and scope of services.

Individual experiences, however, are not difficult to find. One of these, recorded in detail, gives us an extremely interesting picture and may represent a typical reaction. The company was the American Brake Shoe Company, headed by William B. Given, Jr. Addressing a Hygiene Foundation convention in 1947, Mr. Given reviewed the story of his plant medical department, started fifteen years before:

> Looking back, I realize that in that period we had little conception of how far we fell short in giving our people proper working conditions. An earthquake did the trick, and I am still ashamed of the fact that it was a money scare which woke us up. The year was 1933. The company was in red ink for the first time in its history.
>
> Returning from a plant-visiting trip to the Pacific Coast, a telegram was handed to me after the train left Omaha. It read:
>
> THIRTY-FOUR SILICOSIS SUITS TOTALING
> $2,700,000 HAVE BEEN FILED IN BEHALF
> OF CHICAGO HEIGHTS EMPLOYEES.
>
> I had a lot more hours of train ride to think that over! Visualizing the possibilities on the money side—that was only one of our then thirty-nine foundries—our tangible net worth was under $25 million. From the human side, we in management thought we were doing a job of making our plants proper places to work. But the question on the train was: were we? . . .
>
> During the next period of months we did not enjoy those law suits. Today I say they were one of the best things that could have happened to us and especially to me, a fairly new chief. From then on improvements in working conditions began to get top priority in our company.[26]

Things moved rapidly, once that decision was made. Human relations were given greater attention. There were sweeping improvements in the working environment. Medical, hygiene, and safety personnel cooperated to reach common objectives. In 1941 Lloyd E. Hamlin joined American Brake Shoe as medical director. A graduate of the University of Toronto, with long experience in northern Michigan industries, he was given a free hand to develop the company's health program on an even broader scale.

With the continued support of top management American Brake Shoe medical department, in the next decade, grew into a well balanced organization serving ten thousand employees in ten divisions of the company, supervising the activities of an industrial hygiene laboratory responsible for plant surveys and procedural recommendations, and directing a staff of forty-one nurses servicing fifty widely scattered plants. The full program, wrote Hamlin, covered all phases of occupational medicine, including medicolegal and, particularly, the control of hazards due to dust, lead, toxic solvents, and other substances.

Is American Brake Shoe experience of the thirties and forties typical or average? There is no way of averaging. But there is ample evidence indicating that a great many corporation heads, beset by suits, stung by criticism, or impressed by simple facts, re-examined their medical departments organization and services, made careful note of defects, and prayerfully set about remedying them.

If management executives were familiar with the industrial-medical and medico-legal developments of the thirties and were aware of their full meaning, their self-examination would lead inescapably to four conclusions:

1. That occupational diseases and disease hazards were to play a more important part in America's social thinking and in compensation legislation.

2. That an industrial corporation must have consecutive and detailed information about the health of its employees, for business as well as for human reasons.

3. That without such information, in complete and reliable record form, no company could be in a proper position to appraise its medical department needs, control occupational hazards, or defend itself against unjustified compensation claims based on work-connected disease.

4. That adequate records cannot be obtained without physical examinations, not only pre-employment, but job-placement, periodical (adjusted to hazards), and separation (in indicated cases) examinations.

This was unassailable logic, and it led to the great turning point in the road for occupational medicine. For one thing, acceptance of this simple formula completely vindicated the main line of thinking by pioneers in the AAIP&S in their effort to establish the industrial branch of the profession as an indispensable specialty. And (more important) the two principal planks in their original platform, examinations and medical records, eventually provided the practical means by which complex modern systems of occupational health care could be implemented.

XXI

PROSPERITY IN DEPRESSION

Human nature ran true to form in the dark years of the early thirties, as the depression swept like a pestilence across the continent. Reactions followed no set pattern. The strong showed their strength and the weak betrayed their weakness, as always in times of distress or crisis. At different stages and under varying conditions, emotions ran a gamut from fear, panic, and despair to stoic acceptance and stern determination. The loudest complaints came from those who had tried to run shoestring investments into millions. But for every one who mourned the loss of something he had never owned, there were many who faced facts and set about doing what could be done to restore a balanced economy.

Over-optimistic executives in some manufacturing industries tried for a time to bolster sagging business volume by forcing high-pressure tactics on their dealer organizations. But table pounding and pressure selling got exactly nowhere in a market that did not respond because the buying public could not or would not buy anything beyond the bare necessities.

Wise employers recognized the depression for what it was: the "morning after" a period of lush living, the price that had to be paid for the spending and speculative spree of the twenties. Such employers knew that no miracle of salesmanship could turn red ink into black. They radically revised plans and policies, trimmed their sails to the force of the storm, economized wherever economy would help them ride it out.

There is no reason to believe that American doctors fared either better or worse than other professional and business men during those troubled years, or that the situation of doctors in industry differed much from that of private practitioners. The fact is that the entire profession was hard hit. There was less medical business, just as there was less law business and less general business. And it was far less remunerative.

244

Some ambitious studies were made in the thirties, with the idea of determining the effects of hard times on morbidity and mortality. Was the national health improving by reason of a leaner diet and more austere living? Was poverty better for the working man than prosperity? Or were people who needed medical care going without it because they had not the wherewithal to pay?

Such surveys, for the most part, seem to have bogged down in a morass of statistics before they were finished. They produced an enormous amount of information but almost no clear-cut conclusions. For example, a 1933 United States Public Health Service bulletin titled *Sickness and the Economic Depression* and described as a preliminary report on illness in the families of wage earners starts off this way:

> After several years of severe economic distress, the gross death rate has attained the lowest level on record. Infant and tuberculosis mortality have not increased in the country as a whole; on the contrary, they have continued to decline.
>
> These encouraging indications have led to considerable speculation on the part of some as to the possible advantages of "tightening the belt" during hard times, of returning to "simpler and saner living," of the "toughening" regimen of adversity. Others have offered the explanation that any ill effects have been prevented by a marvelously efficient public health system and program of social relief, and are concerned chiefly over the possibility of a breakdown in these efforts before necessary economic readjustments can be completed.[1]

The report, however, almost immediately minimizes the importance of these facts by stating that "the death rate is not an adequate criterion of the extent of sickness and impairment." It goes on to say:

> In fact, fragmentary information also gives a hint of warning that, in certain areas and among certain classes of the population, the situation is not nearly so favorable as gross mortality rates appear to show. Malnutrition among school children apparently has increased, in some localities at least. Higher infant mortality and tuberculosis death rate have been experienced in certain areas of New York City where unemployment was most serious.

Other findings in this report (based on the sickness records and economic history of some 2,500 wage-earning families in three large industrial centers) showed substantially more disabling illness among the entire group between 1929 and 1932 than was suffered prior to that period. The highest rate of illness, whether disabling or not, was found in families that had been in comfortable circumstances in 1929 but had dropped to comparative poverty in 1932. Even the poor who had stayed poor fared better in the matter of health than those whose incomes had been reduced after 1929.

These and other similar statistical findings unquestionably contain both meat and meaning; but the report closes with a warning regarding the significance of the findings; ". . . the writers have purposely refrained from drawing conclusions as to their broad implications and the reader is cautioned to exercise similar restraint."

About two years after the foregoing survey there appeared another USPHS report, entitled "Sickness Among Male Industrial Employees During the Second Quarter of 1935." Like the earlier one, this also sought to appraise the impact of current economic conditions on disease and disability. The report included a detailed tabulation of statistics covering rates of disability from nonindustrial injuries and from specific diseases, over a five-year period.[2]

Also, like the other survey, this seems important for conclusions that can reasonably be deduced from its text rather than for those that can be proved by statistical matter. The meat of its major findings is conveniently boiled down into these few sentences:

> The down trend in sickness frequency which has been manifested during the past five or six years . . . may have reached its nadir, at least for the time being. Progressive increase in the proportion employed on a full-time basis (in 1935) may result in slightly higher sickness rates on account of increased exposure to occupational health hazards.
>
> That a relationship exists between the health of industrial workers and the rate of business activity seems apparent from the changes which have occurred in sickness frequency among industrial employees from 1921 to date.

At the risk of rushing in where statisticians fear to tread, we may draw from such reports a few simple conclusions that are at least tenable and that fairly reflect the conditions faced by the American Association of Industrial Physicians & Surgeons in the early 1930's.

First, there is little convincing evidence of any significant change in morbidity trends during that period, insofar as the over-all health of the nation is concerned. The "medical depression" seems to have been largely a matter of economics. People, on the whole, sought a minimum of self-financed medical treatment and paid out a minimum for medical fees.

Second, any decline in the incidence of occupation-connected disease in the first half of the decade could have been principally due to less exposure to hazards, because industrial employment was at a low ebb.

Third, with business starting its upturn, the later thirties saw the beginnings of a great influx of new metals, compounds, and processes in industry. Growing employment, plus added health hazards, would naturally raise the morbidity rate.

Finally, the extent of the increase of morbidity in any industry would depend very largely on how well the employer fulfilled his obligations, legal and implied, in the way of medical, hygienic, and safety services and precautions.

On this last score, the industries found themselves pulled in opposite directions. On the one side the dismal business picture, demanding drastic economy and retrenchment, brought about a natural disinclination to increase medical staffs and fatten medical services. On the other hand humane, medicolegal and purely fiscal considerations urged larger investments of cash and care in the organization of industrial medical departments.

246

At one stage of the depression there were a good many reports and a great deal of talk in the AAIP&S about employers who, as an economy measure, reverted to the first-aid era, dispensing with medical and surgical directors and turning the entire job over to a nurse or nurses.

It is unlikely that any records were kept to show the extent of this type of economy, especially among smaller plants. But it is certain that, as the thirties wore on, more and more of the important industrial employers were impressed by some phases of the new social thinking, and a fresh realization of the practical value of health in industry, entirely aside from the high cost of neglecting physical examinations, records, and other medical procedures.

The AAIP&S, as the twenties reached their chaotic close, had weathered a world war, a minor depression, and a boom of fantastic proportions. The association's leaders and its members had kept a realistic perspective while the balloon was being inflated, and there was no disastrous aftermath when it exploded.

From an administrative viewpoint, both 1929 and 1930 were difficult years in association affairs. In 1929 the boom spirit was rampant in industry; physicians, like everyone else, were preoccupied with the probabilities of continued prosperity and paid little attention to prognostications that this sort of thing might not go on forever. In 1930, the association, like every other organization, faced a collapsing economy, with no clear idea of what was coming next.

AAIP&S members were saddened in May, 1930, by the sudden death of Guy L. Kiefer of Detroit, a distinguished figure in the fields of public health and preventive medicine and an ardent supporter of organized industrial medicine. Kiefer had served as president of the association in 1928–29, and his was the second presidential death in its history. The organization's resolution in his honor contained the following tribute: "As a diagnostician he had few equals; as commissioner of health of Detroit he gave to his city a department that has always ranked high in the public health field, and to his last post of public service, that of commissioner of health of Michigan, he brought the wisdom of long experience and the unbounded enthusiasm of a true believer in the future of preventive medicine."[3]

Kiefer's principal industrial work was done as medical director of the Michigan Bell Telephone Company, a connection he relinquished in 1924 to enter public health service. His successor at Michigan Bell, Henry S. Brown, was to be elected head of the AAIP&S more than twenty years later.

As association president, Kiefer brought the 1929 annual meeting to Detroit, where he turned the gavel over to C. F. N. Schram, one year, almost to a day, before death ended his own career. Schram, a product of Columbia University College of Physicians & Surgeons, had been chief surgeon for Fairbanks, Morse & Company, Beloit, Wisconsin, since 1917, and in that capacity had developed a shop hospital that was regarded as a model of efficiency. In 1934 he moved to Kingsport, Tenn., to take charge of medical service for 4,000 employees of the Tennessee Eastman Corporation.

A forceful speaker and writer, Schram devoted himself energetically to association affairs. The times were not propitious. AAIP&S finances were still in need of a policy of thrift. Membership figures had seesawed along for ten or more years with no net gain, for many of the founders were gone and others were aging. The number of new members barely offset these losses.

Nevertheless, the association had made real gains in recognition and influence during the twenties; it had preserved the hard, compact core of its membership; it had a nucleus around which vigorous and talented young doctors of a new generation could be rallied. The association rule of *quality* before *quantity* remained inflexible.

One finds nothing in the official proceedings of the association to indicate that its members were particularly worried about the depression, even at its worst. The doctors, by and large, stuck close to their doctoring, facing the bad economic situation as realistically as they would face a crisis in a medical or surgical case.

The 1930 annual meeting, held little more than six months after the stock market crash, opened on an optimistic note. "The association," said V. S. Cheney in his report as secretary, "has had a healthy growth during the past year, having increased both its membership and its reserve by more than 50 percent. This has been due mostly to the membership drive, although quite a number of applications have come in unsolicited owing to the increased interest in industrial medicine that has been aroused by various agencies."[4]

Certainly there was no hint of foreboding in the topics chosen for discussion at the meeting. Members, meeting in Detroit for the second consecutive year, did full justice to a purely medical and surgical program, which included, among the speakers, such men as J. Rollin French, C. O. Sappington, Melvin Henderson (of the Mayo Clinic), Frank Rector, Loyal Shoudy, and John J. Moorhead. The closest approach to the legal aspects of industrial medicine came in an address, "Roentgenologic Findings as Evidence on Medicolegal Problems," by William A. Evans, of Detroit.

One important step in organization progress was taken: a constitutional amendment (previously approved by the Board of Directors) was unanimously passed, creating the new membership classification of "fellow." "A fellowship," the amendment declared, "will be issued only by authority of the Board of Directors to an active member of the association who has been a member for five years, or who has made some definite contribution towards the advancement of industrial medicine and surgery, or performed some special service for the association."[5]

More than a year later, after careful study by a special committee, the *Bulletin* published a list of fifty-five members elected to fellowships by the Board.[6] As far as available records show, these were the first to be so honored for signal service to industrial medicine and its representative association. The list included the then president of the organization, Donald B. Lowe; five past presidents: Otto Geier, William A. Sawyer, "Tom" Crowder, C. F. N. Schram, and Cassius H. Watson; six future presidents: Edward C. Holmblad, Floyd E. Shaffer, Robert P. Knapp, Clarence D. Selby, McIver Woody, and Daniel L. Lynch; and one member who enjoyed both distinctions: Loyal Shoudy, past president for two terms in the twenties and future president, a third term, in 1945–46.

Other names on this honor list, widely known in industrial medicine and association affairs, included those of V. S. Cheney, Sidney M. McCurdy, Henry Field Smyth, James B. McConnaughy, Clarence W. Hopkins, J. Rollin French, Thurman H. Lautenschlager, Rufus B. Crain, Emery R. Hayhurst.

The 1930 meeting chose as president Cassius Watson, who had served as second vice-president during Schram's administration. His associate officers were Donald B. Lowe (B. F. Goodrich Company) as first vice-president, and Edward C. Holmblad (American Railway Express Company) as second vice-president, with V. S. Cheney continuing as secretary-treasurer.

A scholarly man, a wise and helpful counselor to his associates, Cassius H. Watson was one of the founding group of the AAIP&S in 1916 and was the first of several medical directors connected with Bell Telephone enterprises to become prominently identified with association affairs. His first industrial affiliation was with the New York Telephone Company, and from 1915 until his retirement in 1943 he was medical director and adviser for associated Bell System companies, whose personnel aggregated about 300,000.

In a presidential greeting which dealt mainly with new medical developments and problems, Watson spiced his text with this comment:

> I have seen this organization grow from a relatively small group of beginners in the movement of industrial medicine to as compact a body of earnest and well-equipped men as any other professional group in the country. In fact I have a secret conviction, which with due introspection each of you will find personally shared, that this association is several grades above any other sectional[7] groups. . . .
>
> There are few meetings that I attend from which I receive more benefit and inspiration than from those of this industrial group, and this applies equally in a scientific and in a social sense.[8]

The program for the 1931 meeting in Philadelphia was exceptionally rich in professional talent, partly because of the cooperation of the University of Pennsylvania Medical School and participation by its staff. But, despite the growing clamor about the silicosis cases and the compensation claims, there was no formal discussion of industrial lung diseases or of medicolegal complications.

The meeting was momentous for another reason, though the signs could not have been apparent to members in attendance at the time. It was to be the last annual meeting until 1934, by reason of unfavorable business conditions. And members balloting at the 1931 session were, without knowing it, voting their new president into office for a three-year term. Their choice could hardly have been better for a period in which many important policy decisions were necessarily left to association officers and directors, in the absence of annual meetings. Donald B. Lowe, a graduate of Western Reserve University School of Medicine, had spent his entire industrial career as medical director of the B. F. Goodrich Company. He was in his late forties, a man of mature judgment and with a keen analytical mind, who could be relied upon to steer a wise course through difficult times.

Problems of membership (and money) continued to plague the association during that period. How to maintain high professional quality and at the same time achieve a reasonable growth in numbers. Membership requirements were exacting; association services to members were few. It is not strange that growth stopped and interest lagged between 1931 and 1934, when personal correspondence, an occasional bulletin, and a few issues of a new journal were the only links of communication between the organization and its members.

As if he sensed the coming of a letdown, Secretary Cheney ended his report to the 1930 convention in this plaintive tone:

> We ran short of original articles presented at the last annual meeting for publication in the *Bulletin*. This year a stenographic report will be made of the clinics at the hospital and will give us more material for publication. As usual, there was practically no response from members who were requested to write something for the *Bulletin*. It is difficult to publish an interesting *Bulletin* if the members take so little interest in it.[9]

Affairs of the association were indeed approaching a critical phase at that time. After a slight increase in 1931, membership fell off gradually, and in 1935 the combined pressure of internal and external factors reduced the number of active members to its lowest level since World War I. Doctors, under the circumstances, could not be blamed for preoccupation with their own troubles, nor were potential new members greatly impressed by plans, not yet crystallized, for expanding and improving association services. But while the depression continued to hold the country in its grip, strong forces favorable to industrial medicine and the AAIP&S were already at work, foremost among them the plan for certification of medical services, initiated several years before under sponsorship of the American College of Surgeons.

No one need be reminded today that only well-organized and well-run medical departments can attract and hold capable industrial doctors. That requirement was of less importance in the twenties, when emergency treatment of assorted injuries was the chief problem, and a first-aid station staffed by a half-trained man or a practical nurse could, by courtesy, be labeled "medical department." There were still, unfortunately, far too many such "departments," despite the fact that foresighted doctors in industry—physicians as well as surgeons—had long been laboring to raise standards all along the line.

To trace the first steps on the road to certification of qualifying departments one must go back to 1914, when Magnus Alexander, president of the National Industrial Conference Board, established the Conference Board of Physicians in Industry, a group selected to study the special medical problems of the industries and to serve as advisers to the larger board in such matters. This move brought together a most unusual aggregation of talent. All the appointees were M.D.'s; with very few exceptions all were medical directors or chief surgeons of important corporations; all were deeply interested in the same aspects of the same profession. Together, they had charge of medical services for about three-quarters of a million workers.

The extent to which fate took a hand in the future of industrial medicine at that point is indicated by the fact that about half of the members of this advisory Conference Board were destined to become leaders in the policy-making and administrative councils of the AAIP&S.

As a matter of record, the list included such pioneers as W. Irving Clark (Norton Company), W. B. Fisk (International Harvester), George H. Gehrmann (Du Pont), Otto P. Geier (Cincinnati Milling Machine), J. W. Harvey (Tide Water Oil), T. Lyle Hazlett (Westinghouse), Robert P. Knapp (Cheney Brothers), S. M. McCurdy (Youngstown Sheet & Tube), J. J. Moorhead (New York Consultant), Robert S. Quinby (Hood Rubber), Frank L. Rector (government bacteriologist), William A. Sawyer (Eastman Kodak), Loyal A. Shoudy (Bethlehem), Cassius H. Watson (American Telephone and Telegraph), and J. J. Wittmer (Brooklyn Edison).

In August, 1916, only two months after the organization meeting of the AAIP&S, the United States government moved into the industrial medical picture. Anticipating American entry into the European war, the Congress created a Council of National Defense and authorized an Advisory Commission "of not more than seven persons" of special qualifications in civilian life. This Advisory Commission was an august body, its membership consisting of Daniel Willard, Hollis Godfrey, Howard Coffin, Bernard Baruch, Julius Rosenwald, and Samuel Gompers, with Dr. Franklin H. Martin (director-general of the American College of Surgeons) representing the field of medicine and surgery.

Martin was widely recognized as an organizer and leader of men. Of him it has been said: "As a constructive dreamer, he had the courage, tenacity and insight to make his dreams come true." In 1917, with the United States at war and federal boards and bureaus multiplying like mushrooms, he was the prime mover in creating a Committee on Industrial Medicine & Surgery within the General Medical Board of the Council of National Defense.

Chairman of this important committee was Joseph Schereschewsky of the U.S. Public Health Service, and president of the then new AAIP&S. Other appointees included Otto Geier and Harry E. Mock. This committee formulated the noteworthy "Industrial Platform for Conservation of Health of the Industrial Army." Presenting the platform at a meeting in January, 1918, Schereschewsky said: "Such a program will require the earnest cooperation of three groups—the medical profession, the industries, and labor. Labor has in some instances in the past frowned upon medical supervision of the worker. Industry has often been blind enough to object to its cost. The profession has been slow to recognize that the field of the industrial surgeon and physician is legitimate and ethical. . . ."[10]

This was not only sound industrial doctrine but sound AAIP&S doctrine, for the association from its beginning has insisted that, without three-way cooperation, organized industrial medicine could never reach its full potential.

Twice in that same year (1918) Geier expounded the association's philosophy before similar audiences, with enthusiasm and conviction that won many new friends to the cause. These were probably the first occasions on which an association spokesman was given an opportunity to tell the full industrial medical story to such influential groups.

Encouraged by the success of hospital standardization in the United States and Canada, which it had sponsored in 1918, the American College of Surgeons in 1926 appointed a Committee on Traumatic Surgery consisting of members from its own ranks and representatives of insurance companies and of other industrial organizations. Their instructions were to study the situation and recommend specific procedures to improve it. The committee did its work well. From the experience of members and the findings of widespread surveys came a "Minimum Standard for Medical Service in Industry," tailored to fit the needs of any industrial organization regardless of size. It was a forthright document, concisely worded. Its main provisions were and are in substance:

1. That a complying establishment shall have a medical department or service so organized, staffed and equipped as to assure efficient care of the ill and injured.

2. That membership on the medical staff shall be restricted to physicians and surgeons who are Doctors of Medicine from acceptable medical schools, licensed and in good standing, competent in the field of industrial medicine and traumatic surgery, worthy in character and in matters of professional ethics.

3. That there shall be maintained a system of complete and accurate records, making available all information pertinent to cases of illness or injury, or required by statute for compensation claims or other purposes.

4. That patients requiring hospitalization shall be sent to institutions approved by the American College of Surgeons.

5. That the medical department or service shall have general supervision over the sanitation of the plant and the health of all employees.

Accompanying this basic code was a less pretentious program covering the application of the "Minimum Standard" to smaller plants. In setting up procedures for such establishments the American College of Surgeons placed somewhat more emphasis on the employment of professionally qualified medical personnel; the requirement of preplacement and periodic examinations—"to be made only by qualified medical examiners"; the keeping of adequate records; and the maintenance of ethical and cooperative relations with the family physicians of employees, particularly in the matter of referrals.

While these studies were going on, leading members of the AAIP&S were called upon with increasing frequency to take part in the industrial activities of the ACS. Loyal Shoudy was a speaker at the annual meeting of the college in 1927 and appeared in an open forum the following year with A. D. Lazenby (Maryland Casualty Company). In 1929 Shoudy was appointed to the ACS Committee on Traumatic Surgery, a post he held until his death in 1950. Alfred H. Whittaker of Detroit, president of the AAIP&S in 1949–50, was named his successor.

At the ACS meeting in 1929, an open forum on traumatic surgery conducted by Frederic A. Besley turned out to be almost an all-AAIP&S affair. Participating were: Frederick W. Slobe (president, 1944–45), chief surgeon and medical director of several Mid-western companies; C. F. N. Schram, Cassius Watson, V. S. Cheney, Clarence D. Selby (then practicing in Toledo), and Hart E. Fisher (Chicago Rapid Transit Company).

The first series of nationwide surveys of industrial medical services by the college was launched in 1931. They were thorough studies, then, as now, conducted by personal contact and with meticulous care. The work involved was done at no cost to employers. By the end of the following year a total of 174 departments had been surveyed, and the certificate of approval had been granted to exactly 74.

There is no way of measuring with statistical accuracy the immediate effect of this innovation upon management thinking with relation to medical and surgical services in industrial plants. Obviously advantageous to the AAIP&S was the fact that the influential ACS placed its prestige squarely behind objectives to which the association was wholly committed, at a time when such backing and practical help were most urgently needed. Beyond this, the ACS program drew a sharp line between the good and the poor medical departments; gave industry, for the first time, a standard by which to judge performance; and separated the "willing" from the "unwilling" among employers.

But far more tangible results than these were soon to be seen. The ACS Certificate of Approval worked magic of some sort. Industrial corporations wanted it, asked for it, displayed it proudly. It quickly became, and has remained, an envied symbol of progressive achievement.

There was also a seeming magic in the "Minimum Standard" itself, on which the awards were based. Compliance with this code by any industrial organization was on an entirely voluntary basis. There could be no suasion other than a realization, on the part of an employer, that good medical service was good business, plus the added value of ACS approval granted to all departments meeting or exceeding minimum requirements.

Though completely lacking authority to do anything except grant or withhold certification, the ACS board boldly says "shall," not "should." Five times it is used, once for each of five requirements, in a code that contains only 208 words. The imperative, somehow, enhances the value and desirability of the award.

Growth over a period of years is the best evidence of the remarkable success of the plan. In 1934, its third year of operation, the certification program began to show its real potential—the ACS approving nearly 400 medical departments and bringing the three-year total to 518. This success marked the beginning of an uptrend that was to continue unbroken. The college had surveyed a grand total of 2293 departments and certified 1459, when, in 1950, it turned this activity over to the AAIP&S with its blessing.

The distribution, by type and size of company, of certifications granted was as remarkable as the numerical gains. At the end of 1937 there were 843 approvals in effect, divided among about 700 different companies, nearly all of which could be rated as "big business." Of all employed persons in that year, *Industrial Medicine* points out, 30 percent were in manufacturing and mechanical industries and in public utilities. It was in those categories that 80 percent of ACS approvals were given.[11]

Commenting on this enterprise, *Industrial Medicine* declares: "From every angle, in every relation, it is the most important and most significant accomplishment in the history of industrial medicine and surgery. And no small part of its significance lies in the fact that it has been done without publicity, without propaganda, quietly, unobtrusively." And the writer adds: "The college is being increasingly besought by the *smaller* companies: 'Come and give us a survey!' "[12]

Nothing, it now appears, was to prevent organized industrial medicine from keeping its date with destiny, neither wars, nor major economic setbacks, nor basic social changes. The big depression, at worst, only delayed the material progress of the association while at the same time it accentuated the need for its services in a modern society.

The bizarre sequence of events in American life between 1930 and 1935 had an electric effect upon national awareness of and interest in occupational disease hazards and, hence, upon occupational medicine. The legal explosion resulting from the silicosis cases, as we have seen, brought about far-reaching changes in the attitude of industrial employers toward their medical departments and services. There were similar reactions in labor and professional ranks. This transformation, oddly, went on and on through a period in which the fortunes of the AAIP&S itself were at their lowest ebb.

In the association *Bulletin* of October, 1932, appeared the following notice, all set in capital letters to command the attention of members:

THE BOARD OF DIRECTORS VOTED TO POSTPONE THE ANNUAL MEETING OF THE ASSOCIATION FOR THE YEAR 1932. THIS WAS DEEMED ADVISABLE BECAUSE OF THE ECONOMIC DEPRESSION WHICH WOULD PREVENT MANY OF OUR MEMBERS FROM ATTENDING. THE TIME AND PLACE FOR HOLDING THE 1933 MEETING WILL BE DECIDED UPON LATER.

On the next page of the same *Bulletin* was a second notice, urging immediate payment of 1932 dues and offering to extend membership to December, 1933, for all who paid the assessment for the current year. At approximately this time, the association was operating on an annual budget of little more than $1,500, which was met by dues, with a few hundred dollars to spare.

There was spirited opposition in some quarters when, in the following April, cancellation of the 1933 annual meeting was also proposed. In a letter addressed to Edmund C. Holmblad, then first vice-president, J. Rollin French of Los Angeles protested against cancellation, stating his opinion that "it would represent the displaying of a white flag, when courage and perseverance are indicated." French, himself a relatively new member of the Board, sent copies of his letter to the other eleven directors.

In his letter, he declared:

I believe it is reasonable to assume that the depression has reached its low ebb, and if such is the case it is also reasonable to assume that industry will soon start reorganizing. Emerging from the past and looking into the future, it must be admitted that business is approaching a new era. Worn-out customs and traditions formerly adhered to, largely through habit, must now give way to science, reason and common sense.

The new era in business development must not be deprived of the guidance of scientific medical principles. It is my opinion that the American Association of Industrial Physicians & Surgeons, at this particular time, has an added responsibility of aiding industry in formulating its plans and scope pertaining to the physical welfare of its employees for the future. . . .

I feel also that the association owes a responsibility to its members and should aid them during this period of unrest and readjustment. Lay schemes of all kinds are being presented to the doctors, and periodical payment plans and contract practice devoid of ethical tone are being presented almost daily, and for want of professional leadership the doctors are beginning to accept the leadership of promoters. I believe it is our duty to rise to the occasion and start a fight with the idea of aiding our successors in sponsoring scientific medical practice in industry.

There was cogency in French's reasoning. A majority of the Board, however, did not agree that the loss of this personal group contact with members would be disastrous; and, for the second consecutive year, the AAIP&S had no annual meeting.

Evidently individual members, serving industry as medical directors, were able to carry on, effectively representing the association and fighting for its ideals and objectives. True, the depression had its course to run, at great cost in dollars and much want and suffering. But with characteristic resilience and initiative, the people set the economy back on its track and cleared the way to recovery, taking in stride many major changes in social and economic thinking. The outlook steadily improved for industrial medicine as well as for industry itself.

Except for the abrupt drop in 1935, association membership held its own admirably. Losses, due to many causes, were offset by an infusion of new blood, the addition of fine young physicians and surgeons who believed in the future of industrial medicine and in the association as the means of attaining its deserved professional position.

During the depression many young doctors saw in industrial practice not only a coming specialty of great importance but also an immediate and attractive opportunity. In joining the association (at very modest cost) they were banding together with seasoned veterans to assert their economic importance and to win for themselves a share in the future they envisioned.

Industrial medicine, in the thirties, offered a more attractive career than ever before in its history. The AAIP&S experienced during those years an uplift of professional dignity, a notable accretion of respect, esteem, and influence. It was a period, indeed, in which we see the paradox of prosperity in hard times, not money prosperity, to be sure, but a prosperity of over-all progress, marked by extraordinary growth in the association's membership, expansion of services, and real scientific accomplishment.

XXII

PERSONALITIES AND PUBLICATIONS

O N AN early autumn day in 1932 Dr. Volney S. Cheney sat at his desk in Chicago and wrote a paragraph for the October issue of the *Bulletin* of the American Association of Industrial Physicians & Surgeons, the official quarterly publication of which he was editor. He had inherited the job when he agreed to serve as acting secretary of the association in 1928, and, as perennial secretary-treasurer in the thirties, he had retained it, faithfully chronicling medical news and opinion for the membership in a modest four-to-twelve-page leaflet. His paragraph read as follows:

A New Publication

The first issue of *Industrial Medicine* is before me. Its striking green cover is rather attractive. Its contents include a number of articles on subjects of major importance in the industrial medical field. Its "Industrial Medicine Digest" will be of immense value to the busy industrial physician who has the desire but not the time to keep posted on the growth of all the phases of his work. There has never been a publication adequately representing this growing specialty, and in my opinion its appearance is at the psychological moment. If the succeeding numbers maintain the standard set by the first issue its success is assured.

There was little in the current business picture to encourage such optimism. The date should be remarked—October, 1932—not an ideal time, on the whole, for launching new enterprises. The economic barometer was still falling. More establishments were going out of business than were coming in. In the issue of *Bulletin* that told of the founding of *Industrial Medicine,* Cheney announced cancellation of the association's seventeenth annual meeting because of the depression and printed an offer to remit a year's dues to all members paying the regular 1932 assessment.

Nevertheless, the doctor's prediction of success for the new journal proved to be sound. Certainly he was qualified to judge the need for a publication devoted entirely to the professional interests of industrial physicians and surgeons. In four years as a conscientious (and harassed) editor, he had done well with the association *Bulletin,* considering the dearth of money, contributed material, and space in which to print it.

Since the latter part of the twenties there had been an increasing concern, on the part of men interested in occupational health, over the problem of keeping industrial physicians and hygienists even reasonably well informed on the fast moving developments in that field. Cheney had reason to be aware of that concern and to share it.

The problem had been succinctly stated by Carey P. McCord in a letter sent to members of the AAIP&S in June of the preceding year. Since 1920 McCord, an active member of and worker for the association, even at that early date, had devoted a part of his time and talent to serving the Industrial Health Conservancy Laboratories of Cincinnati as medical director. We quote from a copy of his letter received by Edward C. Holmblad, then first vice-president of the association:

> The number of chemical and physical hazards in industry is increasing so rapidly that the busy industrial physician cannot hope to keep fully abreast of developments. A generation ago the better known industrial diseases could be counted on the fingers of the hands. Nowadays, practical hazards may be enumerated in terms of many hundreds of items. The industrial physician, in the midst of his many regular duties, is often called upon to cope with unusual and bizarre physical and mental situations that may or may not be related to employment. . . .

There followed a presentation of advisory services covering an extremely wide range of subjects, available to either individuals or organizations, for private use or for distribution in printed form. The laboratories thus offered a fertile source of reliable research data and related medical information. This material, however, could not be routed to the entire profession through any one publication, for the reason that there was no specialized magazine covering the entire field of industrial medicine.

Despite hard times, there were in the thirties many worthy, well established journals in circulation, representing trade and professional organizations of many types. They were on the whole well edited, purveying material of interest and value to the special audiences they served. The editors were also insatiable in their appetite for newsworthy papers; and able industrial doctors, like speakers and writers of reputation in other fields, were bombarded for contributions. Typical of this competition for good magazine material was a request from the *International Journal of Medicine and Surgery* which Holmblad received in 1931. He was then serving several railroads in surgical capacities, and the editor wrote him primarily as a railway man:

> The fact that practically all the Railway Surgeons' Associations we serve as official organ have, through expediency, postponed their annual meetings this year means

that there is perforce a marked curtailment of the high-class, practical articles that usually come to us through these sources, to publish for the edification of the railway and industrial surgeons in general.

In order not to let down our standard of practical, interesting material that we have published monthly, please permit the writer to urge you to contribute an article soon to the official organ of your own and several other great railway surgical associations—the *International Journal of Medicine and Surgery.*

Of course, a good paper on railway medicine appealed doubly to a railway surgeon, as a doctor and as a railroader. But timely articles on any phase of occupational medicine were of interest not only to him but to every progressive industrial physician, regardless of his company affiliation.

Therein lay the dilemma for the AAIP&S and its members. As industrial physicians and surgeons they had no single journal through which to channel their own literary output or in which to look for the significant work of others with similar interests. Competition for such articles kept circulation widely scattered. AAIP&S members faced the problem of reading an impossibly large number of publications, if they were to keep up with the literature of their specialty.

The need for a publication devoted entirely to industrial medicine was even more acute during the depression than during normal times. The line of communication among industrial doctors, in some of these years, was as thin as the pages of an infrequent bulletin or a form letter. The need and the danger were recognized by several wideawake individuals, both inside and outside the association.

Among the latter was a young Chicagoan, A. D. Cloud. A capable writer and editor, with industrial experience, he established in November, 1930, a small magazine called *Industrial Relations,* a name which, in that era, needed definition and elaboration, as did the term "industrial medicine" itself. Cloud's periodical had to do chiefly with pension systems, but their orientation to the industrial relations field led him into a maze of kindred topics, including bonuses, invitations to thrift, profit-sharing arrangements, welfare policies and, in recognition of the importance of physical fitness, such subjects as health protection measures and medical supervision in employment. Cloud wrote:

> After this journal had been published for something over a year, I met Dr. Durward R. Jones, then medical director of the Sherwin-Williams Company, who told me it was a mistake to consider the medical department in industry as a subordinate part of industrial relations. Instead, he said, I should reverse the picture and put medical supervision first, with nothing else in the whole area of employee relations ranking above it.
>
> Through Dr. Jones I met Dr. C. O. Sappington, who was then identified with the National Safety Council and who for some years had been himself dreaming of a journal devoted to industrial medicine. Persuaded by these two physicians, I changed the name of *Industrial Relations* to *Industrial Medicine,* and directed its editorial policy toward the doctors in industry rather than the so-called personnel

managers. The response was heartening. Thus encouraged we tested the field by putting out three issues, starting with October, 1932.

Again, *1932*—a fateful year in the history of industrial medicine and of the association. It saw the wave of depression-inspired compensation claims shock business into an awareness of the true function and value of medical departments in industry. It saw the first approvals given in the ACS certification program. And now another milestone, the birth of what Volney Cheney frequently called "the only medium adequately representing this growing specialty!" *Industrial Medicine*,[1] Volume 1, Number 1, was a seventy-two-page magazine of conventional format and approximately its present page size. It was published by Industrial Medicine, Incorporated, and its masthead listed D. R. Jones, M.D., editor, and A. D. Cloud, managing editor.

Industrial Medicine had no difficulty in finding an editorial niche all its own in the medical publication field. A seemingly endless number of subjects were calling for exploration. In fact, early issues listed at least two hundred specific topics which the editors considered within their province, ranging alphabetically from absenteeism to workmen's compensation.

The three introductory issues in 1932 were excellent samples of what the publishers had in mind for the future, a balanced combination of feature articles, incisive editorials, association news, and abstracts or reprints of important material from other professional magazines. From the start, the new publication captured the spirit and purpose of the AAIP&S, and set a pattern which, with improvements and refinements, has been followed in essence down to the present.

"Interest in the project was so evident," wrote Cloud, "and the reception among the doctors so satisfactory, that we decided to continue the publication." Launching a new magazine at the time, however, required more than a simple "go" signal. Money was perhaps the scarcest of commodities in 1933. There had to be a working arrangement with the association. Editorial problems needed study.

In April, Industrial Medicine, Incorporated, proposed a plan whereby AAIP&S members would receive the journal monthly. A separate department would be devoted to association affairs, "printing therein such copy as you submit in the form in which you wish it to appear. On a mass order for subscriptions such as yours would represent, we can afford to make a liberal price concession. For the coming year, it would seem that a subscription price of $1.00 per member would cover our extra costs and at the same time save your organization some of the money that would otherwise be spent on printing, postage, etc." The letter closed with this candid comment: "In all fairness, we are making this same offer to other associations whose interests are similar to yours."

Use of the word "liberal" in this offer was decidedly an understatement, even in depression times, since the deal would give each association member twelve issues per year of a full-fledged industrial-medical magazine, thoughtfully planned and expertly edited, at one-third the cost of the old *Bulletin* it published on a monthly basis. An agreement was promptly signed, and in July, 1933, after a lapse of six months in publication, *Industrial Medicine* was once more available to the membership.

Volume 2, Number 1 was a substantial eighty-four-page number. It listed a board of editors consisting of Volney S. Cheney, Otto Geier, Hart Fisher, Donald C. O'Connor, and LeRoy P. Kuhn (prominent Chicago industrial surgeon), with A. D. Cloud as publisher.

Reviewing old files of *Industrial Medicine,* we were struck by the emphasis given, from the very beginning, to fundamental policies and objectives which the association has pursued with almost holy zeal down the years. The matter of physical examinations is a case in point: "Without records, employers have at best a weak defense in many compensation cases. But without examinations there can be no records. Examinations, in turn, require medical departments. And to be effective, a medical department must be under the direction of a trained industrial doctor, supported by adequate personnel and facilities."

This formula, in one variation or another, has been a steady drumbeat through the history of the AAIP&S and the IMA, and its logic remains as cogent as ever. Spearheading the contents of the very first issue of *Industrial Medicine* (October, 1932) was a feature article titled "Periodic Medical Examinations," by Hart E. Fisher, lawyer, doctor, soldier, teacher, writer, chief surgeon of the Chicago Rapid Transit Company, and a valued contributing editor to the association journal for several years.

In this first article Fisher detailed his conclusions about periodic examinations after observing the same group of employees for twenty years. Complete with illustrations, record forms, and statistical data, his article met an acute need in industrial corporations throughout the country. In 1934 Fisher contributed, in serial form, a "Medical Department Manual," a pioneering step in administrative and operational procedures.

These specific literary efforts, two among a total of many thousands covering every phase of industrial medicine, are cited only to point out the utility and value of *Industrial Medicine (and Surgery)* over the years. Not only have individual issues kept open a busy channel of communication between association and members, but cumulatively they have preserved the vigor of objectives, policies, and procedures. The value of the medical information they encompass cannot be overestimated; nor can anyone compute the loss to the present IMA and its members, had they never been published.

Industrial Medicine, from its inception, was fortunate in the matter of editorial supervision. With its first regular issue, C. O. Sappington began his service as editorial consultant. As time went on he became more and more active, and in the spring of 1940 took over the duties of editor-in-chief, an arrangement that continued until his death in November, 1949. At that time, editorship of the magazine (newly named *Industrial Medicine and Surgery*) passed to Jean Spencer Felton, then medical director of the Oak Ridge (Tennessee) National Laboratory (atomic energy) and a lecturer in the sociological department of the University of Tennessee. In July, 1951, Felton resigned from the editorial post and was succeeded by the present editor, Carey P. McCord.

During the quarter-century since the journal was launched, these editors have shared work and responsibilities with a board of associate editors, representative of the membership-at-large. Physicians all, and active in association affairs, they helped in formulating policies, planning editorial content, contributing as writers, or recruiting desirable talent.

The size of this board has increased, along with the scope and activities of the association. Always, this group has included a substantial number of old-timers who have served for many years; yet there is no lack of vigorous young talent to carry on through changing times.

The troubles of the infant *Industrial Medicine* were not over when it started monthly publication under the 1933 agreement. Odds, in a time of depression, were strongly against its survival. Advertisers were hunting bargains, counting pennies, cutting space. Early in 1934, the United States Post Office Department ruled that the journal did not qualify for the second-class mailing privilege but would have to pay the parcel post rate. This ruling was a bitter pill, since it added about six and a half cents per copy per month to mailing costs. But Cloud, though his budget was stretched drum-tight, took the setback philosophically. Reporting to the association's officers, directors and publication committee he wrote: "Please be assured that it is our desire to continue the arrangement with the American Association of Industrial Physicians & Surgeons. We know . . . that, over a period of a year or so, this will adjust itself."

But the financial situation did not soon adjust itself. There was no sudden rush to buy advertising space in an almost unknown new journal. Costs kept nibbling away at limited reserves. And with the mailing of the June, 1934, issue *Industrial Medicine* was forced again to suspend publication for a six-month period. AAIP&S members, however, were as stubborn in their desire for an official journal as Cloud was in his determination to give them one. They liked what they had seen in early issues, and stood loyally behind the editors and publishers. The journal resumed publication in January, 1935. The cycle has never since been broken.

From this modest and shaky start emerged the present *Industrial Medicine and Surgery,* genuinely respected, widely quoted, and commercially successful. In more than a quarter-century of publication it has become one of the leading journals to serve the great medical profession. In the late nineteen-thirties the *International Journal of Medicine and Surgery* and the *Industrial Doctor,* theretofore published in Buffalo, New York, were acquired by, and consolidated with, *Industrial Medicine.*

It may not have occurred to Cheney, when he announced the birth of *Industrial Medicine* in 1932, that he was starting the obituary notice of his own *AAIP&S Bulletin.* The thought would not have disturbed him, for the welfare of the association was ever uppermost in his mind. To emphasize the connection between the new pub-

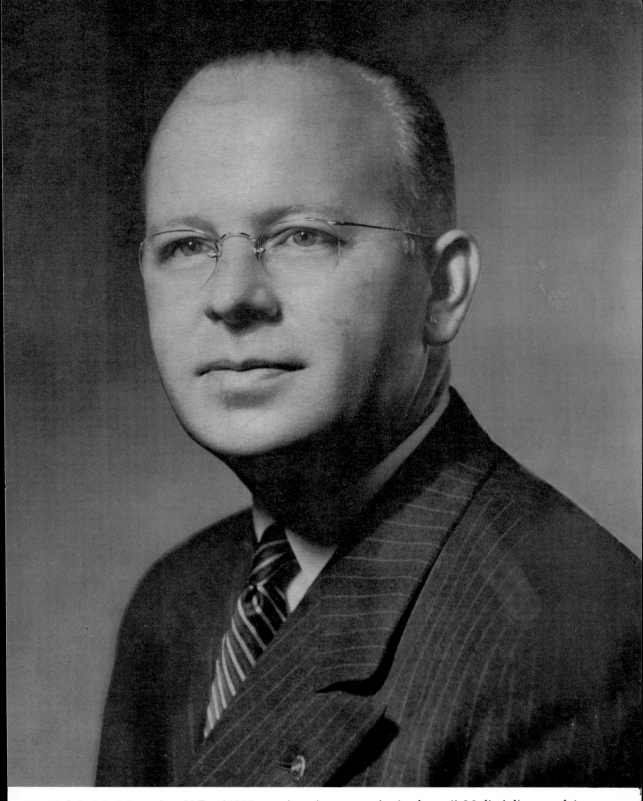

78. *Melvin N. Newquist, M.D.* (1897–   ). *President, AAIP&S, 1945–1946.* Cancellation of the annual meeting in 1945 forced the incoming administration to handle association affairs largely by remote control. As president-elect in 1944, Dr. Newquist automatically took office the following year, but other officers and directors were chosen in a proxy election by mail. Medical director of the Texas Company since 1939, Newquist had conducted, as a field representative of the American College of Surgeons, a first-hand survey of medical services in industry. Despite difficulties his administration also outlined an admirable plan of post-war activity.

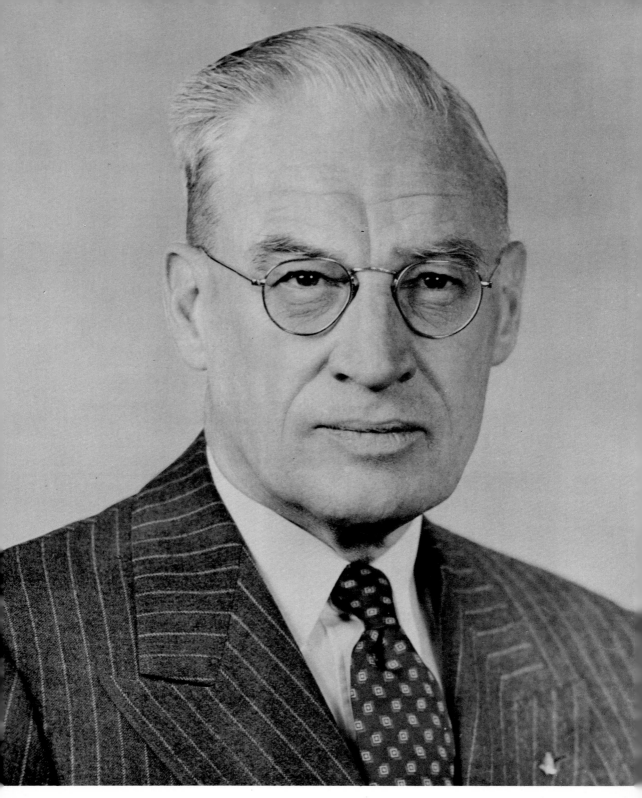

79. *Henry S. Brown, M.D. (1891–). President, AAIP&S, 1947–1948.* From his vantage point as medical director of Michigan Bell Telephone Company (1930–1956), Dr. Brown kept a close watch on the broad trends in occupational medicine and surgery; and as president of the association he maintained pressure on long-range objectives: certification of the specialty, postgraduate education in industrial medicine, and fellowships to encourage specialization. He also sponsored a realignment of component societies and conducted a highly productive membership campaign. He has served on many important IMA committees.

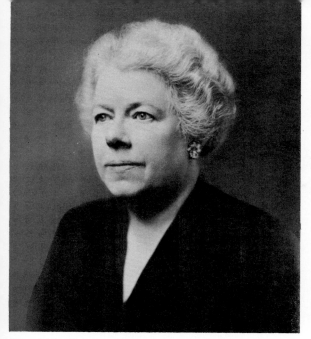

80. *Catherine R. Dempsey, R.N.* A pioneer in the fight for recognition of industrial nursing and first president of the American Association of Industrial Nurses, 1943–1947.

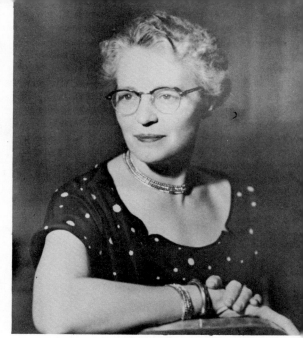

81. *Mary E. Delehanty, R.N. President, American Association of Industrial Nurses, 1947–1951.* In 1948 she told the American Nurses' Association that it was "the hope and desire of industrial nurses for amity and working unity, without duplication of activities between the AAIN and ANA."

82. *Thelma J. Durham, R.N. Third president, American Association of Industrial Nurses, 1951–1953.* She presided over the historic meeting of April 23, 1952, at which the AAIN decided to go it alone as an independent national organization. Her comment: "It was an adult performance."

83. *Sara P. Wagner, R.N. President, American Association of Industrial Nurses, 1953–1957.* Looking ahead, at a congress in Helsinki, 1957, she said: "On-the-job training will become the supplement to more formal education in this special field of nursing. . . . I predict that we will achieve a goal we have desired deeply for many years, namely, that all nurses in industry will have medical direction."

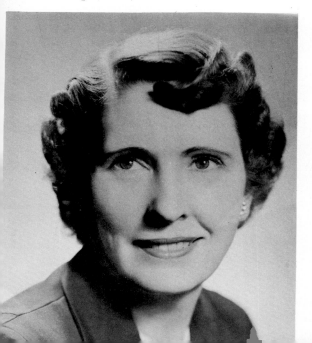

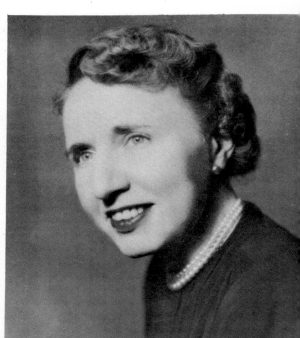

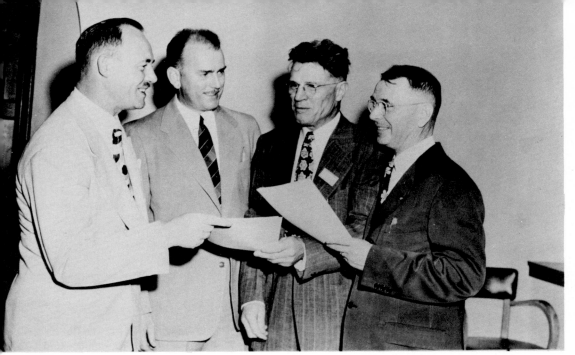

84. *General Motors Citations for Hudson and Sutton.* At a dinner in July 1946, GM honored with special citations the first two full-time physicians the corporation had employed, A. Willis Hudson (1915–1946) and Mahlon R. Sutton (1916–1932). Left to right: Earl F. Lutz (associate consultant, G.M., Detroit), E. J. Nugent (medical director, Rochester Products), Dr. Hudson, Dr. Sutton.

85. *Early Industrial Hospital.* The hospital of the Bradley Mining Company at Yellow Pine Mine, Stibnite, Idaho. A common type of company-owned structure maintained for employees in the early 1900's, especially in remote mining and lumbering areas with no other medical or surgical facilities.

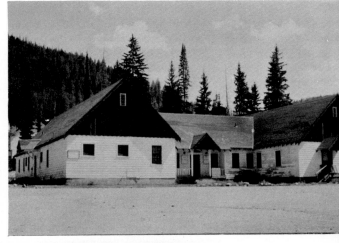

86. *Industrial Nursing of an Older Day.* Early in the 1900's the Crane Company opened for its employees a cottage sanitarium in fifty acres of wooded land on the bank of the Illinois River. To this haven Dr. Harvey sent patients, at his discretion, for recuperation. Cases of contagious or infectious diseases were not accepted.

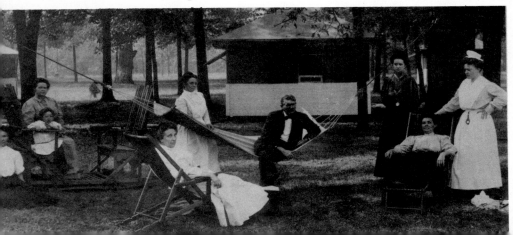

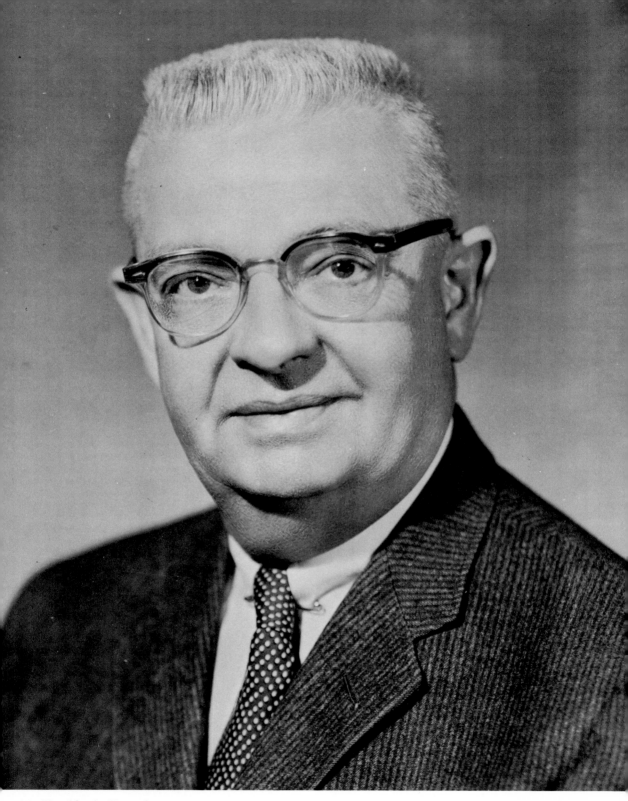

87. *Harold A. Vonachan, M.D. (1898–   ).*
President, AAIP&S, 1948–1949. As president,
Harold Vonachan set about improving standards
of the association and membership selection. He
insisted on "functioning" officers and committees,
encouraged younger men to greater activity, and
campaigned for industrial medical education and
certification as main targets. Vonachan has looked
at the human side of his calling in his many assignments for the AAIP&S and related groups and as
medical director of Caterpillar Tractor Company.
He is noted for his work and writings on rehabilitation, mental hygiene, control of TB and syphilis,
and fatigue and nutrition in industry.

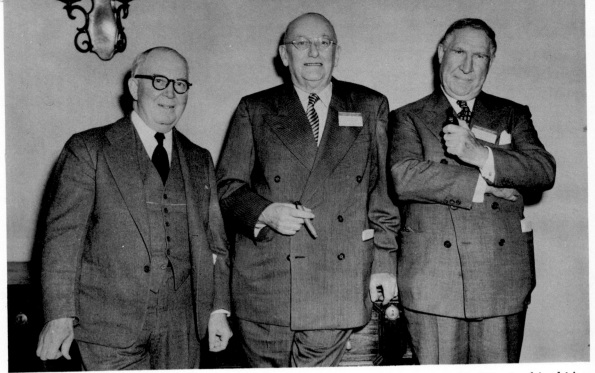

88. *The Three Musketeers of the AAIP&S.* "It's the friendships you remember." Loyal Shoudy, Otto Geier, and Harry Mock hold an impromptu reunion at a mid-century meeting of the association.

90. *Five Old-timers of the AAIP&S.* Taken at the Rochester convention in 1947. Standing, Holmblad, Slobe and Whittaker; seated, Shoudy and Dr. Victor G. Heiser, then consultant in industrial medicine for the National Association of Manufacturers.

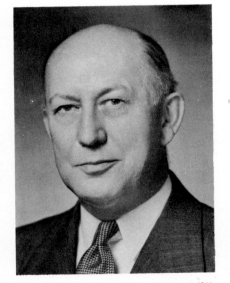

89. *Robert M. Graham, M.D.* Affiliated with the Pullman Company soon after World War I, director of its Department of Sanitation & Surgery since 1942; active in the councils of the AAIP&S—as committeeman, district counselor for the north central states, and member of Board of Directors, 1947–1949.

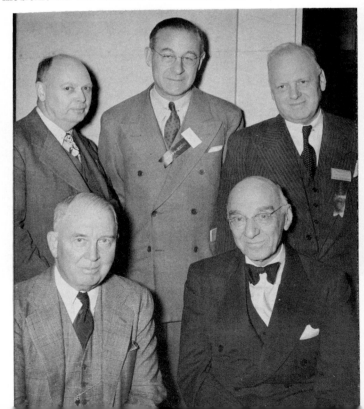

HOSPITALS AND FIRST-AID

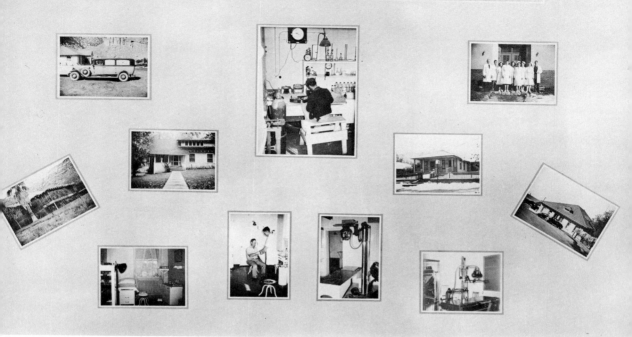

91. *Modern Health Facilities Available to Miners.* Here is reproduced a portion of one of four "Bulletin Board" panels used in a dramatic exhibit of facilities available to American mine workers and their families in modern times. The series, containing more than seventy-five photographs, stresses progress made in four important categories—hospitals and first-aid care, "change-house" facilities, schools and housing, and recreation.

—*Courtesy of the Bureau of Mines, U.S. Department of the Interior*

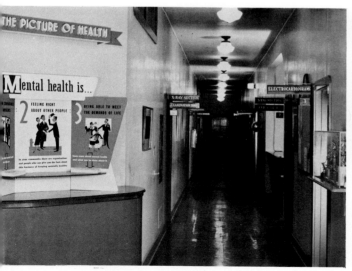

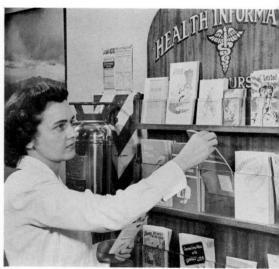

92 & 93. *Mental Health and Health Information at Oak Ridge.* Many progressive employers now carry on continuous campaigns of health education for workers. The displays shown here are part of the program instituted by Dr. Jean S. Felton as medical director of the Oak Ridge National Laboratory from 1946 to 1953. Felton's career includes five years (1940–1945) as a medical officer in the U.S. Army. Since 1953 he has been associate professor in the Department of Medicine and Department of Preventive Medicine of the University of Oklahoma. For almost two years he served as editor of *Industrial Medicine and Surgery.*

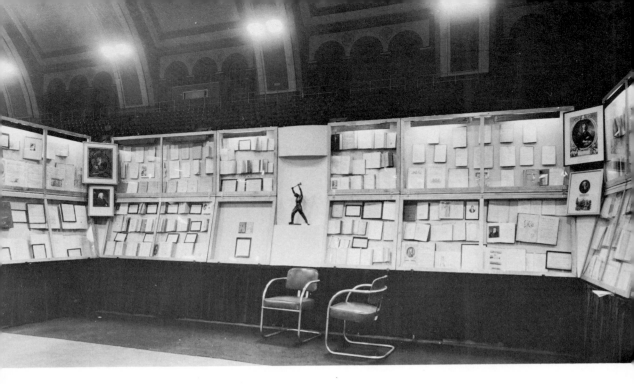

94. *The Whittaker Historical Exhibit, 1947.* This exhibit, outlining medical history from the Greek and Egyptian periods, was a feature of the Hundredth Anniversary meeting of the AMA at Atlantic City and received a special award from the AMA. Arranged by Dr. A. H. Whittaker, largely with material from his own library, it included rare first editions.

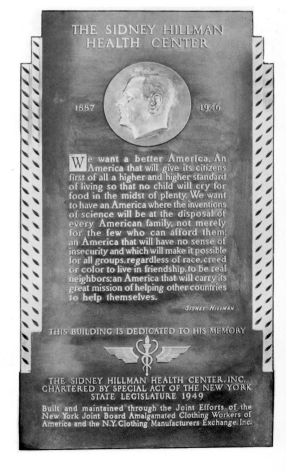

THE SIDNEY HILLMAN
HEALTH CENTER

1887   1946

We want a better America. An America that will give its citizens first of all a higher and higher standard of living so that no child will cry for food in the midst of plenty. We want to have an America where the inventions of science will be at the disposal of every American family, not merely for the few who can afford them; an America that will have no sense of insecurity and which will make it possible for all groups, regardless of race, creed or color to live in friendship, to be real neighbors; an America that will carry its great mission of helping other countries to help themselves.

Sidney Hillman

THIS BUILDING IS DEDICATED TO HIS MEMORY

THE SIDNEY HILLMAN HEALTH CENTER, INC.
CHARTERED BY SPECIAL ACT OF THE NEW YORK
STATE LEGISLATURE 1949

Built and maintained through the Joint Efforts of the New York Joint Board Amalgamated Clothing Workers of America and the N.Y. Clothing Manufacturers Exchange, Inc.

95. *The Sidney Hillman Dedication Plaque.* Formally identifies the huge Sidney Hillman Health Center in New York and keeps alive for millions the memory of a great public benefactor.

lication and the association, he transferred the *Bulletin* masthead and a modicum of news and comment to *Industrial Medicine* as a departmental feature that was continued until late in 1937.

There is a fairytale quality in the story of Volney Cheney's career. Born in 1874, a descendant of seventeenth century Pennsylvania Quakers, he represents the fifth generation of physicians in his family. His early boyhood was spent in an orphanage, but he worked his way through a succession of schools to a medical degree from Northwestern University in 1902. For fourteen years he served many masters on many jobs, before joining Armour and Company as surgeon for the Chicago plant. In 1920 he became the first medical director of the entire Armour organization.

Records indicate that no other individual has yet matched Cheney's official span of service to the AAIP&S—IMA. He was secretary-treasurer from 1928 to 1941, remained as treasurer into 1942, and served as an associate editor of *Industrial Medicine* for many years after he gave up active practice.

Even in retirement, in Las Vegas, New Mexico he soon discovered he could not just take it easy, and in 1950, at seventy-six, he looked around for a second career in medicine. He quickly found it; he became the unpaid school doctor for several thousand Las Vegas children. *Medical Economics* printed the story for its readers in 1952.[2] "He began," it said, "by doing physical checkups, referring children needing attention to their family doctors. Then he helped get a school-lunch program under way." Soon, Cheney started a public campaign for a child health center to provide medical attention for all children whose families could not afford to pay for it. He enlisted civic and other groups to raise funds. Physicians and dentists agreed to handle the children's cases for small fees, and the hospital made beds available at nominal cost. "The new program," the article concluded, "is working fine, and Las Vegans are proud of it. But Volney Cheney, well embarked on his second career in medicine, just keeps busy and looks to the future. 'My plans for the children,' he said, 'will take years to accomplish.'"

The ups and downs of a single trade journal in the early thirties seem trivial, unless considered in relation to the unusual situation existing at that time. It must be remembered that the medical needs of industry, as distinct from the surgical, were just beginning to be recognized. About half of all AAIP&S members bore the title "Chief Surgeon," rather than "Medical Director." Their interests, by training and practice, were primarily surgical.

Many of these, and even more of the newcomers to the industrial field, knew relatively little about the respiratory and skin diseases common to certain kinds of employment or about the new toxic hazards that were constantly appearing in industry. With the so-called "dust diseases" (and particularly silicosis) causing national concern, with compensation suits clogging court calendars and threatening industry with staggering losses, there was a rocketing demand for medical and medicolegal information and opinion.

There is irony in the fact that the National Safety Council was pressed into service as an information center for industrial medical data. Under the heading "Silicosis Important," the October, 1932, *AAIP&S Bulletin* printed this notice:

> From an economical and medical viewpoint, the present silicosis situation is without precedent in the history of occupational disease in American industry. It is of great importance that industrial physicians be prepared with technical information, so that they may be of definite assistance to the various industries in which such problems may arise.
>
> The National Safety Council has been in a position to gather a considerable amount of information on this subject, through its national contacts, the work being carried on by C. O. Sappington, director of the Division of Industrial Health. It is understood that Sappington will gladly assist any industrial physicians or industrial organizations by giving them the benefit of this accumulated experience.

This offer was, of course, a gracious gesture on the part of the National Safety Council, and it made important silicosis data available where it was needed. But it was an ironic coincidence that the notice appeared in the industrial doctors' own *Bulletin,* in the same issue that announced the coming of their journal, *Industrial Medicine.* Further than this the information offered was to be supplied by Sappington, who was shortly to become editorial chief of the new journal.

Such incongruous situations, however, were a commentary on the sad lack of liaison within the profession rather than a reflection upon its members. In the years of greatest need for large-scale information services, the AAIP&S was forced to cancel its annual meetings, normally an open forum for discussion of special medical problems in industry. The journal *Industrial Medicine,* was not launched until late in 1932, and at the end of that year was still on its trial run. Medical schools, in that period, had no more than scratched the surface in their approach to specialized education for industrial practice.

Health agencies, universities, and individual doctors, however, were doing what could be done. While American business, in the early thirties, was realigning its forces and planning "better things" through technology, medical research was on the march along its entire frontier. The doctors wrote assiduously of their findings and published them through such media as were available. Legge, from the eminence of a half-century as a witness and historian of industrial medical progress, points to "distinguished researches" by the United States Public Health Service on the problem of radium hazards, aftermath of the tragic poisoning of women watch dial painters. *Industrial Medicine and Surgery* reports that in 1932 "it seemed only minor that sulfanilamide, previously a dye, was rediscovered as a drug,"[3] the first of the antibiotics. There were important new findings on lead poisoning by George Gehrmann (Du Pont Company) and pioneer studies of other toxic metals and compounds. From Henry Field Smyth (University of Pennsylvania School of Medicine) came a prophetic study on noise in industry. Perhaps more, and more penetrating, research was accomplished in the field of pneumoconiosis during the thirties than in any comparable period in history, despite the scantiness of individual health records and supporting x-rays in most industries. Such investigators as Carey McCord and the father-and-son team of Lewis and William Gregory Cole made many new contributions, after the Gauley Bridge episode, to the already immense literature of the dust diseases.

The middle thirties produced study and discussion of the entire silicosis problem. In June of 1934, '35, and '36 the important Saranac symposiums instituted by Leroy U. Gardner, director of the Saranac Laboratory, were held in the Trudeau School of Tuberculosis at Saranac Lake. These brought together a notable group including Henry K. Pancoast (University of Pennsylvania), whom Lewis Cole called the foremost roentgenological authority in the country, E. P. Pendergrass, another eminent radiologist (University of Pennsylvania), Anthony J. Lanza (Metropolitan Life Insurance Company, Royd R. Sayers (USPHS), later president of the AAIP&S, Henry K. Kessler (New Jersey Rehabilitation Commission), Roy R. Jones (USPHS), Homer L. Sampson (Trudeau Sanatorium), Philip Drinker (Harvard University), W. S. McCann (University of Rochester), and D. M. Brumfiel (Saranac Laboratory).

In June, 1935, there was also a silicosis symposium in Wausau, Wisconsin, organized and widely publicized by the Employers Mutuals of Wausau. Medical interest in silicosis seemed to know no bounds. Government concern was indicated by the appointment, in 1936, of four committees to head a cooperative campaign "to lessen the ravages" of the disease, to which a half-million workers were said to be exposed.[4]

Playing a prominent part in the studies and reports that followed was the Committee on Medical Control, with R. R. Sayers as chairman. Sayers headed a group of physicians that included Lanza, McCann, Gardner, and Pendergrass, Cassius H. Watson, president of the National Safety Council, J. Norman White, of Scranton, Pennsylvania, and Beverly L. Vosburgh, medical director of General Electric Company.

Silicosis literature poured from the presses during those eventful years. C. O. Sappington called the disease "a top problem," so important that "no less a person than the chief officer or president of any corporation should take the responsibility for the proper handling of it."[5] E. R. Hayhurst commented on the ease of diagnosis.[6] Michael H. Barsky produced a valuable study in which he analyzed the results of a thousand pre-employment examinations, observing the amount of physical impairment from varying degrees of exposure to silica dust.[7] Thomas L. Dwyer, of Chicago, in a detailed review of the literature of silicosis, cited a bibliography of at least fifty contemporary references.[8]

The dust diseases represented only one category of subjects that clamored for attention. The mounting interest in toxic hazards from metals and chemicals of every type heralded the fantastic new era of technical progress soon to come. Discussion of these and other immediate problems was seriously handicapped by a depression economy that restricted publication enterprises and curtailed business and professional conventions.

It is certain that a great deal of useful, even vital, industrial-medical news and research data produced in that period failed to reach those who most needed authoritative material for study and reference. Many urgent inquiries went unanswered because they were not directed through the right channels or because the answers were not available in printed form.

There could have been no more forceful reminder of the necessity for the development of broader and better information services within the profession. Leaders of the AAIP&S also realized that more frequent personal contacts among the membership were required, for debate and decision on current issues. But if industrial medicine was ever to win its place in the sun, specialized education must be made available in the medical schools at both undergraduate and postgraduate levels. A long-range problem, this last, not to be solved in a year, or a decade!

XXIII

INDUSTRIAL MEDICINE AT THE

CROSSROADS

By the spring of 1934, there were signs of improvement on the business horizon. Directors of the AAIP&S called the nineteenth annual meeting for June 11 and 12. It was the first general session to be held since June, 1931, and members flocked to Cleveland, eager to greet old friends and get at unfinished business.

The convention atmosphere was reminiscent of a college reunion, though the association had little to boast about in the way of material prosperity. Membership, in a process of turnover, was barely holding its own, and nearly one in every six members was delinquent in dues. The meeting was a down-to-earth affair, without frills. The program itself was a mimeographed sheet, a time-and-money saver. But no one minded; the association was inured to economy. Following the trend of the times the medical sessions heavily accented silicosis and related problems, which were discussed in a carefully prepared symposium, with E. R. Hayhurst and C. O. Sappington among the speakers.

The year 1934 might be considered a crossroads for the association, a meeting point of old and new. One era was ending; another beginning. Many of the early members were approaching twenty years of active association work; younger doctors, in increasing numbers, were getting into industrial practice. There was promise in the air. This was a time for forward thinking and forward looking.

At the business session D. B. Lowe retired from the presidency after three years of depression-time service, his ears ringing with the applause of his associates for a difficult job well done. He was succeeded in office by Edward C. Holmblad, an experienced industrial surgeon, and a fellow of the ACS, the AMA, and the AAIP&S.

267

He had been increasingly active in association affairs for several years and had served as first vice-president since 1931.

Like many another prominent member, Holmblad came into the industrial field as a railroad surgeon. A graduate of Rush Medical College, he completed a twenty-seven-month internship at Cook County Hospital in 1920 and soon built a busy practice, serving several railway and insurance companies. Through membership in the Central States Society of Industrial Medicine and Surgery, and through service on its Board of Governors, he became interested in the opportunity offered for contacts at the national level in the AAIP&S.

The Central States Society was an outgrowth of the Illinois Society of Industrial Medicine and Surgery, which was founded in 1924 but changed its name and broadened its scope in 1931, to include members from neighboring states. It has the distinction of being the first official component society of the AAIP&S(IMA), a distinction announced in 1937, a few months before the same status was accorded the Association for the Advancement of Industrial Medicine & Surgery.

The latter was a New York organization whose announced purpose was "to disseminate accurate medical knowledge in reference to the diagnosis and treatment of all conditions arising out of and in the course of employment." At the time of its affiliation with the AAIP&S its president was John J. Wittmer, medical director of the Brooklyn Edison and Consolidated Edison and affiliated companies. Heading the Central States Society in the same year was Frederick W. Slobe, of Chicago. Both men, in the 1940's, were to be elected to the presidency of the AAIP&S.

With Holmblad on the 1934 ticket, Robert P. Knapp (Cheney Bros.) was elected first vice-president and Philip K. Brown (Southern Pacific Railway) second vice-president. Retained on the Board of Directors were five from the 1931 list—Watson, Smyth, McConnaughy, Shaffer, and French, and one, C. F. N. Schram, who had served since 1930. With these six, to round out an able and experienced Board, Don Lowe, A. Girard Cranch (National Carbon Company), Donald Guthrie (Lehigh Valley Railway), Royd R. Sayers (USPHS), L. A. Shoudy (Bethlehem Steel Company), and Peter A. Bendixen, of Davenport, Iowa, were named for two-year terms. The death of Bendixen, medical director of a group of insurance companies, was announced before the end of the first year.

A critical period in the life of the association lay just ahead, as the new administration was well aware. This was no time for either apathy or complacency. Problems arising from technological progress already were challenging the best medical brains in the country. Organized industrial medicine, or, specifically, the AAIP&S, had to set the pace or follow it. If it did not show leadership, others surely would.

Never, during the latter thirties, was the attitude of association members or their elected officials in doubt on this point. They stood solidly behind the upgrading of association services, the upbuilding of membership, the strengthening of finances, the demonstration of leadership both in medical research and in the discharge of medical department responsibilities.

There was little oratory in support of these and other goals, but individuals and groups went to work in earnest. One of the early acts of the 1934–35 administration was to create the office of president-elect, a foresighted move which not only gave the association an added pair of shoulders to carry current work but assured for each succeeding president a year of practical training as preparation for the duties of that office. This change was incorporated in the constitution at the next annual meeting.

In 1934, too, a committee composed of President Holmblad, Secretary Cheney, and John W. Harvey made a study of the journal *Industrial Medicine* to arrive at a satisfactory basis for continuation of its activities as official journal of the association. Assured of good editorial coverage and continued publication, the association approved a new agreement to re-establish it as a vitally needed service. In June, 1934, *Industrial Medicine* had published the program for the Cleveland meeting; in early 1935 issues, it printed papers and proceedings from the 1934 convention.

Old-time members have never quite forgotten the 1931 annual meeting in Philadelphia, a memorable affair which included two days at the University of Pennsylvania Medical School with Charles H. Frazier and Alfred Stengel and their staffs. Loyal A. Shoudy was one of those who remembered. Reminiscing many years later, he said: "In 1935 I went back and asked Dr. Frazier and Dr. Stengel to take us again. They both said, 'Shoudy, that is the finest group of men we ever talked to. Bring them back.' So back we went to the University of Pennsylvania."[1]

A committee consisting of Loyal Shoudy (chairman), George M. Piersol, medical director Bell Telephone Company of Pennsylvania, Henry Field Smyth, and Mervyn R. Taylor, also of Pennsylvania Bell Telephone, labored long and hard to make the 1935 meeting another memorable success. A letter in Shoudy's files throws an interesting sidelight on the process of getting suitable speakers and papers for such an occasion. It was written in response to a request from Shoudy by Dr. E. H. McIlvain, personnel manager of the Budd Manufacturing Company, and it said in part: "There are certainly enough subjects to concern lots of us, but as most of them are confined to relations with labor, it would hardly be a fitting topic for the attention of physicians and surgeons." *O tempora! O mores!* A letter from President Holmblad to Shoudy late in May said: "Thanks for your efforts in arranging such a splendid program," and went on to inform him that letters of information and invitation were being sent to member and non-member physicians, and that the American College of Surgeons was mailing one hundred copies of letter and program to the management and medical directors of large corporations.

Impetus was given to a sustained drive for membership. The association's attitude, in substance, was this: "Come and see us at work—then you can decide whether this organization deserves your active support."

Those who went to Philadelphia were not disappointed. Attendance was large. Visitors were impressed by the professional tone of the meeting and by the range of industrial medical subjects covered in morning, afternoon, and evening sessions. These included eye protection, dust diseases, fatigue, neuroses and dermatoses, and toxicological hazards. There was a round-table discussion of physical examinations, a symposium on fractures.

The speakers list was impressive: George M. Piersol (medical director Bell Telephone Company of Pennsylvania), Dr. Mervyn R. Taylor (also of Pennsylvania Bell), Pendergrass, Gehrmann, Smyth, C. O. Sappington, R. R. Sayers, C. H. Frazier, Alfred Stengel, Robert A. Kehoe (University of Cincinnati), H. H. Kessler (medical director New Jersey Rehabilitation Commission, and many more.

It was at one of the sessions in Philadelphia that Shoudy made his now famous report on heat cramps. Investigating cases among Bethlehem Steel foundry workers several years before, he noted that men who ate pretzels and drank beer at lunch time had no cramps. Others who used peppermints or oatmeal water suffered relatively little from heat. Shoudy's clinical findings resulted in the adoption of salt-and-dextrose tablets as a preventive treatment. His researches on "Heat and Muscular Work" were published in 1937.

The 1935 meeting marked the beginning of a pronounced upturn in the fortunes of the AAIP&S. The stimulating effect of personal contact upon the members and the educational value of medical papers and discussions cannot be overestimated. The program, setting a procedural pattern for succeeding meetings, clearly demonstrated the association's capacity for service to the profession, to labor, and to management. Beyond this, it was a potent invitation to prospective members.

AAIP&S membership at the time was at low ebb, but morale had never been higher. The association had little money, but it was solvent. With an operating budget set at $1,500, it had spent slightly more than $1,000 during the fiscal year.

Retiring from the presidency at Philadelphia, Holmblad urged more intelligent and equitable treatment of partially disabled workers and the wider use of placement examinations to determine the type and amount of work they could perform.

At the business session Floyd E. Shaffer (Bethlehem Steel Company) was elected president for 1935–36 and Robert P. Knapp was named president-elect. In addition to four holdover directors from preceding terms, the association called on three veteran members to serve on the Board: Andrew M. Harvey, a moving spirit in founding the association twenty years before, and Edward C. Holmblad and William A. Sawyer. Three new directors—all presidents-to-be—were also added: Alfred H. Whittaker of Detroit, fellow of the ACS and the AMA, then serving as surgeon and consultant for a number of insurance companies; McIver Woody, fellow of the AMA and medical director of the Standard Oil Company of New Jersey; and Daniel L. Lynch, fellow of the AMA and medical director of the New England Telephone & Telegraph Company.

Shaffer was a graduate of Johns Hopkins, and his interests were primarily surgical. His first and only industrial connection has been Bethlehem Steel. While still serving Bethlehem at Sparrows Point, Maryland, and at Baltimore, he was considered as the logical successor to Shoudy in the corporation's top medical post. When the appointment eventually came, he said that his chief loss was in not seeing his patients personally. And workers quickly learned that when he visited Sparrows Point they could count on finding him in front of the plant at lunchtime to say, "Hello."

In his year as AAIP&S president Shaffer found himself facing the agreeable task (as he has described it) of "planning activities for a large and growing organization." Realizing that the future promised a rapid increase of interest in industrial medicine, he centered the efforts of his administration on promotion of a program that would lead the way to such development rather than follow in its wake.

Throughout the 1930's the association (always its own severest critic) kept a watchful eye not only on problems close at hand, but on long-range plans and objectives as well. Some of the appraisals and reappraisals in that period are of historical interest, since they reflect the thinking from which the present IMA has emerged.

Shortly after the market crash that ushered in the great depression, J. Rollin French, president of the Western Hospital Association, commented bitterly on a situation that reduced many industrial physicians and surgeons to positions subservient to the heads of minor departments. Scornfully he referred to "the days of the so-called 'company doctor' who assumed only sufficient responsibility for the physical welfare of employees to appease public sentiment." Declaring that there was "too great a tendency to confuse industrial physical service with traumatic surgery," he urged a complete overhaul of industrial medical procedures, "to inject standardized business methods into a standardized practical system of physical service."[2]

In his first address as president of the AAIP&S in 1931, D. B. Lowe declared:

> I say the name has never adequately described the association, because it [the association] differs in character from any I have ever known. There is a friendliness among those who attend [an annual meeting] that marks it apart from the stereotyped convention. . . .
>
> The continuation and further development of this spirit . . . throughout the years to come is an ideal we should always keep in mind. It will aid us as industrial physicians to advance industrial medicine and keep it on the highest plane.
>
> There should be no misunderstanding of the term "industrial medicine." It can mean nothing but the application of good medicine and good surgery to those employees of industry who are unfortunate enough to be injured during the course of their employment or to suffer from occupational disease. . . .
>
> Far and wide, for a long period of time, the industrial physician and surgeon has been supposed to be a combination civil, mechanical, heating, lighting, ventilating and chemical engineer; economist, welfare worker, athletic director, public health officer, insurance expert, and sanitary policeman, not to mention a few other conferred titles.
>
> It is my opinion that few of us are qualified in this way, and that it will be far more beneficial to industrial medicine if we confine our activities to the one thing we were trained for, and that is the practice of medicine.[3]

In 1933, another prominent industrial physician and teacher commented constructively on the scope and procedures of the profession, particularly with respect to toxic hazards. W. Irving Clark (Norton Company), declared it the duty of the industrial physician to be versed in the action and danger of every chemical and physical health hazard *in his own factory*. Clark detailed various procedures necessary for the "control of the environment" and strongly urged not only employment and periodic examinations of workers but periodic examination of working conditions in various departments and the transfer to non-hazardous work of any worker showing signs of industrial disease.[4]

Thus, by a process of self-criticism, the association broadened its thinking, raised its sights for the future, and at the same time established practical procedures for attainment of its goals. Here a writer, there a speaker, introduced a bit of relatively new thinking, and each new concept strengthened the foundation on which industrial medicine rested and enhanced the value of the services it rendered.

One must not conclude, however, that there was no criticism of the specialty from outside the association. At least three times in the thirties the ever old, ever new issue of "contract medicine" broke prominently into print. On no occasion did an open feud develop, but there was a considerable amount of spirited verbal fencing.

In the secretary's report to the Board of Directors of the AAIP&S in June, 1930, Volney S. Cheney wrote: "In an editorial in the *Journal of the American Medical Association*, January 4, 1930, industrial medicine has been officially recognized as a challenging specialty that is threatening to disturb the smug complacency of organized medicine; that plans must be considered for curbing its activities and it must confine those activities to its 'just and proper domain' and relinquish those functions which are 'beyond its legitimate field.'"[5]

Because it throws light on an interesting phase of inter-association relations, the editorial in question will bear some further quotation. After considerable preliminary comment, the writer made the following statement:

> The foremost objectives of industrial medicine are: (1) to fit every person to types and quantities of work according to his ability to perform such work continually without undue impairment, without injury to himself or his fellow workmen, and with profit to himself and his employer; (2) to procure and maintain fitness for work through efforts applied to the worker as an individual, to groups of workers, and to the work environment; (3) to educate the worker to a comprehension of the value and significance of physical and mental well being and, in particular, of personal hygiene and accident prevention; and (4) to reduce all loss of time, absenteeism and short work spans in industry the cause of which may be related in any way to health.[6]

There was nothing to offend anyone in this rotund statement of objectives, nor could it be seriously criticized even today, for it was broad enough to cover almost any constructive activity. The barb was in the statement that followed: "With these boundaries, much so-called industrial medicine is revealed as quite beyond the legitimate field."

The editorial went on to blast the medical care of "entire communities" through contract arrangements, a practice aimed, it declared, at "the confounding of compensation cases" for profit to the casualty companies. "The need is great," said the writer, "for organized medicine (1) to mark the just and proper domain of acceptable industrial medicine, (2) to stimulate a demand for the truly qualified industrial physician, and (3) to limit industrial medicine wholly to the boundaries set forth."

It is to be inferred that the above mention of "organized medicine" was not intended as a reference to the AAIP&S, and it seems clear that the suggested limiting of boundaries was to be done by the AMA.

Commenting on the editorial in his report, Cheney (never a man to mince words) had this to say:

Industrial medicine, after many years of a tolerated existence, is at last coming into its own. Its recognition is due not to the employment of bombastic methods or the assumption of "holier than thou" attitudes, but because its devotees, and I use the word "devotees" with premeditation, have gone ahead and done those things unusually well that industry has required of them and gradually and subtly proved their superior ability, over that of the general practitioner or any other group of medical men, in solving the medical problems of industry.

Having delivered this riposte, Cheney urged the association to act definitely upon standardization of industrial medical practices, to establish minimal qualifications for doctors in industrial work, and to strive for better instruction in the specialty in our medical schools. Thus he found himself in agreement with the AMA, at least insofar as objectives were concerned, and upon this note, available records indicate, the verbal tilt ended.

About two years later, contract medicine again invited the wrath of critics but for a different reason. They became aroused when the Washington (State) Hospital Association adopted a plan "to apply the principle of insurance to the modern problem of maintaining health, expressed in the motto: 'A large number paying a small amount to guarantee complete medical care for those who require it.' "

This plan was the basis of a contract between the hospital association and a local brass foundry, signed in May, 1928. For some strange reason, however, this agreement did not come to the attention of the AAIP&S until four years later, when a copy was sent to the editor of *Industrial Medicine* just in time for the first trial issue of that publication. The editor printed the text of the contract in full, along with an editorial calling attention to the fact that the name of the clinic handling the foundry clients was being withheld by special request of the hospital association. "The staff members," said the editorial, "are afraid that old-line members of the medical profession may seek to oust them from the medical societies for taking cases on a contract basis. The feeling within the ranks of the profession is rather apprehensive, hence the recipients of the work, although they are glad to get it, desire to keep the facts under cover."[7]

In December of 1932 the Committee on the Costs of Medical Care made its final report, which was widely-publicized, then disbanded. Michael M. Davis, Ph.D., director of medical services for the Julius Rosenwald Fund, explained in an address, on February 7, 1934, before the Philadelphia College of Physicians:

> The majority recommended a fuller planning and organization of medical practice and an extensive use of the principle of insurance as a means of distributing the uneven and unpredictable costs of medical care so that they would not fall with crushing weight upon some of the people every year. . . .
>
> But the *Journal of the American Medical Association,* in an editorial appearing in December, 1932, just after the committee had disbanded, attacked the majority report as a plan which would turn doctors into hirelings and treat sick people like robots. . . . The editorial denounced the plan as "socialism and communism, inciting to revolution," contrasting "on the other side the organized medical profession of this country urging an orderly evolution guided by controlled experimentation." [8]

The Washington Plan and the type of contract medicine under fire in the thirties were, of course, phases in the evolution of the Blue Cross and Blue Shield services which have eventually come to affect millions of workers in every kind and at every level of employment. Casual involvement in this battle was one of the earliest contacts of the AAIP&S with the complex problem of health insurance, which remains controversial and an issue of increasing concern to the industrial doctor today.

Four years, almost to the day, after the text of the Washington Hospital Association contract appeared in *Industrial Medicine,* that is, in October, 1936, the *Journal of the American Medical Association* launched another editorial attack on the "evils of contract practice," which it described as being "born of geographic and social necessity" for the servicing of isolated districts (mining, lumber, etc.) unable to extend medical facilities in any other way. "Most modern types of contract practice," said the *Journal,* "lack this excuse of necessity. . . . Contract systems are now operated more often to reduce compensation costs, absenteeism, labor turnover, inefficiency, and wage payments, than to supply needed medical service."

The editorial went on to declare that the features of contract plans for which their founders fight hardest were those "most profitable to industry but not always most helpful to the patients. . . . Contract practice is at present almost universally accompanied by advertising, commercial bargaining, underbidding, subletting, coercion or plain racketeering, and all of these are destructive ingredients in medical service." It concluded as follows: "It is too much to expect that commercial interests, having no knowledge of the principles of medical ethics, and no understanding or appreciation of the personal and private relationships that should exist between patient and physician, should devise and administer a system of medical care devoted alike to the interests of the public and of the medical profession."[9]

This analysis of industrial practice appears to have left the AAIP&S puzzled, rather than disturbed. It brought a temperate editorial rejoinder from *Industrial Medicine,* stating that differences in the quality of medical service were a reflection of differences in attitude and understanding on the part of employers rather than the ethics and objectives of the doctors. This editorial concluded: "The best that medical science can bring to bear upon the injuries and the diseases of occupation is the most profitable. Being so, it will ultimately be the rule rather than the exception, even in the smaller employment situations."[10]

It so happened, however, that at its annual meeting in Atlantic City early in October, 1936, the AAIP&S had debated at great length the problem of ethical cooperation between industrial physicians and physicians in private practice. And the article in the *Journal of the American Medical Association* produced a far stronger, if less publicized, retort from a former president of the industrial association.

In a letter to Loyal Shoudy and a dozen other prominent members, C. F. N. Schram indignantly declared:

> To my way of thinking it is such articles that build up in the minds of private practitioners the thought that we are outside the pale of decency, and those who do not and will not learn the real facts regarding an industrial practice talk loud and long, not only to other physicians but also to patients who, when well, work in industries medically served by us. They use the term "contract doctor" with all the venom at their command and quote such articles from the AMA to prove their points.
>
> Such shotgun write-ups are offensive, breed discontent, are uncalled for, and when applied to salaried physicians in industry are untrue. . . . I would not ask for a retraction because there is no need for controversy, but this is not the first article of this nature which has been called to my attention by private practitioners who were even more critical than I. Possibly I am making a mountain out of a molehill, but if I am, we sure wasted a lot of time at Atlantic City.

Thus another word battle came to a close. The issue, at the time, was of real importance. In the eyes of many industrial physicians the AMA—even if trying only to purge medicine of an actual abuse—was in effect tarring all organized industrial practice with the stigma of "contract medicine."

Happenings, however, are not always entirely explicable. Mixed motives may have influenced all parties to this particular dispute. Or, it may have been just another instance of business—mankind's strange habit of fighting an issue through to the last bitter word, then using the controversy as the foundation for a lasting cooperative friendship.

It is certain that while the AMA was rattling the skeleton of contract medicine, it was moving steadily toward the establishment of a section within its own organization which would serve the medical profession in matters concerning industrial health. From its planning came the Council on Industrial Health, an official AMA agency whose activities are largely designed to improve and maintain standards of professional competence and procedure in the industrial field.

First steps toward organization of the council were taken at a meeting of the

AMA House of Delegates in May, 1936. At that session a resolution was passed calling for further study of industrial diseases by the AMA, the objective being passage of uniform compensation laws by the states. Ten months later an investigating group of physicians strongly recommended establishment of an industrial council, to function as a standing committee of the AMA. With approval of the house, the Board of Trustees acted promptly, and the new organization was formally launched at a meeting in December, 1937.

At the eighty-ninth annual meeting of the AMA in June, 1938, Robert T. Legge talked bluntly but constructively about the association's industrial activities. In his address as chairman of its Section on Preventive and Industrial Medicine and Public Health, he reviewed developments in this field:

> The American Medical Association took a rather conservative or possibly badly advised attitude toward early recognition of the importance of industrial medicine. It was even late in developing a dual section for preventive medicine and public health, a section which now includes industrial medicine. . . .
>
> The association, through its new Council on Industrial Health, now has its greatest opportunity to be a benefactor to American industrial medicine: to promote by research and uplift by education and mutual cooperation the humanizing of industry by preventive medicine.
>
> Its aim should be not only a wholehearted program in the study and prevention of occupational diseases but also to strengthen a loyal cooperative spirit to support medical practitioners who are so engaged. It must stimulate the consciousness of all industrialists to the need for the application of modern industrial medicine entailing the service of competent physicians and the development of standardized health services in which preventive medicine and surgery as they have been outlined in this address will be scientifically practiced.
>
> The fear that industry desires to engage in so-called corporate medicine is shared by some; while it is true that the organization of medical protection in a plant contributes to the cost of the service by necessity, it also involves vital interests in the prevention of disease and avoidable accidents. The new Council on Industrial Health must not fail in the new order of medicine. It has the opportunity, with the greatest group of our population, the worker and the industrialist, to forestall a political form of medicine with which the organized profession is not in sympathy.[11]

Historically, the AMA indicated some interest in the industrial phases of medicine many years before an industrial council was dreamed of. Activities, however, developed slowly. The dual Section on Preventive Medicine and Public Health mentioned by Legge was formed in 1909 and was itself the outgrowth of a long succession of similar groups stretching well back into the 1880's. C. D. Selby, in addition to his many public health activities in Ohio, was appointed secretary of the section in 1920.

Two years later, by the simple inclusion of the word "industrial" in its name, this group became the AMA Section on Preventive and Industrial Medicine and Public Health. Among its members was Andrew M. Harvey, one of the co-founders of the AAIP&S. Several years later Royd R. Sayers served as its chairman in a subsequent period.

When it set up the Council on Industrial Health in 1937, the AMA gave the problems of occupational disease a great deal of mature thinking as well as the experience of highly capable, widely respected physicians and surgeons. Yet, as a matter of record, membership of the council in its early years included very few physicians engaged in active practice in manufacturing and other production industries which accounted for a high percentage of occupational disease hazards in that period. Almost without exception the experience of officers and members alike was in contiguous fields—public health, hygiene, medical education, etc.—rather than in day-to-day medical contacts in manufacturing and processing plants.

Stanley J. Seeger, of Milwaukee, first chairman of the council, who remained in that office through the 1940's, was a consulting railway surgeon. A. D. Lazenby, vice-chairman until his death in 1939, was chief surgeon of a Baltimore insurance company. His successor, Raymond Hussey, was associate professor of medicine at the University of Maryland at the time of his appointment. The secretary, Carl M. Peterson, whose long and loyal service was ended by a fatal accident, had no special background in industrial practice.

But members active in the AAIP&S (and strongly approving its viewpoint and objectives) were appointed from time to time. Harvey Bartle, an indefatigable worker in the association and its president in 1943–1944, was one of the original nine members appointed to serve on the council in September, 1937. Others included Leverett D. Bristol (then health director, American Telephone and Telegraph), Lanza and Selby in 1938, Legge in 1939, William A. Sawyer in 1944. As the association grew in size and importance, its council representation likewise increased in a reasonable ratio, a factor that has contributed greatly to harmony of thought and action.

The later experience of the AMA Council on Industrial Health, in the words of *Industrial Medicine and Surgery,* "has been one of the gradual expansion of functions, of a growing realization of the vast scope of industrial health and welfare, and of sharpened focus on those medical relationships which stand out as of fundamental importance. . . . [The council] has worked closely with other councils, bureaus and sections of the AMA to upgrade standards of industrial medicine, surgery and hygiene, and to intensify interest in health education and legislation."[12]

The acrimonious disputes of bygone years, concerning industrial medical ethics and standards and problems of jurisdiction, may perhaps be best appraised in the light of these later developments, indicating as they do the growth of a healthy and realistic relationship between the AMA and the IMA.

From a professional viewpoint the mid-thirties saw dramatic developments in the surgery of trauma. This was the result of industrial expansion as well as improved surgical techniques. Developments of this sort were widely discussed in the periodicals of the day, a review of which brings to light the following engaging commentary from the January, 1936, *Industrial Medicine:*

> Industrial injuries have been reduced considerably, according to some authorities to an almost irreducible minimum, during the past ten years. The fact is that most traumatic surgeons at the present time are depending for their clinical material largely upon the results of public accidents, especially automobile accidents. . . .
>
> It may be assumed that for some time to come there will be a considerable number of public accidents resulting from the misuse of the automobile, though in some quarters this is vigorously denied. Granting that there have been many improvements in making roadways safe, providing adequate and properly working traffic signals and traffic supervision, and making the automobile as a mechanical unit as foolproof as it is possible to do, there will still be what is called "the human element." And probably this factor will be the cause of a great number of casualties for many years to come.
>
> Nevertheless, it is sensible to believe that there will be a material reduction in the number of public accidents in the next five years, for the public is becoming thoroughly aroused to the necessity of cutting down the enormous number of casualties and deaths from this source. Moreover, it is not impossible . . . that the amount of automobile travel may be materially reduced, this having a desirable effect upon the decrease of automobile casualties and deaths.
>
> It may be assumed, therefore, that the material afforded for traumatic surgery may reasonably suffer a considerable decline, and with the increasing number of traumatic surgeons developed, will accordingly cause a disproportion of material and men.[13]

As a picture of coming conditions and events in the sphere of public safety, the foregoing predictions were wide of the mark on almost every count. Trends in the latter thirties, whether recognized or not, proved to be unmistakably favorable for the industrial doctor as an individual and for industrial medicine as a profession. AAIP&S members, to a man, seem to have been aware that their association had reached a turn of the road and that better things lay ahead.

Nothing else could explain the growth of interest among young doctors in industry as a field for specialization; and the remarkable revival of activity by older members of the association, many of whom had helped win its first battles twenty years before. As Floyd E. Shaffer points out, the IMA owes much to this latter group for their aid in the difficult task of preparing and financing important programs in the depression and post-depression years.

The list of old-time members who came forward to give their experience, energy and influence in the drive of the thirties is too long to print here in anything like entirety. One finds them serving as officers, directors, editors, committeemen, policymakers: Andrew M. Harvey, "Tom" Crowder, Geier, Cranch, Sawyer, Shoudy, Lowe, Watson, Lynch, and many more.

At the Atlantic City convention in October, 1936, the AAIP&S met with the Industrial Health Section of the National Safety Council and shared a balanced program devoted to discussion of industrial accidents and the prevention of common industrial diseases. The medical sessions included a round-table led by A. J. Lanza and papers by Selby, and B. L. Vosburgh.

It is of more than passing interest that among the speakers was Burrill B. Crohn, of New York, whose talk was titled "The Relation of Industrial Life to Gastrointestinal Disease." Crohn, a well known gastroenterologist, was cited at some length a few months later in a feature article published in *Industrial Medicine*.[14] The writer was R. G. Johnston, of New Kensington, Pennsylvania, and his subject was "Regional Ileitis." That disease, which was the object of considerable research in the 1930's, was to become page-one news around the globe twenty years later when President Eisenhower underwent surgery for ileitis just before the opening of the 1956 presidential campaign. Johnston's findings, since they cover some points which were made an issue in that election, are given verbatim as they appeared in *Industrial Medicine* of February, 1937:

Conclusions:

1. Ileitis occurs most frequently in young adults in any part of the small intestines.

2. The etiology still remains unknown.

3. Early diagnosis and surgical removal carry a low mortality and little morbidity.

4. Medical treatment cannot arrest this ulcerating, necrotizing, and cicatrizing process.

5. Multiple-stage operations carry a high mortality.

At the 1936 meeting the association installed the president-elect, Robert P. Knapp, in office for the ensuing year; named Royd R. Sayers as president-elect; elected Clarence D. Selby first vice-president and McIvor Woody second vice-president. The Board of Directors again included a preponderance of former officers and members of long standing.

Knapp was a product of Syracuse University and Columbia College of Physicians & Surgeons. After serving overseas as a captain in World War I he joined Cheney Brothers, of Manchester, Connecticut, as medical director, and held that post throughout his entire industrial career. As president of the AAIP&S he pushed the association's expanding program forward with efficiency and success, as records of the period attest.

The late thirties were full and eventful years in the history of industrial medicine, with interest mounting and activities of the association gaining momentum.

It was in 1937 that the association established the first special committee to study and report on the problem of certification, the opening gun in a militant campaign for official recognition of industrial medicine as a specialty. Many of the association's long-standing objectives were in the process of attainment; *now* seemed the time to drive for the most desired goal of all, certification of physicians and surgeons in industry by an American board of occupational medicine. The battle was to be long and hard fought. We shall hear more of it in later chapters.

It was in 1937, too, that the association's concept of annual meetings was broadened to open up a new and inviting vista. Largely through the efforts of a committee consisting of Selby (consultant, General Motors), McCord (consultant, Chrysler Corporation), and J. J. Prendergast (medical director, Chrysler), members were offered "two great attractions for the price of one" for the week of May 3–8.[15]

The occasion was the twenty-second annual meeting of the AAIP&S, held jointly in Detroit with the Midwest Conference on Occupational Diseases, under the auspices of both the American and the Michigan Associations of Industrial Physicians & Surgeons, the Michigan and Wayne County Medical Societies, the Michigan and Detroit Boards of Health, and the Engineering Society of Detroit.

The conference brought together, for the first time in representative numbers, important figures in industrial medicine, public health and industrial hygiene. Doctors who crowded the meeting rooms were well rewarded with a star-studded program covering almost every phase of occupational medicine and hygiene.

In addition to the three Detroit committeemen, the list of speakers figuring prominently in group and general sessions included Harry Mock, Otto Geier, Robert T. Legge, and Loyal Shoudy; C. F. Kettering (vice-president in charge of research, General Motors) and Detroit Health Commissioner Henry F. Vaughan; E. R. Hayhurst and C. O. Sappington (then a Chicago consulting hygienist); A. J. Lanza, McIver Woody, and J. J. Moorhead (Columbia Post-Graduate Medical School).

Industrial medicine had indeed progressed since the small group of dedicated physicians and surgeons met in Detroit in 1916 to launch the first industrial medical organization of its kind in history. In 1937 several of the same men were present in the same city to help write the preface to a new chapter on progress. So successful was the first Midwest conference that it was renewed in Chicago in 1938. These joint gatherings led, thereafter, to the merging of other industrial and medical interests in joint annual meetings of national scope and importance.

At the business session in 1937 Knapp yielded the presidency to Royd R. Sayers; and the association named Selby as president-elect, with McIver Woody (medical director, Standard Oil Company of New Jersey), and D. L. Lynch (New England Telephone and Telegraph Company) as first and second vice-presidents, respectively.

Sayers, educated at Indiana University and the University of Buffalo School of Medicine, brought to the presidency an enviable record in the fields of military and industrial medicine, public health, and industrial hygiene. His diverse experience had convinced him that cooperative effort by agencies interested in occupational health and hygiene could accomplish more than scattered, independent action. To that end, his administration concentrated on the development of closer relations with other associations and societies and on the expansion and financing of the AAIP&S. Again the pace of programmed activities quickened.

Among the many milestones of the following year was the first Medical Conference of General Motors' Physicians, May 19–20, at Flint, Michigan. Its importance lay not only in the high-grade content of the program but in the declaration by a leading industrial corporation of the value it placed upon plant medical services. Nationwide and international interests of the corporation were represented at this meeting. Professional papers were presented by medical directors of most General Motors divisions, including M. R. Sutton, J. S. Lambie, M. M. Shafer, R. D. Mudd, Henry Snow, C. D. Selby (consultant), Max Burnell, A. L. Brooks, Fred Irwig, L. H. Childs, William J. Fulton, G. L. Bird, and A. A. Tower. Other speakers included President Sayers of the AAIP&S and C. F. Kettering. *Industrial Medicine* recognized the occasion with an issue devoted almost exclusively to the conference, with abstracts of important papers, which were described as "fourteen presentations of very unusual value."[16]

General Motors again made news in June, 1938, at the annual meeting of the AAIP&S in Chicago. There, in an unobtrusive statement by William S. Knudsen, the W. S. Knudsen Award was announced, to be made annually (starting in 1939) "for the most outstanding contribution to industrial medicine." Said Mr. Knudsen:

> There is no argument about the value of medical service in industry. The more we improve health conditions in plants, the more we improve health conditions in general. The man who has the benefits of a health maintenance program in his work must inevitably carry some part of what he learns there home with him.
>
> Many years ago I, myself, was the entire first aid department of a plant where eight hundred people were employed. The progress since those days has been tremendous, as we in industry know. With the desire to concentrate and crystallize the attention of the industrial and medical world on the wonderful progress that has been made and is being made in industrial medicine, I am glad to announce an award to be given to the industrial physician making the most outstanding contribution to industrial medicine.[17]

Education, too, was headlined in the industrial medical news of 1938, with the introduction of what T. Lyle Hazlett has described as "the first intensified course in industrial medicine" given under the auspices of the Graduate Education Committee of the Allegheny County Medical Society and the Department of Industrial Hygiene, University of Pittsburgh School of Medicine.

Many among older physicians in industry will remember that Emery Hayhurst lectured on military and industrial hygiene at Ohio State University as early as 1917, but formal preparation for industrial practice was almost nonexistent during the next twenty years. The revival of interest in the late thirties started a new cycle which has brought industrial medical education to the forefront among present-day goals in this field.

The course at Pittsburgh, consisting of a series of lectures for senior medical students, was made possible by the establishment of a Department of Industrial Hygiene in 1936, with Hazlett as director. The time allotted, in an overcrowded curriculum, was necessarily brief, but it permitted effective coverage of the commonest health hazards in industry and instruction in control and preventive measures.

At the same time the Department of Hygiene and Public Health at the University of Michigan was offering, primarily for graduate students, a more general course in industrial hygiene, comprising two one-hour periods per week for one semester each year.[18]

By the middle of 1938 there were unmistakable signs that industrial medicine and the AAIP&S had indeed "turned a corner" and were headed toward a brighter and better future. In attendance and enthusiasm the annual convention in Chicago duplicated the success of the previous year. Again it was a joint meeting with the Midwest Conference on Occupational Diseases, offering an impressive program made possible by the collaboration of Illinois, Ohio, Michigan, and Wisconsin health agencies.

At annual meetings prior to that year there had been occasional experiments with scientific exhibits as a convention feature, but at Chicago in 1938, displays became a major attraction. A distinguished committee (Sawyer, Mock, Geier, Lautenschlager, Wittmer, and Cheney) produced a total of fifty exhibits, divided almost evenly between scientific and commercial displays. It was an important venture in association history, as subsequent events have proved.[19]

It was at this meeting that Clarence D. Selby, who since 1935 had headed the medical staff of General Motors Corporation as consultant, took over the presidency of the AAIP&S. The officers elected included McIver Woody, president-elect, Daniel L. Lynch, first vice-president, and Lloyd Noland (Tennessee Coal, Iron & Railway Company, second vice-president. A directorate composed almost entirely of veteran members rounded out the administration.

Selby's active career, dating back to 1905, had given him an unusually diversified experience in "mass medical" practice—with the military in World War I, in the public health services, and in the organization affairs of both the AMA and the AAIP&S.

Under his administration the AAIP&S struck out boldly along lines that would expand and strengthen its services, advance its prestige, maintain quality while increasing numbers. It is significant that its membership, which had slipped back to a seven-year low in 1935, registered a net gain of 350 in 1938–39, the largest recorded in a single year up to that time.

Another milestone in the march of industrial medicine appeared in January, 1939, when the first Congress on Industrial Health of the AMA held the stage for two days in Chicago. It was a momentous occasion, the first substantial activity of the new AMA Council on Industrial Health. A noteworthy program was presented, in which many doctors prominent in the AAIP&S participated as speakers and group leaders.[20] The Industrial Health Congress has since become a major annual event in organized medicine. Its influence and success are evidence of what may be accomplished by constructive cooperation among all agencies and organizations within or bordering on the field of occupational health.

In June, 1939, the AAIP&S journeyed to Cleveland for a meeting with what was termed, in that year, the "American Conference on Occupational Diseases and Industrial Hygiene." This departure was another step in the evolution of multi-purpose meetings with various health agencies in the industrial field.

The Cleveland program, in which more than a dozen Ohio organizations took part, had many impressive moments, not the least of which was the presentation at the annual banquet of the first Knudsen Award, by Knudsen himself. The Award Committee previously appointed by President Selby consisted of Loyal A. Shoudy (chairman), McIver Woody, and C. F. N. Schram, who had had under consideration for several months books and scientific studies submitted in the competition. The committee withheld the name of the recipient until the night of the presentation, thereby setting a precedent followed in subsequent years. The honor of receiving the first of the Knudsen plaques, symbolic of the award, went to C. O. Sappington, distinguished consultant in occupational diseases and industrial hygiene, "for the contribution he has made to the literature of industrial medicine in his book entitled *Medicolegal Phases of Occupational Diseases.*"[21] Acknowledging the honor, Sappington commented as follows upon the significance of the award: "It seems to me that it means that a great industry and a great association of medical men have realized that the two groups have a common ground of objectives and purposes, and that through this mutuality it is possible for them to provide the basis for recognition and encouragement which is vital to progress."

It is of interest to IMA members that the family of Sappington has since donated to the association the original plaque awarded to him for preservation in its archives.

At the business session in Cleveland McIver Woody formally took over the presidency of the AAIP&S. A graduate of the University of Richmond, he received his medical degree from Harvard School of Medicine and held a fellowship in surgery there from 1914 to 1920. For the next two years he was dean and professor of surgery at the University of Tennessee Medical School. When elected to head the AAIP&S, he had been since 1926 medical director of the Standard Oil Company of New Jersey, responsible for medical service to some thirty thousand employees.

Other officers for 1939–40 were D. L. Lynch, president-elect, Lloyd Noland, first vice-president, T. Lyle Hazlett, second vice-president, with Cheney still serving as secretary-treasurer. As if in preparation for times of great necessity, an exceptionally strong Board of veterans members was provided for this administration: Sayers, McCord, McConnaughy, Wittmer, Slobe, Shoudy, Holmblad, Sawyer, Prendergast, Selby, Bartle (Pennsylvania Railroad), and R. C. Engle (Republic Steel Corporation).

Woody's long experience in organizing medical services for large industrial groups, and that of his officers and directors, was soon to find employment, for catastrophic world events were in the making. Overseas the misnamed "stalemate" war was smoldering ominously, ready to burst into disastrous eruption. The thirties, a decade of great happenings, were hurrying to their close, as if eager to merge with a strange new age for science, industry, and medicine.

PART SEVEN

THE ATOMIC AGE

A NEW HORIZON—NEW FRONTIERS
FOR INDUSTRIAL MEDICINE

History is the voice of the past, reciting its lessons
for guidance of the future.

XXIV

MILITANT—AND MILITARY—

MEDICINE

O<small>N</small> J<small>UNE</small> 6, 1940, members of the American Association of Industrial Physicians & Surgeons, assembled in New York from every section of the country, paused in the routine business of their twenty-fifth annual meeting to endorse unanimously, by acclamation, the following resolution:

> Whereas, many parts of the world are now engaged in bitter warfare; and
>
> Whereas, for twenty-five years the American Association of Industrial Physicians & Surgeons has devoted itself to a study of occupational diseases and industrial accidents; and
>
> Whereas, the medical directors of the nation's leading industries have had an extensive experience in supervising the health of millions of workers; and
>
> Whereas, epidemics and occupational diseases and industrial accidents would materially impair the nation's productive efficiency; therefore, be it
>
> Resolved: That this day the American Association of Industrial Physicians & Surgeons express to the President and to the Congress of the United States its wholehearted willingness to assist the federal government in strengthening our national defenses.

It was almost exactly eighteen months before the Japanese attack on Pearl Harbor when the association voiced this pledge of cooperation. The average American citizen was not yet convinced that his country would be drawn into the conflict; the hope still lingered that international differences could somehow be patched up. But there was expectancy in the air, and mounting tension. Business and pro-

287

fessional organizations across the land were passing similar resolutions, offering their services for whatever might eventuate.

The months preceding Pearl Harbor offered a parallel with the period just before the United States entered World War I. In 1916 the cry was for "industrial preparedness"; in 1940 it was for "national defense." The two terms, in effect, were the same. They called for a quick evaluation of the nation's production potential, a reappraisal of its available manpower, and a rapid upbuilding of its neglected military machinery.

Many long-time members of the AAIP&S knew from personal experience the meaning of warfare on a 1914–1918 scale and were in a position to realize the magnitude of the burden that a second and infinitely more devastating global war would lay upon production industries and their working forces. Nor did they have any illusions regarding the responsibility of industrial medicine in the maintenance of national health.

In the somber setting of world events the New York meeting in 1940 gained an importance out of proportion to its size. Every official action or decision of the association was freighted with consequences. Members were well aware that this was the time for them to assume and exercise leadership of organized industrial medicine or, as a likely alternative, forfeit the right to such recognition.

The convention itself was unusual in many respects. It was the first annual meeting of the AAIP&S to be held jointly with that of another national industrial health organization, the American Industrial Hygiene Association. This sharing of programs was neither accidental nor incidental. It was the logical result of an interesting series of events involving several different health agencies, governmental and private, in that extraordinary decade, the 1930's.

In the early years of the century industrial hygiene as a science had progressed slowly; it was scarcely recognized professionally as a field for specialized practice. True, by 1930 the American Public Health Association had its Industrial Hygiene Section and the National Safety Council, its Industrial Health Section, each capably performing highly important duties in its own sphere. But in both parent organizations the strictly industrial aspects of health were subordinated to broader mainline activities.

Relatively few industrial concerns had established special hygiene units to keep watch on environmental factors and forestall, where possible, dangerous exposures. The great majority of employers did not believe that the size of their plants or the incidence of disease justified such action. They were content to leave to their medical departments the task of recognizing health hazards and dealing with them. This was in line with a comfortable theory which, in effect, declared that there was nothing to worry about unless or until the doctors could produce actual cases of job-connected disease in substantial numbers and of considerable severity.

Even the most prevention-minded physician, with this hurdle in his path, found it difficult to eliminate an environmental disease hazard even when he had the means

288

of detecting it. And plant safety engineers often had trouble with proposals for new accident safeguards, simply because there had not been enough injuries to demonstrate the need.

Long before the thirties there had been plenty of voices to challenge this time-honored custom of relying on occurrence of cases as the criterion in judging industrial health hazards. The AAIP&S had, since its earliest years, preached prevention; individual members practiced it where circumstances were favorable. The association's persisting fight for adequate examination procedures was part of the same program.

Again and again, prior to 1930, tragic outbreaks of occupational disease had roused the American people to indignation and brought demands for action. There was phosphorus poisoning in the match industry, outlawed at last in 1912. Dust diseases flourished in the twenties, after the introduction of pneumatic rock drills. There were the tetraethyl lead cases in the automobile industry and the radium poisoning of watch dial painters.

Each of these catastrophes shocked the nation (for a time) and pointed unmistakably to the need for preventive measures. Each produced action, of one kind or another. All exemplified history's way of repeating itself. For none of the diseases was new. Only the circumstances were different; the causes and effects were as old as man's contacts with materials from nature's storehouse.

There was rapidly growing medical interest, in the late twenties, in the relationship of working environment to industrial health, and a dawning recognition of the fact that a new type of industrial hygiene was necessary for effective control of occupational disease.

The wave of silicosis claims that flooded the courts in the early thirties greatly stimulated the demand for scientific research. Facts were needed. Without them there could be no remedies, no prevention. Suddenly, as if by common plan, industrial hygiene groups and agencies sprang up in every part of the country. Their aims and activities were as diverse as their locations.

It was the silicosis situation specifically that brought representatives of a score of important industrial concerns to Pittsburgh, to the Mellon Institute, in 1935, seeking research assistance on their problem. The project also had the active backing of the United States Public Health Service and the Bureau of Mines, which had launched industrial health programs of their own many years before.

Under existing circumstances, participation of these governmental agencies in the silicosis research plan was of special interest to members of the AAIP&S. Anthony J. Lanza (of the USPHS), distinguished for his pioneer work in the investigation of industrial dust hazards, had been chief surgeon of the Bureau of Mines until 1920. At that time the bureau formalized all its health work under Royd R. Sayers, who also headed its Safety and Health Branch. From 1933 to 1940 Sayers served as senior surgeon of the USPHS.[1]

As this text has amply testified, both Sayers and Lanza had been prominent in the

289

activities of the AAIP&S since its early years, in addition to their signal services in other health fields. Actually, the silicosis research project proved to be the prelude to a cooperative relationship between the AAIP&S and the industrial hygiene agencies, a liaison that was to affect importantly the role of both groups before, during and after World War II.

The industrialists who took their silicosis problems to Pittsburgh in 1935 soon found that they had come to the right place for a sympathetic hearing and prompt action.

The Mellon Institute, founded in 1913, was the first organization of its kind in the country. It was (and is) a privately endowed, non-profit institution, incorporated in 1927 for long-range research in pure and applied science, financed under a fellowship system. Sanitation and control of industrial hazards were well within its field of operation, along with many other types of enterprise for the public welfare.

From the very first closed-door discussion at the Pittsburgh meeting there emerged a new organization, the Air Hygiene Foundation, established in 1936 by a group of large industries, the United States Public Health Service, the Bureau of Mines, and the Mellon Institute. By 1941 its field of activity in environmental control had so broadened that the name was changed to Industrial Hygiene Foundation. It has since continued to expand and to contribute increasingly to the advancement of occupational health through research.

Though the new foundation flourished from the start, though individual groups of hygienists were being formed on every hand, there still was no central, national organization representing all types and all aspects of industrial hygiene. Various attempts were made to launch such a body, but engineers, chemists, and other groups could not seem to agree on questions of scope and affiliations.

While these matters were being argued, governmental industrial hygienists, in 1938, started an organization of their own to promote education and information in the field. Then, in September of the following year, came the first public announcement of the American Industrial Hygiene Association. Its prospectus, a single mimeographed sheet, declared:

> The object of the association is the advancement and application of industrial hygiene and sanitation through the interchange and dissemination of technical knowledge on these subjects; the furthering of study and control of health hazards through determination and elimination of excessive exposures; and the correlation of such activities as conducted by diverse individuals and agencies throughout industry, educational and governmental groups; and the uniting of persons with these interests.

This statement left no doubt as to the broad and inclusive base on which the new association planned to operate. Elaborating, the prospectus continued:

> Provision has been made to enroll in various classes of members any person interested in the field of industrial hygiene. Among those groups which we hope to

include are persons whose nominal titles may be listed as engineer, physician, safety inspector or engineer, chemist, nurse, personnel, or executive, whenever such persons have industrial hygiene problems which lead to an active interest in the subject. It is believed that only through such a broad organization can information be brought to the smaller units of industry where the full time of an industrial hygienist is not warranted.

At its organization meeting in Cleveland the Industrial Hygiene Association named as president William P. Yant (Mine Safety Appliances Company, Pittsburgh); as president-elect Warren A. Cook (Zurich Insurance Companies, Chicago); and as secretary-treasurer Gordon C. Harrold (Chrysler Industrial Hygiene Laboratories, Detroit).

The value of such an organization in the industrial structure became more and more evident as time went on. It was needed for many reasons: for the effective pooling of information and effort, to eliminate duplication and overlapping of services, and (highly important) to assure proper representation for industrial hygiene in its relations with other agencies in the health field.

The matter of such relations was recognized in the constitution, which contained a provision that the association should, when possible, meet with other organizations. And from discussion and negotiation in this direction came the agreement that the industrial hygienists should convene with the AAIP&S at its annual meeting in 1940. Thus was another important precedent set in the history of the AAIP&S. The joint-meeting arrangement has continued down the years, and was fortified, in the 1940's, by the addition of still other participating organizations.

Thus too, was another link forged in the working alliance between industrial medicine and industrial hygiene, an alliance that has been fruitful for both associations and for the objectives they hold in common. The effectiveness of this cooperative effort was to be tested sooner than either of the parties could, in all probability, have suspected.

While these interorganization developments were taking place, the federal government was becoming increasingly interested in both industrial medicine and industrial hygiene, largely because of growing uneasiness over the international situation. Since the turn of the century the Public Health Service had operated a hygienic laboratory for the investigation of infectious and contagious diseases and other matters concerning the public health. In 1930 its activities were considerably broadened, and its name was changed to the National Institute of Health.

After July, 1939, when the USPHS was transferred from the Treasury Department to the newly created Federal Security Administration, the National Institute of Health was one of eight subdivisions of the Service administered by Surgeon General Thomas Parran. It was housed in six new buildings on the outskirts of Bethesda, Maryland, about ten miles from Washington. And one of its own nine divisions was devoted to problems involving industrial hygiene.

So the stage was set when the AAIP&S gathered in New York in June, 1940, for its twenty-fifth annual meeting, and the young Industrial Hygiene Association came for its first. Unquestionably the gathering was one of the most important in the history of either group.

The broad scope of the program required four days of meetings, starting early each morning and often lasting well into the night. Yet every minute was crowded by agenda which included papers, reports and discussions covering no less than forty major medical and technical subjects, in addition to the transaction of association business. This meaty program was carried out to the letter, with a smoothness that bespoke expert preparation.

The big news of the convention, however, in point of public interest and professional importance, did not stem from any of the formally scheduled events. It was, in fact, made known before the general sessions were even well under way. At a meeting of the Board of Directors, held the morning of June 4, Shoudy called the attention of his confreres to a telegram received from Surgeon General Parran of the USPHS, asking that the AAIP&S appoint a committee "to cooperate with the Division of Industrial Hygiene of the National Institute of Health in developing and applying plans or programs for coordinating the health needs in industry" in connection with the national defense program.

A better spot for the government's request or the association's reply could scarcely have been chosen, with the national leaders of both industrial medicine and industrial hygiene assembled in Manhattan and to some extent already in the public eye. Despite the appearance of casual, almost impromptu, action, such an agreement must have been preceded by many unrecorded hours of sober thought, detailed discussion, and careful decision.

Consideration of the surgeon general's request by the officers and directors of the association was brief and to the point. President Woody pointed out that inasmuch as this was a war measure he wanted authorization by the Board before appointing such a committee. Sayers, who within the year had been elevated to the post of director, United States Bureau of Mines, remarked that he had "made a recommendation" six months previously. A motion was made, and carried.

The following day (June 5), in a telegram to Parran, the AAIP&S released a news story announcing that the "medical men of industry" had "enlisted for national defense." It quoted Woody's reply to the surgeon general, listing the personnel of the new committee approved by the Board of Directors.

It was a strong committee by any standard, seasoned by professional and administrative experience, fully representative of the various divisions of industrial health, and eminently fitted for their assignment:

Royd R. Sayers (chairman), past-president and a director of the AAIP&S; chairman, AMA Section on Preventive and Industrial Medicine and Public Health; influential in the APHA and the USPHS.
Clarence D. Selby, also past-president and director of the AAIP&S; first secretary,

AMA Section on Preventive and Industrial Medicine and Public Health; consulting hygienist, USPHS, in World War I; author of the famous *Bulletin 99.*

Edward C. Holmblad, likewise director and past-president of the AAIP&S; fellow, American College of Surgeons; medical director, American Railway Express, Chicago.

Daniel L. Lynch, president-elect AAIP&S (1940); medical director, New England Telephone and Telegraph Company; chairman, Industrial Health Committee, APHA.

T. Lyle Hazlett, second vice-president, AAIP&S (1940); medical director, Westinghouse Electric Corporation; head of the Department of Industrial Medicine, University of Pittsburgh Medical School.

William P. Yant, Mine Safety Appliances Company, Pittsburgh; first president (1939–40), American Industrial Hygiene Association.

Philip Drinker, Industrial Hygiene Department, Harvard University School of Public Health.

In announcing the appointment of this group, President Woody said:

> Our prompt response to the request of Surgeon General Parran is possible because we specialists in industrial medicine have managed, through the years, to build up a genuine *esprit de corps,* freely sharing with each other special knowledge and techniques, as acquired. Thus, when the emergency arises, it finds us no longer raw recruits.
>
> Industrial physicians and surgeons have been devoting their best efforts to this field for the past twenty-five years. Consequently, industrial medicine is mature and has a vast store of unwritten knowledge acquired by the physicians and surgeons who have extensive experience in this special field of medical practice.

At the close of this momentous session President-elect Lynch was formally installed as president, along with Vice-Presidents Lloyd Noland and T. Lyle Hazlett, and a new directorate. Daniel L. Lynch had attended Boston College and graduated from Tufts College Medical School in 1907. For thirty years he had served the New England Telephone and Telegraph Company as medical director for some 35,000 employees.

The story of occupational health in World War II is the story of the AAIP&S —and related national organizations in action. Even the over-all picture of their task, however, is not one that can be drawn clearly in a few simple lines. For governmental organization, in peace or war, involves a maze of agencies and activities which must be dovetailed together like pieces in a giant jigsaw puzzle. Reduced to simplest terms, what the federal government wanted (and got) from organized industrial medicine in 1940 was an advisory committee capable of developing specific programs, of whatever type, which would best serve industrial health needs in the national emergency. The committee was to refer its programs to the proper authorities, working through the Industrial Hygiene Division of the National Institute of Health of Bethesda, Maryland. The assignment, at the very outset, was little more specific than this. Its effects, however, were to be far-reaching, in many directions.

The Advisory Committee took its instructions from a chain of command headed by the Federal Security Agency and continuing through the USPHS to the National Institute of Health, under the surgeon general's office. From the latter, under date of June 25, committee members received notice of the first meeting to be held July 9 at the institute headquarters. These instructions were formalized, typically, in the following directive from Parran, dated July 3:

> You are hereby authorized to proceed on or about July 9, 1940, to Bethesda, Maryland, in connection with field investigations of industrial hygiene. Upon completion of the duty enjoined, you will return to (name of home city).
>
> In carrying out the foregoing orders, you will be allowed actual and necessary transportation and $5.00 per diem in lieu of subsistence.
>
> You are authorized to use your personally owned automobile for the travel directed and will be reimbursed therefor at the rate of three cents per mile, it having been administratively determined in advance that the allowance at that rate for all or any portion of the authorized travel will be more economical and advantageous to the government than travel by common carrier.

To view in true perspective the role of medicine in World War II, and the problems to be met, one must accept the statement of L. D. Bristol,[2] an authority on public health, who pointed out that there was not much of wartime precedent or experience on which to base a national defense industrial health program in 1940. The problems, in short, were fundamentally different.

The immediate situation, said Dr. Bristol, was one in which "our chief defense will be our industrial skill"; and to keep the availability of that skill and its continuity of application at their maximum, the medical profession, which in the first World War was mobilized for repair, was in 1940 mobilizing for prevention. The problems, he declared, were "the preservation of expert workers . . . the development of additional skilled workers . . . reducing lost time due to occupational and non-occupational illness and accidents."

Obviously, a task of such gigantic scope could not be performed by any single organization, private or governmental, or by all the organizations in any single field of health activity. It required the coordination of *all* agencies, concerned with any and all aspects of health. Because of the preventive angle, it called in particular for effective integration of industrial hygiene with industrial medicine wherever possible.

Speaking on this subject early in 1940, a prominent industrial hygiene engineer, H. G. Dyktor, said in part:

> I want it understood that I regard industrial hygiene as meaning an official industrial hygiene unit and industrial medicine as meaning a plant medical unit. . . .
>
> The main reason for the existence of an official hygiene unit is the presence of occupational health hazards in industry. Therefore its objective is the elimination or control of these hazards. These two fundamental considerations are clear-cut in the case of the official agency. . . .

As regards the status of the industrial physicians, I cannot do better than to refer you to a paper read before the Second Annual Midwest Conference on Occupational Diseases held in Chicago in 1938. In that paper Selby expressed himself to the effect that it was difficult to understand how any except full-time physicians could be in a position to assume appreciable responsibility in industrial hygiene in a plant.

The extent to which they do depends on their knowledge, vision, professional ability and capacity to organize or fit into the organization that employs them. Here, too, the prospects are good because of the interest in industrial hygiene exhibited by the profession as a whole.[3]

Dyktor's viewpoint could well have been adopted as a platform for the government's program of manpower conservation, its approach being basically the same as that of the USPHS. And the Advisory Committee setup was a perfect example of effective, workable liaison between industrial medicine and industrial hygiene.

The July 9 meeting at Bethesda took place as scheduled, with Assistant Surgeon General L. R. Thompson, director of the National Institute of Health, as chairman, and with the entire committee present. The day's agenda were broad in scope and extremely complex, but the group handled its task with swift precision. There was a minimum of discussion and no bickering over matters of jurisdiction or precedence.

Many a veteran member of the AAIP&S, receiving reports of this meeting, thought back with satisfaction to 1917, when Geier, Schereschewsky, Mock and others fought publicly and privately through official Washington for some recognition of their infant organization and for an opportunity to serve the nation in wartime.

Vastly different was the atmosphere at Bethesda in 1940. The Advisory Committee was accepted for exactly what it was, a mature body of experienced professional men, representing the best thinking of the time on industrial medicine and hygiene and a good deal of thinking that was ahead of its time. "The specialty" had come far in a quarter-century.

At the very outset the committee recorded in the minutes its own attitude toward the project: *There is a safe job for every worker, provided we utilize the knowledge already developed in the field of industrial health.*

The extent, the nature, and the value of the work entrusted to the Advisory Committee are indicated by a partial list of its major recommendations to the surgeon general as a result of that first meeting. These included:

Determination of existing health service facilities in industry.

Selection of important industries for immediate medical and engineering control of existing and potential health hazards.

Determination of methods for absorption of handicapped persons into vital industries.

Mobilization of all existing laboratories for investigation of hazardous materials to be employed in industries concerned with national defense.

Preparation and dissemination of information on toxic materials and processes for the practical protection of the health of workers.

Training of personnel for both industrial medicine and hygiene.

There were other recommended activities of comparable importance, all bearing directly on the industrial health of the nation and hence upon its potential production. Upon these recommended measures, in the aggregate, the success of the entire manpower program might well depend.

Fortunately, in view of the urgent need for industrial health statistics, the USPHS had, between 1936 and 1939, made a comprehensive survey in fifteen heavily industrialized states, embracing nearly 17,000 plants of types considered most important in the build-up of national production, and employing nearly 1.5 million workers. This survey included studies of such environmental factors as general sanitation and hygiene, as well as the incidence of disease, degree of exposure to various occupational hazards, and efficacy of plant health services.[4]

Available, too, were the findings of another, smaller survey made by the National Industrial Conference Board,[5] covering 301 establishments employing more than 600,000 workers. This survey showed that in 1940 most small plants still provided only a minimum of emergency medical service, though three out of four of them employed either a physician or nurse, or both, and in 88 percent of the plants workers were given pre-employment examinations by physicians.

The federal Division of Industrial Hygiene at Bethesda also had access to reports and other data made available by the American College of Surgeons, then responsible for the certification of medical services in industry. And *Who's Who in Industrial Medicine,* issued in 1936 by Industrial Medicine Publishing Company, gave detailed information about approximately a thousand physicians and surgeons practicing in that field.

In the summer of 1940 the Council on Industrial Health of the AMA was also gathering data on medical preparedness from all United States physicians. Five of eighty items on the AMA questionnaire pertained to industrial medicine; and the council was contemplating a special survey among physicians doing full- or part-time work in industry. Such fact-finding activities by federal and outside agencies gave the government a substantial backlog of information on the status of industrial health services and made it unnecessary to conduct further time-consuming studies in that particular area.

This saving of time also enabled the planners to speed up the all-important manpower conservation program, which was the special province of the Advisory Committee representing the AAIP&S and the Industrial Hygiene Association. In that effort the committee had the counsel and active help of the National Conference of Governmental Industrial Hygienists.

Medical organizations from coast to coast were simultaneously mobilizing for action. The AMA, veteran of many wars and emergencies, had size, prestige, experience, facilities, and gave generously of all. State and county medical societies, the

American Dental Association and affiliates, nurses and technicians, all joined in the common effort.

Quickly the National Institute of Health reached a cooperative agreement with the Division of Labor Standards to launch an accident prevention project that blanketed the country. Working under a committee appointed by the secretary of labor, an army of voluntary safety experts in eight regions set about carrying to even the smallest plants operating on government contracts the type of accident control exercised by the largest and best managed industries. These same safety men, when they encountered occupational disease hazards not receiving attention, were authorized to seek the services of state industrial hygiene units.

Similar working arrangements were made with important units of organized labor, with individual industries, universities and medical schools, foundations, and research organizations.

In these and other related enterprises, the industrial medical Advisory Committee was deeply immersed from the day of its appointment in June, 1940. A sub-committee on the training of medical personnel for industry, consisting of C. D. Selby (chairman), T. Lyle Hazlett, and Philip Drinker, started work immediately on the knotty problem of supplementary education for physicians and hygienists so urgently needed in industry. In August it submitted a plan which was successfully followed throughout the war in the emergency training of such personnel.

Coordination was the watchword of the day. Irvin Abell, chairman of the Health and Medical Committee of the Council of National Defense, told the Third Annual Congress on Industrial Health of the AMA (January, 1941): "The successful outcome of military activities depends upon the proper coordination of various resources. . . . Lost time must be regarded as comparably important to casualties."

He also said: "Physicians in industry should not be assigned to strictly military service unless there is obvious necessity and emergency. Short intensive courses should be given for physicians, while other professional men will develop through experience and training."[6]

Not many months before this meeting of the AMA Council, an important but little publicized change had been made in the government's emergency health setup which gave the AAIP&S and its co-workers in industrial hygiene a far larger role to play in the selfsame "coordination" discussed by Dr. Abell.

Soon after the New York convention at which appointment of the Advisory Committee was announced, its chairman, Royd Sayers, had personally presented to Surgeon General Parran, in outline, its comprehensive recommendations for development of industrial medicine and hygiene in relation to national defense. Parran accepted the plan as it stood, and it was promptly put into effect by the creation of a new sub-committee operating under the Committee on Health and Medicine, of which Abell was chairman and which was the responsible agency in directing over-all health activities pertaining to the national defense program.

By this step, industrial phases of the work were split from the main committee, and the Subcommittee on Industrial Health and Medicine took over the task of co-ordinating activities specifically involving industrial manpower. The new group, in short, was charged with carrying out the procedures recommended by the original Advisory Committee.

Four of the seven members of the original committee, Selby, Holmblad, Yant and Drinker, were able to accept duty with the new group. The remaining three posts were filled by the appointment of A. J. Lanza, Lloyd Noland (Tennessee Coal, Iron & Railroad Company), and George M. Smith (Department of Anatomy, Yale Medical School). When, in the spring of 1942, Lieutenant Colonel Lanza resigned because of the pressure of other work, Robert A. Kehoe, director of the Kettering Laboratories, joined the group.

With Selby as permanent chairman, the new committee held its organization meeting in Washington, November 6, 1940, with representatives from the top echelon of the health services in attendance. Presenting the agenda, Selby stated that the "foundation function" of the group was "to control, insofar as possible, those conditions that are sources of inefficiency and losses of time that arise out of ill health."

It soon became apparent, however, that the committee was to be a multi-purpose body, able and willing to grapple with any problem related to occupational health. When the National Research Council created a Committee on Medical Research in the autumn of 1941, Selby's group (with William A. Sawyer serving in place of Lloyd Noland) collaborated on industrial phases of the work. When the Procurement and Assignment Service was established just before Pearl Harbor, the Industrial Health and Medicine Committee was part of the central organization.

Selby himself described its objectives as follows: "The Subcommittee on Industrial Health and Medicine is an advisory coordinating agency whose principal purpose is to inspire progress in as many directions and through as many channels as possible, in order that the health of the workers in war industries may be safe-guarded."

How shall we recount the wartime roles of the doctor in any but very general terms? The subject is one that calls for many volumes of text, rather than brief chapters.[7]

One thing is certain: In the closing years of the 1930's and the early years of the 1940's, industrial medicine attained maturity. It became militant medicine, assuming added responsibilities, setting higher goals and marching confidently toward them, while it prepared to meet the wartime demands of military medicine.

McIver Woody sounded a keynote in his address as retiring president of the AAIP&S meeting in 1940: "Now that the parent organization has a membership equal to nearly 1 percent of all the physicians in active practice throughout the country, its future would seem to be secure, provided it measures up to the needs of the hour."

At the same meeting Carey McCord pointed to the responsibility resting on industry and industrial physicians for the conservation of manpower in the stepping up of production. Congestion, epidemics, acceptance of older persons and the handicapped, the use of new processes and materials, he declared, were problems that must be solved.

A year later Daniel Lynch, in his address as outgoing president of the association, eloquently described its defense obligations, and concluded: "We must pledge ourselves to this cause—that no blood is spilled, nor tears shed, where it can be prevented."

In July, 1942, *Industrial Medicine* editorially paraphrased a national motto in these words: "United, we're on the move."

Officially, as an organization, the AAIP&S made its most significant contribution to the war effort through committees working closely with government agencies. Yet for every member required at that level there were scores who served, inconspicuously, on sundry boards and committees of every size and degree of importance, everywhere in the land.

Members of the parent association and its affiliates in active military service on various fronts numbered into the hundreds. Who can weigh, or even estimate, the value of their contribution? Or that of the many who increased the nation's might by their research and their writings?

Yet by all odds the largest, most decisive battle fought by industrial medicine was waged in another theater, the manufacturing plants of America. There, in the maelstrom of unprecedented production, amid new hazards to life and limb, the industrial physician and surgeon first "faced up" to the modern future of his profession.

XXV

WAR—AND A CHALLENGE TO MEDICINE

Ｉn actual time, little more than twenty years separated the cease-fire of World War I, which was to "make the world safe for democracy," from the declaration of World War II, "the war to end war." The two conflicts might well have taken place a century apart, so greatly did they differ in the scale of operations, in the deadliness of weapons, and in the utilization of manpower. Moreover, correspondingly great differences soon became apparent in the functions and duties of industrial doctors, and the degree of their involvement, in the second war.

Science, within a single generation, had made incredible strides toward the conquest of distance. Suddenly, it seemed, our vast, mysterious globe had become one small world, girdled in an imperceptible moment by radio and in a matter of hours by aircraft. Oceans and mountain ranges no longer offered security; they were merely hurdles to be leaped. Faraway nations, hostile or friendly, became next door neighbors.

This telescoping of communications, by itself, had profound effects on the strategy of war and the economy of peace. But many more, and equally revolutionary, scientific miracles were to come. With the means of rapid, long-range transport at hand, industry set about producing lighter but deadlier weapons, in larger volume.

In primitive times, when man's radius of operation was a forest, a valley, an island, or even a continent, wars were isolated. Half the world did not know how the other half lived and died; or, if they knew, they regarded distant strife with complacency. But now, in this most enlightened of centuries, entire populations had the status of combatants in fact if not in name.

Even in America, unscarred by actual attack, men, women and children lived in

300

terrible intimacy with the conflict abroad. American boys were fighting on many fronts. America was "the arsenal of democracy." What happened at Guadalcanal or Iwo Jima, on the beaches of Europe or the deserts of Africa, had immediate repercussions in the fields, the mines, the laboratories, and the factories of America.

Since war had became *total,* attention naturally was focused on many things that were of little importance in World War I. In the final analysis all problems sifted down to one problem: manpower and its conservation: not only the fitness and readiness of men to fight but the fitness and readiness of people to work and produce as never before. And, since health is the province of the physician and surgeon, the ranking problem in industrial medicine was the availability of doctors for industrial duty, and their fitness and readiness to discharge the added responsibilities thrust upon them.

Looking ahead in the summer of 1940, when each day was bringing word of disasters overseas, McIver Woody summed up the situation and the problem with these comments at the annual meeting of the American Association of Industrial Physicians & Surgeons:

> Now, just as in 1916, the military powers of Europe are locked in a life and and death struggle, the outcome of which no man can foretell. This much is sure, no matter who wins in the end, medicine as a profession will never be quite the same again. Medical books will have to be rewritten, and the rules of the medical profession may have to be revised. . . .
>
> Even if we doctors wished to do so, we could not insulate ourselves from the turmoil and change going on in other countries which are so affecting our own. If we are to be of real use to industry, we must have some regard to the environment in which industry operates; we must be aware of the fact that a new and cheaper source of raw material discovered on the other side of the globe may have a profound effect on a whole branch of industry at home; that remedies and new ideas born of frontline emergency needs may change accepted techniques in a few short months. . . .
>
> We are not at war, no, not yet, but the effects of the war are already being felt in every factory and office in our land, both physically and mentally. Whether these people can be restored to usefulness as workers in industry, whether they must be hospitalized or placed on relief, only the trained physician can know. Production must go on regardless of human suffering. . . .
>
> Would that we doctors could cure nations duped by delusions of grandeur as often as we can the individual.[1]

Yes, there was complete agreement that production must go on. And indeed, industrial medicine had to gear itself to constantly changing techniques dictated by front-line needs. But the doing was not so simple as the saying. There were at least three major hurdles to be cleared if industry was to meet its production quotas: the precarious manpower situation; new health and accident hazards in industrial plants; and the need for more and more physicians with industrial experience.

301

Even in the earliest stages of "defense" preparation the manpower shortage was acute, and it grew steadily worse. Not only was there substantially less total manpower available to industry, but it was, on the average, substantially less fit for the work at hand. Early in the war Lowell S. Selling, a Detroit psychiatrist experienced in public health service, warned plant physicians of a phase of this situation already encountered by most of them.

"In peace times," he said, "particularly in times of depression, the labor pool is so deep that one can pick and choose according to his own likes and dislikes in order to find the kind of personnel he wants for his plant. In wartime the opposite is the case. No longer can the problem individuals be thrown out because they are mental problems. As a matter of fact the army has taken and will continue to take the best of American manpower, throwing back to the occupations behind the lines those who are not considered fit for military service."

It would be necessary, he added, for plant physicians to add some psychiatric work to their other responsibilities as the war continued. At least they would be called upon to practice "medical psychology" to the limits of their ability, since fewer and fewer psychiatrists would be available for civilian duty.

In conclusion he commented: "The plant physician, while not a psychiatrist and hence more likely to make a number of psychiatric errors . . . is in a position to utilize the knowledge available from this branch of the profession in a competent fashion. He is better off to use what little knowledge of mental medicine he can acquire and apply than to ignore the whole subject in times like these when every available man must be utilized."[2]

Of the unfit for military service, of course, only a minority were mental problems; but whatever the cause for rejection it was important that the employability of men in this class be determined and that they be placed whenever possible on jobs suited to their capabilities. Naturally, final decisions as to the physical and mental fitness of applicants became a responsibility of the medical directors.

There were many questions to be answered before workable procedures could be set up to meet the manpower crisis. How much potential production was being lost and from what causes? What was the health situation in different industries and in specific plants? How efficient were existing medical services? What could be done to improve them, quickly?

The war emergency revealed a deplorable lack of reliable statistics on industrial health in its many ramifications. Available information was, on the whole, insufficiently detailed to serve as a guide for industry-wide procedures; classifications of occupational disease—with respect to source, incidence, severity, etc.—were generally inadequate.

Federal and state governments, as well as private industries, seemed suddenly awake to health needs that had existed for many years without general recognition. Plant services and procedures long advocated by organized industrial medicine now held the limelight. The medical and hygiene teams sent out by the National Institute of Health, from Bethesda and from state health departments, were a potent force in tightening hazard controls, particularly in government arsenals, proving grounds, and supply depots. Many large industrial corporations, through their medical and statistical departments, contributed much-needed surveys of health conditions in individual plants. Influential business associations made similar studies, broader in scope.

Unquestionably, the most intimate knowledge of, and the most concentrated experience in, industrial medicine were to be found in the membership of the AAIP&S. Individually, in groups in the government services, and in committees of their own association, they went to work for the common cause, at the tasks they could do best.

Whether in large plants or small, and regardless of the type of industry involved, fact-finding research teams were unanimous in naming the factor chiefly responsible for holding industrial production consistently below its potential. Absenteeism was the culprit, an elusive and a formidable enemy. It is doubtful that the full extent of industrial absenteeism was realized until World War II. And it is of historical interest that, despite continued improvement of working environments and procedures, it is still among the chief problems plaguing industry and industrial medicine.

Wherever they turned in their wartime studies of production, researchers found the shadow of absenteeism overhanging American factories. Figures, as would be expected, varied widely because of differences in record-keeping systems and the purposes for which they were used. Nevertheless, there was a remarkable amount of agreement on important points.

Speaking at the annual meeting of the AAIP&S in 1939, William S. Knudsen said that industrial absenteeism, on the average, amounted to more than ten days per year per employee, while occupational disease and accidents caused less than half of one day's absence. In other words, ordinary disease accounted for nearly twenty times as much loss of time as trade hazards and accidents combined.[3] These figures he credited to Victor G. Heiser, consultant in industrial health for the National Association of Manufacturers.

At the organization meting of the Defense Council's Subcommittee on Industrial Health and Medicine in November, 1940, Clarence Selby, as chairman, laid the problem of productive manpower squarely before his group in terms of absenteeism and disability.

Analyzing the health situation among workers he said:

The best index is in the time losses, of which there are two sources—occupational and nonoccupational. The nonoccupational account for 95 percent, and the occupational for 5 percent. The nonoccupational are in ordinary sicknesses and injuries outside of employment, such as might occur in any adult group. These are treated entirely by the general practitioners of medicine.

The occupational sources are in the conditions which result in occupational injuries and occupational disease. Eighty-five percent of the workers are in plants that employ general practitioners on part-time or call basis for the treatment of these conditions. Therefore, inasmuch as the general practitioners of medicine treat 100 percent of the nonoccupational disabilities and 85 percent of the occupational, the problem of removing the sources of ill health in industry is predominantly in the hands of the general medical profession. Any effort to obtain maximum results by way of health maintenance in industry must be through them.

At least as early as 1938, realizing the direct bearing of sickness on national productivity, the AAIP&S had a special (and extremely active) committee at work on studies of industrial absenteeism. In that year the group appointed by President Selby included Sayers (chairman), William A. Sawyer, D. L. Lynch, John J. Wittmer, J. B. McConnaughy (Aluminum Company of America), and R. D. Mudd (Chevrolet Grey Iron Foundry). This committee continued its work for several years with slight changes in personnel, A. W. Schoenleber (Standard Oil Company, New Jersey) replacing McConnaughy and Wittmer in 1939. Important among its reports was a recommendation submitted in June, 1940, outlining a simple record system which would provide industrial management with vitally needed information on absenteeism due to all forms of illness, whether or not of occupational origin.[4]

A few months before the Japanese attack on Pearl Harbor an all-important AAIP&S Committee on National Defense was appointed by the new president, T. Lyle Hazlett. Its chairman was Dan Lynch, perennially occupied with association activities, who had just retired from the presidency. Other members were Henry S. Brown (Michigan Bell Telephone Company), D. O. Hamblin (American Cyanamid Company), and Charles-Francis Long, an authority on the problems of tobacco workers.

In the summer of 1942 this committee released the results of an exhaustive study, known as the Lynch-Brown report, of wartime health problems and a detailed program for industrial management, designed to minimize the effects of possible enemy attack. It was a militant, and confident, presentation, but the over-all picture it painted of manpower losses through accident and illness was far from encouraging.

Citing National Safety Council accident statistics for 1941, the committee said: "Although it would appear from these data that occupational deaths and disabling injuries may not have increased in the same degree as employment, it still seems clear that the sacrifice of life and vital man-hours was not lessened appreciably. The reported 18,000 deaths and 1,600,000 disabling injuries represent a tremendous wastage of manpower, and a continued challenge to everyone concerned in saving lives and saving this nation."[5] Accident figures such as these were indeed shocking to contemplate, yet they were only an echo of much older industrial statistics. The rate of fatal and nonfatal injuries had followed a seesaw course for many years, showing no conclusive trend in either direction. The situation was one which led Sayers to comment: "In spite of the spectacular achievements which have been made in safety work, special studies still show that we have not reached the irreducible minimum in accident rates."[6]

Comparisons with later periods are of more than passing interest in this connection. During 1955, according to figures cited by a large weekly magazine, more than 1.9 million men and women suffered on-the-job accidents; and of them 1,200 were killed and more than 75,000 injured permanently.[7] If there is encouragement in such figures it is to be found in two facts: the number of men and women employed in industry increased enormously in the decade following the war, and death and injury totals would unquestionably have been far greater were it not for improved safeguards and more efficient medical services.

Turning from trauma to illness in industry, the Lynch-Brown report concluded (from partial data) that in 1941 disability due to occupational disease had increased faster than employment: "In view of the great influx of new employees into industry, the use of many new substances and substitutes and work processes, and the heavier usage of known inherently dangerous chemicals, the increase over the country may not be of real significance. But again it does not appear that we have made real progress in the prevention of occupational disease."

Wherever researchers delved into the causes of absenteeism and lost production they found a common stumbling block in the problem of *non*occupational illness, often unrecorded except on time cards and even more frequently unexplained. The experience of Lynch's committee was no exception. "The fact remains," it concluded, "that nonoccupational illness resulting in lost time in industry continues to be a major problem, that it will adversely affect production, that we do not seem to be making much progress against it, and that lost time, reportedly but not actually due to sickness, appears to be increasing." Although statistics on nonoccupational sickness among workers were neither complete nor altogether trustworthy, reports did not differ greatly in estimating its frequency as compared with disability for other causes.

Presenting the William S. Knudsen Award to Royd R. Sayers in 1941 for his studies of sickness absenteeism,[8] Selby dwelt briefly on this frequency, citing statistical data from General Motors records. The corporation, he said, had an average of 187,000 hourly-rated employees in 1940, who lost a grand total of nearly 830,000 hours from nonoccupational causes. He quoted figures showing that of all sickness disability almost 83 percent (in days lost) was due to nonoccupational illness and slightly over 17 percent to occupational.

Although General Motors records on absenteeism in later years have been broken down in greater detail and on a somewhat different basis, the distribution of total time lost in 1951 showed 86.3 percent due to nonoccupational sickness, 11.3 percent to nonoccupational injuries, and only 2.4 percent to occupational diseases and injuries combined.[9]

The great increase in the number and percentage of industrially employed women in the 1940's had an appreciable effect upon medical statistics. Their in-

305

vasion of the mechanical production trades resulted in a succession of studies dealing with their selection and training, their working hours and environment, their susceptibility to fatigue and other hazards. Writing on their problems in 1942, Milton H. Kronenberg (Illinois Division of Industrial Hygiene) quoted press releases predicting that more than 18 million women would be employed in the United States by the end of 1953—over 200,000 of them in munition plants. "It has been reported," he wrote, "that sickness absenteeism among women in industry is high. A daily absence of 10 percent is not unusual. Their annual rate exceeds that of the men by approximately 60 percent and their disability periods are correspondingly higher."[10]

The special health problems of women workers came into prominence in wartime, but they did not disappear with peace. Speaking at a symposium on industrial medicine at the Harvard School of Public Health in April 1953, George F. Wilkins, medical director of the New England Telephone and Telegraph Company, and president-elect of the Industrial Medical Association, quoted USPHS statistics dealing with this phase of absenteeism. For the year 1950 alone, he pointed out, the number of absences per thousand persons (on account of nonoccupational sickness and injury disabling for eight consecutive days or longer) was 116.8 for males and 258.4 for females. If these frequency rates are applied to the (approximately) 55.5 million employees in nonagricultural industry, said Wilkins, "it is found that each year more than 4.25 million men and more than 4.75 million women are absent from work for eight consecutive calendar days or more as the result of illness or injury not related to their occupation." Then he went on to quote Robert Collier Page (president of IMA, 1954–1955) as authority for an estimate that the total cost of nonoccupational absenteeism might amount to as much as 1.8 percent of the total payroll of the industry, the estimate being based on a ten-year study of absence in a large oil industry, completed in 1948.

Data on industrial absenteeism, as typified by the foregoing, are cited here not for their statistical value but to underscore the importance of, and the growing emphasis on, nonoccupational sickness in its relation to the nation's productivity. The problem intruded as a controversial topic in wartime, and it still awaits satisfactory solution.

All studies (and they could be quoted at great length) seem to bear out the fact that, as a source of lost man-hours, nonoccupational illness outweighs job-connected disability from all causes by a very large margin. It appears, moreover, that absenteeism due to common adult ailments is a relatively bigger problem in large corporations which, by highly efficient medical and safety programs, hold occupational accidents and illnesses to a minimum.

The important point in this situation, however, is not the exact ratio of one type of absenteeism to another but the fact that the scope of industrial medicine has steadily expanded to include many areas formerly considered entirely outside its province.

There is general agreement today that industrial disability, whether partial or total, temporary or permanent, whether due to accident or disease, of occupational or other origin, must be considered as a single, over-all problem which cannot be handled piecemeal. Its solution is a task for all health agencies, working cooperatively with management and labor. And the industrial physician, even if he should be so minded, cannot ignore or slight any aspect of it.

Nevertheless, though he has been made an active member of the public health team, the industrial doctor's primary responsibility as a specialist is still the treatment, control, and prevention of occupational trauma and disease. This is the practice for which he is peculiarly fitted by training and experience. This is the profession to which the employer looks for the protection of his workers. This is the area in which compensation laws and the dictates of humane business policies are fully operative.

It is a matter of common knowledge that the second great war loosed upon the world a sudden deluge of new materials, alloys, and compounds, along with a new body of industrial science for their manufacture and processing. It is doubtful, however, that most people understand the full extent of this technological revolution, or the transformation it has wrought in the lives and affairs of men.

The outpouring of new applied science from laboratories and factories, if it can be dated at all, may be said to have started, almost as if by pushbutton control, at the outset of the so-called "defense" production in this country. It continued to gain volume and momentum not only through the war period, but in the following years. It is still accelerating, and the man would be brash indeed who would predict when it may end or slow its pace.

Statistics dealing with this outpouring (from whatever source we take them) challenge credulity; yet certain key figures are well authenticated. To establish dependable criteria in this connection, we quote from the editorial page of *Industrial Medicine and Surgery* in September, 1953:

In the pharmaceutical world, of all drugs sold over the druggist's counter, 90 percent have appeared in the past fifteen years. The majority of older medicaments, little useful, have been relegated without precise disappearance to a state of unimportance.

So in the world of diseases many, while always threats, seldom are seen. Where is typhoid fever, or small pox, or pellagra, or tuberculosis? Replacements, although replacements are unwanted, spring from industry.

At the present time there are 600,000 named organic chemical compounds, as lately mentioned by Gustav Egloff before the Chemical Specialties Manufacturers' Association. He said: "The possibilities are almost limitless when one considers that there are now 600,000 organic compounds and in a few years there may be over a million. Not only are new chemicals continually being introduced, but new specialty applications are being found for products already in use."

Loosely stated, there have been just 600,000 work days since the beginning of our time year, A.D. 1. Without consequence, that means one new organic chemical compound for every day of the Christian era. But, some 500,000 of these compounds have been man-made since 1900.

The same type of figuring reveals thirty-one new compounds created on the average for every day of the past fifty-three years. In stark conservatism, at least one of these thirty-one is demonstrated to possess toxic properties or is potentially damaging. It follows that on this basis 15,900 chemicals are suspect, or, to be bolder, are damaging when manipulated without protective controls.[11]

The time is past when industry could introduce chemically active substances into manufacture without knowledge of their properties or develop production procedures likely to expose workers to undue hazards. If for no other reason than that it is "good business," wise management is more interested in the ounce of prevention than the pound of cure. And it has become part of the routine business of industrial physicians, along with hygienists, safety personnel and public health officials, to keep both a telescopic and a microscopic eye on the constant flow of new materials and techniques in industry.

Discussing the application of the so-called new chemicals at a New York Safety Council meeting in 1951, Thomas W. Nale, well known industrial toxicologist (Union Carbide & Carbon Corporation), made this pertinent comment:

> It is generally recognized that any chemical whatsoever can be produced and applied safely. Precautions in handling are expensive and should be recommended only if they are truly necessary in order to protect health. Once safe ways of operating are defined, cost accountants and marketing experts can decide whether the need for a chemical in its probable application is sufficiently pressing to justify the cost at which it must be sold and the expense of using it safely.
>
> No chemical or application of a chemical can be successful if it injures health or if precautions to avoid injury are more burdensome than is justified by the utility of the compound.[12]

Necessity, however, dictated many undesirable compromises in time of war, and, in spite of heroic efforts to protect plant workers from occupational health hazards, the swelling tide of new toxic materials and the reappearance of old ones soon created an extremely serious problem.

Lieutenant Colonel W. J. McConnell (United States Medical Corps) in November, 1943, at the eighth annual meeting of the Industrial Hygiene Foundation in Pittsburgh, reported:

> Industrial absenteeism under war conditions has become alarmingly high and at times has seriously interrupted the production of greatly needed material. . . . Accumulated evidence points to sickness as the most frequent cause for absence from work. Although the truly occupational diseases account for only a small percentage of the total cases of illnesses, they are tremendously important in particular types of work and their incidence has never been so great as at the present time. How-

ever, their early recognition, and the improvement in methods of controlling harmful exposures have greatly diminished their seriousness.

This same absenteeism problem was uppermost in the mind of T. Lyle Hazlett when, as retiring president of the AAIP&S in 1942, he addressed the association at what he termed the most important meeting in its history.

> We were charged with keeping men fit. We are the medical field marshals for the Army of Production. These men who fight behind the lines in mines, mills, and factories cannot go on losing an average of eight days per year because of illness. Occupational accidents claimed approximately 20,000 lives last year, a gain of 8 percent over 1940; nonfatal injuries totaled about 1.75 million, a 14 percent increase.
>
> The Gallup Poll estimates that throughout the United States 24 million man-hours of work were lost because of illness in the four-week period of last November 24 to December 20. This is in approximate agreement with findings from the study of sick absenteeism which is being made by the Industrial Hygiene Foundation and the United States Public Health Service, in which our association is collaborating.[13]

It was greatly to the credit of the "shock troops" made up of industrial medical, hygiene and safety personnel, entrusted with the protection of munitions workers, that despite the tremendously increased power and volume of explosives produced, handled and shipped, there was no major disaster in United States munition plants during the war or in ensuing years.

It is true that many years earlier, in peacetime, a $50 million blast destroyed the Picatinny Arsenal at Dover, New Jersey, touching off 5.5 million pounds of TNT, wrecking two villages and taking twenty-three lives. Only the fact that it occurred on a week end holiday, July 10, 1926, saved hundreds of workers. The explosion, triggered by lighting during a violent electrical storm, was second only to the disaster in Halifax, Nova Scotia, in 1917.

The research staff of the National Institute of Health vigorously pursued studies of the toxic properties of TNT in 1940–41. Editorially, in October, 1941, *Industrial Medicine* warmly complimented the Bethesda group for its progress in control of TNT vapor and dust, responsible for serious outbreaks of jaundice in the first World War.

Nor could the hazard hunters of the forties find the counterpart of the "canaries" encountered by Alice Hamilton in her World War I research at nitrous plants along the Eastern Coast.[14] Safeguards had long since banished the clouds of noxious vapor that ate away the clothing and dyed the skins of workers orange-yellow.

Nevertheless, contact with tetryl, TNT, DNT, and other materials in the explosives industry remained a common cause of dermatoses; and dusts, fumes and vapors, unless constantly checked and adequately controlled, could easily reach atmospheric concentrations sufficient to make them dangerously toxic. Munitions manufacturing, however, has had no more than its share of health hazards during and since World War II, and, as in other industries, tested and proved protective measures have kept them well under control in most factories.

It is patently impossible to include in this work even a representative list of the potentially toxic metals and compounds either contained in common industrial products or used in processing them at the present time. For one thing, their number and identity change every day or even every hour of every day. Old hazards are constantly being overcome but are replaced by new. Ancient enemies sometimes reappear in different guise.

White phosphorus, it will be remembered, was banished from the match industry after the full exposé of its pitiful ravages among workers. As a result, phosphorus necrosis as an occupational disease practically disappeared. Yet, thirty years later, an article in *Industrial Medicine* recalled this public scandal and commented as follows: "Several cases arose later in the manufactures of firework implements in this country, and a few, and milder, cases still arise in the factories producing phosphorus and in factories using it in the production of certain alloys. In the growing war industry this danger must be remembered, insofar as phosphorus may be used in alloys."[15]

Likewise, the status of an industrial material, with respect to its toxicity, may change as the result of research. In 1941 John M. McDonald, director of Baltimore's Bureau of Occupational Diseases, published in *Industrial Medicine* a detailed discussion of a dozen toxic metals, their properties and those of their commonest compounds. He closed his report with this statement: "The following metals are generally considered to be nonpoisonous insofar as industrial use is concerned: tin, aluminum, gold, silver, copper, cobalt, iron, barium, and titanium."[16]

Writing editorially twelve years later in the same journal, Carey McCord commented on the fact that the last named of McDonald's "exceptions" (titanium), as well as its most important derivative, titanium dioxide, had long been credited with being almost entirely innocuous. He then ventured this cautious surmise: "Since the recent advent of metallic titanium into industry, scattered complaints have appeared among workers alleging nausea, headaches, and malaise. It is deemed prospective that a titanium metal fume fever does occur and that the expectable manifestations would be similar to those from zinc or magnesium metal fume fever."[17]

The unqualified safety (in industrial use) of at least one other metal on McDonald's non-poisonous list has been questioned to some extent. There was considerable talk around airplane plants, during the second World War, of so-called "aluminum poisoning." Of it, A. Fletcher Hall, consulting dermatologist at Douglas Aircraft, had this to say: "Dural poisoning, aluminum poisoning, and like expressions have been popularized by aircraft workers and threaten to find their way into medical parlance as haphazard diagnosis." Actually, in a series of 202 cases of occupational dermatitis subjected to analysis in Hall's own report, only 5 percent were found to be due to dural and only 2 percent to aluminum. In short, "sensitivity" reactions of this type were relatively few and not particularly severe.

Forrest E. Rieke, medical director of the Oregon Shipbuilding Corporation and Kaiser Company, relates the following instance in a noteworthy article that throws an interesting light on some of the medical problems involved in a not unusual type of war contract. Late in 1944 his company received an order for construction of four thousand aluminum pontons for the army. As soon as specifications were at hand (meticulously detailed like all army authorizations), engineers, medical staff and hygienists went into action, analyzing the production processes required, studying all materials entering into manufacture, and, finally, estimating the health hazards involved and the means of combating them. The army pontons were constructed mainly of aluminum, alloyed for the most part with small quantities of other metals (duraluminum). Not more than a half dozen medically important chemicals were used in processing the materials for assembly. Following is Rieke's terse description of the resulting health problem:

> Health difficulties had arisen in association with degreasing, etching, and painting aluminum, and in subsequent drilling and machining of painted aluminum. Our main assistance to plant engineers consisted of counseling on selection of the least hazardous etch process and paints and proper ventilation, locker space, and bathing facilities.
>
> We then turned to the chemistry, toxicology, and health hazards connected with our materials and processes and outlined protective and preventive measures to assure safe and healthy workers and working conditions.[18]

The doctor's simple summary certainly does not overemphasize the amount of careful study and planning required to safeguard the thousands of workers on this particular contract. Yet the type of production involved seems fairly representative of conditions to be found in industrial plants of many types across the country.

Not until we had pored over discussions at directors' meetings of the Industrial Medical Association and studied closely the files of *Industrial Medicine* did we fully realize the immensity of the task of keeping industrial physicians constantly informed as to potential hazards stemming from materials used in industry, making certain that they are provided with chemical data on resulting diseases and are well posted on modern methods of control and prevention.

Scores of important papers on various aspects of dermatology alone, by eminent research scientists and practicing specialists, appeared in *Industrial Medicine* during and after the war. No single journal would undertake to name and describe all the materials and compounds that are suspect in this connection, for they are as the leaves of the trees. But one journal can cover adequately the main types of skin irritants and the diagnosis and treatment of infections.

More serious, if not so numerous, are the hazards presented by poisons that enter the body by ingestion, inhalation or penetration through the skin. During the era of industrial expansion launched by World War II, *Industrial Medicine* has rendered a distinguished service by its coverage of industrial toxicology.

John M. McDonald, in his study of metallic poisons,[19] discusses a dozen important offenders, old and new, among them lead, antimony, chromium, arsenic, mercury, manganese and selenium. His estimates indicate that more than a million United States workers were exposed to these seven metals and their compounds at the time of the study. The others on his list, for which exposure statistics were not available, are cadmium, thallium, zinc, phosphorus and radium.

Radium, since the dawn of the Atomic Age, of course, has come back to haunt the dreams of humanity around the globe. But the very name of this awesome substance, in an industrial connection, recalls the tragedy of the watch dial painters thirty years before the first atomic bomb. McDonald, in passing, issued a warning that this original type of radium hazard in industry might again need close scrutiny, since it was again being used to illuminate airplane instruments for night flying.

Such lists, however, scarcely scratch the surface of the subject. There are beryllium, magnesium, plastics, DDT and other insecticides, gallium, fluorine, industrial cyanides, even toxic woods. These and many other known and suspected hazards are grist for the mill of *Industrial Medicine,* as is the discussion of hazards peculiar to specific industries, such as aircraft, rubber and petroleum.

All the areas listed in the foregoing inventory lie within the industrial physician's special and immediate field of practice, entirely apart from broader collateral problems such as absenteeism, alcoholism, disability, geriatrics, noise, and air pollution (public as well as industrial). There will be commentaries on these and other related responsibilities later.

Nor does this listing take into account the requirement imposed upon those specializing in industrial medicine as a profession to meet its future personnel needs by doing all that can be done to promote a special education and training that will insure a succession of able physicians and surgeons in industry. This, too, is the business of the industrial physician.

Here, in sum and substance, is the challenge issued by the age in which we live, a challenge to medicine in general but to industrial medicine in particular, and hence to the official organization representing the specialty, the Industrial Medical Association.

Many have written authoritatively about the abilities and training required by the individual, if he is to reach the top of this profession in modern times. Seldom, however, has the topic beem summarized more eloquently than by Daniel Lynch (past president, AAIP&S) in 1942:

> [The physician in industry] should possess a knowledge of the detection and control of occupational diseases, and be able to locate hazards, and to study the earliest exposures caused by them.
>
> He should become experienced in case finding in communicable disease and its control.
>
> He should possess a knowledge of administration, which includes industrial relations, because many of his problems are personal as well as medical.

312

He should know job analysis, to assist in the proper placement of new workers and in the rehabilitation and proper placement of the injured, of the worker with arrested tuberculosis and of those handicapped by heart disease, hypertension, arthritis, and other chronic diseases.

He should have a knowledge of factory laws and records, of compensation laws, of plant sanitation, ventilation and illumination, of accident prevention and safety, of humanitarianism.

He should have had special training quite beyond the field of private practice.[20]

Such an array of requirements may well have been greeted with skepticism in some quarters at the time, but it is likely that most present-day medical directors, particularly in large industries, would agree that the objectives suggested are not only desirable but attainable. Indeed, it must be acknowledged that since the early forties all these items, and many more, have come well within the purview of the industrial specialist, by self-imposed discipline.

"Certainly during the war," wrote Morris Fishbein in his *History of the American Medical Association* "industrial health rose to its highest level of recognition and acceptance."[21] This statement summarizes in a nutshell the gains made by industrial medicine up to that time. But it could as truthfully have predicted that the pace of its progress was to quicken beyond all parallel in the subsequent decade, as industry unleashed the full power of its new technology in production.

XXVI

THE INDUSTRIAL DOCTOR
AT THE APPROACH OF
THE CHEM-ELECTRIC ERA

Mₒₛₜ readers of the old *Bulletin* of the American Association of
Industrial Physicians & Surgeons (and there were not a great many of them) probably spent a minute or two in perusal of the following item, printed in the January
1931 issue under the headline "The Old, Old Story." And some of them may have
done something about it.

> There are many physicians, at least a thousand, doing industrial medical work
> in the United States, who are eligible for membership in the American Association
> of Industrial Physicians & Surgeons and do not know that such an organization
> exists.
>
> One or two of them may be your next door neighbors and, as a member, you
> owe it to the association to see that they know something about it. Will you not
> see them personally, and invite them to join us? Or, if you prefer, send their names
> in to the secretary and he will do the rest.
>
> Our influence in medical affairs will depend upon the quality of our members,
> but the extent of that influence and our strength in exerting it will depend upon
> the quantity or number of members we have to back it up.

By an interesting coincidence C. O. Sappington (then connected with the Division of Industrial Health of the National Safety Council) launched a similar query
in April 1931, in addressing the Michigan Association of Industrial Physicians &
Surgeons at its sixth annual meeting in Detroit. Said the doctor:

With approximately 50 million persons gainfully employed in the United States, and the loss from illness in industry totaling $10 billion a year, there must be definite reasons why industrial medicine has not assumed a more important place in our national life.

Speaking conservatively, there must be approximately 20,000 industrial physicians and surgeons in actual practice, and yet after fifteen years a representative national organization in industrial medicine and surgery has approximately a membership of only 325.[1] Three other official and unofficial organizations have sections on industrial medicine the membership and attendance of which has never reached more than 100 each.[2]

We need not be concerned about the wide discrepancy between the two estimates of the number of physicians in industrial practice. Trustworthy statistics simply did not exist, and one man's guess was as good as another's. Obviously it was the *Bulletin* editor who was conservative and Sappington who was liberal; the true figure was somewhere between one and twenty thousand. The really pertinent fact was that the membership of the AAIP&S in 1931 was nearly one-third smaller than in 1921, and that it was to fluctuate aimlessly at about the same level for another six or seven years. And, as Sappington remarked, other industrial medical groups were having the same trouble.

This was indeed an "old, old story." Among the earliest and most active of AAIP&S standing committees were those concerned with membership. They worked hard and incessantly. But, while the association suffered many tribulations during its first fifteen years, it had never known the exquisite anguish of growing pains.

Why this apparent stagnation in the matter of membership? What was the drag retarding a normal and reasonable growth? Depression was not the answer, for membership maintained a higher level in the troubled thirties than in the booming twenties. Nor can the emphasis on quality be considered an impediment. Association leaders may have been tempted at times to expand the roster at whatever cost, but they steadfastly rejected the thought, knowing that any lowering of standards was a sure road to professional suicide.

Perhaps the most valid reason for the continued slow progress was the fact that the AAIP&S needed a great deal of good publicity in the right places. Outside its own circle of membership the great majority of people did not seem to know what an industrial doctor was, or wherein his functions differed from those of any other doctor. There were still medical men who, even when face to face with industrial medicial audiences, were prone to inform them blandly that no such specialty existed and that an industrial physician was simply one whose practice, or part of it, came from specific industrial employers.

Then, as the thirties neared their close, the drift of industrial medical affairs changed abruptly. Up, up went association membership, not by tens or scores but by hundreds each year. The coveted 1,000 mark was passed in 1940, and at the annual meeting in Pittsburgh in May, 1941, delegates greeted with loud applause the announcement that membership had reached a total of 1,200. Hard working committees, of course, were entitled to much credit for these gains, but there had been well organized, sustained drives before, with no such results.

One may ask again—Why this sudden turn in the fortunes of industrial medicine and of the association officially representing it? What could occasion, after a generation of constant struggle, an increase in AAIP&S membership from about 250 in 1935 to more than 1,600 in 1945, and steady, continuing gains of comparable size in the after years?

The easy answer is the outbreak of World War II in 1939, huge defense production in this country, followed by America's entry into the conflict. No one can quarrel with this conclusion, but to go no further is to ignore many factors of great significance as well as of general interest.

Beyond question, industrial management at large acquired a new viewpoint toward plant medical departments during the prewar and war periods. The events of those years laid at the doorstep of industry a great many problems other than those having to do with the technical aspects of production. In their dealings with manufacturers holding government contracts, federal agencies made it clear that maximum production meant far more than any previous maximum, up to and including goals thitherto considered impossible of attainment.

A corollary of that demand was the necessity for conserving manpower to the utmost. Every available worker must be fitted to some sort of job, or jobs be adapted to the capacities of available workers. That process, in turn, called for physical examinations on an unprecedented scale, detailed medical records, therapy wherever indicated, and careful consideration of the abilities of job applicants with relation to the work to be done.

Much of this was unfamiliar ground to the rank and file of manufacturers, particularly among the smaller companies. Suddenly, physical and mental health had become recognized as the key to urgently needed industrial production. At every turn, facts rose to confront employers with the realization that adequate medical services were not only desirable but absolutely necessary under the conditions prevailing.

Management officials were deeply impressed by a monumental survey made by the Committee on Healthful Working Conditions of the National Association of Manufacturers, industry's own official organization. The study, which covered 2,064 plants employing 1.9 million workers, disclosed an enormous amount of statistical data on the frequency of accidents and occupational disease, labor turnover, and man-hour losses. This was language which American business understood and heeded.[3]

Guiding the NAM committee in technical matters was an advisory committee of industrial physicians and hygienists, a group in which the interests of the AAIP&S were fully represented. And the association, through many other channels, helped spread the gospel of "industrial health for industrial production."

Addressing the new Western Association of Industrial Physicians & Surgeons as its first president, in May 1941, Robert T. Legge quoted a statement by Victor G. Heiser (a leading figure in the NAM survey): "The apparent inexhaustibility of the German war machine is due particularly to the carefully planned industrial health program of the Nazis."[4]

As for the economic aspects of the NAM study, *Industrial Medicine* commented in its October, 1941, issue: "The exhibit of a balance sheet showing, on the basis of actual figures from operating concerns, that a health program saves the average five-hundred-employee plant $5,611 net per year is indeed stimulating. In fact, this amount includes much more than the bare profit element; it incorporates a substantial conservation of material and manpower."

Clarence Selby's governmental advisory Subcommittee on Industrial Health and Medicine pounded away without respite on the need for a new approach to the entire question of plant medical services. In a report to the Board of Directors of the AAIP&S at its annual meeting May 5, 1941, in Pittsburgh, Selby asserted that the bottleneck of the whole defense program was the participation of physicians who should serve in the small industries engaged in production for national defense.

To further this end, he said, the AMA Council on Industrial Health was co-operating with the committee by contacting and registering physicians for industrial duty. The Selby committee also kept teams of two, an industrial physician and a hygienist, constantly on tour to visit war production plants and survey each situation. And it was ready with a complete program of procedures for organizing and operating medical departments in line with approved standards.

Potent among industrial surveys then were those dealing with the causes and effects of absenteeism. Employers looked at data compiled by General Motors and other large corporations and did not like the figures. Such waste of manpower and man-hours was compatible neither with the wartime conservation policy nor with good business practice.

The net result of this kind of health crusade and this brand of business logic was a steadily growing interest, on the part of employers, in the human side of management-labor relations. More and more corporations heads came to realize not only that keeping workers well and on the job was a desirable social end in itself but also that it actually paid dividends in quality and volume of production.

In the national emergency, it was not exceptional for forward-looking employers to call in their medical directors and tell them, in effect: "Don't ask us what we want you to do. Tell us what you think ought to be done." Such a receptive attitude was, of course, warmly welcomed by the profession.

Among the older members of the AAIP&S there were many who had pioneered in reconstruction and rehabilitation work during and after World War I. The concepts of placement and periodic physical examinations and the complete recording of histories had been, as we know, dominant among association policies for a generation. In the broad-scale programming of modern industrial medical services all members, young and old, saw the possible fruition of long-range plans which were the heart and soul of the association's mission in American life.

Almost the first words spoken to the membership by T. Lyle Hazlett, as incoming president at the Pittsburgh meeting in 1941, were these: "I feel that there has never been a time when this association has had a responsibility such as it has now, and I think we should accept that responsibility. We have a responsibility in guiding medical practices, and with all these new plants and this new wave of production, there is a tremendous amount of guidance that we can do this year." But the association was busy stepping up the tempo of current enterprises and activating other agreed-upon policies. By the summer of 1941 a dozen new committees were functioning, at least half of them directly connected with some phase of the emergency program.

At the first directors' meeting (Chicago, January 12, 1942) after America's declaration of war Daniel Lynch, as chairman of the Committee on National Defense, reported to the Board that in the course of his committee's survey of wartime health problems he was developing a pattern of civilian defense procedures for large industries and that Charles-Francis Long had developed a similar plan for small plants.

This committee was chiefly concerned with equipment and procedures for first aid squads in event of enemy air attack or similar catastrophes. There were medical problems to be ironed out and differences to be settled between manuals published by the United States Bureau of Mines and by the Red Cross as guides in dealing with such matters as shock, hemorrhage, artificial respiration and transportation of the injured.

These matters again came up at a meeting three months later (Cincinnati, April 15), when Royd R. Sayers was a guest of the Board and President Hazlett called upon him to speak. Sayers pointed out that in his sixteen years as chief surgeon of the United States Bureau of Mines his department had done a great deal of work on all types of first aid and that Shoudy and other AAIP&S members had played an important part in the preparation of manuals and would be needed again in the current emergency. The Bureau, he said, had trained more than a million people in the mining industry in first aid, among them some 14,000 certified instructors, who were being used by the Office of Civilian Defense. As for first aid manuals, he reported that the Bureau and the Red Cross had agreed that a certificate from either body should be recognized as satisfactory for first aid and air raid work.

At this meeting the Board of Directors received and unanimously approved a significant resolution presented by the Defense Committee. As dispatched to Dr. Frank H. Lahey, chairman of the government Procurement and Assignment Service, it read in part:

Whereas—This nation is now engaged in war to preserve its existence as a free nation; and

318

Whereas—The President of the United States has said that "this war will be won by industrial production"; and

Whereas—The deflection into the armed forces of physicians and surgeons trained and experienced in protecting and maintaining the health of these workers will jeopardize all-out production: Be it

Resolved that this association bring to your attention the urgent necessity that physicians and surgeons engaged in essential war industry be deferred as long as possible from active military service because their greatest contribution to the success of the war will be in their continued efforts to protect the health of the workers in industry.

Just how this communication was received in Washington is not recorded, but apparently little was done to ease the situation, for soon afterward industrial medicine found itself facing a critical manpower shortage of its own. Again the feasibility of seeking some governmental relief in the interests of industrial health was thoroughly debated at a long and important meeting of the AAIP&S Board of Directors, at Chicago.

The date was October 29, 1942, about six months after John J. Wittmer (New York Edison Company) had taken over the presidency of the association from T. Lyle Hazlett. A graduate of Long Island College of Medicine and an outstanding physician and administrator, Wittmer served the AAIP&S zealously in many capacities over the years. Although seriously ill at the time of the Chicago meeting he made the trip, but collapsed in his hotel room and was forced to return home.

In consequence, chairmanship of the Board meeting was divided between President-elect Harvey Bartle and Vice-President Frederick W. Slobe. It was the latter who introduced the question of deferment for certain key physicians in industry. He said:

It is our duty to try to clarify that situation at this time so that some immediate action can be taken.

The doctors are torn between two fires, one of patriotism, which would indicate that everyone should go into the armed forces irrespective of affiliations, and that would apply to many of us here. At the same time, we all know that one of the big keynotes in the last few years is industrial health and efficiency, conservation of manpower. But we haven't done much about the conservation of the physician who is responsible for this.

He went on to cite United States Procurement Service rulings on "essential" and "nonessential" classifications, stating his belief that they needed clarification with respect to men serving small industries.

We all know how much small industry needs, and how backward it has been so far as industrial management is concerned. Small industry is going to be hit very much harder by an indiscriminate program of taking all physicians into the army than the large groups that are so much better organized. . . .

I think definitely that when a group of physicians band together and service a

319

large number of small plants, they are entitled to the same consideration as one individual who occupies a key position in one large plant. At the present time procurement branches do not consider them in the same category.

Frank T. McCormick, of Detroit, a Board member, spoke strongly against what he considered the "shortsighted" policy of taking doctors away from industry without regard to industrial health needs. "In Detroit," he said, "we have been hit very hard right along the line of small industries."

On the heels of McCormick's protest, several other speakers rose to corroborate his testimony, citing the plight of specific doctors, serving groups of small plants, whose offices had been stripped of professional personnel by procurement boards made up of men with neither experience nor interest in the industrial aspects of medicine.

Alfred H. Whittaker, of Detroit, strongly urged action by the association to resolve "an acute problem" resulting from the existing policies. Said Dr. Whittaker:

> I discussed this with the procurement man in Wayne County, and he said he was sorry, but he felt that the men in industry were high class first aid men and there was no reason why they should be deferred.
>
> Three weeks ago we had a meeting with the procurement officers and doctors representing the larger plants in Wayne County. Prendergast and Selby and the industrial committee of our county medical society were there. I was astonished at the attitude of the procurement officers.
>
> They were frank to state that the only thing of importance at the present time was the war. They said that for every thousand men going into the service, six doctors would be taken in; and, while they felt sorry the public would be neglected, they would go in regardless of what happened.
>
> Yesterday in Congress, the Senate woke up to the fact that an acute situation in this country has developed, and they are appointing a lay committee to take this out of the hands of the military as far as possible. I believe now is the opportune time for this society (and we should work with the American Medical Association) to contact our senators and say we are 100 percent behind them to have this put through Congress so it will be better handled.
>
> Everybody gets excited and wants to do something for the army, but they must sacrifice their desires and stay where they are if they are in a key position in industry.

On this note the Board meeting ended—with the passage of a motion authorizing dispatch of an appropriate letter to the Procurement and Assignment Service in Washington and a copy or similar letter to the Senate committee and state procurement chairman.

Lynch's casual reading habits were responsible for the appointment of another important emergency committee in 1941. At the directors' meeting in Pittsburgh, May 5 of that year, he reported as outgoing president that he had read "in some magazine" that there was a great deal of eye injury in industry, that employers were responsible for it, and that they were not doing all that could be done to control it. He had forthwith contacted the National Society for the Prevention of Blindness. As a result of correspondence an AAIP&S Committee on Prevention of Blindness was appointed to serve in an advisory capacity to combat the hazard.

At the next annual directors' meeting (Cincinnati, April 13, 1942) this committee, consisting of John J. Wittmer (chairman), N. E. Eckleberry (Consolidated Edison Company, New York), and Harry Spaulding (New York), reported that monthly meetings had been held throughout the year with the corresponding committee of the Society for Prevention of Blindness. An illustrated manual and primer had been prepared for national distribution through employers. The committee was also working closely with national health and safety organizations to extend among plant employees everywhere a dramatic educational program for the protection of industrial eyesight.

Because expanded production inevitably called for maximum working hours, employers immediately wanted to know how many hours men could work efficiently and safely. Obviously, that question could not be answered in generalities, or by averaging statistics, since the effects of long hours would vary widely in different trades and different types of industry. The problem was complex, particularly in view of the large number of women seeking factory employment.

To help arrive at usable standards, the AAIP&S established a Committee on Fatigue, consisting of J. M. Carlisle (Merck & Company) as chairman, M. H. Heilman, and Mack M. Shafer, which had at its disposal a large amount of data from fatigue studies made by association members and was empowered to collaborate with university fatigue laboratories in their investigations.

At the April 13, 1942, directors' meeting Carlisle reported satisfactory progress in the work of this committee but warned the Board that widespread publicity for the findings would be impossible because the project was largely under control of the National Research Council, which opposed release of the information for security reasons.

High on the agenda of the Research Council was the question of the dietary needs of workers employed on defense and war projects, and in 1941 the AAIP&S added a Committee on Nutrition to study those needs and collaborate with government agencies to see that they were met. At the Cincinnati Board meeting in April 1942, this committee, consisting of William A. Sawyer (chairman), A. G. Kammer (Carbide & Carbon Chemicals Company) and H. H. Fellows (Metropolitan Life Insurance Company), reported the start of a nationwide educational campaign utilizing printed matter produced by the council. Thus another link was forged in the chain of information made available through industrial medical directors for the guidance of employers and plant workers.

At the annual directors' meeting in Rochester, N.Y., in May 1943, Chairman Sawyer reported that the work was going ahead smoothly under direction of a Nutrition Committee of the National Research Council, with which his own committee was cooperating. Since Sawyer was also a member of that committee he was able to maintain close liaison with the NRC, which was supplying the funds.

This problem of nutrition became increasingly important as the war went on, and association members were called upon to give close personal attention to the educational program. Frederick W. Slobe, incoming president of the AAIP&S in 1944, stressed this responsibility at the annual directors' meeting in St. Louis (May 10), when he urged that "medical departments emphasize problems of in-plant feeding to the point of supervising them, if necessary, for adequacy of diets."

War, with its multiple dislocations of normal living and readjustments to constant crises, brought in its wake (as we have seen) a rash of new behavior and personality problems in industry. Large-scale psychotherapy among large numbers of factory workers was impossible. The situation, however, demanded immediate study, and the AAIP&S in 1941 appointed a Psychiatry Committee to recommend a course of action.

After months of investigation and discussion, its chairman, Loyal Shoudy, at the April 1942, meeting asked and received permission of the Board of Directors to mail the following letter to every member of the association:

> It is with reluctance that I add to the already heavy burden of the industrial physician. However, the stringency of war conditions makes it imperative that I bring to your attention the work our committee is mapping in the field of the highly important industrial psychiatry.
>
> While the time is short, we are making every effort to avoid the "too little and too late" fault in a branch of medicine which has proved itself so highly effective under war conditions abroad.
>
> Therefore, doctor, this preliminary appeal is being made to you with the conviction that whatever program can be evolved should, in the final analysis, be administered or supervised by you or your colleagues.

There followed a detailed quotation from Clarence Selby's report on the handling of employees' personal problems, submitted to the National Research Council in the preceding year. In that report Selby's advisory committee outlined ways in which plant medical directors could help disturbed or poorly adjusted employees, but made it perfectly clear that there was to be no encroachment on the private practice of medicine.

The association's Psychiatry Committee was soon renamed the Committee on Psychosomatic Medicine and carried on its work, intermittently, into the 1950's, with E. A. Irvin and then John L. Norris following Shoudy as chairmen. Among the committee members, at various times, were Clarence Selby, Cassius Watson, Harvey Bartle and C. F. N. Schram, as well as neuropsychiatrists Lydia Giberson (Metropolitan Life Insurance Company) and L. E. Himler and G. A. Eadie (both associated with General Motors).

"Medicine of the mind" has, of course, grown phenomenally in latter years, and research steadily extends its frontiers. In the same period personality and behavior problems, the individual and family worries of workers, have demanded more and more attention from industrial medical departments. As a result, we find medical directors increasingly concerned with human relations, helping confused or maladjusted workers to the extent that simple psychology can be effective and recommending special treatment where it is indicated. Here, at least, is a constructive approach to a problem that is still far from final solution.

We cite these samples of AAIP&S committee activities because they indicate in a general way the extent and variety of extra duties laid upon industrial physicians in the early 1940's. The time-consuming nature of these special projects, the thoroughness and the seriousness with which they were discussed, the amount of aid they contributed to the war effort come to light only by painstaking study of the minutes of directors' meetings. Little or nothing of the give-and-take of those sessions, often dragging on through the day and deep into the night, has been recorded anywhere else.

Yet most of this emergency work had only an indirect bearing on the industrial doctor's chief responsibility, the treatment and control of occupational sickness and injury. Far weightier than the extracurricular duties stemming from the manpower crisis was the burden imposed by the new technology that sparked what we may call the "Chem-Electric Era" in American industry.

New metals and alloys, chemicals, and compounds pouring into industry have made possible spectacular advances in production, but they have also posed many grave health problems. Upon the medical director, with the hygienist and engineer, has devolved the task of determining the hazards inherent in these new processes and taking measures for their control.[5] And it goes without saying that vigilance in the matter of older health hazards can never be relaxed.

Of equal importance is the fact that science, while revolutionizing the techniques of manufacture, has been likewise diligent in improving the weapons, equipment, and procedures of medicine and surgery. The epoch that first used atomic fission for destruction has made at least some progress in harnessing atomic power for beneficent ends. It has discovered that radium the killer has unguessed potentials as radium the healer. It has developed radioactive isotopes for beneficent purposes.

To the aid of medicine in its curative function, chemistry has brought the antibiotics, penicillin, aureomycin, streptomycin, etc.; the long and well known list of the sulfa drugs; cortisone, ACTH, and other hormones. Physiological research has developed the magic of blood transfusion and shown the way to completely new techniques in shock treatment.[6]

The list goes on and on. There is no end—may never be an end. The advances are not for war but for peacetime, for the future of mankind. And no physician or surgeon, in whatever type of practice, needs to be reminded that he also must, through his medical journals, by discussions at his medical meetings, by clinical experience, keep fully abreast of the progress, always.

Even after Nagasaki and Hiroshima had shocked the world into an uneasy truce, scientific and technological progress continued its swift acceleration. There was no promise or sign that either industry or industrial medicine could look forward to a return of the slower pace and lesser pressures of pre-World-War-II years. On the contrary, many new medical problems were in the making and many new burdens in the building, largely as the result of physiological studies which had been steadily coming to the forefront for a decade or more.

There was the challenge of the old and the aging, the spectacular increase in their numbers, the puzzle of their status in modern society. The word "geriatrics" was coming into the popular vocabulary and with it the need for more knowledge of that sphere of living in which (too often) the feared Four Horsemen are loneliness, poverty, age, and pain.

Noise was demanding more and more attention not only in industry, but from public health agencies seriously disturbed by its potential shattering effects on human bodies and minds.

With manhours and production under constant analysis, problem-drinking became of increasing concern to employers, and hence to the industrial medical profession.

Since industry was at least in part responsible for destructive, sometimes deadly, smog, industrial medicine was called upon for help in its possible control.

There was more, and ever more, to be learned and done in the field of atomic medicine. And the frontier of the industrial physician not only was extended to include aviation but moved on—into space.

In the net, the Chem-Electric Era substantially increased the size and prestige of the AAIP&S, magnified its role in society, multiplied its responsibilities, intensified its interdependence with labor and management, and, beyond these, made necessary basic and extensive changes in its organization and procedures.

XXVII

THE ASSOCIATION RAISES
ITS SIGHTS

Even in the early 1940's it became apparent that the American Association of Industrial Physicians & Surgeons was about to reach one of its long-sought goals, a membership large enough to assure a reasonable degree of stability and security, along with the quality upon which its leaders had always insisted. Steady growth, past the first 1,000 and beyond the 1,500 mark, gave the association a very satisfactory ranking in the matter of size, at least among national organizations representing highly selective professional specialties. And as for personal qualifications, the caliber of new applicants left little or nothing to be desired.

With medical services and facilities expanding rapidly under the urge of the emergency, the industrial field beckoned to a larger number of able, enterprising young physicians and surgeons than ever before in history. But for one important safeguard, membership might well have set a runaway pace, to the detriment of the association. Bylaws, however, imposed upon applicants exacting requirements as to their experience in the industrial field and the percentage of their total practice devoted to the specialty. These provisions, while they barred many fine doctors, placed a proper premium upon experience in handling industrial health problems.

It is worthy of note that through this trying period of growth and readjustment the AAIP&S remained the "friendly association" of older and even more trying times. Perhaps because of the close community of aims and interests among members, perhaps by a process of natural selection, like has always attracted like to this association. And it is seldom, even at the present writing, that the prized tradition of friendliness throughout its ranks is not referred to at annual meetings by one speaker or another.

Members of the AAIP&S, flocking to New York for the twenty-fifth anniversary meeting in June 1940, came prepared for momentous happenings. Because of the war threat and swift expansion of the defense program, interest in this convention ran high. It has been called the "first big meeting" of the association, and the program justified the description. Presence of the industrial hygienists, holding their first joint sessions with the physicians and surgeons, not only swelled the total attendance but added tremendously to the amount of work involved.

Even before the convention was called to order it was clear to the officers and Board of Directors that 1940, for them, was to be a year of decision. The growing complexity of association affairs, plus continued emergency demands upon personnel, made it evident that the situation called for revision of administrative procedures from top to foundation. No longer was it possible for a handful of officers and directors personally to study all problems, adjudicate all issues, make all decisions. Operation on a broader base and a larger scale was required if the association was to fill its projected role.

The 1940 meeting of the Board ushered in a period of years in which there appeared to be no end to the business demanding deliberation and action and in which entire week ends devoted to day and evening sessions became a common-place—as fat typewritten records of minutes attest.

Quite by chance, at the very opening of the 1940 Board meeting, Cassius Watson and Loyal Shoudy dropped in and, as founding members of the association, were asked to speak. Watson indicated his awareness (probably shared by the others present) that the organization was entering a new and radically different era. Contrasting the simplicity and informality of an older day with the elaborate planning and programming of the New York convention, he recalled the slimly-attended fifth annual meeting at New Orleans in April, 1920. At that time Harry E. Mock was president, F. D. Patterson (Pennsylvania Health Insurance Commission) was secretary, and Shoudy was chairman of the Publicity Committee. As Watson explained it:

> The first section of the meeting was held in the old Cafe Louisianne. As we went up to the hotel, we found nobody had arranged any particular meeting place. So Patterson, Harry Mock and myself scurried around and got some chairs and put them in front of a table, at which he presided in a very dignified fashion.[1]
>
> Those early meetings were very delightful. As these things grow (and there is evidence of developing a still greater number), older members may be somewhat overcome by the magnitude of the projects they originate. I think both Shoudy and I are glad we are not going to be presidents conducting this organization through the devious paths of the years to come. . . .
>
> In the early days we tried to have organized medicine recognize us, and they were rather scornful in their statement that there was no such thing. We then agreed with them that industrial medicine was nothing more or less than good medicine applied to industry. Now the time has come when the American Medical Associa-

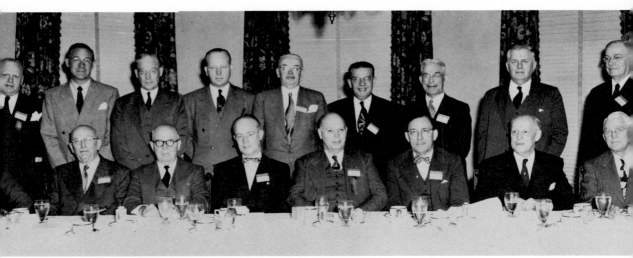

96. *Past Presidents Luncheon, Detroit, 1949.* Left to right, seated: Harry E. Mock (1918–20), Otto P. Geier (1920–21), Loyal A. Shoudy (1923–25, 1946–47), William A. Sawyer (1926–27), Edward C. Holmblad (1934–35), Floyd E. Shaffer (1935–36), Royd R. Sayers (1937–38), Clarence D. Selby (1938–39); standing: Alfred H. Whittaker (1949–50), Frederick W. Slobe (1944–45), Henry S. Brown (1947–48), Melvin N. Newquist (1945–46), T. Lyle Hazlett (1941–42), Harold A. Vonachan (1948–49), Daniel L. Lynch (1940–41), McIver Woody (1939–40), Harvey Bartle (1943–44).

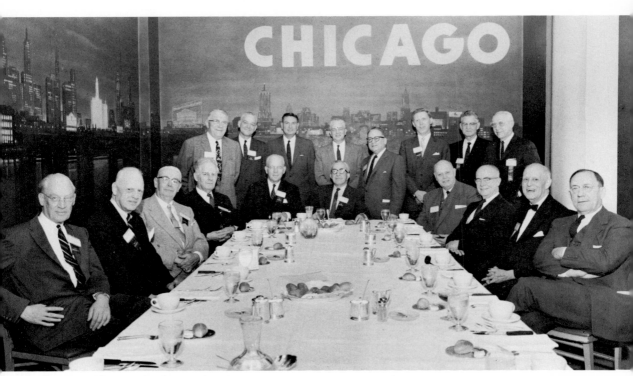

97. *Past Presidents Luncheon, 1959.* Seventeen IMA past presidents were the guests of Hans Lawrence (seated at head of table) at this 1959 luncheon in Chicago.

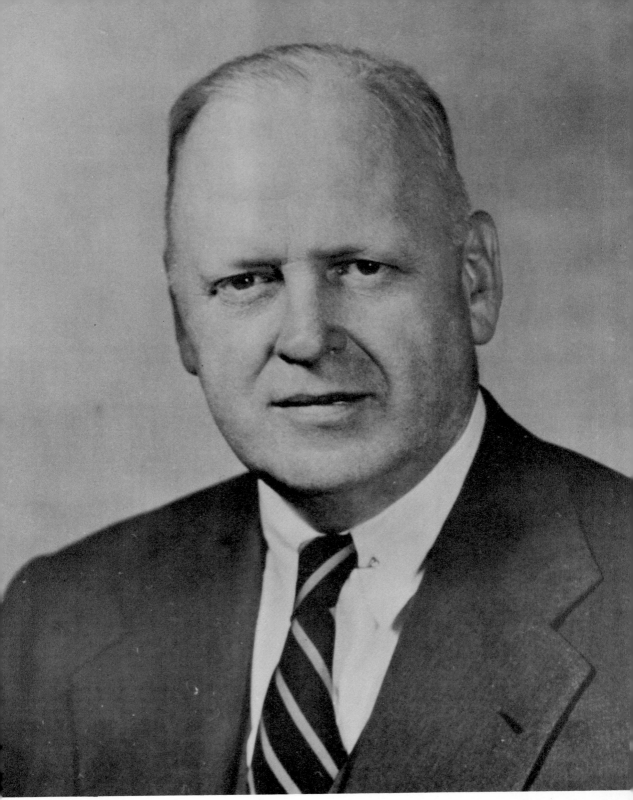

98. *Alfred H. Whittaker, M.D. (1894–   ).*
President, AAIP&S, 1949–50. In a career started
during World War I, Whittaker has had three
consuming interests: surgery (particularly the
surgery of trauma), occupational medicine and
surgery as a specialty, and the history of medicine.
As president he pursued broad policies aimed at
improving medical services and increasing the
prestige of the association—in the period of its
sudden growth. Whittaker's activities in the
AAIP&S date far back and have continued through
the 1950's. He has written extensively on historical
and clinical subjects and has been continuously
active in civic organizations.

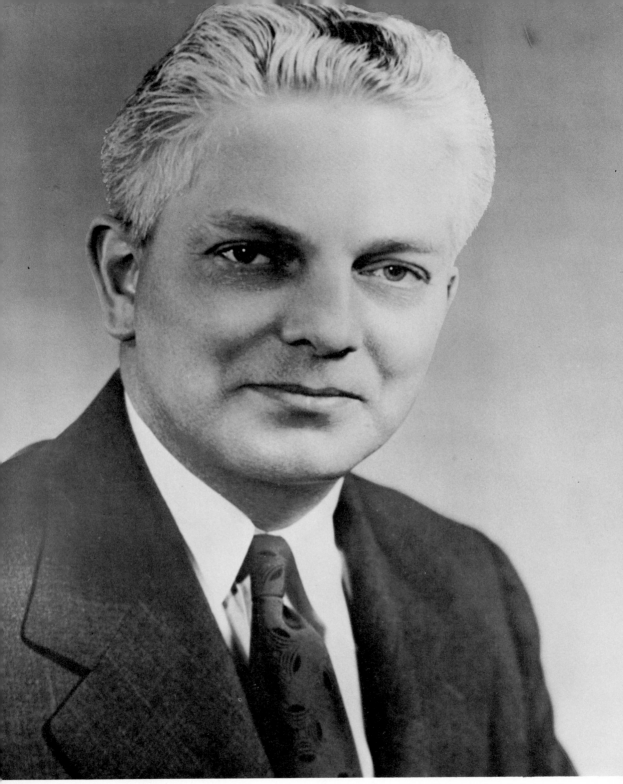

99. *Edward H. Carleton, M.D. (1904–   ).*
President, AAIP&S, 1950–1951. A medical graduate of the University of Louisville (1932), Carleton
joined the Inland Steel Company in 1937 and became general medical director in 1953. As president he saw the need for a still larger and more
active membership as a means of improving the
status of industrial medicine. His administration
strengthened the district counselor group to stimulate local activities; started reorganization of the
(now) Occupational Health Institute to facilitate
fund-raising for scholarships. To Carleton, in April
1951, fell the honor of announcing the change of
name to the Industrial Medical Association.

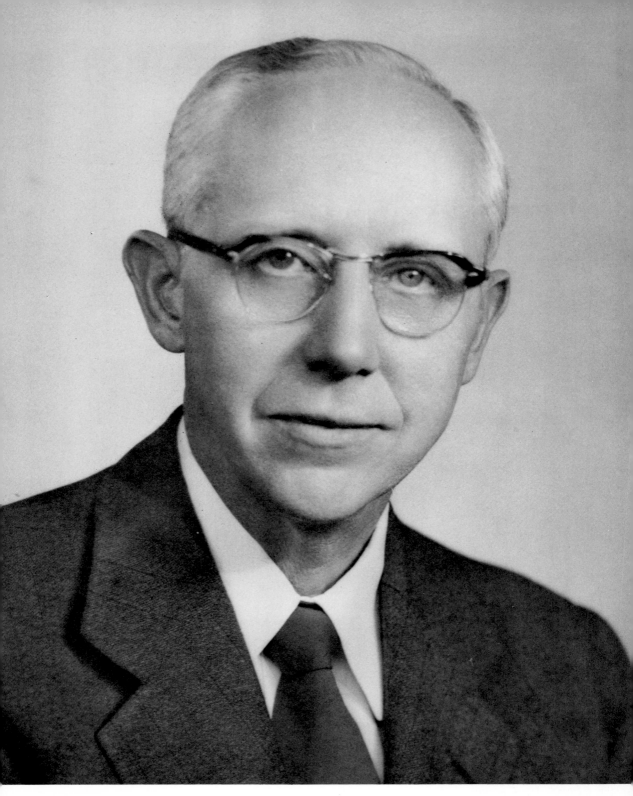

100. *Adolph G. Kammer, M.D.* (1903–   ).
President, IMA, 1951–1952. Kammer brought to
the presidency a background made to order for a
period of great expansion. He had been chairman
of the IMA Committee on Education and Training and a member of the Atomic Energy Commission Committee on Industrial Medicine. He was a
medical professor at the University of Pittsburgh
and a fluent writer and skilled administrator. His
policies aimed at the delegation of responsibility
to junior officers, development of strong executives, and the transfer of the program of medical
department evaluation to the IMA. He is now
editor of the new *IMA Journal of Occupational
Medicine.*

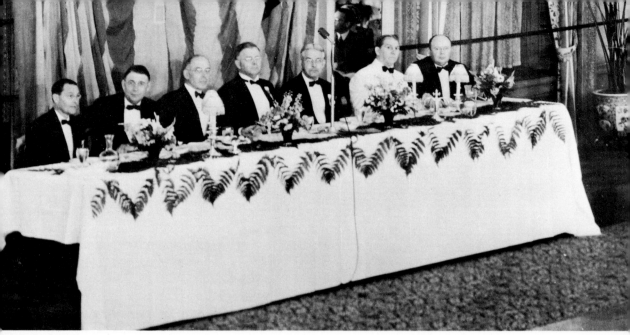

101. Speakers Table, 1940.

AAIP&S Annual Banquets. The growth of the AAIP&S is reflected in the difference between the seven at the speakers table in 1940 and the thirty-six at the table in 1950.

102. Speakers Table, 1950.

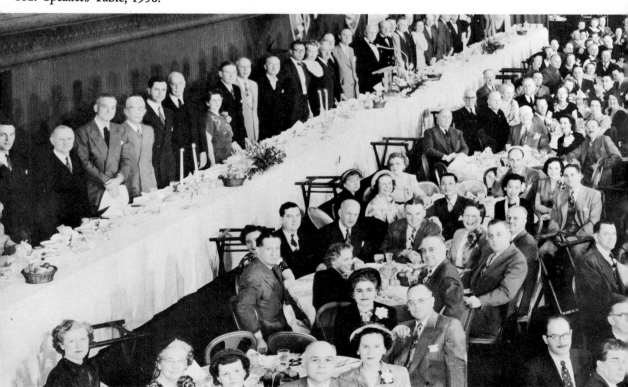

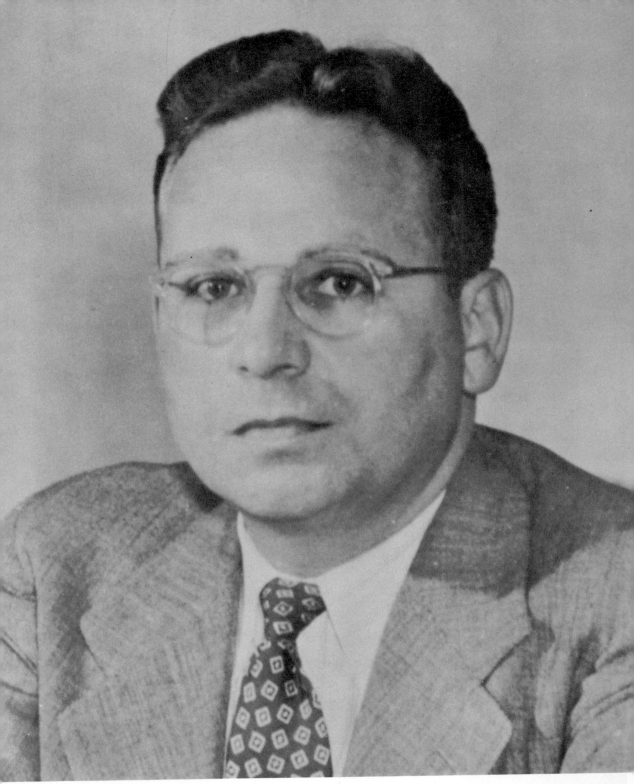

103. *Earle A. Irvin, M.D. (1908–). President, IMA, 1952–1953.* Irvin made his first industrial connection in 1934, a year after graduation from the University of Michigan Medical School, and just twenty years later he became medical director of the Ford Motor Company. He is known as a tireless worker for things he be-

lieves in and, on occasion, as a tough opponent. He championed the IMA name change and, as president, he fought for certification, campaigned for members, and sought closer working relations with medical schools. He developed for Ford a model medical record system.

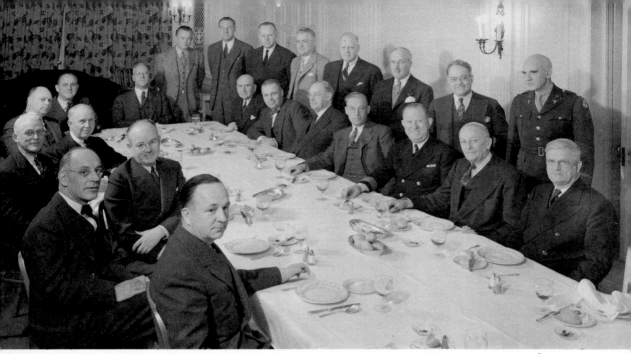

104. *AMA Council of Industrial Health, Chicago, February 12, 1945.* Progress was made toward AMA Board status for occupational medicine at this meeting, at which officers and directors of the AAIP&S were dinner guests of the Council on Industrial Health. Left to right; seated: S. G. Seeger, L. U. Gardner, W. A. Sawyer, C. D. Selby, L. A. Shoudy, E. C. Holmblad, C. M. Peterson, A. J. Lanza, Henry Sensenick, R. F. Kurz, Harvey Bartle, Henry S. Brown, Henry J. Kessler, O. P. Geier, Don B. Low; standing: F. E. Poole, F. W. Slobe, M. N. Newquist, R. P. Bell, A. H. Whittaker, E. P. Heller, C. O. Sappington, Col. Raymond Hussey.

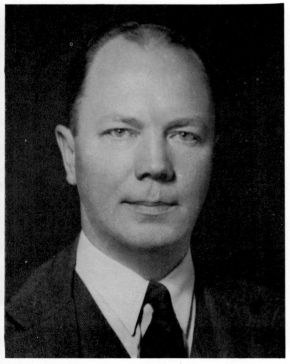

105. *Melville H. Manson, M.D.* A career man in Bell Telephone enterprises; medical director and advisor of A. T. & T. since 1943; member of AAIP&S Board of Directors, 1946–1948, a valued contributor to medical literature.

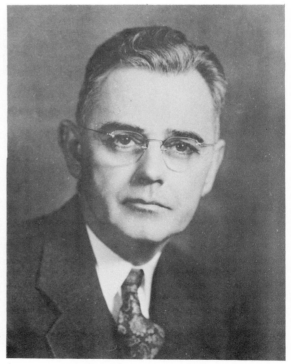

106. *George H. Gehrmann, M.D.* His long career as medical director of E. I. Du Pont was interrupted by active service in the British Army, 1917–1918. His scientific investigations were invaluable to the AAIP&S during the transition into the chemical age in industry.

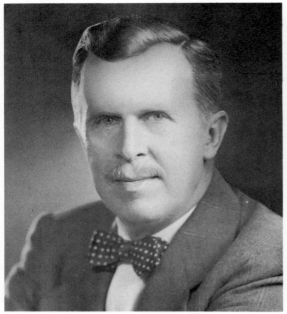

107. *James H. Sterner, M.D.* An authority on nutrition and toxic reaction, he was appointed in 1946 to the interim medical advisory board of the Atomic Energy Commission. He has served on many important AAIP&S and IMA committees and on the Board of Directors, 1949–1952.

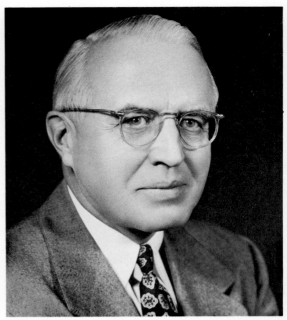

108. *Max R. Burnell, M.D.* Organized the medical department of the AC Spark Plug Division of General Motors at Flint, Michigan, in 1931 and served as its director for many years. The department won national praise for its model system of placement for World War II veterans. Burnell was appointed medical consultant of General Motors in 1949, served as a director of the IMA, 1950–1952.

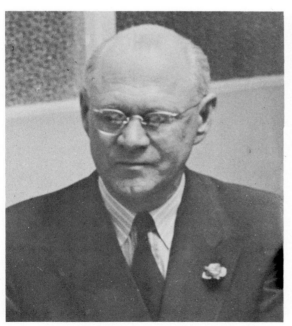

109. *Russell G. Birrell, M.D.* A graduate of University of Toronto Medical College, Birrell joined the staff of Standard Oil (New Jersey) in 1929. After many years as physician-at-large, he became medical director of Imperial Oil Ltd., Toronto. As a Director and district counselor, he has done much to stimulate Canadian interest in the IMA.

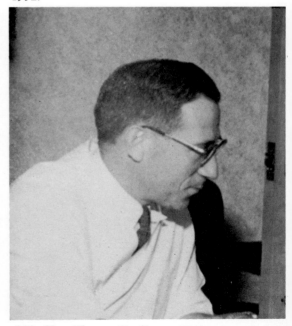

110. *H. Glenn Gardiner, M.D.* Served the AAIP&S for many years in many ways, during an industrial career that started in 1936 and has led him, successively, to posts as medical director of Foote Brothers, Sears, Roebuck & Company, and Inland Steel Company. In 1954 he started four years of service as secretary of the IMA.

tion recognizes this field of industrial endeavor and wants to have a going concern in its own fold.

Continuing, he commented briefly on the problem of affiliation with other branches of organized medicine and mentioned the possibility of "some kind of integration" with the AMA. "But, that," he said, "remains for the members of this organization as they come one by one, year by year. I don't believe we humble members who have now grown old and are about to be placed on the emeritus list should do this. We want to see the younger group going ahead."

This incident, in bald narration, appears trivial. Actually, however, it was a keynote for far more serious discussions later on, in which the status of old-time leaders, and the amount of official responsibility they should be asked to assume in administering the active affairs of the association, was to become a debated issue.

The first big step in the reorganization (and modernization) of the AAIP&S came in the spring of 1941, with the creation of an entirely new post in the association, that of managing director. Available records do not indicate that the precise duties and responsibilities of the office were ever stipulated. There was no doubt, however, as to the qualifications of the occupant, Edward C. Holmblad, who had served the association as a vice-president, a president, a director for several terms, and a member of important committees.

Holmblad was elected managing director at the Pittsburgh meeting (May 1941) in which Hazlett took over the presidency, heading a ticket that included Wittmer as president elect, Prendergast and Bartle as first and second vice-presidents, respectively, and Cheney as treasurer.

There proved to be no difficulty in accumulating work of the type and importance implied by Holmblad's new title. The managing directorship was a magnet for tasks, large and small, that needed doing. Appointed first as a part-time staff member, the doctor changed to a full-time basis in 1945. And he has continued, year after year, to discharge the exacting duties that have accrued to the office, with a success which might not have been possible for an incumbent less mindful of the manners and uses of authority.

Increased membership, of itself, brought about some improvement in the financial condition of the association. At least the wolf at the door retreated to a safer distance, much to the gratification of old members who had fought deficit financing for a generation. But at the same time, growth created new problems that demanded money as well as time and attention.

For one thing, the simple bookkeeping that sufficed in earlier times, when the association was small and cash assets were perennially close to the vanishing point, would not do for a large and rapidly growing organization whose activities were expanding in every direction. At the 1941 meeting the directors examined the balance sheet of the previous year and decided that the organization needed strict budgetary control, along with more detailed accounting records and a professional system of auditing.

After a long discussion of detailed procedures, the Board referred the entire problem to the Finance Committee for study and recommendations. Action was prompt. At the meeting of directors in October, Chairman Slobe reported that the accounting system had been completely overhauled by an outside firm, the books placed on an accrual basis, and adequate controls set up to meet all foreseeable needs.

These desirable reforms, however, merely provided proper checks on outgo; they did nothing to build up organization income. And more revenue was needed, to carry increased overhead, pay for new services, finance surveys and other professional projects. To be sure, the association's current needs were modest, but so were the budgets of that time, and increased expenditures had to be matched by increased receipts.

One example of higher costs was furnished by the rental (at long last) of headquarters for its exclusive use, at 28 East Jackson Boulevard, Chicago. The AAIP&S moved into these quarters February 1, 1941. Equipment—some furniture and a rented typewriter! Personnel—a permanent stenographer and the managing director! The same quarters, with adequate equipment and a larger staff, are still the home address of the Industrial Medical Association.

In their study of the association's financial affairs, officers and directors were attracted by the potential value of technical exhibits at the annual meetings. Little attention had been paid to this field until the late thirties. About twenty-five suppliers to industrial medicine had displayed their equipment and service at the 1938 meeting, and a few more had been added in the following four years. With the upsurge of technical and product development, interest in commercial exhibits of this type became widespread, and in the fall of 1942 the association contracted with Stephen G. Halos (then advertising manager of *Industrial Medicine*) to promote and sell display space.

It was apparent that exhibits could serve several highly worthwhile ends, providing a productive advertising medium for suppliers to the profession, keeping physician abreast of the latest developments in this field, and producing much needed income for the association itself. Subsequent events are described in greater detail elsewhere in this volume.[2]

While plans for expansion were still in a preliminary stage, the officers and directors found themselves facing a most peculiar predicament, brought to light by the sudden discovery that, as the result of a series of commonplace legal maneuvers, the AAIP&S was no longer a corporation under Illinois law. The story, as spread on the records at a Board meeting in October 1942, brought out the fact that when federal Social Security legislation became effective (January 1, 1937), the government required from employers such financial information as was necessary for administration of the law. The Illinois legislature, as a matter of routine, enacted a statute calling for the filing of annual reports and payment of a nominal fee. The strange factor in the incident is that thousands of corporations in the state—either unaware that such a law was on the books, or misinterpreting its provisions—filed no reports. Among them was the AAIP&S. There was no particular blame attached to this delinquency, but the state courts in due course dissolved the corporations for noncompliance, thus depriving the association of the benefits of corporate organization.

The AAIP&S chose the simplest and most direct way out of this dilemma. On May 2, 1942, an application for reincorporation was filed with the Illinois secretary of state, and five days later the association was again certified as a nonprofit corporation. In due time its status under Social Security regulations was cleared up, and it also became eligible for certain income tax exemptions. The reincorporators signing the application were Holmblad, Slobe and Sappington, chosen because all were in Cook County, and it was convenient to have their signatures notarized at the same time and forwarded with the necessary papers.

There was, however, a considerable amount of other red tape to be cut, and at the October meeting the Board patiently went through the business of transferring the assets and liabilities of the unincorporated association to the new corporation, reelecting the officers, reenacting the bylaws, and passing sundry other required resolutions. The lapse in corporate existence had affected the validity of activities carried on in the interim period, for the organization automatically functioned as an unincorporated association, much like a partnership in status. The directors, however, could breathe easier after reincorporation, since it relieved them of the personal liabilities inherent in partnerships. Thus was an abiding lesson in jurisprudence etched upon the ledger of experience of the AAIP&S.

Among the new members who came into the association on the rising tide of the post-depression period were many men of exceptional attainments and capabilities, men who had become immediately active in association affairs and were plainly marked for leadership. Though they could be expected to conform, on the whole, where long-term objectives were concerned, they were destined to shape the organization of the future rather than to be shaped by it.

No one was more sensitive to the emergence of these new personalities, and to their likely impact upon the association, than the handful of old-time members who had devoted their entire professional careers to the upgrading of industrial medicine and the battle for its recognition. They realized that big changes were on the way, that these denoted progress and should be not only accepted but also promoted by the older generation.

This line of thinking came out into the open at the annual business meeting in Cincinnati, April 15, 1942. Daniel L. Lynch, with the full approval of the outgoing president, Lyle Hazlett, asked the Board of Directors to consider and formally vote upon a question involving the extent to which older members should participate in the executive management of the association. Said Lynch:

> Those of us who have had the honor and privilege of being president of this association have recognized that we were members of the Board before we assumed

office, that we were honored with the presidency for a year; and then we went back as members of the Board for two years, so that we were in office for practically five years, denying the opportunity, probably, for some younger men to come forward in this association. Our bylaws provide that the retiring president shall automatically become a member of the Board of Directors.

Mr. President, may I present a motion to the effect that the bylaws be modified so that the compulsion of making the retiring president a member of the Board be stricken out, and that there be substituted a clause to the effect that the retiring president shall, *ex officio,* be a member of the Board of Directors?

It will thereby afford an opportunity for some new men to come on the Board and to help with the advancement of the welfare of the association.

Though Lynch's idea had been privately discussed at some length, his motion (promptly seconded by Sawyer) provoked a lively debate at the directors' table. The chief dissenter was Loyal Shoudy, who believed the older men wanted to keep on serving and didn't believe they should be barred. "We must work," said he. "A man needn't sit back on his haunches just because he is an ex-president. He has to work a couple more years because you did, and I did, and all the rest."

A majority of the Board sympathized but didn't agree, and Lynch's motion was carried. As events proved, however, this little exchange of pleasantries, and the ensuing vote, were to have interesting consequences. The change in election procedure could not be effected without constitutional authority, and extensive revision of the bylaws happened to be a very live project at the time. Shoudy was to have another chance to keep past presidents busy at useful work for the association.

This rewriting of the bylaws was at best a long and tedious task, not to be hurried. Any change in the method of choosing directors had to wait for other decisions. Nothing more was heard, in fact, about the problem of past presidents until February 1944. Then, in his report at a Board meeting in Chicago, Edward C. Holmblad mentioned a suggestion from several members that "some certificate of acknowledgment of service be issued to presidents on their retirement." President Bartle submitted the idea to the meeting, and the Board promptly authorized him to appoint a special committee "to prepare an adequate certificate." This group, known as the Committee on Past Presidents, turned out to be also a Committee *of* Past Presidents, including Shoudy (chairman), Selby, Wittmer, and Lynch.

Harvey Bartle was again in the chair when the Board next met at the annual meeting in St. Louis, in May, 1944. The Committee on Past Presidents, in the interim, had been working hard on its report and was ready with recommendations that went far beyond the certificate of acknowledgment originally suggested.

Reasoning that little progress was being made with the AMA in the matter of certification for industrial medicine as a specialty, and that this issue was not likely to be settled for several years, the Committee on Past Presidents urged boldly that the AAIP&S take matters into its own hands and watch reactions.

Specifically, the committee proposed that the association award to its ex-presidents a degree of Master of Industrial Medicine and that they serve as the association's own certification board, to be known as the American Board of Industrial Medicine. Beyond this the committee suggested that the past presidents (or masters) comprise an advisory council to the president and that there be formed within the AAIP&S an American College of Industrial Physicians, roughly corresponding to the American College of Surgeons in its field, consisting of masters and fellows of the association.

This unexpected feature, which Shoudy credited largely to Selby, produced mixed reactions from the Board. Most members liked the idea of a bold step in the direction of certification, and no one questioned the fitness of past presidents to serve as examiners for a specialty board. On the other hand there was strong opposition to the idea of conferring master's degrees, which could well be confused with honors and degrees from established universities and medical schools. After considerable debate President Bartle disposed of the question by proposing that it be referred back to the committee with instructions to confer with the Committee on Certification and make further recommendations.

Back again to a directors' meeting in October, 1944, came Chairman Shoudy. None of his committee could be present, but he brought a revised plan which, he said, was based on a suggestion made by the new president, Frederick W. Slobe. The section concerning master's degrees had been completely deleted. The new program provided for organization of a permanent Past Presidents Committee consisting of all former presidents who were still active or honorary members. It specified that they should be invited to attend Board meetings, with the privilege of discussion, but no voting power, and they were empowered to serve as a certification board. There were, said Shoudy, eighteen former presidents then living.

In the absence of his colleagues on the committee, he came armed with written comments, portions of which he read:

From John J. Wittmer: "I think that an organization of past presidents could be the guiding spirit in the whole association and could be in time powerful enough to watch any unusual move that the younger group with any radical tendencies might try to inject into the association. It could act as a sort of inner council to advise the Executive Committee and in a way help the workings of this group."

From Clarence Selby: "I should like to see something more done about certification along the line that we proposed at the last meeting, but I think it can be assumed that this would be a function of the Past Presidents Committee when organized."

From Daniel Lynch: "As far as I can remember, past presidents of the association have always been welcomed at meetings of the Board of Directors, particularly at convention time, and have spoken their minds freely and helpfully. I still feel some unusual and special recognition such as was proposed by our committee at St. Louis is preferable if it is possible. . . .

"As usual, I find myself on the opposite side of any given proposition, for I do not believe it is wise to establish a committee of past presidents to advise with the Board of Directors. The committee is merely a perpetuation of officers in another form, and if I were a director I believe I would feel such advice as might be available to the past presidents could be given to the Board without having a super organization to pass on it."

Present at the meeting, it chanced, was the oldest past president then living— Otto Geier. Asked his opinion of the prosposed committee he stated his belief that it could be very useful and could recreate renewed interest in some of the oldsters who have something to contribute. He did not, however, think any brakes on the younger men were needed; and as an ex-president he expressed some embarrassment "in the matter of our pinning roses on ourselves and making ourselves so particularly useful to the association."

There was little more discussion. Shoudy's report and motion were put to a vote and approved. This action fitted nicely into the schedule of the important Committee on Constitution and By-Laws Revision, whose labors were drawing to a close. If the new laws were to become effective in 1945, a long list of basic changes and refinements had to be agreed upon early in the year.

The committee in charge of this project was representative of the type of new blood that was being infused into the directorate in the forties. Its chairman, Rudolph F. Kurz, was thoroughly experienced in both industrial and aviation medicine. He had served his industrial apprenticeship with the Cincinnati Milling Machine Company (managed by the Geier family), had been a flight surgeon in the Army, and was, in 1945, a medical referee for the Travelers Insurance Company, St. Louis. Robert A. Kehoe, widely known educator, medical director, and consultant in pathology and physiology, had served since 1930 as director of the Kettering Laboratory of Applied Physiology, Cincinnati. B. L. Vosburgh (medical director, General Electric) was distinguished for his special work on toxicology and silicosis.

At a night meeting February 11, 1945, the committee presented its final report to the Board. Revisions were examined and discussed in detail and approved for submission to the association membership. With its acceptance, June 22, 1945, the new document became effective, and, except for minor amendments, has remained intact. Along with other important changes, the Shoudy committee's proposal relating to past presidents became part of the bylaws. Provision was also made that the most recent past president should be a member of the Board, but as an addition to the twelve elected directors and to serve for only one year.

So, and by such a devious route, the Past Presidents Committee of the association came into existence. Shoudy, in the end, had his way, but so did the dissenting Lynch. Retired presidents were given a considerable amount of responsibility and useful work to do, while room was made at the same time for a younger man on the Board each year. By and large, the old guard of the association has shown an understandable reluctance to bow out of aministrative duties, and have shown, over the years, a deference for the rights and opinions of others that has won the respect and affection of their junior associates.

The Past Presidents Committee continued to follow the elder statesman tradition, but it is a matter of record that its original members wasted no time in starting to function as an advisory group. The Board of Directors reconvened early in the afternoon of February 12, 1943, having approved the new bylaws the night before. The past presidents, however, had met even earlier, and Shoudy appeared at the Board meeting with a specific plan demonstrating one type of service they could render. The plan was that the past presidents should personally contact the management of corporations they were serving, discuss with them the long-range policies and plans of the association, and report to the Board industry's reaction to the contemplated plan. The idea, it seemed, was feasible and constructive, and the Board formally accepted it with due appreciation.

This story has been told at some length because it illustrates a way of working that has remained characteristic of the association, a probing patiently to the heart of a problem, a reduction of it, bit by bit, to simplest terms before passing judgment. Association leaders have consistently clung to original principles, but they have readily voted for change when its benefits could be demonstrated. And because the association has so seldom acted in haste, it has had to do remarkably little repenting at leisure.

During the early part of 1942 the association had gone along steadily with its internal reorganization plans. Extra work imposed by prosecution of the war was spread to the best advantage among special committees. The piecemeal task of rewriting the By-Laws went on and on. Volney S. Cheney, who had wished for a year or more to retire, finally made his resignation as treasurer effective in January 1942. "I haven't time to do all the supervisory work that should be done," he told the Board. "Another thing—I'm getting old." A testimonial of appreciation was voted and was ready for presentation at the next meeting in April. Illness kept Cheney away, and the plaque was formally awarded *in absentia*. The headquarters office had already taken over his secretarial duties (in 1941), and Edward Holmblad now added the treasurership to his other responsibilities.

Cheney, at the time, was sixty-eight years old, and his period of service to the association, in official capacities, dates back to the middle twenties. Nevertheless, though relieved of his onerous duties, he did not give up his active practice until nearly six years later. Then, on October 1, 1947, he retired to make his home in Las Vegas, New Mexico. At its next meeting the Board of Directors awarded him an honorary membership. President Henry S. Brown described him as "one of the fine old gentlemen of industrial medicine."

*   *   *

As World War II settled down to a grim pursuit of victory by destruction of lives, depletion of resources, and attrition of materials, the association continued its multiple activities on both home and battle fronts. Very early in the war the question of long-range planning began to assume importance not only in industry but also in the medical aspects of industry.

Holmblad voiced the opinion of many members when, at the 1943 annual meeting in Rochester, New York he introduced the question in his report as managing director. Commenting on the rapid changes in membership figures and personnel, he said: "As one follows the roll call from year to year . . . one recognizes the desirability of some committee or group of men whose purpose should be to develop plans for continuing the life and membership of this association. It might even be a broader group, a planning committee the purpose of which would be to look into the future, planning such features and programs as would be beneficial for this specialty and this association."

At the business session that followed, President Wittmer asked for a discussion of Holmblad's suggestion. It was pointed out that the association had an Executive Committee consisting, under the bylaws, of five elected officers, and the Board thereupon supported a motion making it a specific function of that committee to set up a planning program. The Executive Committee, at the time, was buried in current agenda and unable to give immediate attention to future problems.

In the following months, however, the need for planning on a broad basis was brought before Board meetings. Loyal Shoudy, for example, in November 1943, wrote to Holmblad as follows: "I think it is high time that we began to consider just what is the future of industrial medical practice. I mean, what will it be when the war is over and we begin to scramble for some of those idealistic things which, want them or not, are going to be forced on us? Just as we are not certain as to what is going to happen to medicine and the practice of medicine, neither are we certain as to what is going to happen to the industrial practice. I admit I do not know how to do it, but I do feel that we ought to be thinking along lines of what our future is to be."

A copy of this letter was duly included in Holmblad's next report to the Board of Directors in February 1944, and it served as a reminder that concrete thinking on plans for the future was still a part of unfinished business. Moreover, the Executive Committee, though formally entrusted with the preparation of a long-range program, had no time for such a task. Its hands were already full of pressing duties, and future planning was a subject requiring concentrated, uninterrupted attention.

It was, in fact, almost impossible to plan at all, with any assurance, in the years from 1942 to 1946. Travel restrictions grew steadily tighter: federal priorities, necessarily, limited civilian activities in many directions. At the October 29, 1942, meeting of the Board, one of the first items on a full calendar was the question of whether the annual meeting in 1943 should be cancelled because of war conditions.

Reporting for the industrial hygienists, who were planning to continue their joint meetings with the AAIP&S, Robert A. Kehoe and Warren A. Cook, both of whom were directors of the American Industrial Hygiene Association, expressed the opinion that such a meeting might prove more valuable in war than in peacetime. Governmental industrial hygienists, they pointed out, had vital reasons for conferring with their civilian colleagues, and an interchange of information with the industrial physicians and surgeons would be fruitful for all concerned.

In the main the AAIP&S directors concurred in this reasoning, provided the program was limited to essential business and week-end travel was avoided insofar as possible. After long discussion the Board voted that the 1943 meeting be held "if at all practicable and possible," but left the final decision to the Executive Committee.

The Executive Committee, in turn, approached that decision with caution. There was a great deal of work involved for a great many men. There were matters of space commitments to be considered, and the possibility of slim attendance. They wanted to avoid the experience of the American College of Surgeons, which had a meeting planned for Chicago, decided suddenly to transfer it to Cleveland, and, about two weeks before it was to be held, was forced by circumstances to cancel it entirely.

As it turned out, the twenty-eighth annual convention of the AAIP&S, in Rochester, New York, May 24–27, 1943, was a great success in every particular: in attendance, with 569 persons registered; in quality of speakers and papers; in general interest and enthusiasm. Further, all space available for commercial exhibits was readily sold. An immense amount of routine work was pushed through at a six-hour Board meeting, but the business session was brief. The incoming president, Harvey Bartle (then chief of medical service, Pennsylvania Railroad), formally took over the office for 1943–44. Frederick W. Slobe (Chicago) was named president-elect; Melvin N. Newquist (New York), first vice-president; Loyal A. Shoudy (Bethlehem), second vice-president. Among new directors added to the Board at this meeting were Beverly L. Vosburgh (General Electric), Edward P. Heller, a general and industrial surgeon serving many important companies in Kansas City and extremely active in committee work of the association, Henry S. Brown, medical director of the Michigan Bell Telephone Company and likewise active in association affairs, and T. L. Story, of Southbridge, Massachusetts, medical director of the American Optical Company.

The new president, Harvey Bartle, received his medical degree at the University of Pennsylvania in 1902. A prominent consultant in general industrial health, he was a veteran in the railway field, serving the Pennsylvania system for many years as chief medical examiner. He was an original (and influential) member of the AMA Council on Industrial Health and was equally active in the affairs of the AAIP&S.

Bartle found in the presidency plenty of problems on which to exercise his administrative talents and experience. "It was," as he says, "an important year in expansion of activities in allied groups." There were jurisdictional disputes to be

335

cleared up, and the long campaign to win certification for industrial medicine as a specialty was entering a new phase, in which Bartle's good offices were extremely useful.

Opening a Board meeting in February 1944, he told the directors: "The industrial physician has come into his own rightful place in his chosen field of service. The medical service in industry has been definitely established as a going concern. Its status has been greatly strengthened during the prodigious industrial expansion era incident to a global war, by federal directives." He urged consideration of three "musts" in the further development of industrial medicine: 1) the medical profession should assume the leadership; 2) the medical profession, management and labor should collaborate in principle and work out amicably a general plan for a satisfactory service to be rendered, with proper personnel, acceptable and satisfactorily remunerated; 3) the dignity of personality should not be violated—the service must be personalized; human fellowship cannot be feigned, and disregard of it will do violence in any industrial medical service.

These were in perfect accord with the thinking of the middle 1940's, which may be described as a period of expansion of industrial medical services and reorganization within the AAIP&S. The efforts of at least four successive presidential terms were concentrated on those two objectives and upon improvement of the relations between the association and other agencies interested in industrial health.

Expansion and reorganization, above all else, called for high-level planning, a task that could best be handled by special committees, each responsible for the necessary research, analysis, and recommendations involved in a specific problem. Prior to the forties few committees were required—one on membership, one to arrange each annual meeting, one or two others for special purposes. The officers and directors were able to carry most of the load, with little outside help.

Emergency demands at the outset of the war made committee organization necessary on a much larger scale; and, once introduced, the committee system remained as the backbone of administrative procedure. There were more AAIP&S committees at work on policies and projects in 1947 than at the height of the war, although most of the emergency committees had been disbanded by 1945.

In succeeding years the number of committees required has varied from fifteen or twenty to thirty or more, to meet existing needs. Indicative of the stature and maturity of the association is the fact that it has been able throughout a period of unparalleled change to produce men of sufficient caliber, in the needed numbers, to make the committee system a productive and economical working tool.

Matters of policy and planning filled the air in May 1944, when the AAIP&S convened in St. Louis. This was the meeting at which Frederick W. Slobe took over the presidency, the remainder of the ticket including Melvin N. Newquist, president-elect, L. A. Shoudy, first vice-president, and Henry S. Brown, second vice-president. Among new names on the Board were those of H. A. Vonachen, of Peoria, Illinois, and A. H. Whittaker and E. A. Irvin, of Detroit, all of whom were later to serve as presidents.

Slobe, who received his degree from Rush Medical College in 1917, served with the United States Medical Corps in World War I. His early interest was in general and traumatic surgery, but in 1921 he entered the industrial field, and built an extensive practice as chief surgeon and medical director of numerous concerns in the Chicago area. In 1949 he turned this industrial practice over to his associates to become medical director of the Illinois Medical Service (Blue Shield) and Blue Cross Plan for Hospital Care.

At a long and dramatic Board meeting that opened the 1944 convention, both the outgoing and the incoming presidents, Bartle and Slobe, took the platform to urge early and decisive action on plans for the future. Following the line of thought he had discussed with the directors at their winter meeting, Bartle re-emphasized the need for special undergraduate and postgraduate education as a prelude to industrial practice, the development of preventive medicine, certification of industrial physicians, and steps to solve the "tremendous problem" of rehabilitation and placement of the handicapped. Commenting on the necessity for an enlarged financial program to match the scope of association activities, he pointed out that no such plan had been forthcoming. "There is need," he said, "of definite measures outlining policies, methods and practices, involving the ever expanding standards of medical service in industry. We can advisedly coordinate our efforts with other groups that are actively interested in similar projects, out of which will stem directives in the vast field in which our association is naturally the leader."

Slobe was equally forthright in his address as the incoming president, and his basic views were in agreement with those expressed by Bartle. "It seems to me," he said, "that we are at the crossroads, requiring a choice as to which course to follow, whether we wish to adhere to our past policy of confining our activities largely to the holding of an annual convention or whether we wish to enter into the many fertile fields of exploration which are beckoning along the road to better industrial welfare."

Slobe left no doubt as to what his own decision would be. Reiterating the importance of a Board of Certification for physicians and surgeons in industry, and the need for training in industrial health as a prerequisite for certification, he continued: "Facilities for that training should be available in representative medical schools throughout the country. Fellowships must be established in order that those facilities may be utilized. Such fellowships require a stipend of approximately $6,000 for the three-year period. Postgraduate refresher courses, likewise, need to be developed in more cities."

He went on to characterize the education of management in industrial health problems as one of the association's greatest fields of endeavor and to suggest that a survey of medical services might well be within its province. "What organization," he asked, "is better qualified to do it? How can we better demonstrate our altruistic motives than by making such a survey and giving advice as to needed improvement?"

Like Bartle, Slobe accented heavily the association's obligation to take an active part in the absorption of war veterans into industry. "But," he added, "the field is so broad in its scope that the mere participation in it to the extent of appointment of an appropriate committee would only scratch the surface."

Further, Slobe pointed out the possibility that many physicians, after demobilization, might seek fellowships in graduate training to prepare them for industrial practice. This suggestion provoked, at the close of his talk, a spirited debate on the problem of financing fellowships and the part that the AAIP&S should play in that activity. This was one of the earliest open discussions of a fund-raising project for educational purposes, and though the directors took no immediate action, interest grew steadily and led, eventually, to establishment of the American Foundation of Occupational Health, a name later changed to the Occupational Health Institute.

These, then, were the principal problems that came into sharp focus in the middle forties: extension of industrial health education in medical schools; certification of the specialty; expansion of industrial medical services, with emphasis on rehabilitation; and the clarification and improvement of AAIP&S relations with other organizations having interests in common.

All these objectives were of major importance. All demanded action. But, though each presented its own peculiar problems, they were so closely interrelated that none could be approached without reference to the others. How the objectives were met will be described later.

As 1944 progressed, however, there arose at closer range a problem which, from a practical viewpoint, transcended all others. For it became apparent that, barring a miracle, the association would have no annual meeting in 1945. The nation's transportation system was loaded to its limit, and civilian travel was reduced to a minimum.

As an immediate result of the 1944 meeting a new Committee on Policy and Planning had been appointed, consisting of F. E. Poole, medical director of the Lockheed Aircraft Corporation (chairman), H. A. Vonachen, and Harvey Bartle. This committee reported to the Board on October 3, 1944, summarizing at considerable length the knotty problems involved in long-range planning and recommending continued study of all factors.

In the discussion that followed, the question of money bobbed up at every turn. Without sufficient funds how could anything be decided? Alfred H. Whittaker spoke for a majority when he said: ". . . most of these matters coming up for consideration depend on the broadening out of the activities of the society, and they in turn are contingent upon a bigger income. I think perhaps somewhere in the agenda there should be time spent in the definite determination by the Board of Directors

338

as to what the future activities are to be." Upon that note, and with no conclusive action, the session ended.

Nor was there an opportunity for further discussion of distant objectives at the next Board meeting, February 1945, for in his opening remarks President Slobe officially announced cancellation of the 1945 convention. The association had presented its case to the government with reasoned emphasis on the importance of industrial health problems to be dealt with at such a meeting, but the Office of Defense Transportation, besieged by requests from every side, said "No" with firmness and finality. In fact, Edward Holmblad reported, only two of more than two hundred applications acted upon had been approved.

Said Slobe: "We all rejoice in this from a sense of cooperative patriotism; but it also causes keen regret because of the loss of continuity of our annual conventions, the loss of time and energy expended by those who have made extensive preparations for this meeting, and the loss of personal contact with our membership."

Naturally, a tremendous amount of work already done was undone by this ruling. Medical and other addresses relating to the war effort could not be delivered. Only a small fraction of their text could be printed in *Industrial Medicine,* and discussion was impossible. In Chicago, the largest amount of commercial exhibit space ever contracted for in the association's history had to be canceled, along with other arrangements.

These setbacks were to be expected. But there still remained the problem of transacting essential business by remote control.

So began the long-to-be-remembered year of "proxy meetings," by means of which American industrial medicine carried on its top-level planning and activities, in the interests of a membership scattered to every corner of the nation.

XXVIII

COMPONENT SOCIETIES, INDUSTRIAL NURSING, AND INDUSTRIAL DENTISTRY

THERE is a great deal that appears commonplace in the year-by-year chronology of most organizations and very little which, standing alone and out of context, if of great significance. That was, at least, true of the American Association of Industrial Physicians & Surgeons in the 1940's. The successive events that marked the association's progress toward midcentury were not always, to the contemporary eye, clearly related to a composite whole. Out of them, however, at the end of World War II, the outline of a larger picture began to appear, much as the shape of a mountain range or a broad sea vista emerges from a lifting fog.

For the trial and error of former years, the seemingly slow forward steps of the AAIP&S were the light tracings from which came the image of today's industrial medicine. And, just as surely, the policies and plans of the Industrial Medical Association of today will evolve into the industrial medicine of tomorrow.

Several important pieces of the organization puzzle were fitted together in 1945, under handicaps that severely taxed the resourcefulness of the officers and directors. Putting first things first, as was their custom, they concentrated at their February meeting upon ways and means of enacting essential measures without a meeting of the membership to ratify their action.

Among those first things was a revision of the bylaws—important because the proposed new laws redefined the qualifications required for different classes of membership and changed to some extent the regulations governing organization and operation of the association. Also needed was a plan whereby the annual spring election of officers and directors could be held under conditions which permitted no large meetings and few small ones. At a Sunday night session (February 11, 1945)

340

the Board discussed at length the question of its authority in certain policy matters. It then went patiently through the proposed bylaws, paragraph by paragraph, making final revisions. Before adjournment, the directors approved publication in *Industrial Medicine* of the bylaw changes, as required by the original constitution.[1] The question of a membership vote was left for later consideration.

On May 6, the directors gathered at the headquarters office in Chicago, prepared to act upon a resolution officially convening the annual meeting then and there and listing in proxy form the items of business to be transacted. They had also obtained legal assurance that association members, under existing regulations, were permitted to vote by proxy. This resolution authorized the immediate issuance of absentee ballots providing for a membership vote on officers and directors for the ensuing year; adoption of new bylaws to supersede the old constitution and bylaws; creation of a trust or corporation for educational purposes in connection with industrial medical research and education (American Foundation of Occupational Health, later known as the Occupational Health Institute); and a $500 contribution by the AAIP&S to such a trust. The proxy plan was carried out as scheduled, with a representative number of members voting. Directors and officers were duly elected, and all proposals approved. But most important, in over-all effect, was the fact that the administrative heads of the association were enabled to proceed with basic programs that called for immediate action.

Because of the cancellation of the regular annual convention for 1945, there had been a disposition at the February Board meeting to retain the same officers for another term, a step strongly opposed by President Slobe. "I do not believe," said he, "that perpetuity in officers is a sound thing, and the directors also should rotate periodically."

Learning, however, that a proxy election was permissible, a nominating committee went ahead with the usual procedure, and the approved candidates took over their duties as soon as returns from the field had been duly tabulated. As president elect, Melvin N. Newquist automatically succeeded Slobe; Shoudy became president elect, with Henry S. Brown and Harold A. Vonachen as first and second vice-presidents, respectively.

Urged by his associates, Slobe consented to extend his long service to the association by taking over the duties of secretary, an office with no incumbent at the time. Interesting, too, was the addition of five new members to the Board: A. G. Cranch (Union Carbide & Carbon Corporation and AAIP&S member since 1917) F. G. Barr, veteran medical and public relations director (National Cash Register), James A. Carlisle (Merck & Company), J. N. Shirley (Arrow Mutual Liability Insurance), and A. L. Brooks (Fisher Body Corporation).

Wherein, one may ask, lay the urgency and importance of those proxy-year activities? The answer is found in the rapid growth of AAIP&S membership and the extraordinary expansion of association services and contacts. By the middle forties the AAIP&S was collaborating closely with many organizations in the field of industrial health and had interests in common with many others. The problem of its relationship to, and relations with, such organizations had become an ever sensitive and frequently controversial issue. How, and how soon, such problems were resolved might materially influence the future course of industrial medicine.

The so-called "component" societies offer a case in point. Far back in the 1930's the AAIP&S committed itself to a federated type of organization, in which the national association is affiliated with completely autonomous regional or local groups. Members of the parent organization carry their memberships through these component societies wherever possible. Only in areas not serviced by components are national memberships carried direct. Under this policy the component societies pass upon the eligibility of their own applicants, and the decisions are accepted so long as membership qualifications and governing regulations are not in conflict with those of the national association.

Many regional and local organizations devoted to industrial medicine and surgery received their earliest national mention in the thirties through the columns of *Industrial Medicine,* under an arrangement that entitled them to group subscriptions and gave them editorial representation in the columns of the magazine. Among such groups, in 1937, were:

The Central States Society of Industrial Medicine and Surgery, which drew its membership mainly from Illinois, Indiana, Iowa, and Wisconsin. Its president (1937–1938) was F. W. Slobe, of Chicago, and its secretary-treasurer, Frank P. Hammond, then medical director of Blue Cross in the area.

The Association for the Advancement of Industrial Medicine & Surgery, whose membership was centered in Metropolitan New York. Its president was J. J. Wittmer; its purpose, "to disseminate accurate medical knowledge in reference to the diagnosis and treatment of all conditions arising out of and in the course of employment."

The New York State Society of Industrial Medicine, representing out-state industrial medical interests and headed by E. A. Vander Veer, of Albany, surgeon for the New York Central Railroad.

The Michigan Association of Industrial Physicians & Surgeons, whose president was, in 1937, Alfred H. Whittaker, of Detroit.

Such regional groups as these were quick to recognize the advantages of affiliation with the association that represented their professional specialty on a national scale, and the AAIP&S warmly welcomed contacts with and support by active affiliates at local levels. Yet there was little news of editorial comment when, in its December, 1937, issue, *Industrial Medicine* listed the Central States Society and the Association for the Advancement of Industrial Medicine & Surgery as components of the AAIP&S.

Interest in component societies increased steadily, as did their number. Two were added in 1939: the Association of Railway and Industrial Physicians & Surgeons, of Kansas City, headed by M. J. Owens, division surgeon, Atchison, Topeka & Santa

Fe Railroad; and the New Jersey Association of Industrial Physicians & Surgeons, whose president, Donald O. Hamblin, was nationally prominent as medical director of the American Cyanamid Company, and an active worker in the AAIP&S.

In 1940 two more state societies became affiliated: a Michigan unit (R. H. Denham, of Grand Rapids, president) representing industrial volume and numerical strength sufficient to maintain an active component apart from the Central States Society; and the Georgia Association of Industrial Surgeons, under R. L. Rhodes, of Augusta, as president.

Notable advances were made in 1941. The Hawaiian society, accepted as a component in January, has remained the only such affiliate outside the continental territory of the United States. Originally designated as the Hawaiian Society of Industrial Physicians & Surgeons, it became in 1944 a unit of a new territorial organization which has since been listed among components as the Territorial Association of Plantation Physicians. Its overseas members, though numerically few, have enthusiastically supported the programs of the parent organization, insofar as they have been applicable.

Also in 1941, two large and important regions were given representation in the national structure, with acceptance of the Western Association of Industrial Physicians & Surgeons and the New England Conference of Industrial Physicians as component societies.[2] And Florida, Maryland and Milwaukee associations were added to the roster. The Georgia society, along with the Maryland and Milwaukee units, withdrew after brief periods, having found member support in wartime insufficient to justify participation in national activities.

It is of interest that personal representatives from seven of eleven components of record in 1941 were welcomed at the annual meeting of the Board of Directors in Pittsburgh on May 5. Of the other four the Hawaiian Society was deterred by distance, and the newly organized Western Association had held its first annual meeting on the preceding day. Its president, Robert T. Legge, sent a telegram of greeting and explanation to the Board in Pittsburgh.

There was no question, even at that early date, as to the value of active component societies in advancing the cause of industrial medicine, nationally as well as locally. They were in constant touch with both large and small industries and were thoroughly familiar with local medical programs. By monthly or quarterly meetings they kept interest alive and stimulated productive activities while, at the same time, furthering the aims and policies of the national organization.

On the other hand, development of the components presented several disturbing and difficult problems. There was a good deal of confusion and misunderstanding as to the status of a component society within the AAIP&S. The components, naturally, wanted no second-class membership. They did want a share of major responsibilities, and reasonable representation on the Board of Directors. They asked for clear-cut decisions as to dues, membership qualifications, rights and privileges.

These and other issues were aired at great length at the association's 1940 meeting in New York. Present, to speak for the New Jersey society, was D. O. Hamblin; for the Georgia association, Richard E. Newberry, its president; and for the Michigan association, the incoming president, Frank T. McCormick, of Detroit. Michigan was also represented by such AAIP&S stalwarts as Selby, McCord, and J. J. Prendergast (medical director, Chrysler Corporation), a former vice-president of the association.

As events proved, components had no reason to worry about representation on the Board of Directors. The association settled that question later by naming both Newberry and McCormick as directors for the 1941–43 term. Discussion of membership status soon developed the fact that the main problem lay in the lack of uniformity of standards and policies set up by local and regional societies, and, sometimes, opposition from other medical organizations.

By way of example, R. C. Engel, of Cleveland, spoke of the difficulties encountered in efforts to form an industrial medical group in Ohio. Daniel Lynch explained the conflict of membership qualifications that had delayed approval of a New England component. Indicating, on the other hand, the extent of interest in the industrial phases of medicine, William Sawyer cited the establishment of a Section on Industrial Health by the Philadelphia County Medical Society, one of the earliest, if not the first, of its kind at the county level.

Obviously, the complexities of the "component problem" could not be ironed out at a single directors' meeting. The Board adjourned without action. There was, however, unanimous agreement on one point—that solutions must be found and final decisions must be incorporated in a crystal-clear code stipulating the classes of membership and requirements for each. This was the compelling reason for the painstaking, time-consuming revision of the association by-laws that followed.

As an immediate result of the 1940 meeting, a special Committee on Components was appointed to study the entire membership structure and submit recommendations. This committee represented widely scattered sections of the country. With Alfred H. Whittaker (Michigan) as chairman, it was made up of R. E. Newberry (Georgia), prominent industrial surgeon; Christopher Leggo (California), medical director, California Hawaiian Sugar Refining Corporation); W. W. Lasher (New York City), later surgical director of Lloyd's of America; J. A. Simpson (Texas), representing insurance and utility companies; and Don W. Deal (Illinois), a general and industrial surgeon with widely varied interests.

The committee's first step was to divide the country into industrial areas and assign one member to each of these sections—six in number. In October, 1941, Whittaker reported to the directors that his group was engaged in collecting all available information as to the standards and qualifications expected of the men who wished to become members of component societies. Again, an old motto of the association, "Quality is more important than quantity," was emphasized.

Once more, at the spring meeting of the Board, in April, 1942, developments in the affairs of the components were exhaustively reviewed. Whittaker laid before the Board two main issues for discussion: Should membership applications be processed by the components or by the association without going through the components? and 2) Should applicants from component societies be eligible for active membership or limited to associate membership? Answers to these questions were of the utmost importance, for, unless decisions completely satisfactory to both the components and the AAIP&S were reached, the association's entire long-range program for expansion and activity might well be shattered. The problem was debated long and earnestly. Then, at the suggestion of Whittaker, it was referred to the Board for further study and action.

Two noteworthy developments in this situation were launched at the next directors' meeting. Reporting in October, 1942, Whittaker told the Board that his group, while studying standards and membership qualifications among regional and local industrial medical societies, were so widely separated geographically that they could not possibly function as a committee. His opinion was that the only practical way to build up a strong and active component organization was to delegate responsibility to one man who had time to devote to that purpose, Dr. Holmblad. "Have him travel around the country," he said, "and contact key men personally. Have him stay in a locality long enough to get groups together and form component societies where there are none at present. I should like very much to see this work carried on by the association in such a way that it will be representative of the country as a whole, rather than just some central localities. I hope the Board will accept our suggestion that the central office be asked to take it over in the future, without adding too much to Holmblad's already big job."

This proposal led to a lively discussion, in which representatives from scattered sections of the country described the local needs of their respective component societies. F. E. Poole (Western Association) predicted that a considerable number of new applications of industrial medicine would come from the rapidly growing aircraft industry on the Pacific coast and urged the association to foster programs that would appeal directly to the self-interest of lay management. "We can't sell our services to the plants," he said, "until they are thoroughly familiar with what we have to offer them." Other speakers included Frank P. Hammond (Central States), E. P. Heller (Kansas City), D. L. Lynch (New England), and R. E. Newberry (Georgia). Their comments covered various situations, but on one thing all were agreed—the need for closer contacts between the AAIP&S and component societies and between components and industrial employers and more frequent meetings with management executives for the presentation and discussion of papers on subjects of special interest in regional industries. At the close of the discussion the Board voted to accept the committee's report and its recommendation. In effect, this approval was a long step in the direction of more practical, more productive, relations between industrial management and industrial medicine.

No one, perhaps, at that directors' meeting in 1942, noticed that Whittaker, in referring to the members of the Committee on Components, spoke of them as "counselors representing the association in different districts of the country." At any

345

rate there was no comment on his choice of words. The term "district counselors" may have appeared now and then in casual conversation, but officially there was no such office. Yet here were six members (including Whittaker) functioning as district counselors on a committee assignment.

It is unlikely that any of the directors at the meeting in question recalled that Guy L. Kiefer, of Detroit, in his speech accepting the presidency of the association in 1928, made this announcement: "We decided last night in our Board of Directors meeting that there should be appointed some regional chairmen in different parts of the country who shall look for other desirable members for this association."[3] Here, at least in embryo form, was a plan for establishing a nationwide organization of district counselors within the AAIP&S. The project was discussed from time to time but, like many an innovation, it was repeatedly shelved as unfinished business.

Whittaker had been for some time deeply impressed by the potential value of such an organization in strengthening membership and stimulating activity in the "home" districts they represented. He remained a perennial champion of the plan and pressed for its activation on every occasion. Yet, though there was little or no opposition to the program, progress was slow. It was difficult to find, among over-busy doctors, men who, however willing, could take on the added duties involved.

Final results, however, more than justified the time and energy spent. Fully developed, the district counselor organization has become an almost indispensable link in the association's chain of liaison with component societies and, through them, with the nation's industries. We shall hear more, in another chapter, of its growth and the expansion of its functions.

Though relieved of field contacts, the Committee on Components was not dissolved but continued in an advisory capacity as a three-member group, with Whittaker as chairman. Holmblad's traveling schedule increased substantially in the next few years, for meeting with other AAIP&S officials and representatives of local societies. Bit by bit, as a result of discussions with groups, a satisfactory membership policy for components took shape. It was a task that required infinite patience and the full cooperation of the committees on Components, Bylaw Revision, and Membership.

Reporting to the Board on this phase of the problem Holmblad commented: "It is but common sense and good reasoning that the qualifications for membership should be identical and that anyone not acceptable to a component society should not be taken in as a member of the parent organization, and *vice versa.*" This approach found ready support both in the AAIP&S and in the components. It was, as we have seen, the policy that prevailed in the final version of the revised bylaws, officially adopted in the summer of 1945.

In the fall of 1944 Whittaker, urging action on the district counselor program, called to the Board's attention the fact that current reports were emphasizing more and more the importance of component societies. Increased interest and activity in various sections gave ample evidence of that trend.

The Rhode Island society, small but active, applied for a component status but, though wholly acceptable to the AAIP&S, later decided it would be in a better position if it functioned as a section of the New England Conference, to which it was geographically joined.

During 1944 a progressive group of Canadian industrial physicians expressed great interest in forming an affiliate of the association in Ontario. Extensive correspondence followed, and Holmblad attended a meeting in Toronto to discuss the plan. The proposed union did not materialize, mainly because of a fear that such an affiliation might bar the group from becoming an industrial section of the Canadian Medical Association. It goes without saying that Canadian doctors in industrial practice have been welcomed to direct membership in the American association and, as a unit, have been consistently active in its affairs.

Midway in the forties the trend toward component affiliations was greatly stimulated by developments in New York. In 1944 the strong and long established New York State society applied for component status. However, the war situation, coupled with the still-pending revision of the bylaws, repeatedly delayed final action, and it was not until 1947 that all arrangements had been completed.

In the spring of that year one of the oldest of all AAIP&S components, the Association for the Advancement of Industrial Medicine & Surgery, was dissolved and a new corporation formed to take over its assets and membership, along with those of the upper New York state society. The new component, promptly accepted by the parent association, was incorporated as the New York State Society of Industrial Medicine.

At that point the AAIP&S policy with respect to components had become fairly well stabilized. Individual units, over the years, have had their ups and downs. There have been some losses, but they have been offset by gains. In 1949 the Association of Mine Physicians was admitted as a component. In the next year the Industrial Medical Association of Philadelphia was enrolled, to be followed in 1955 by the Industrial Medical Association of Pittsburgh.

Under that policy the association has achieved nationwide representation mainly through a small number of large units with broad regional influence. Notable exceptions are found in a few highly industrialized areas of great importance. Only New York, of all states, has within its borders two strong and active component organizations: The New York State Society of Industrial Medicine and the Western New York Society of Industrial Medicine & Surgery, which achieved component status early in 1955. The original development and subsequent success of this group were very largely due to the efforts of John L. Norris (Eastman Kodak Company), an outstanding authority on problem drinking in industry, who has served the association as a director and as chairman of important committees.

The long-term effect of components upon association membership was strikingly illustrated in a report made January 1, 1948, a decade after the plan was started. On that date the AAIP&S had a total of 1,516 active members; of them, 1,100, or nearly 80 percent carried their memberships through the (then) nine components, the four largest of which alone accounted for almost exactly 800: New York (Eastern), 283; Central States, 263; Western, 143; Michigan, 109.

Throughout the entire 1940's, one notes, the association devoted a great deal of time to studying, adjusting and strengthening its relations with other organizations having allied or collateral interests. In fact, the revision of the bylaws and other changes in internal policy were largely actuated by a desire for harmony in those important professional relationships.

Obviously, no one type of cooperative arrangement could be expected to apply in all cases. The component society program, once membership qualifications had been standardized and financial questions settled, proved mutually satisfactory and rewarding. The industrial hygienists, of course, were in another category. While their objectives were in full harmony with those of the physicians and surgeons, their interests and their functions were basically different. Yet, as members of health teams working on common problems in the same industries, both medical and hygienic personnel could expect to benefit greatly from frequent discussion and interchange of ideas.

There were, naturally, dissident opinions and controversial issues involved in this relationship, but they were brought out into the open, freely discussed, and reconciled in good time. As we have seen, the first joint meeting of the American Industrial Hygiene Association with the AAIP&S (New York, 1940) gave promise of success that has long since exceeded expectations. As a consequence of this step the National Conference of Governmental Industrial Hygienists joined their colleagues at the wartime meeting of 1943 in Rochester, New York.

The reciprocal benefits of this type of arrangement were important. Presence of the hygienists substantially increased attendance at AAIP&S annual meetings, added interest in and support for commercial exhibits, made available joint sessions that have been a steadily growing attraction over the years. It would be difficult to estimate how much these and other features have contributed to the present stature of industrial medicine and to the prestige of organizations devoted to the improvement of industrial health.

Thus, well before the close of the forties, we find long-range programs beginning to yield a double harvest: first, in a flourishing network of component societies, and second, in a conference type of annual meeting for consideration of all the many-sided problems of industrial health. Affiliation and participation! It was apparent that both had come to stay, among the basic policies of the association.

At the St. Louis meeting in May 1944, the American Association of Industrial Nurses, the third participating group to join forces with the AAIP&S, made its official debut, conducting a program of its own and taking part in joint sessions with the physicians and surgeons. Although a newly organized unit, the AAIN had behind it a long and honorable tradition. In fact, as Whittaker remarked at a directors' meeting in that year, the industrial nurses were active in this country before the industrial doctors.

In their own official chronology the nurses recognize 1895 as the birthdate of their specialty. Bethel J. McGrath, R.N., in her well documented history of industrial nursing,[4] assigns to that year "the first record in America of nurses being employed and paid by industry to help guard the health of an employed group."

Mrs. McGrath credits this notable innovation to the humane interest of a Vermont man, Fletcher D. Proctor, in the health of employees in his Vermont Marble Company. In this early service, says she, "little" emphasis was placed on the care of injuries. It was essentially a home visiting service. Calls came through physicians. Service was free to employees of the Vermont Marble Company and their families, and to the needy in the town who were unable to pay.

The first nurse employed for these peripatetic duties was Ada Mayo Stewart, then twenty-four years old and an 1894 graduate of the Waltham (Massachusetts) Training School. For her first year's work, it is recorded, she was paid $900 "partly in money and partly in paid expense," and she got a $100 increase in her second year. She and her sister commonly rode bicycles on their visits to neighboring villages.

In view of the multiple, and often highly specialized, duties of today's industrial nurses, it is interesting to note that from 1896 through 1898 obstetrical cases topped the list in the Stewart sisters' records, with medical cases a close second, and surgical cases few.[5] Actually, the "industrial" nurse of that time was a general nurse; she took what she found in the homes she visited, and did what she could for her patients.

There were other early ventures of similar type, among them that of the Wanamaker Company, of New York, which hired a nurse in 1897 to visit sick employees and to see that its benefit association funds were distributed fairly. By 1900 the idea was attracting somewhat more attention, first among stores, then in a few industries scattered across the country.

At best, however, progress was slow and irregular, seeming to follow business cycles and the trends of employment. Available records indicate that in 1914 only sixty firms in the country were offering nursing services; yet by 1918 there were 871 companies employing 1,213 registered nurses. The United States Census of 1930 reported 3,189 trained nurses employed in industry and commerce, but the number dropped precipitately as the depression deepened. In the middle thirties, came an upturn, and surveys in 1941 and 1943 showed, respectively, 6,244 and 12,838 industrial nurses registered, the majority of them active.[6]

The evolution of organized industrial nursing was, in some ways, similar to that of organized industrial medicine. In the pioneering years, doctors came into industry along with the safety movement; their primary interest was in trauma and the surgery of trauma. The industrial nurse was, at the outset, a general nurse; usually she gravitated into industry from public health nursing.

The nursing profession as a whole was, of course, bound together by a large and influential national organization, the American Nurses' Association; yet the thousands of young nurses who wanted careers in the special field of industry received little in the way of recognition or representation at the national level before the 1940's. There were, it is true, some encouraging developments. The influential National Organization for Public Health Nursing created an industrial nursing section in 1920—to stimulate interest in special industrial problems, to promote good standards in industrial nursing, and to provide a forum for discussion. This group also served the National Safety Council from 1930 to 1943, when the council established a similar section of its own. Not until 1944 was an industrial section formed within the American Nurses' Association, and it did not become fully active until 1946.

Though eager to conform to the highest standards of ethics and procedures in their profession, the industrial nurses were not entirely satisfied with a "sectional" status for their special field. They welcomed the support and practical help of the ANA, the NOPHN, and other related organizations, but they believed that industrial nursing needs justified more consideration, more detailed study, than they would receive under such an arrangement.

Even more, perhaps, they wanted administrative independence that would enable them to work out their own future, build their own organization, and write the policies under which it would operate. To make their voices heard, to achieve self-determination (within the accepted codes of nursing), they founded the AAIN in 1942, much as the industrial physicians and surgeons (within accepted medical codes) had established the AAIP&S in 1916.

What can one write, in estimation of nurses and nursing, that is not already widely known? Of the nurse in industry, Mrs. McGrath had this to say in 1946: "It is to the credit of the Nightingale tradition and the stuff of which nurses are made that she has, on the whole, done well. . . . Although some of her activities have caused head-shaking on the sidelines, there is no question that she has answered a real need in industry where she started fifty years ago, a field where unproductive expense is not tolerated."[7]

Certain it is that, first as an attending nurse in the emergency rooms of factories and later as a trained and registered assistant to the industrial physician and surgeon, the industrial nurse has come far. And it may be added that her code, like that of the doctor, has been shaped and perpetuated in a rigorous mold of self-discipline.

In a brief history of industrial nursing Katherine M. Holmes, of Detroit, describes the unusual chain of events that led to the organization of the American Association of Industrial Nurses. The story starts with a Mrs. Anna M. Staebler, a Boston graduate in public health nursing, who, after completing her course (about 1914), made a leisurely tour of nearby factories to inspect nursing procedures. In the course of personal interviews with the girls employed as nurses in various industries Mrs. Staebler inquired particularly into their experience and their attitude toward the profession they had chosen. She was surprised to learn that their interest, in most cases, did not extend beyond the administration of first aid. "The majority of the nurses," wrote Miss Holmes, "were not selected because they were particularly qualified to do this kind of work but because of some service they had rendered in the employer's family as private duty nurses."[8]

More than a little shocked by this lack of training, and the girls' limited understanding of their opportunity, Mrs. Staebler started recruiting members for an industrial nurses' club for discussion of current problems and future activities. The plan appealed both to the nurses and to employers and was promptly put into effect in the Boston area. Stenographic notes were taken at monthly meetings, and printed summaries were mailed to all members.

So successful was this local club that it quickly grew into a state-wide organization, and then into a New England association. As usual, success invited competition, and in 1916 another organized group of industrial nurses appeared in Boston. Known as the Factory Nurses Conference, it admitted to membership only graduate, state-registered nurses belonging to the American Nurses Association. For many years the Conference enjoyed great popularity. Branches were established in quick succession, and in 1922 the combined groups became the first American Association of Industrial Nurses. This association continued into the thirties; then economic pressure asserted itself, and, with the number of nurses in industry steadily dwindling, the American Association merged with the original New England Industrial Nurses Association.

This group weathered the economic storm and in 1938 demonstrated its vitality by joining the New York, New Jersey, and Philadelphia groups for the first of a series of annual conferences to consider the affairs, problems and future of industrial nursing. It was at such a conference in Philadelphia, with the Detroit Industrial Nurses' Association also represented, that several hundred delegates voted the present American Association of Industrial Nurses into existence. The date was April 19, 1942.

Ten years later, the *AAIN Newsletter* commented as follows on that historic decision: "In 1942 several roads were invitingly open for the young, promising field of industrial nursing was beginning to find its place in the American health scene. We could affiliate with industrial medical associations, or we could become a section in one of our professional nursing associations. Or we could decide to go it alone, at least until the field of industrial nursing had taken surer form and its principles and practices were understood by our allies as well as ourselves."

They did decide, dramatically, to "go it alone," and before adjournment they scheduled a meeting for August 15 to consider a constitution and bylaws, and voted to hold their first annual meeting in New York in May, 1943. The new association, their announcement stated, would be "open to all graduate registered nurses actively engaged in industrial nursing."

At their business session, delegates elected as the first AAIN president Miss Catherine Dempsey (Simplex Wire & Cable Company, Cambridge, Massachusetts), a pioneer in the fight for recognition of industrial nursing. Other officers were Elizabeth Sennewald (Dolphin Jute Mills, Paterson, New Jersey), first vice-president, Polly Acton (*New York Times*), second vice-president, Martha Purcell (Thompson Products, Incorporated, Detroit), treasurer.

While insisting upon freedom to direct their own activities, the industrial nurses saw the need for some sort of working arrangement with other organizations in related fields. In 1943 they petitioned the ANA for a meeting at which recognition of the AAIN would be considered. They received the following reply:

> The American Nurses' Association recognizes the National Organization for Public Health Nursing as the national association concerned with public health nursing, and that association has created a section on industrial nursing. Therefore, it seems inadvisable for the ANA to recognize a second national nursing organization which is concerned with one special phase of public health nursing only, particularly as provision for this type of nursing has been made by the National Organization for Public Health Nursing.[9]

This viewpoint remained unchanged even after the ANA had organized its own industrial section, although nurses appointed as members of that section also asked that the AAIN be recognized as the national association representing industrial nurses and industrial nursing. Opinion polls were taken, correspondence and discussion continued, but the stalemate went on and on. The ANA took no decisive action; the AAIN clung to its position, which its president, Mary E. Delehanty, said in 1948 was characterized by "the hope and desire of industrial nurses for amity and working unity, without duplication of activities between the AAIN and the ANA." They would, she commented, "like to remain in the ANA as members.[10]

In October, 1941, a full six months before the AAIN was officially established, the problem of a professional affiliation for industrial nurses came up for discussion at a directors' meeting of the AAIP&S. A committee was appointed, consisting of Daniel L. Lynch (chairman), J. M. Carlisle, and J. J. Wittmer, "to consider what the association might do to help and guide the nurses employed in industry." At the next annual meeting in Cincinnati (April, 1942), just six days before the industrial nurses officially launched their own national association, Lynch's committee made a full report to the Board, commending the nursing organizations for their "noteworthy progress" and recognizing "the parallel relationship between the work of the nurse in industry and the physician in industry."

Commenting on the fact that membership in the AAIP&S was limited to duly qualified physicians, and must remain so, the report made the following recommendations:

"That nurses in industry be encouraged to develop their national organization, and that this association assist, as far as may be possible and proper, toward that end.

"That the national organization of industrial nurses be invited to hold its annual meeting each year with this association and be invited to take part in its program."

So, after necessary formalities had been completed, another large related group joined an annual assembly which has become increasingly important, year after year, as the arbiter of standards and procedures in the field of industrial health.

Time did not permit the AAIN to participate fully in the 1943 meeting, which was labeled as a Wartime Conference on Industrial Health, but close to fifty industrial nurses were present as guests of the AAIP&S. There was, however, an enthusiastic response at the St. Louis conference in 1944 to a call which read as follows:

"This will be the first big industrial nurses' meeting to be held in the Midwest, and we are looking forward to welcoming industrial nurses from every state. We earnestly urge every industrial nursing group to send representatives to these sessions, at which many important nursing problems will be discussed."

The nurses' program at that meeting, as in subsequent years, showed a full awareness of the obligations assumed by the AAIN in 1942, when it announced simply that its objective was "to improve the standards of nursing practice in industry." At the time the association was established it represented perhaps 300 industrial nurses; as this is written its membership is approaching 5,000. And the annual meeting in Chicago in 1954 attracted a nurse registration of more than 500.

The objectives, the purposes, of the industrial nurses' organizations? They were quoted (1957) from national and state bylaws by Evelyn M. Johnson, president of the Michigan State Association of Industrial Nurses, in a message to members:

> To maintain the honor and character of the nursing profession.
> To improve community health by bettering nursing service to workers.
> To develop and promote standards for industrial nurses and industrial nursing services.
> To stimulate interest in and provide a forum for the discussion of problems in the field of industrial nursing.
> To stimulate industrial nurse participation in all nursing activities, local, state, and national.
> To do within the limits of law all things necessary, proper, incidental, suitable, useful and conducive to the complete accomplishment of the foregoing purposes.

The American Association of Industrial Nurses, like the Industrial Medical Association, has been fortunate in its leadership. The dynamic Catherine Dempsey served as president from 1943 to 1947. Mary E. Delehanty, her successor (Equitable Life Assurance Society), was elected to two consecutive terms of two terms each (1947–1951). Thelma J. Durham (Continental Can Company) served as chief executive from 1951 to 1953, when she was succeeded by Sara P. Wagner, for many years on the staff of Standard Oil Company of New Jersey.

The AAIN underwent the severest test of its unity and stability in 1952, when it was called upon to decide whether or not the organization should be dissolved as a prelude to merger with the National League for Nursing. The momentous question was presented to the membership in essentially this language: "Shall we join organically with our allies or continue to go it alone? Shall we trade our present right of decision in an independent organization for limited autonomy in a larger and stronger interdependent organization?"

Delegates to their 1952 conference discussed this proposal at length—then asked: "What do our doctors think?" They received their answer immediately (April 22, 1952) in the form of this resolution by the IMA directorate, also in session at Cincinnati: "The Board of Directors of the IMA look favorably upon continuation of the American Association of Industrial Nurses as an organizational entity. This is based on recognition of excellent contributions that the AAIN has made to the specialty of industrial nursing."

In a historic standing vote at their business session the following day, almost exactly ten years after their association was launched, the nurses rejected the dissolution proposal by a majority of thirty to one. Their decisive action was not only an expression of unqualified faith in the future of occupational nursing but a vote of confidence in the organizational aims and procedures of the IMA. Of this meeting, at which President Thelma Durham officiated, the *AAIN Newsletter* commented: "It was an adult performance, an event of unforgettable drama and sober democracy."

Thus, another large and capable group successfully worked out a pattern in partnership with other professional and technical associates, who, in modern industrial medical departments, have been welded into alert and resourceful teams, functioning with skill and precision that match hospital standards.

What is the future of industrial nursing and its representative organization? Members, on the whole, would perhaps agree with the opinion of Evelyn Johnson (General Motors Technical Center), who wrote:

"The constantly changing pattern of industry presents new and exciting challenges to the industrial nurse of today. To do an effective job of nursing care, she must keep abreast of new trends in medicine as well as in industry. The changes to automation, radioactive isotope development, the stress and strain of modern living, create new conditions which must be recognized if the specialty of industrial nursing is to progress and maintain its pace with the industrial health team."[11]

The executive viewpoint is well summed up in these words from President Sara Wagner's annual report in 1956:

> If industrial nursing is to make a serious impact on the future development of nursing, if it is to meet the challenge of the expanding industrial health field, it must continue to grow. If industrial nursing has real vitality, its history is a ceaseless evolution. If development is to be intelligent, final goals must be clearly defined and dependable gauges of progress must be found. For unless our job is measurably reaching its objectives, it is moribund. . . .
>
> What the future requires is a gradual perfecting of what we now have. What we build must be devoted to the end of raising our real work to higher levels of

distinction. On no other basis can we proceed with conscience and sincerity. Ours is not an experiment in need of bolstering against imminent collapse but a permanent institution with a mission for a distant future.[12]

*   *   *

The minds of men, in the latter forties, had become acclimated to an atmosphere of continuous crisis, or so it seemed. Change followed fast on the heels of change. The times were freighted with problems that had no precedent, all demanding immediate decision. Industrial medicine, like every other business and profession, had its share of these. Soon to come were revolutionary developments in applied science, technology and production, all vitally affecting health programs in industry.

The AAIP&S had served well, and fared well, during the war emergency. Its president in the "proxy" year of 1945–1946, Melvin N. Newquist, had amply demonstrated the value of his training and experience as an administrator. The officers and directors had managed not only to take care of essential current business but also to make substantial progress in important postwar planning. The proxy election had gone smoothly. Bylaw revisions had been approved. The Foundation of Occupational Health (Occupational Health Institute), as authorized by the ballot, was officially established June 22, 1945, and started operations soon afterward with a nest egg of $1,600 in gifts.

A graduate of the University of Nebraska College of Medicine in 1924, Newquist practiced general surgery for several years. He made his mark in industrial medicine in the thirties, as assistant director of the appraisal of medical services in industry by the American College of Surgeons. In 1939 he became medical director of the Texas Company. During his long membership in the association he has been extemely active in its affairs. A tireless crusader in the campaign for certification of industrial medicine as a specialty, he strongly supported plans for the Foundation, development of which was one of the chief objectives of Frederick Slobe's administration. Newquist has also served as a member of the Editorial Board of *Industrial Medicine.* Retiring from the presidency in April, 1946, he made a stirring appeal for an adequate program of rehabilitation, improved medical services in small plants, and recognition of the needs in industrial medical education.

When cancellation of the 1945 annual meeting became a certainty, near the close of President Slobe's term, there was much speculation as to how much, if any, of the elaborate program already arranged for that occasion could be salvaged, and how much interest there would be in the 1946 convention, provided it, too, did not become a war casualty. Those questions came first on the agenda at a long session of the Board in February, 1945.

As events proved, there need have been no worry about the drawing power of the postponed meeting. The Chicago conference in April 1946, was the largest up to that time, and one of the most successful. Clinics at St. Luke's and Cook County hospitals, planned for the year before, reappeared on the program. So did joint sessions with the hygienists' associations and a well-planned panel discussion with the industrial nurses.

There also was an important new attraction, for the American Association of Industrial Dentists, carrying out a long considered plan, added its contingent to the organizations participating in the annual conferences of the AAIP&S. This was the beginning of another valued and productive alliance within the structure of industrial health agencies.

The American Association of Industrial Dentists came into being under highly favorable circumstances. From the start it had the blessing of the strong and solidly established American Dental Association, and it has been actively supported by that organization's Council on Dental Health. It was, in fact, the ADA Committee on Economics which called the first meeting of United States Dentists practicing in industry to discuss the need for a permanent organization. This was in 1942, but cancellation of the annual ADA convention caused a postponement until February, 1943.

Like many another milestone in America's crusade for health, organization of the industrial dentists was a war-born project. Announcing the meeting, the ADA *Journal* said:

> The dental health problems created by the rapid expansion of the population in the centers of war production have given impetus to the development of industrial dental health programs to meet emergency needs. . . . The industrial program is now at a critical stage, and careful guidance is needed to assure that the interests of public health and the rights and interests of the dental profession are properly served.
>
> No group is better qualified to assist in giving this needed guidance than the men who are themselves engaged in the practice of dentistry in industry. At present, however, there is no channel through which industrial dentists and others concerned with the development of this industrial program can be heard as a group.[13]

The importance of oral health as a factor in general health had of course been understood, and the universal need for dental care had been recognized, long before such industrial programs were even considered. It must be remembered, however, that dentistry itself progressed very slowly in a younger America. For many generations it was regarded as a craft or trade and did not attain the dignity of a modern profession until after the turn of the twentieth century. Early dentistry, or what passed for dentistry, had little in the way of scientific authority to recommend it. It has been said that a dentist of the 1850's usually did one of three things for a patient: extracted aching teeth (none too gently), pounded fillings into cavities, or capped them (where a smile would reveal them) with gold foil.

Dentistry, like medicine, was given great impetus as a profession between 1910 and 1915, largely as a result of the Flexner survey which triggered a reappraisal of medical and dental education and extensive reforms in teaching methods. Writing in

Industrial Medicine and Surgery in 1951, Edward R. Aston, a former president of the American Association of Industrial Dentists and a powerful advocate of industrial dental programs, states that oral health in industry was discussed by authors as early as 1920.[14] The first professional paper on industrial dentistry to be scheduled at an AAIP&S convention ("The Scope of Work in an Industrial Clinic") was delivered at the 1923 annual meeting in Buffalo by a Cleveland physician, Ralph W. Elliott.

There was, however, a considerable lag between discussion of industrial dental problems and productive action toward their solution, if the pages of the official journal of organized industrial medicine may be taken as a criterion of interest on the part of employers and their medical departments. The great expansion of industrial dental literature seems to have started in the 1940's, contemporaneously with the war and the rise of the AAID.

Brief excerpts from a few of many major papers, published in *Industrial Medicine* during that decade, represent typical findings as to the extent and seriousness of dental troubles among industrial workers of that time, and indicate their importance as a factor in absenteeism and loss of production.

In an article published in 1940 on the health of workers, for example, Royd R. Sayers (USPHS) cites one of the findings of A. G. Kammer, who examined 6,100 old employees and 3,900 applicants for employment in a steel plant. "The most common type of defect among the old employees," he says, "was dental impairment, 42 percent against 14 percent for new employees."[15]

Outlining a dental program in 1941, Ernest W. Miller (chief surgeon, Milwaukee Electric Railway & Light Company) wrote: "It may truly be said that a large number of conditions which come to the attention of the internist or gastro-enterologist are primarily the result of some dental pathology. Needless to say, the theory has long prevailed that much of our gastric pathology, as well as gall bladder disease and even the common appendicitis, may be attributable to a focus of infection in the mouth."[16]

Under the intriguing title, "You Are Only as Healthy as Your Teeth," Lon W. Morrey, D.D.S., then publications director of the ADA, wrote in 1944: "A survey conducted by the University of Illinois College of Dentistry shows that war workers in particular are subject to certain specific mouth troubles. Dust, gases, and acids are the principal mouth hazards."[17]

Writing on "Industry's Toothache," originally published in *Oral Hygiene* in 1946, Dr. Ernest Goldhorn (Pullman Company, Chicago) affirmed: "Of the many factors that influence health, mental and physical fitness—such as nutrition, recreation, sanitation, and housing—dental ill health is probably the most constant and affects far greater numbers in all branches of industry and occupations."[18]

To what extent do oral impairments contribute to absenteeism? Dr. H. A. Hooper, Chicago dental consultant, wrote in 1942: "There is authority for the statement that at least 25 percent of employee absenteeism from nonoccupational illnesses is directly traceable to oral conditions. . . . Their majority prevalence in the general population has been common knowledge, especially since World War I. They caused more rejections at that time than any other physical defect."[19]

Writing on the same subject ten years later, Dr. James M. Dunning, lecturer on public health dentistry at Harvard, emphasized the seriousness rather than the amount of such absenteeism. "The dental absences," he states, "are a relatively small proportion of the total, but they assume an importance well beyond their frequency for three reasons: 1) the dental absences so listed are only those referred quite locally to the teeth and gums and do not include the more remote sequelae of dental infection; 2) they are usually associated with a need for corrective treatment beyond the mere abatement of acute symptoms; and 3) are preventable to a surprising extent."[20]

Perhaps the most critical problem of industrial dentistry in its early years lay in the fact that a very large percentage of young men and women, applying for their first jobs in industry, had only the vaguest notions about oral hygiene and had had little or no regular dental care. Because of neglect, dental impairment progressed unchecked, often resulting in deep-seated and serious effects on general health.

Broad-scale action to improve dental conditions in industry was spurred by the manpower situation very early in the 1940's. The federal health services were gravely concerned about the rate of rejections by the military services for dental reasons. Among outstanding men in the dental field who attended the meeting of February 22, 1943, were James M. Dunning, then dental director of the Metropolitan Life Insurance Company; L. D. Heacock and G. L. Nevitt, representing the USPHS; Carl M. Peterson, Secretary of the AMA Council on Industrial Health; and Ernest Goldhorn, of Chicago.

About sixty dentists from all sections of the country were present at the preliminary meeting. It was agreed that they should constitute a temporary organization, pending the final establishment of a permanent association and the adoption of a constitution and bylaws. The organization meeting was scheduled for October, 1943, in Cincinnati, scene of the annual convention of the ADA in that year.

An alliance with the industrial dentists was first discussed by the Board of the AAIP&S at a meeting in May, 1943. Edward Holmblad reported that the new dental group was still in the process of organization. Loyal Shoudy stated that he had talked with a past president of the ADA, who had told him that the new industrial group "would like to meet with us" and would assume part of the program.

In February, 1944, Holmblad reported a letter from the AAID that spoke encouragingly of "joining," and described a scientific exhibit representing the "dental viewpoint on industrial diseases" which the dentists hoped to display at an AAIP&S convention when available. In that year, with necessary agreements negotiated, the dentists were welcomed officially as a participating organization.

Cancellation of the 1945 convention naturally came as a great disappointment to the new association. At the Board meeting of the AAIP&S at which it was announced, Goldhorn represented the AAID. In its second year, he said, membership

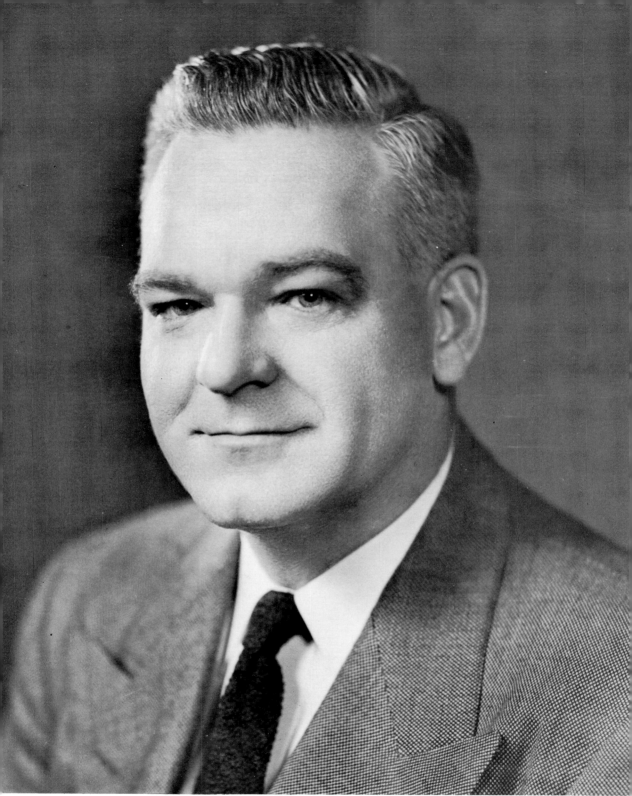

111. *George F. Wilkins, M.D.* (1907–   ). *President, IMA, 1953–1954.* Two main objectives —"Board" status for occupational medicine and provision of necessary education in the specialty —were in the spotlight when Wilkins took over the presidency. He vigorously advanced both objectives, insisting that specialists be of highest caliber and industrial medical standards above criticism. Wilkins joined the New England Telephone & Telegraph staff in 1937 and became medical director in 1948, after four years of active service in World War II. He is a widely recognized authority on absenteeism and the rehabilitation of alcoholics.

—*Photo, Fabian Bachrach*

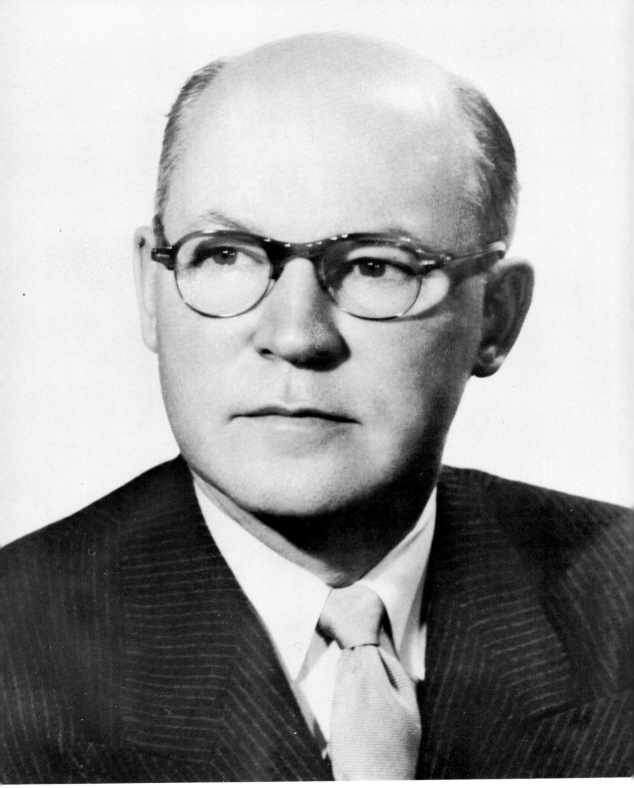

112. *Robert Collier Page, M.D.* (1908–   ). *President, IMA, 1954–1955.* Page entered the industrial field in 1939, when he left the staff of Northwestern University Medical School to join Standard Oil (New Jersey) as assistant medical director. After war service—as command surgeon of the First Air Commando Force—he returned to Standard Oil in 1946 as general medical director, responsible for global services available to 120,000 employees, and in 1955 was appointed chief medical consultant. Since 1949, he has been associate clinical professor of industrial medicine at New York University. He has written extensively on preventive medicine and health maintenance.

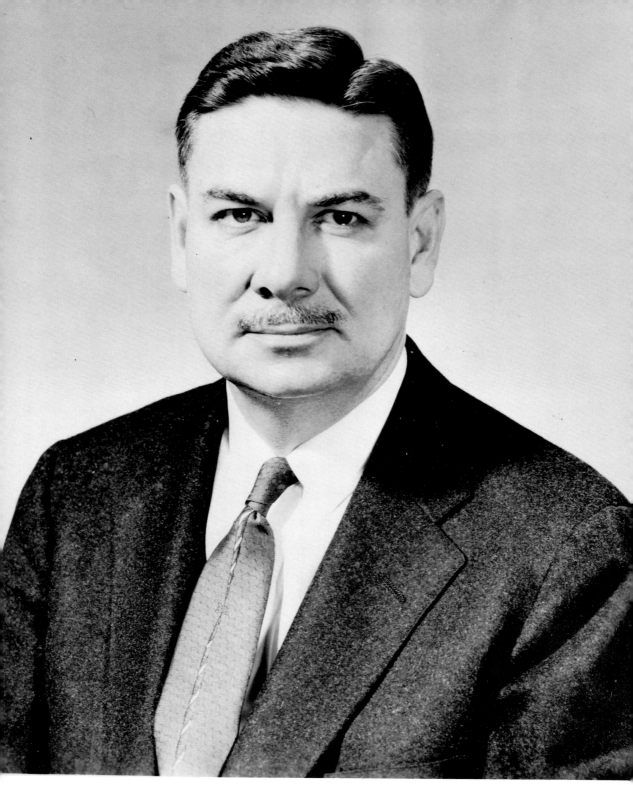

113. *Kieffer Davis, M.D. (1913–   ). President, IMA, 1955–1956.* Problems of industrial medical education and certification headed agenda for the meeting at which Kieffer Davis—medical director of the Phillips Petroleum Company since 1947—took over the presidency. As chairman of a special committee on OHI affairs he was intimately familiar with all aspects of the certification issue, now completed. He dedicated his administration to the task of gearing IMA machinery to rapid growth, and to "the enlightenment of many more of our professional colleagues to the true meaning of occupation health."

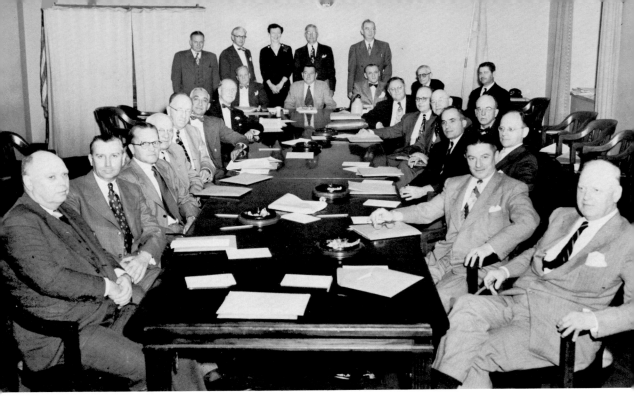

114. *President Truman's Conference on Occupational Safety.* The co-ordinating committee of the President's 1951 Conference in session at Washington, D.C. By Presidential invitation the IMA was represented by two members: E. C. Holmblad (left front), A. H. Whittaker (right front).

Late Presidents of the IMA

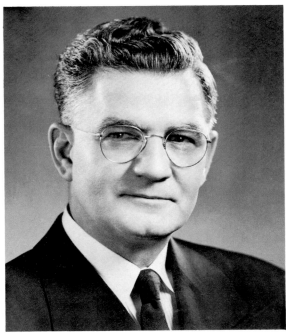

115. *President: Eli S. Jones, M.D., 1956–57,* Hammond, Indiana.

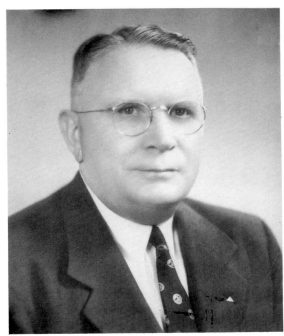

116. *President: Jerome W. Shilling, M.D., 1957–58,* Southern California Telephone Company, Los Angeles 27, California.

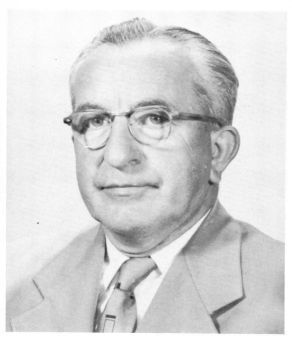

117. *President:*
Hans W. Lawrence, M.D., 1958–59,
Procter & Gamble Company,
Ivorydale 17, Ohio.

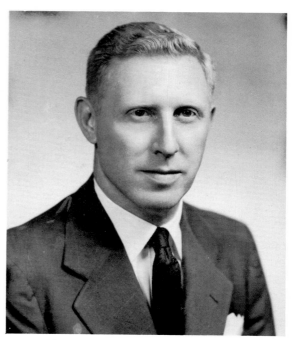

118. *President: John D. Lauer, M.D., 1959–60,*
Hilton-Davis Chemical Company,
National Lead Company,
Cincinnati, Ohio.

Officers of the IMA, 1960–61

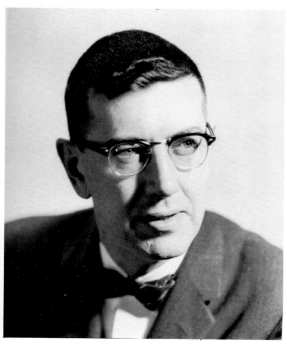

119. *President: R. E. Eckhardt, M.D., 1960–1961,*
Esso Research & Engineering Company,
Linden, New Jersey.

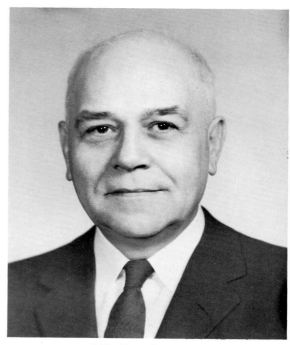

120. *President-Elect:*
Gradie R. Rowntree, M.D., 1960–61,
Fawcett-Dearing Printing Company,
Louisville 1, Kentucky.

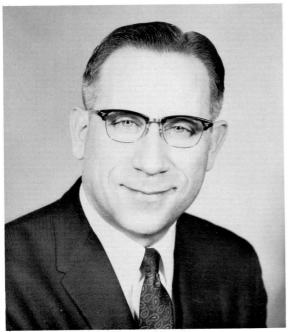

121. *First Vice-President:*
H. Glenn Gardiner, M.D., 1960–61,
Inland Steel Company,
East Chicago, Indiana.

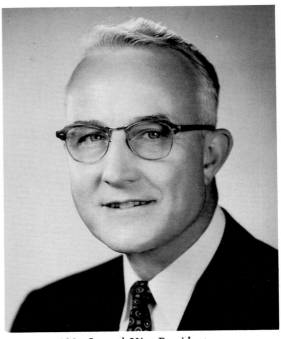

122. *Second Vice-President:*
John L. Norris, M.D., 1960–61,
Eastman Kodak Company,
Rochester 4, New York.

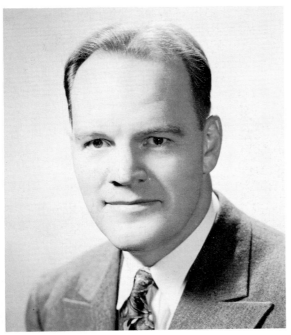

123. *Secretary: Leonard Arling, M.D., 1960–61,*
Northwest Industrial Clinic,
Minneapolis 14, Minnesota.

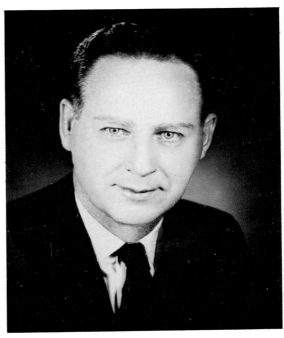

124. *Treasurer:*
Jermyn F. McCahan, M.D., 1960–61,
Western Electric Company,
Chicago, Illinois.

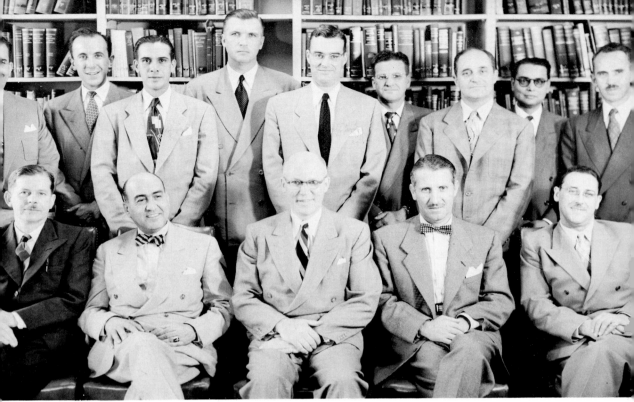

125. *International Staff, Standard Oil of New Jersey.* To companies maintaining worldwide organizations, occupational health demands uniform medical standards and procedures in all quarters of the globe. Physicians representing holding and affiliated companies in a dozen countries are shown here, attending a medical indoctrination course conducted by Dr. Robert C. Page as general director of Standard Oil of New Jersey. Standing, left to right: **Dr. Fernando Diaz, Brazil;** Dr. Enrico Aonzo, Italy; Dr. T. E. Aramburu, Cuba; Dr. F. J. Rummel, Massachusetts; Dr. J. M. Daley, New York; Dr. R. M. Adams, Louisiana; Dr. Guillermo Gorbitz, Peru; Dr. R. Majumder, India; Dr. Gordon Sinclair, Canada; seated, left to right: Dr. E. H. Capel, England; Dr. Alfonso Bortone, Venezuela; Dr. R. C. Page, New York, Dr. F. V. B. Dumoulin, Indonesia; Dr. J. J. L. Garelly, France.

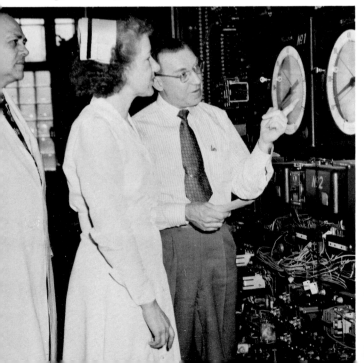

126. *Instruction in Plant Operation.* Gradie R. Rowntree, medical director of the Fawcett-Dearing Printing Company, Louisville, Kentucky, believes all medical personnel should be thoroughly familiar with plant operations. Dr. Rowntree ('at left) and nurse are being briefed on electrical equipment.

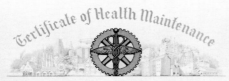

Certificate of Health Maintenance

The
OCCUPATIONAL·HEALTH·INSTITUTE
HAS·APPROVED·THE·MEDICAL·SERVICE·OF

WHICH·HAS·COMPLIED·WITH·THE·STANDARD·FOR·MEDICAL·SERVICE
IN·INDUSTRY·AS·ESTABLISHED·AND·APPROVED·BY
THE·INDUSTRIAL·MEDICAL·ASSOCIATION

I
THIS establishment has an organized medical department with competent medical staff, including consultants. It has policy, procedures and facilities for adequate emergency dispensary and hospital needs and personnel to assure efficient care of the ill and injured.

II
MEMBERSHIP on the medical staff is restricted to doctors and/or nurses who are (a) graduates of acceptable schools of learning with degrees of Doctor of Medicine and Registered Nurse respectively, in good standing and licensed to practice in their respective states or provinces, (b) competent in the field of medicine and nursing as applied to industry, (c) worthy in character and in matters of professional ethics.

III
FACILITIES are available for the performance of competent preplacement and periodic medical examinations in keeping with existing needs of the organization.

IV
A system of accurate and complete records is maintained. Such records include, particularly, a report of injury and illness, description of physical findings, treatment, estimated period of disability, end results, as well as other information pertinent to the case or required by statute for Workmen's Compensation claims and other purposes. All medical records are regarded as confidential material filed under medical supervision, and maintained only in the medical department.

V
EMPLOYEES requiring special care are referred to competent consultants.

VI
THE medical department has general supervision over the sanitation and industrial hygiene of the plant which has to do with the health and medical welfare of all employees.

This certificate is hereby granted

_____ to

Chairman, Board of Trustees

District Counselor

127. *OHI Certificate of Health Maintenance.* Issued by the Occupational Health Institute to organizations in which complete medical department surveys indicate compliance with standards of medical service in industry established by the IMA.

128. *The Knudsen Award Plaque.*

WILLIAM S. KNUDSEN AWARD
GEORGE HOWARD GEHRMANN, M.D.
FOR THE
MOST OUTSTANDING CONTRIBUTION
TO INDUSTRIAL MEDICINE
1954   1955

INDUSTRIAL MEDICAL ASSOCIATION

had about trebled, but the association had to work out ways and means of keeping that membership interested and intact.

Alfred Whittaker, as a director and chairman of the AAIP&S Committee on Component Societies, replied: "I think you should have 2,000 members instead of 200. I think the doctors should do all they can to stimulate interest in industrial dentistry, because the workmen's teeth are in bad condition, and most of the larger plants should have more dental service than they do. I hope we can help you to enlarge your membership."

At its first joint meeting with other industrial health agencies (in April, 1946) the industrial dentists presented a very creditable two-day program, which included two joint sessions with the industrial doctors, a spirited round-table discussion, and papers by Edward R. Aston, dental consultant of the Pennsylvania Department of Health, and C. O. Sappington, editor of *Industrial Medicine.*

Officers of the AAID in that year were James M. Dunning (Cambridge, Massachusetts), president, R. M. Walls (Bethlehem, Pennsylvania), president elect, E. R. Aston (Harrisburg, Pennsylvania), vice-president, and Lyman D. Heacock (USPHS), secretary-treasurer.

Some fifteen years after its organization, the AAID finds that deep-seated dental troubles of long standing are still a continuing problem. As one writer remarked, industry cannot wait for job applicants to have all dental impairment corrected before they are hired. Years of accumulated neglect, when discovered, usually call for extensive work, and many industrial workers, even today, indicate that they cannot afford the treatment they should have.

The profession, of course, is in agreement that the ideal way to dental health would be to start with baby teeth and continue with regular inspection and prophylaxis for life. Since this cannot usually be assured, the dentists accept the alternative of starting as early as possible and doing what can be done. The accent, nevertheless, is on preventive rather than corrective dentistry.

There is, however, a bright side in the industrial picture. As Edward R. Aston, one of America's leading authorities on industrial dentistry, points out, dental programs in industry provide an excellent means of evaluating the various programs for children, by examining industrial workers "as they graduate from these programs and are absorbed by industry."[21]

Further, in summarizing the results of a formidable study of dental health in Pennsylvania industries, made by the state Department of Health in the late forties, Aston found that "more than two-thirds of those examined were in the habit of obtaining dental care every year or less, indicating that in the younger age groups, school dental health groups were effective."[22]

More recently Aston cited insurance statistics based on records of 1,000 employees with good mouth conditions and 1,000 with poor conditions as evidence that the latter group had a greater incidence of ailments that resulted in absence from work. "Current surveys also corroborate this statement," he comments, "revealing an average of four and a half days per employee per year are lost from work because of toothache or some dental ailment. From this figure it is easy to see that the dental disability rate is an industrial liability."[23]

Summing up the Pennsylvania dental health campaign, which may be regarded as a thoroughly modern approach to this industrial problem, Aston says: "The three major objectives of the program are, first, to detect dental diseases of occupational origin, second, to ascertain the dental health of the employees, and third, to educate employees in the importance of dental health."[24]

For dental services industry depends upon three professional groups: the full-time industrial dentists who make industrial dentistry their specialty, those engaged on a part-time basis, and dentists on call as needed. Actually, industries may use only one, or combine all three, of these arrangements. Departments vary widely in size and system, ranging from highly organized programs (such as that of the Du Pont Company or the cooperative enterprises exemplified by the joint plan of textile mills in Wyomissing, Pennsylvania) to first-aid stations entirely dependent on dentists on call.

Another effective type of dental service is found in the huge River Rouge plant of the Ford Motor Company, employing more than 70,000 workers. Ford's first industrial emergency hospital, at the Highland Park plant in 1916, included a complete dental department, and the company has since given a certain amount of non-industrial care because of wartime or economic emergencies. At the close of World War II, however, dental staff services were again concentrated at the Rouge plant.

Describing the problems of dentistry in so large a plant, Grant MacKenzie, Ford dentist and a former president of the AAID (1954–1955), states: "I wish to reiterate that while we did not then and do not now provide full dental care in forty different plant locations, we do arrange facilities so that all Ford employees are given full *industrial* dental care."[25] With respect to general, personal care, the procedure provides for examinations on request, and referral to family dentists.

During the early years of the chemical era industrial dentists were repeatedly warned of the dangers of contact with certain acids and gases. Armed with a list of such hazards and their oral manifestations, prepared in 1949 by C. O. Sappington, MacKenzie consulted the records of his department. "I find," he reported, "that while a number of our employees work with many of the chemicals Dr. Sappington named, the controls on these chemicals developed by our safety and industrial health departments have reduced the hazards of working with them to the point of nonexistence."[26]

There is every indication, as this is written, that industrial dentistry is rapidly coming into its own. There have been no serious roadblocks in the path of progress, other than the inevitable hurdles of financial problems and difficulties of increasing personnel and extending programs in industry.

The AAID has fostered good public relations in every direction, cooperating closely with other associations and with medical departments in industry. Its parent organization, the ADA, sees a great future in the industrial field and a need for many more dentists. More and more employers are recognizing the value of modern dental programs as a matter of sound management. And dentists in private practice are reassured by the AAID's endorsement of the following policy adopted by the ADA in 1942: "We feel that work done on company premises should be limited chiefly to preventive measures and emergency treatment, referring all corrective work to the private practitioner as a stimulus to private dental practice."[27]

*   *   *

In those busy years of growth and progress at the close of World War II there were sad, as well as pleasant, duties to be performed within the AAIP&S. During the presidential administrations of Melvin Newquist and his successor, Loyal Shoudy, an unusually large number of prominent members came to the end of their service to their profession. Among the deaths recorded and announced were the following:

In 1945, C. F. N. Schram (aged sixty-one), distinguished industrial surgeon and president of the AAIP&S in 1929–1930; A. W. George, of Detroit (at sixty-two), chief surgeon of the Packard Motor Car Company and for many years a director of the AAIP&S; and Donald B. Lowe (aged sixty-two), who served as president of the association from 1931 to 1934.

In 1946, Francis D. Patterson (at seventy), special medical consultant for the Pennsylvania Railroad, distinguished both in medicine and in public service; Frank T. McCormick (at sixty-six), a director of the association, chairman of important committees, and a man of many talents and activities; and Richard E. Newberry, of Atlanta, Georgia (in his fiftieth year), whose keen interest and work as a director added substantially to the prestige of the association.

The passing of these men of the old guard seems, a decade later, symbolic of the end of one era and the beginning of another. For the AAIP&S—its internal reorganization nearing completion, entered a new stage of activity of great historical importance to the future of industrial health.

XXIX

BIG BUSINESS
AND BIG LABOR

NOT long after American ironclad ships had proved their prowess in the Civil War, Henry Adams, impressed by their performance, wrote from London to his brother Charles at home: "I tell you these are great times. . . . Man has mounted science and is now run away with. I firmly believe that before many centuries more, science will be the master of man. The engines he will have invented will be beyond his strength to control. Some day science may have the existence of mankind in its power, and the human race commit suicide by blowing up the world."[1]

Surely Henry Adams knew nothing of nuclear fission; nor could he possibly have visioned very many of the engines men were to invent, but he was not far from the mark. Brother Charles may well have regarded the prediction as an idle dream and dismissed it with a smile. In these times, however, when many a youth scarcely of shaving age can recite abstruse mathematical formulae as glibly as scholarly lads a few centuries ago did their Greek and Latin, Adams' offhand comment seems like a spectacular bit of forecasting.

Well before the start of World War II it was evident that great developments in research and industrial production were on the way, but no contemporary fiction came even close to the truth that was soon to appear. The knowledge for which men had groped in the half-light of the late 1800's and early 1900's unfolded swiftly, like an opening flower, in the glare of mid-twentieth-century science.

As a banquet speaker at the New York meeting of the AAIP&S in June, 1940, General Amos A. Fries, of the United States Army, talked of lessons learned in World War I and pictured the task that lay ahead for industrial medicine in America.

In summary he remarked that "everything done in peace is applicable to war, only it is intensified."[2]

What was true of the first World War was doubly true of the second, whether judged by enormously increased industrial production or by the strides made in medicine and surgery. The cease-fire, however, brought no slackening of activity in industrial engineering or in medical research; on the contrary, the pace steadily quickened. General Fries could, with equal truth, have made his statement in reverse, pointing out that knowledge gained in war is likewise applicable in peace, though the objectives are different.

It was, at best, an uneasy peace that followed the surrender in the Pacific, but manufacture of civilian goods was quickly resumed and on a huge scale. Moreover, hostilities in Korea (1950–53) gave new impetus to research and production of every type; and, sadly, the Korean armistice was but a prelude to a "cold" war. The entire period will be remembered as one which produced more medical and surgical triumphs than had ever before been crowded into a comparable span of time. Obviously, even a bare enumeration of those accomplishments is impossible in this text, yet no story of industrial medicine in our time can be complete without mention of the interests that industry and medicine hold in common, and some discussion of their interlocking problems.

Improvements in the techniques of surgery and postoperative care alone have been of such scope and importance as to challenge credulity. They have enabled the surgeon, teamed with anesthesiologists and special-duty nurses, to make amends in a hundred new ways for nature's missteps and mankind's blunders. And each day's news, it seems, adds to the list.

Within a few brief years we have seen the successful introduction of a score or more of different operations for the repair of damaged and defective hearts. Equally advanced are new techniques in stomach, brain and lung surgery. We have seen successful kidney and cornea transplants in human beings, with hope held out that further insight into the mysteries of transplantation may one day permit broader use of this procedure to save life and conserve health. Mid-century science has worked wonders with prosthesis for amputees. Surgery has to its credit the growth of new human tissues from grafts and has successfully replaced bones and joints by the use of substitute materials.

Concurrently, progress in medicine has been equally impressive, if not perhaps so spectacular. The same period has seen the promise of antipolio vaccine at least partially realized, strengthening the probability that the dread disease may eventually be bracketed with diphtheria and smallpox, as a conquered enemy. Immunizing agents aimed at ancient killers—malaria, typhus, cholera, and many more—have been constantly improved and their fields of usefulness extended. Cancer research grows steadily in volume and effectiveness, and hope grows with it.

While most of the research is in the field of public or general health, its benefits extend to all strata of society and to all age groups, from very young children to very old adults. And, be they sick or injured, partially disabled or otherwise handicapped, organically sound or suffering from some impairment, industrial employees share in the rewards of medical research along with the rest of the citizenry.

If anything, progress in medicine and surgery may be even more important to workers in industry than to those in other occupational fields, because of the very nature of their work and the conditions of their employment. The relation of health to productivity has become increasingly apparent to employers of labor in every decade since the turn of the century. The result of this awareness has been their increasing willingness to support both medical research and industrial medical services.

Beyond their growing interest in the day-to-day health of plant workers, leading manufacturers in a score of great industries have called upon the best of available talents and skills to evolve new mechanical and electrical devices to meet the needs of modern medical science. Chemists, physicists, and engineers; pathologists and surgeons; radiologists, anesthesiologists and other specialists, have teamed together in the task. The twentieth century has been, indeed, an age of weighty problems, but it has likewise been an age of inspired and inspiring solutions, as an unadorned list of a few of its marvels testifies:

The Centri-Filmer, produced by General Motors with researchers at the Michael Reese Foundation. This is a complex rotary machine capable of high-speed operation to sterilize vaccines, serums, or blood on a large-production basis.

The Photoelectric Oxyhemograph, a triumph of GM and Henry Ford Hospital research. It monitors the oxygen blood count of patients during surgery and produces a continuous pen-and-ink recording of conditions that the anesthetist can read at a glance.

The Electric Stethograph, another GM product, inspired by Charles F. Kettering, which so amplifies even faint heart sounds that they can be reproduced visually. It is, in essence, a combination of the doctor's stethoscope and a surface gauge used in automobile production.

The Breathophone, developed at Lutheran Hospital in Baltimore, an ordinary hearing aid of the transistor type, adapted for use in anesthesia. The tiny microphone is removed, inserted in a small T-tube, and placed in the breathing circuit of the unconscious patient. From that point it "broadcasts" clearly to the doctors a continuous record of breathing conditions, including sounds that are normally inaudible.

In the spotlight, too, is a new aid to hospital dietetics, an ingenious pump driven by a small, silent motor, which delivers to the stomach of a patient precise amounts of liquefied natural food at any desired rate. This improved method of tube feeding was pioneered at Ford Hospital by Dr. James Barron and was built by Chrysler engineers.

So goes the list, on and on, typifying the spirit of the age and the rewards of its research. In the sphere of experimentation new products and projects are legion. And lest seemingly fantastic ideas be too lightly dismissed, let us bear in mind that today's experiment may well revise tomorrow's scientific truth.

Already, exploratory science bids fair to strip the human digestive tract of its mysteries, one by one. We read of a tiny "radio pill" developed by RCA engineers. In reality a miniature broadcasting station, it can easily be passed through the stomach and intestines and is expected to transmit valuable information regarding pressures, contractions, acidity, and temperatures.

Matching this device, the University of Michigan has announced the Fiberscope, a flexible cable equipped with lens and lamps, which, its inventors believe, will make possible not only visual observation but detailed still and motion pictures of the stomach walls. This diagnostic aid, in its experimental stage, is likewise the result of cooperative effort by physicians and physicists.

Such products as these, in whatever stage of development they may be, are cited here, not because they are especially adaptable to industrial medicine, but because they emphasize the fact that clear lines can no longer be drawn to separate medical research on the one hand from industrial research on the other. In brief, industry is already a full partner in medical research, not alone through the numerous endowed foundations it sponsors or finances but as a collateral of its mainline activities.

The story of lithium offers an example. This element, the lightest solid known, was discovered in 1818, yet its only important use 125 years later was in storage batteries for mine engines and submarines. Then, suddenly, came a tremendous demand from the military in World War II. Because of its low freezing point and strong affinity for water, lithium became a strategic material, invaluable, among other things, for air purification, the de-icing of airplane wings, and the manufacture of all-weather lubricants. Within a dozen years American plants had increased their capacity to process lithium to nearly 50 million pounds per year. Moreover, the future of this strange element may be even more sensational, since many experts predict it will be indispensable in the production of high-energy atomic fuels on a large scale. Such successes are not, of course, uncommon in this age. Of more than passing interest is the fact that scientists, while studying the behavior of lithium, discovered that its compounds were valuable in the production of synthetic vitamin A and antihistamines and for scores of other seemingly unrelated purposes.

We have also seen a great expansion in the use of aluminum and of less well-known metals which, because of lightness and strength and other characteristics, have suddenly become industrially important. Countless compounds have emerged from chemical obscurity. A surprising number of these have, in one way or another, made important contributions to both medicine and surgery. Thus is medical science profiting from basic industrial research, regardless of what its primary target may be.

This intimate association of industry with general research, in its own plants or through institutes and foundations which it supports, is beyond question an outstanding phenomenon of our time, of great economic and social significance. Such activity requires far more than lip service to science. It calls for huge sums of money, organization at the highest professional level, and (also important) the will to carry on broad and penetrating research beyond the limits of business expediency or the hope of immediate returns.

It is axiomatic that contemporary statistics, for purposes of historical comparison, must be used with extreme caution, not because they are unreliable, but because they may represent short-term activities rather than long-term trends. Nevertheless, a few key figures serve to indicate the scale on which industry is engaging in scientific research, and the way in which it has integrated research expenditures with long-range planning.

One of the earliest industrial research laboratories in America was established about 1890 by E. I. DuPont de Nemours Company, but such research got its first real impetus from the organization of the National Research Council in World War I. In 1921 the council listed 575 of these laboratories; in 1927, more than 1,000; in 1931, a total of 1,620, with about 30,000 scientists and technologists engaged and $200 million per year spent for research.[3]

In contrast, we find one expert, Sumner H. Slichter, Lamont university professor at Harvard, writing in 1954: "Actually the expenditures on organized research in industry in the eight years beginning with 1946 have been more than twice as large as the total for all previous years up to 1946."[4] Industry's investment in research before 1946, he says, totaled a little more than $4,600 billion; while $9.5 billion was spent in the period from 1946 to 1954. Slichter adds that government spending for research in the same eight years was likewise more than double all corresponding outlays prior to 1946.

Reporting on what it called "a zooming expenditure for research and development unique in all history," Newsweek commented (in 1955) that an estimated 15,000 companies were engaged in research activity of some sort and that nearly three-fourths of such work in the United States was performed by 160,000 research men employed by industry.[5]

Obviously, expansion on such a scale could be sustained only in a vigorous and growing economy, and by 1940 an army of forecasters in every walk of life was busily trying to figure out what fate had in store for the nation. By mid-century, however, actual developments had dramatically demonstrated the futility of predicting social and economic trends far in advance. The majority of the 1940 seers, in fact, were almost as wrong as they could have been in charting the future of birth rates and population, production and national income, employment and prosperity. Predicted declines in population turned into increases. Estimates of national income and employment for 1960 were exceeded, in most cases, in the early 1950's.

Late in 1953 the United States Department of Commerce reported that even with figures adjusted to take account of price changes, total national production had risen from a "constant dollar" level of $149 billion in 1929, to $307 billion.[6] Yet, despite this 105 percent increase, the Joint Committee on the Economic Report some twenty-seven months later declared that a $405 billion estimate of the gross national product for 1956 was "a minimum."[7]

These over-all facts and figures give a fairly clear picture of the economic backdrop against which the drama of industrial medicine in the chem-electric era has been played. And beyond this, they underscore the even more remarkable fact that research expenditure in the United States has increased at a much faster rate than the national output itself.

Sumner Slichter referred to a study of 191 large companies which showed that about 44 percent of their research expenditures were for the purpose of creating new products and processes.[8] As he points out, such expenditures necessitate more scrapping and replacement of plant equipment, more rapid obsolescence of consumer goods, and an increased demand for new and improved products, which in turn creates more employment.

Needless to say, capital spending by industry on such a scale is a new economic force in American (and world) history and one exercising a powerful influence on the business cycle. It is equally clear that this expansion, the outpouring of billions rather than millions of dollars per year for development, could not fail to affect profoundly both the health services in industry and the professional organizations responsible for them.

The spirit of inquiry and invention was everywhere in the 1940's, and corporate management found itself in closer accord than ever before with the objectives sought by organized industrial medicine. Industry's own stupendous programs, in fact, were predicated to a considerable extent upon the maintenance of the labor force at the highest level of fitness and efficiency. Moreover, cumulative records in individual industries were clearly demonstrating to employers that the over-all health of workers had substantially improved as a result of safeguards and remedial measures already in operation. This improvement received official confirmation in an elaborate study of United States health, published in 1952 by The Brookings Institution.

One measure of the health and safety progress in industry is the fact that between 1926 and 1950 the rate of injuries and diseases from occupational causes, as reported by the United States Bureau of Labor Statistics, dropped from 24.2 to 14.7 per million man-hours in the manufacturing industries.

Substantial numbers of the companies in the 1951 health survey of the National Association of Manufacturers credited their health and safety programs with reductions in accidents, in the incidence of occupational disease, and in compensation insurance premiums.[9]

Members of the American Association of Industrial Physicians & Surgeons were wide-awake to the opportunity and the challenge of the times when, at the April 1946 annual meeting in Chicago, they elected Loyal A. Shoudy president and launched a vigorous program of postwar activities. Elected to office at the same meeting were Henry S. Brown (Detroit), as president-elect, Harold A. Vonachen

(Peoria, Illinois), first vice-president, Alfred H. Whittaker (Detroit), second vice-president, with E. C. Holmblad continuing as managing director-treasurer, and F. W. Slobe again agreeing to serve as secretary.

It was Shoudy's third term in three decades of service. He was in his 66th year. He had carried heavy responsibilities during the war and had been one of the leading proponents of long-range, large-scale planning for the association. Responding to his introduction as incoming president he told the membership: "I thought that this year they ought to let me step down and out, and let a younger man step in. They wouldn't listen to it. I counseled with some of my own boys and they said no. So I am to be your leader for the next year." Despite this protestation, his eyes were on the future. He devoted his administration to upbuilding the association's staff services to its members and to strengthening its financial position in the face of increasing activities. In this program he had the ardent support of officers and Board.

The forward look in association affairs was reflected in new faces and new viewpoints among the directors elected for 1946–48: M. H. Manson (New York), medical director, American Telephone and Telegraph Company, G. Frederick Oetjen (Jacksonville, Florida), an industrial surgeon serving many oil and insurance companies, Edward H. Carleton (Chicago), well-known orthopedic surgeon, affiliated with the Inland Steel Company, Oscar A. Sander (Milwaukee), an authority on occupational diseases of the lungs, Rutherford T. Johnstone, a specialist practicing occupational medicine in California industries, Frank R. Griffin, a general practitioner of industrial medicine in Toronto.

Times, indeed, were changing. Industrial physicians and surgeons in America had seen their professional specialty grow steadily in responsibility and recognition. Membership in the AAIP&S, little over 500 in the latter thirties, was crowding the 2,000 mark ten years later. The number of medical departments whose services bore the coveted ACS Certificate of Approval had shown a highly satisfying ratio of increase. Industrial practice was attracting more and more young doctors each year.

Cooperative handling of industrial manpower problems during the war had taught valuable lessons. Writing in *Industrial Medicine* late in 1945, Forrest E. Rieke, medical director of the Oregon Shipbuilding Corporation and Kaiser Company, made this astute comment on the postwar situation:

"It is most important that the medical profession recognize that this shared wartime experience of labor, management and the profession in the field of health has given the former two groups a much wider insight into medical matters. They now share an aggressive determination to continue expanded health services; they have every expectation that physicians will exert a vigorous leadership in continuing and enlarging health maintenance work after the war."[10]

The mood of members who flocked to the Buffalo meeting, of the AAIP&S in 1947 was in thorough accord with Rieke's line of thinking. At a seven-hour session officers and directors plunged into a detailed discussion of expansion plans and ways and means of winning industry support for a fellowship program to provide post-graduate education in occupational medicine. There was full agreement on the fundamentals of this plan, but there was also recognition that a long and difficult task lay ahead, calling for effective promotional work with foundations and in-dividual industries throughout the country. These problems were left for con-tinuing study by various committees, from whose findings the program of the associa-tion's Occupational Health Institute emerged in the 1950's.

The meeting was a conspicuous success. Interest in the specialty and in the as-sociation was at a new high. Edward Holmblad reported an actual registration of well over 600, with a total attendance probably close to a thousand. Since easing up on his work in the preceding year, he told the directors, he was able to spend more time in conference with working committees of the association and in talking to young medical students and interns about the opportunities presented by industrial specialization.

There was conspicuous evidence of more thorough planning and better publicity for programmed features. President-elect Henry Seabury Brown, chairman of the Committee on Arrangements, reported that hospital facilities were severely taxed by the number of members wishing to attend scheduled clinics. Alfred Whittaker described elaborate preparations made for a surgical panel discussion conducted by Henry C. Marble, of Boston, the participants attending a special luncheon before the session to go over the subject matter in minute detail. Holmblad announced that 25,000 copies of the preliminary program for the meeting had been sent out during the year. "Such activities," he said, "are beginning to bear fruit."

At this meeting President Shoudy formally stepped down, after thirty-two years of service, during about thirty of which he was active in some official capacity. Brown was duly installed as president, Vonachen as president-elect, Whittaker, as first vice-president, Edward P. Heller, prominent Kansas City industrial surgeon, as second vice-president. Recognizing important services to the association, the follow-ing were elected as directors for 1947–49: A. G. Kammer (South Charleston, West Virginia), F. E. Poole (Glendale, California), L. E. Hamlin (Chicago), E. A. Irvin (Detroit), Robert M. Graham, long affiliated with the Pullman Company (Chicago), and Louis R. Daniels, medical director of the Hood Rubber Company (Watertown, Massachussets) since 1916.

Brown, a native of Providence, Rhode Island, was educated at Brown University and Tufts Medical School. Early in his career he started a general and industrial practice in Detroit, became affiliated with the Michigan Bell Telephone Company in 1924, was appointed medical director in 1930, and served in that capacity for more than twenty-five years. One of his innovations at Michigan Bell was the adoption of an annual course of health instruction "to give female employees an opportunity to learn how to live." A strong proponent of industrial nursing, he had developed in

Detroit a visiting nurse program which attracted widespread attention in industrial centers, and he collaborated closely with the Industrial Nurses Association in its formative years.

Clearly, officers and directors in 1947–48 were agreed that the time had come in AAIP&S affairs for concerted action toward objectives that had been repeatedly stated and thoroughly discussed in preceding years, with emphasis on the certification of occupational medicine, establishment of industrial curricula in the medical schools, and the financing of fellowships through the American Foundation (Occupational Health Institute).

Addressing a joint meeting of industrial medical societies in Ontario and Quebec October 2, 1947, President Brown summed up the administration's policy in these words: "There is still much pioneering work to be done, both in showing young men the tremendous opportunity in the industrial medical field and in demonstrating to management the dollars-and-cents value of a complete medical program. That is the challenge of industrial medicine. Whether organized medicine will meet the challenge or sit idly by, permitting the government or the public health service to take over the work, remains to be seen."

The year 1947 saw honorary memberships in the AAIP&S conferred upon four of its ranking members in point of age: Otto P. Geier, then seventy-three years old, one of the pioneer founders; Henry Field Smyth, of Pennsylvania, eminent teacher of industrial hygiene, who supported the plans and activities of the organization at the time of greatest need; John F. Kenney, who started his industrial practice in Rhode Island in the earliest years of the association; and J. A. Simpson, a veteran among member railway surgeons in Texas.

Such awards were a subtle reminder of the need for constant replacement of manpower in the ranks of a virile and growing organization. There were other reminders. Brown was greatly impressed by the industrial expansion in Canada and the interest in occupational medicine displayed by doctors in the populous provinces. Though the American association could not well establish a component society north of the border, friendly contacts have led many fine Canadian doctors individually to join the AAIP&S (IMA), while maintaining active membership in their own national and local organizations.

Profoundly affecting the course of the specialty in the United States was a strong new trend toward a wholesale geographical shift in industry after the war. Burgeoning of the aircraft, petroleum-chemical, and other great industries in the South and far West not only created new occupational hazards, but immediately brought the problems of industrial health to the forefront in areas where they had been relatively unimportant.

A concentrated drive for new members in 1947 caught this favorable trend as it gained strength. Brown set a total association membership of 2,000 as the goal in this drive, conducted by a committee consisting of E. A. Irvin (chairman), N. E.

Leyda, of Dayton, and Charles F. Shook, of Toledo. The drive missed its objective by a narrow margin, but membership at the end of the administration year had jumped from 1,671 to 1,915, the second largest net gain in the history of the association to that time.

Along with growing membership came marked increase in attendance at annual meetings, which in turn complicated not only the problem of physical accommodations but also the programming of professional activities. Among developments in the late 1940's were notable improvements in convention planning, to provide more time for obtaining key speakers and more care in selection of subject matter.

At the April, 1947, session of the Board of Directors, Boston was approved as the 1948 meeting place, and President-elect Vonachen, as chairman of the Convention Committee, was enabled to start work immediately, with a full year to complete a program. At that same session Alfred H. Whittaker (first vice-president) put in a strong bid for Detroit as the 1949 convention city, assuring the Board of full cooperation of the three big automobile companies, the support of a strong state component, and adequate clinical facilities. The selection was tentatively approved, subject to later confirmation.

Opening the annual business meeting in Boston (April 1, 1948) Henry S. Brown, as outgoing president, remarked on the promise of the times. "I think right now," he said, "we are at the threshold of great things. We have one of the finest and best attended meetings we have ever had."

Secretary Slobe's report reflected the progress of the five preceding years. The component societies were developing into a well-balanced network, effectively covering the main industrial regions of the country. Formation of counselor districts in the United States and Canada was a forward move of much potential value. Long strides had been taken toward certification of the specialty. The Foundation (OHI) had been incorporated. Graduate training in industrial medicine and funds for fellowships remained the two most pressing problems.

At the Boston meeting acceptance by the association of two new annual awards was also announced: one a citation for excellence in medical authorship, donated by *Industrial Medicine* and designed to raise the quality of literature in this field; the other, known as the Health Achievement Award, also given by *Industrial Medicine,* for presentation by the association to an industry making the most significant contribution to health services.

Among members who had labored unceasingly for the success of the Boston convention was Daniel L. Lynch, nearing retirement after more than thirty years of service with the New England Telephone & Telegraph Company. He was given a noisy, rising vote of thanks by the assembled membership. "He was worried," remarked the chairman, "that we would not get a dozen people in the two hospital amphitheaters the other day, and they were both jammed to the roof."

Taking over the presidency at the close of the meeting, Harold A. Vonachen said: "I agree with Dr. Brown that this association has reached a point where we have a tremendous obligation to go forward and a beautiful opportunity in the coming year to do things." Specifically, he stressed again the necessity of educating younger men in industrial medicine and of providing fellowship funds to assist them in postgraduate work.

Educationally, Vonachen was a product of St. Viator College, Bradley University, and St. Louis University Medical School. Professionally, he had served since 1927 as medical director of the Caterpillar Tractor Company, his first industrial affiliation. He was a member of the AMA Council on Industrial Health from 1948 to 1952 and in 1951 was appointed to the Advisory Committee of the USPHS Division of Industrial Health. A man of dynamic personality and marked administrative ability, he has won distinction as an authority on rehabilitation, serving on the Federal Security Agency's Medical Advisory Committee on Rehabilitation, Forest Park Foundation. For his work in this field he had received the Knudsen Award at the 1944 meeting of the AAIP&S.

Installed with Vonachen at the 1948 business session were Alfred H. Whittaker as president-elect, Edward H. Carleton (medical director, Inland Steel Company) as first vice-president, and Adolph G. Kammer (medical director, Carbide and Carbon Chemicals Corporation) as second vice-president. There were new names on the Board of Directors for the 1948–1950 term: George F. Wilkins, medical director, New England Telephone and Telegraph Company, Harold M. Harrison, a native Canadian practicing industrial medicine in Toronto, Earl F. Lutz, associate medical consultant for General Motors Corporation, Robert C. Page, medical director, Standard Oil Company of New Jersey, James M. Carlisle, medical director, Merck & Company, and Edward P. Heller.

From its first full meeting in June, 1948, the new administration concentrated on improving standards of association services and of membership selection. Vonachen was a firm believer in "active and functioning committees," and, in the months that followed, the committee system was measurably strengthened; reports by chairmen and district counselors were discussed in great detail at all Board meetings.

Lines of communication within and without the AAIP&S were greatly improved in January 1949 by distribution of a new association directory listing both alphabetically and geographically the names and addresses of the more than 2,000 members and containing other important data. Also, to improve liaison among members, needed additions were made to the secretarial staff at the Chicago headquarters, a step which later led to the appointment of Mrs. Rita Packer as executive secretary of the association.

Growth of membership and changes in administrative procedure were, however, only straws in a wind that was blowing toward a single, central objective. As outgoing president in April, 1949, Vonachen touched upon it briefly in his final statement to the Board of Directors. "I feel particularly," said he, "that there is one thing we must do more and more in this organization, and it cannot be accomplished in a single year. We have to become more closely associated with management; let management know our problems; let them understand what we have to offer them, and what the future of their organizations is insofar as health is concerned."

Already, in the latter 1940's, a new pattern in the practice of industrial medicine was beginning to take shape. As we have seen, the upsurge of science and technology during and after the war loosed a flood of new chemical compounds and other materials for use in industry, thereby multiplying the health hazards to be identified and held in control. But the change was even more fundamental than this. As management began to see more clearly the value of fitness in the labor force, the total working environment of employees in every major industry became the target for closer analytical study. Any condition that contributed to good health or to ill health was within the purview of the doctor, the hygienist, and the safety engineer.

According to that concept, industrial medical practice called for a sustained attack upon health problems stemming from the subtlest of physiological, psychological, and environmental factors. The problems involved were of many sorts; each, moreover, had characteristics of its own; they could not be grouped in conventional categories or handled by routine procedures.

There were old problems, of industrial fatigue, nutrition, and noise, for example, which were passing through new phases. There was that ancient enemy, tuberculosis, recurring unpredictably and demanding constant vigilance. There were newer hazards rising from radioactive substances, from air pollution, and from man's experiments in flight. These and similar hazards were not necessarily connected with in-plant practice, but nonetheless they required studious attention from the industrial medical profession along with other health agencies.

There were also challenging problems in the new specialty called, as one chooses, "gerontology" (the study of senescence) or "geriatrics" (the medical treatment of the aged), a science which promises much for the comfort and security of the old but which (fortunately or unfortunately) cannot be expected to restore lost youth. This special field received little recognition until 1945, when the American Gerontological Society was organized. The *Journal of Gerontology* was started in the following year, and in 1951 the federal government established a Committee on Aging, now part of the Department of Health, Education and Welfare.[11]

Though none of the foregoing problems or hazards has become of critical importance in industrial medical practice, there was a sharp upturn of interest in these and other related subjects during the 1940's and early 1950's. The trends then, and the reasons for them, are covered in greater detail elsewhere.[12] Studies in environment and its influence, significant research in physiology—coming as they did at a time of great advances in science and technology—imposed added burdens of responsibility upon medical departments in all industries.

Here was the Scientific Revolution reaching an undreamed of peak of momentum and force. Its total impact upon industry, medicine, and labor is as yet immeasurable.

Addressing postgraduate students of industrial medicine at Long Island College of Medicine late in 1944, the New York industrialist Howard Coonley, then director of the Conservation Division of the War Production Board, said:

> In the application of synthetic organic chemistry to preventive and remedial medicine, in methods of treatment of wounds and sickness, the advances made in these few years may ultimately outweigh many times even the staggering losses of the worldwide conflagration.
>
> Yet the usefulness of all these gains in resources depends upon an advance in human relations. It requires an increasing degree of organization and cooperation to utilize this expanded productive capacity, as well as to distribute the products where they are needed.
>
> It requires organization and cooperation, beyond any ever achieved before, to keep the market in such balance that exchange of goods and services will be continuous, that producers may use one another's product, and that all may go on producing." [13]

The broad problem of economic balance is not, of course, new. The dangers of imbalance have been expounded in every era of our history. They were repeated again and again after the war, and they gained new urgency as American production continued its upward spiral.

Industrial medical departments had never before been in so good a position to handle the health services required in a rapidly expanding economy. Employers, fully aware of the problem, were more receptive than ever to plans that would help in the maintenance of a healthy and productive labor force. Industrial practice was attracting capable physicians and surgeons in satisfactory numbers. And for the first time the "health team," at least in the larger and more progressive industries, was on its way to becoming a strong and well-balanced professional unit.

In the postwar period, too, the "participation" plan was bearing fruit in the form of better understanding and closer liaison among related health organizations. The precedent, it will be remembered, was set in 1940 by the American Industrial Hygiene Association, first of such organizations to hold its annual meetings jointly with the AAIP&S to discuss common problems, policies, and plans. Similar participating arrangements with the governmental hygienists (1943), industrial nurses (1944), and industrial dentists (1946) have proved equally successful.

The value of plan-sharing with such associates was emphasized by W. J. Fulton, medical director of General Motors' central office, in an address at the Ninth Congress on Industrial Health in January, 1949, under the auspices of the USPHS and the AMA. In a time-and-job analysis of medicine in industry, he said:

> Not only the full-time industrial physicians should plan, but also that right arm of the physician, the full-time industrial nurse, has planning potentials of equal im-

portance. Included also should be the industrial hygienists, the safety engineers, personnel administrators, and others engaged in human relations activities. . . .

Medicine standing alone in industry is not self-sufficient. While it may and should take the lead, it nevertheless needs the cooperative help of and can give valuable cooperative help to those other agencies.

Fulton went on to voice "a near conviction that perhaps the whole political future of medicine may depend more upon good human relations than upon excellence in the specific art."[14]

A great deal was written about human relations in the 1940's, and the subject was widely discussed in both management and medical circles. There was considerable confusion as to terminology, jurisdiction, and procedures and much duplication of effort. In 1941, for example, the National Association of Manufactures had a committee on health and working conditions, and the AAIP&S a committee on records, personnel, and procedure, both committees being concerned with practically the same problems. The NAM was contemplating a report covering specifications and layouts for medical departments. The United States Public Health Service and the AMA were planning similar studies.

There was also, in the war period, some hysterical thinking with respect to in-plant activities. In 1941 at least one union was reported to have forbidden its members to take part in a nutrition experiment, the suspicion being that the test might prove a worker could live on so little that he would not need any increase in wages.

All such matters required adjustment—the important and the unimportant, the reasonable and the absurd, the strictly medical along with the purely emotional. Clear lines of responsibility had to be drawn, and duplication of effort and of records eliminated. Industrial health personnel had on their hands a difficult task of rectifying relationships within their own groups, as well as with management workers.

The 1940's, in fact, may be considered the dawning period of serious attention to what we now describe as human or personnel relations. And it was in the years around mid-century that the greatest strides were taken to establish the plant medical director as a middleman in industry, responsible to management, but serving impartially the best interests of both employer and employee. Indeed, the niceties of terminology are not important. Human, or personnel, or industrial relations, in the sense in which the terms are used here, can mean no more and no less than relations with the men and women employed in industry and business, since it is for their health and well-being that all these plans and programs have been devised.

"What is needed in a plant," wrote wise Otto Geier in 1916, "is a doctor to look after the human machinery, to study the stresses and strains on it, to give warning of a probable breakdown, to advise easing up on the load until the human mechanism has been adjusted, to do the hundred and one things that make for comfort of mind and body."[15] Also, in 1920, a year of widespread labor unrest, he wrote: "In conserving the body and mind of the worker, the industrial physician is able frequently not only to add to the earning capacity of the man but also to change his attitude toward his job."[16]

We are mainly concerned, in our book, with management-labor relations insofar as they have a bearing on the health and productivity of workers in American industry. Nevertheless, the role of industrial medicine in furthering those ends is better understood if the broad social and economic trends of the past century and a half are kept in mind.

There is scarcely a shadow of resemblance between the jobs, working environments, and living conditions of the industrial employee in America today and those of his English prototype in the period when power machinery was coming into general use. The British worker then was usually ignorant and impoverished. More often than not he lived in squalor, and he was regarded and treated as a chattel. In a comparable period his counterpart on this side of the Atlantic was, in some respects, better off. His was a newer, roomier land, with vast untouched resources, needing workers of every kind, and offering opportunity to all who would pioneer. Yet modern Americans, with their eyes fixed on miracles of invention and production, often need a reminder that labor, as an entity, made small progress in this country until the twentieth century, and that its important gains have come in relatively recent years.

In the forty years following the outbreak of the Civil War the stage was set for the entry of Big Business on the American scene. It was an era of open exploitation of men as well as of national resources. Power and money were being concentrated in the hands of a few individuals, who have been described in terms ranging from "empire builders" and "public benefactors" to "robber barons" and "malefactors of great wealth." What we still conveniently classify as "labor" won very little in the way of recognition or material rewards during that period.

The lot of even skilled workers was far from enviable in 1882, when the first Labor Day was celebrated. The press of the day reported that union members were warned that they would lose their jobs if they took part in the festivities, but some 10,000 turned out to march through the heart of New York, led by a band and a contingent of white-aproned bricklayers. The outlook for organized labor was not promising four years later when Samuel Gompers, with a kitchen table and soapbox chair for furniture, opened his office as president of the (then) National Federation of Labor. And it must be remembered that records from the early decades of the twentieth century were indelibly stamped with the dark history of child labor in mills and mines, sweatshop conditions in many industries, and serious health and accident hazards in many more.

The extent of labor's gains, and the swiftness with which they have piled up in our time, can be indicated by mentioning a few important milestones. According to federal labor statistics, the average work week in the United States in 1850 was 69.8 hours, by 1900 this had been cut to 60.2 hours, a reduction of 9.6 hours in fifty years. But by 1955 it had been shortened to 40.2 hours, a further reduction of 20 hours in fifty-five years. As this is written the five-day week has become general in industry, and there is serious agitation for a standard four-day week of 32 hours or even less.

It will be noted that the period of sharpest reduction in working hours was also the period in which mechanized mass production enjoyed its greatest expansion and employment its greatest growth. With those trends came a corresponding increase in the strength and power of organized labor. Figures from the United States Bureau of Labor Statistics show that union membership (in non-agricultural establishments) jumped from less than 2.75 million workers in 1913 to between 14 and 16 million in 1952.[17] Such figures mean that only about one in every fifteen such employees belonged to unions in 1913 as against an average of roughly one in every four in the early 1950's.

At no time in their entire history have American labor unions taken their eyes from their oldest objectives: higher wages, shorter hours, and improved working conditions. These, though they have been substantially achieved, still remain the primary planks in labor's platform. Strategy, however, has changed; public attention and private negotiation are now centered largely on special programs that do not involve direct wage-and-hour demands but that assure equivalent benefits. Typical, in this category, are health and welfare, pension, and insurance plans, in large numbers and of infinite variety.

A few red-letter years serve to mark the road followed by American labor in its march to power. The calendar may well start with 1926 and the passage of the Railway Labor Act requiring railroads to bargain collectively. The Norris-LaGuardia Act in 1932 prohibited federal injunctions in most labor disputes, and in 1935 the National Labor Relations (Wagner) Act[18] extended collective bargaining to all industry. All wage-and-hour workers won a smashing victory in 1938, when the Fair Labor Standards Act provided minimum wages and time-and-a-half for overtime.

The first big health-welfare fund in industry was set up in 1946 for the United Mine Workers, a step which, because of the size and importance of the organization involved, greatly stimulated other similar projects. The fund was financed by the coal operators with per-ton payments, and the first medical services under its provisions were given to paraplegic employees. Later in 1949, the steelworkers were granted a pension plan, a significant gain.

There were also, in this sequence, two significant events which represented a new long-range approach to wage problems. The first, in 1950, was the signing by General Motors and United Auto Workers of the so-called "escalator" contract in which the wage scale was keyed to the cost of living. The second was the Ford agreement in 1955 on a modified guaranteed wage plan, the Ford Motor Company's answer to the demand for an outright annual wage guarantee.

In this list of innovations the steps that led to full-scale collective bargaining were of the utmost importance. Collective bargaining gave to organized labor

377

exactly what the term implies, the right to meet with management on an equal footing, for expression of its collective views on pertinent issues, and for the discussion and settlement of differences. There can be no doubt that the intent of laws ensuring and regulating such rights has been to substitute orderly negotiation for the hatred and violence so often engendered by strikes.

Common sense, backed by legislation, has indeed gone far toward establishing peaceful procedure in industrial disputes, but obviously no means have been found to do away with recourse to strikes, which American labor traditionally regards as a right under the Constitution. And while strike action itself is widely deplored, the danger is ever present. As someone has said: "The request becomes a demand; the demand becomes a threat; the threat becomes a weapon." So strikes remain on the industrial scene, including that strange hybrid known as the "wildcat" strike, unauthorized and disclaimed by union management but still persisting. We are interested in these work stoppages, here, only with relation to their effect on productivity; and simple statistics show that they have been widespread and extremely costly in almost any period selected.

Addressing the Society of Automotive Engineers in Detroit in 1946, Henry Ford II said: "The Department of Labor shows that a total of 216 million man-days were lost between 1927 and 1941 as a result of strikes alone. I am not here concerned with the justice of these strikes or their injustice. I am saying that some 216 million man-days of work were lost. This idleness was expensive, to the strikers, to the companies, and to the nation."[19]

Entirely aside from participation in or reliance on strikes as a weapon, organized labor has steadily extended the frontiers of collective bargaining ever since that principle became part of American policy, and results have amply proved its potency as a means to union ends. Complete financial reports are not available, but official figures from individual unions indicate that labor treasuries in the mid-fifties contained funds totaling nearly a billion dollars collected in dues and other fees, plus pension and welfare funds estimated at more than $25 billion.

Thus, at this writing, Big Labor has come to sit with Big Business at the conference table. There are differences between them to be reconciled, but the gulf has been substantially narrowed within a few decades. And it is certain that management-labor relations of the future will be worked out by negotiation, as indeed, in the final analysis, they have been in the past.

"I believe," said Mr. Ford in his address, "that management must take the initiative for developing the relationships between labor and management. Labor has a great opportunity to achieve stature through assuming greater responsibility. But I consider that management is in charge, that management must manage, and that the test of management is whether or not it succeeds."[20]

Relatively new in American economic thinking is the concept that management can in a measure control, or at least substantially influence, the business cycle, generally by the exercise of its new sense of social responsibility and specifically by its individual long-range decisions as to new products, prices, and marketing policies. A corollary to this concept is the idea that labor, too, can materially affect economic trends by its collective exercise of restraint or lack of it.

Gone from this country is the primitive, top-heavy capitalism of the nineteenth century. In its place there is solidly entrenched an economy in which the producer is also the consumer of goods and services on an immense scale and in which production is dominated and regulated by the needs, tastes, and desires of consumers at large. It is an economy of almost unlimited potentials, but it succeeds only when it is kept in balance, and it is extremely sensitive to both inflationary and deflationary forces. From this fact stem the repeated warnings of highly regarded economists against excesses on the part of management, labor, or government that might impair the delicate balance required.

With a beneficent system in effect, it seems like an anachronism from the distant past to observe a recurring belief that machines can put men out of business and the fear that some day they will do so. This has been the reaction, in some quarters, to the growth of automation in American industry. Automation has, within a few years, created an enormous literature of its own, and needs no explanation here. Dramatically illustrating the extent to which automatic machinery has penetrated business is the statement that if telephone companies were to go back to the manually operated system that preceded dial phones, there would not be enough women of eighteen to forty years old in the entire country to handle present telephone traffic. Equally dramatic examples are to be found in practically every industry of any importance.

Addressing America's newspaper publishers in New York (April 25, 1955), Henry Ford II said of automation and its effects on business:

> We should remember that technological progress is the very life force of our system, a wave of the future so elemental that, in time, it surely must overwhelm all opposition. The social manipulators—the reactionary men and the systems that oppose technological progress—must some day answer to the poor and hungry masses of the world.
>
> I do not mean to suggest that technological improvements do not ever create problems. Any change involves problems. Machines do constantly eliminate certain kinds of jobs. . . .
>
> Nor is there any direct way I can imagine to avoid by private means the dislocations which come from technological obsolescence. Coal put firewood out of business, and then along came gas and oil. Now it's atomic energy, and one day it may be solar radiation.
>
> Obsolescence is the very hallmark of progress. The faster we obsolete products, machines, and antiquated, costly ways of working, the faster we raise our living standards and our national wealth.[21]

This ideology is, as every student knows, a purely American product; and, since it is the formula by which American business has operated in periods of greatest prosperity, one may fairly assume that most people consider it sound. Nevertheless, as the new technology of production made itself felt in industries of every type, there came, from some segments of organized labor, loud and continued predictions of disastrous unemployment as a result of what we call (for lack of a more inclusive term) automation.

This clamor against mechanization was strangely reminiscent of the cry of the weavers in early nineteenth-century England that steam power would condemn them eternally to idleness and pauperism. Seemingly, those who echoed that fear in the mid-twentieth century were overlooking the fact that increased production at lower cost has been in this country a highroad to prosperity, that no other workers in history have ever been so well cushioned against unemployment and, in general, that there is no absolute economic security short of slavery.

"I, for one," said Henry Ford in his address to the publishers, "am highly impatient with the reactionary thinking of some union leaders, who stand resolutely against progress, who resist the introduction of new machines and methods, who seek to preserve obsolete trades and skills, who generally are wedded to the mean and miserly concept of a mature economy that is going nowhere—in short, the advocates of guaranteed stagnation."

Employers were quick to concede that progress in industry was inevitably attended by some technological unemployment, but they also pointed out that improved machinery and methods were tools which, in the long run, workers could use to increase their productivity and earning power. At the same time they considered it significant that while some plants reported satisfactory increases in output per manhour, time studies in other plants indicated a slowdown in many operations. Here, it appeared, was another issue to be settled by discussion and negotiation—another test, on a broad scale, of management-labor relations.

What, one may ask, have all these technical and economic developments to do with industrial medicine? The question can be answered briefly. Let it be clear, however, that industrial medical directors, in their official capacity, have no partisan interest in labor disputes or negotiations as such. Their concern is with working conditions as they affect health; their job is to promote and conserve health by every practical means. On that basis the professional interests of an industrial physician rightly extend to any aspect of health that interrupts production by the working force or impairs its quality.

Currently, business as a whole is deeply disturbed by the extent of absenteeism and the dangers of an upward trend in it. It has been the subject of elaborate studies by General Motors and other large corporations; it has been thoroughly discussed by national, state, and local medical societies; it is the largest single source of lost manhours and lost production.

Physical examinations, and the resulting medical department records, touch the problem of absenteeism at many points, whether absences are due to job-connected accident or disease or to nonoccupational causes. Medical records provide evidence in compensation cases. They help determine degrees of disability and capacities for work. They are essential to both remedial and preventive medicine. They are useful even in exposing the malingering absentee.

Industry, unfortunately, is periodically plagued by work stoppages (usually "unauthorized") in which the chief issue is the physical ability of men to perform certain tasks or work a certain number of hours. More often than may be supposed, such strikes involve a protest against physical examinations or a refusal to submit to them. The role of the industrial physician in such disputes is self-evident.

In a far broader sphere the potentials of industrial medicine have become more and more evident with the advent of the new scientific age and of new social attitudes. The problems of employment for older workers, for the handicapped and the partially disabled, are already in the forefront and are certain to demand greatly increased attention in the future. The study of capacities and limitations, the physical and mental aspects of placement, are of course mainline functions of the industrial medical team.

Specialization, in industry as well as in business, has grown enormously in our century. It was said in the early 1950's that the Ford Motor Company recognized some 2,400 different job classifications among its employees. The number is bound to grow rather than diminish. Automation demands new skills in many plant operations. Already, plans are under way for new training and retraining. Again, training and placement problems concern the industrial physician and his associates.

These examples indicate some of the ways in which modern science and technology are changing the course of industrial medicine, broadening its horizon, increasing its burden of responsibility. We shall see, in closing chapters, how organized industrial medicine has geared itself by planning and by action to meet the changes.

XXX

HEALTH INSURANCE PLANNING

So SPECTACULAR was the parade of world events in the midyears of the twentieth century that many developments of great significance were overshadowed and lost much of their impact upon the American public. Were it not for that fact, the period starting with World War II and stretching on into the 1950's might aptly be called the Era of Health Insurance, for it saw the flowering of medical care plans on a grand scale.

These projects were of every sort, and in the aggregate they affected to some extent the well-being of virtually everyone living under the American flag. They provided for group as well as individual insurance—voluntary and compulsory, military and civilian—underwritten by the government at various levels, and/or by commercial insurance carriers, as well as by organizations of the Blue Cross and Blue Shield type.

Important prepayment health programs were sponsored by the medical profession, hospitals, and other organizations operating on a nonprofit basis. In an entirely different category were the compulsory disability benefits provided by workmen's compensation laws. From organized labor, in the same period, came far-reaching proposals asking that health and welfare provisions be included as fringe benefits in union contracts with industrial employers.

This intricate web of health care projects evolved quite naturally from the trends of the time: the swift advance of science, the enormous growth of industry, the rising costs of medical care, expansion of the labor force, and the emergence of new social attitudes. Health—curative and preventive medicine—has become an American obsession, and every aspect and phase of the subject has implications of importance to the future of industrial practice.

Contrary, perhaps, to popular belief, the ideas underlying modern medical care plans are far from new. France, scourged by incredible poverty and want in the late 1700's, enacted a series of laws aimed at the same objectives. This legislation was part of an answer to the protest of a people who believed that every human being, regardless of his estate, was entitled to employment, food, shelter, and medical care. There were of course differences between the old French and the new American programs. The former, for example had to rely on government for finance and administration, there being no industrial or private enterprise to support such activities. As for content, there is a remarkable similarity between the eighteenth-century French and the twentieth-century American plans—a fact brought out by George Rosen in a scholarly paper published under the title "Hospitals, Medical Care, and Social Policy in the French Revolution."[1] On the eve of the Revolution, in a time of national tension, suspicion and fear and in the face of widespread food riots, the French passed laws providing comprehensive medical care for the "sick poor." Says Rosen: "Basic to the plan was the premise that from the cradle to the tomb, man henceforth in the new France would be an integral member of a maternal and provident society."

One law (1793) established the basis for a national system of social assistance; it also "envisaged a national social insurance fund based on voluntary contributions." Unfortunately, the entire French program never reached fruition. France had neither the resources nor the political stability to attain that goal. But the thinking remained in operation for future generations to follow.

America, in the 1940's, had never known the want and suffering endured in France a century and a half before, but it had had periods of deep depression and widespread unemployment. And the health planning of that period was born of a conviction that the benefits of modern medical science should be made available to people at every social and economic level. Plans based on that belief were incubating well before the forties. But actual programs in operation before the second world war were a mere scratching of the surface by comparison with the activities that followed.

Only by studying the detailed minutes of directors' meetings of the American Association of Industrial Physicians & Surgeons can one get a clear picture of the drama that went on behind the scenes in the period under consideration, the interplay of social, political and economic forces; the conflict of ambitions, motives and beliefs. And the depth and breadth of the association's interest in health plans of every type may surprise those who were not close to its inner councils.

At a Board meeting of the association directors in February, 1945, President Slobe commented:

> Prepayment medical service plans are more and more in the public interest, and it is my desire to appoint a committee to cover this important subject. Were such plans in effective operation throughout the country, there is little doubt that the development of socialized medicine would be retarded or even prevented thereby.
>
> The preferred plan appears to be one limited to complete medical care in the

hospital, payments being made directly to the physician. Where Blue Cross hospital plans are in existence, a tie-up with them would appear to be mutually advantageous. Since most of this insurance will be written for industrial groups, should we not be active participants in this rapidly expanding field?

The answer to Slobe's question was an emphatic "Yes." There had been compensation and insurance committees in the association before this, but they were small, and they dealt for the most part with routine affairs. At this point association policy underwent extensive changes. A new Committee on Prepayment Medical Service Plans was appointed to explore the problem and recommend a course of action. It consisted of Frank P. Hammond, of Chicago (chairman), a veteran of industrial practice and an authority on prepaid and other types of health insurance, R. F. Kurz, of St. Louis, a director of the association and a medical referee in insurance cases, and J. J. Prendergast, of Detroit, medical director of the Chrysler Corporation and a former vice-president of the AAIP&S.

On May 6, Chairman Hammond made a preliminary report to the Board.

It is quite universally believed by the medical profession that doctors must awaken and cooperate with one another and with hospital people now, to plan, organize, and promote voluntary prepayment medical care plans. Unless full understanding of this need develops soon, national legislation embodying compulsory health insurance will become an accomplished fact. It is difficult to exaggerate the importance to medicine of immediate action.

Medical care plans operating in conjunction with *hospital* care plans are beginning to take root; actually these plans are now [1945] in operation in nineteen states. They are serving the needs of 1,800,000 Americans to the satisfaction of the patients, the doctors, and the medical societies. But their growth is not rapid enough, nor does it give assurance that tomorrow there will be a sudden mushrooming of these plans and participants in numbers so large that the threat of federal operation of medical practice will vanish. [The italics are Hammond's.]

Association reaction to this kind of thinking was immediate and enthusiastic. Interest in, and zeal for, the promotion of medical service insurance spread like a benevolent epidemic among officers and membership. Committees became larger and more important; their field of activity broadened steadily. During the next ten years a distinguished coterie of industrial physicians and surgeons gave their services to a succession of workmen's compensation and insurance committees, which at times kept eight or nine active members well occupied with investigative and advisory duties.

For several years, workmen's compensation and prepaid medical care were treated as separate subjects in the association's agenda, and were assigned to different committees. Actually, however, it was difficult to discuss one field without reference to the other. There was much overlapping of interests and some duplication of effort; and in 1948 the two groups were merged into a single Workmen's Compensation and Insurance Committee.

A compensation committee headed by Slobe reported in December, 1945: "The present compensation laws are a form of social insurance designed to remedy and replace the only previous recourse, which was through common law action. The objectives of these laws are to provide medical care for injuries and occupational illnesses and to provide payment for lost time, permanent functional impairment, specific loss, and death."

There was no lack of experienced personnel to represent the AAIP&S (and subsequently the IMA) in matters pertaining to compensation and health insurance. Following Slobe and Hammond, J. Daniel Willems, of Chicago, a recognized authority in both fields, headed an outstanding committee whose report on work-men's compensation legislation won high praise in the spring of 1948. Another notable figure was Carl T. Olson, also of Chicago, whose industrial practice kept him in constant touch with compensation and health insurance problems. In practically a decade of committee service for the association, he was chairman during the period of greatest activity in those fields.

The strength of these committees was to be found in their rank-and-file membership as well as in their leadership. Personnel was representative of the nation as a whole, and included many men thoroughly versed in indemnity law and practice. Listed on committees of the 1940's and 1950's one finds such men as Thomas W. Nale (Charleston, West Virginia), John N. Shirley (Boston), T. I. Boileau and John E. Caldwell (Detroit), Ben M. Frees (Los Angeles), James S. Chalmers (Tulsa), and J. T. Scott (New Orleans). Also active on compensation committees at various times were several former presidents of the association, among them Wittmer, Slobe, and Whittaker.

The prestige and influence of the association in this sphere extended, however, far beyond such official activities. Individual industrial medical directors, in the day-to-day routine of administration, found themselves called upon more and more frequently for decisions and services related to health insurance programs or medico-legal problems. Inevitably, too, there was a steady increase of reciprocal assistance between governmental and civilian agencies in medical research projects of many kinds.

In 1946 the United States Department of the Interior undertook an exhaustive medical survey of the bituminous coal industry under the direction of officers assigned from the Navy Medical Corps. From the facts brought out by a voluminous report, released in 1947, came the pattern used in working out the far-reaching operations and procedures for administering the huge Mine Workers Welfare and Retirement Fund in ensuing years. By 1952 a potential of 1.5 million miners and their dependents were eligible for its benefits, and in that year about $50 million were spent for medical and hospital care.[2]

Among the physicians participating in this important study was Dr. John M. Shronts, then an officer in the Naval Reserve, to whom was entrusted the task of compiling the chapters on industrial medicine and public health in the final report.

In 1947, this document finished, Shronts became medical director of General Mills, Inc., Minneapolis. Active in IMA affairs, he was elected to the Board of Directors in 1955. It is interesting to note that while the coal mine study was under way no mention was made of the uses to which the findings might be put. "This development," wrote Shronts, in a letter to the IMA History Committee, "came as a total surprise to those of us who took part in the survey, and was a good demonstration of the ingenuity of John L. Lewis."

Proceedings at directors' meetings of the AAIP&S give some idea of the time and thought officially devoted to workmen's compensation and medical service plans in the latter half of the forties. Transcribed minutes show that such problems were among the leading topics of discussion at practically every executive session from 1945 through 1950. And committee reports on the same subjects add a substantial literature to the total.

Public interest in medical care programs had been growing steadily for several years prior to that period. By 1938 the American Medical Association was already fighting "to stem the tide in behalf of socialized medicine," according to Morris Fishbein, then editor of the *Journal of the American Medical Association.* "That movement," wrote the doctor, "really swelled in earnest with the report of the Committee on the Costs of Medical Care and the passing of the Social Security Act."[3]

As a counter-measure the *Journal of the American Medical Association* published an editoral, in January, 1938, calling upon the medical profession "to initiate, develop and put into practice a comprehensive system of medical care for all the people according to the American plan of medical practice."[4] This proposal met with favorable reactions in both medical and labor circles, but progress beyond that point lagged discouragingly.

In June, 1943, the House of Delegates of the AMA established a Council on Medical Service, which, three months later, reaffirmed approval of "voluntary prepayment medical service under the control of state and county medical societies," and spelled out the reasons for professional opposition to compulsory health insurance. In the following year the council adopted a fourteen-point "Constructive Program for Medical Care," one section of which approved programs to defray the costs of hospitalization, "such as the Blue Cross plans," and prepayment plans for medical care, "such as those developed by many state and county medical societies."

It is safe to say that the uncompromising stand taken by the AMA Council on Medical Service against any form of compulsory health insurance met with the approval of a majority of American doctors, a fact evidenced by endorsements at national, state, and local levels.

Among the strong and active supporters of that stand was the Association of American Physicians & Surgeons, a national non-profit organization founded in 1943 by a group of Indiana doctors. Successful from the start, it grew steadily to a membership of several thousand (including many members of the AAIP&S), who viewed with favor the objectives announced by the new organization. The program set forth by this association was concise and unequivocal. With the stated belief that medicine could not long remain free in a "sea of socialism," it provided for careful scrutiny of all medical care plans, study of proposed legislation concerning medicine in a free economy, education of the profession and public in such matters, the alerting of sympathetic groups to the dangers in current legislative developments, and the coordination of action to preserve private enterprise.

Since 1944 the association has continued to pursue these objectives by the use of news letters and pamphlets from its Chicago headquarters, by appealing to the people to express their views to Washington, and by providing professional testimony before congressional committees if necessary.

It was in the mid-forties that the AAIP&S first showed serious official interest in these projects, the development of which was bound to be of great consequence to industrial workers. In a general report to members President Slobe pointed out that by 1945 there were eighteen million people enrolled in Blue Cross hospitalization plans, and that about five million were being added every year. Turning to prepayment medical service (as distinct from hospitalization), he called attention to pioneer projects inaugurated in Michigan and California and remarked that similar plans were already operating in eighteen states. It was from these programs, sponsored by state and local societies, that the Blue Shield medical and surgical service plans later evolved.

"It appears," said Slobe, "that insurance coverage of this type is inevitable in this country, and we have the choice of government operation or operation controlled by the medical profession. Hospitals and Blue Cross have made a great success of their plan; so why not have the doctors make a similar success of theirs, working in harmonious relationship with the other plans? It appears that neither can or could survive without the other."

While signs indicated an overwhelming sentiment, on the part of the medical profession, in favor of voluntary insurance covering both hospitalization and medical-surgical benefits, they exposed the necessity for organization on a countrywide scale. Blue Cross was not yet operating as a national unit; nor could the various medical care plans at that time provide uniform agreements or benefits outside their own geographical areas.

At the May 6, 1945, directors' meeting of the AAIP&S Frank Hammond, speaking for his committee, strongly emphasized the need for national coordination.

National employers have got to have something that will cover their situation. They want a plan that will enable national employers in Cleveland to insure their employees in Dallas, in San Francisco, or in Chicago. And you might be interested to know that 65 percent of the employed people, excluding agriculture and domestics, are employed by national employers.

The time for thinking and talking about national sickness benefit plans has passed and the time for action is here. There is no alternative; disinterest and procrastination may mean nonsurvival for voluntary hospitals and invasion of professional independence. Unyielding cooperative action now means universal health benefits, voluntarily subscribed to, and under the control of medical and hospital people.

An unusual opportunity presents itself for our association to take the lead in organizing and promoting a prepayment medical care plan. It should be national in scope, under its own sponsorship and supervision, operated not for profit, and voluntary rather than compulsory. It should assure the individual free choice of a physician, with no interference with the professional relationship between physician and patients or between physician and hospitals.

The directors promptly approved Hammond's committee report "as a preliminary declaration of the association's attitude and inclination in connection with the establishment of a national medical care plan."

There lay ahead, however, many hours of amicable but not altogether conclusive debate as to exactly how far the association could or should go in organizing and assuming responsibility for such a plan. The question being asked on every hand was not whether a nationwide program, offering uniform benefits at standard rates, was needed but who should sponsor it, finance it, operate it, and meet all consequences, good or bad. Was it a task for insurance companies? For medical associations and societies? For an entirely new organization? Or for government? The answer to these questions was obviously of the utmost importance.

A great many individuals and groups regarded the AMA as the ideal agency to take over this problem and direct the action needed to solve it. The AMA was fully representative of the medical profession; its Council on Medical Service had done a great deal of work on voluntary prepayment medical insurance. Patently (and naturally) the AMA wanted a decisive role in working out the medical policies to be followed by a national coordinating organization. In fact, the House of Delegates had already set up a code of minimum standards for both indemnity and medical service plans.

By 1945, various medical groups were urging the AMA to take the entire problem into its own hands and get a program started. The Medical Service Plans Council, of Kansas City, published a policy statement to the effect that it was "looking forward to the time when the AMA will form a national coordinating agency." Dr. Roland George, of New York, attended a meeting with the AMA committee on Medical Care to present a similar proposal on behalf of the United Medical Service, which was operating under the sponsorship and direction of the New York Medical Society.

Replies to these overtures were, on the whole, noncommittal; for the AMA walked warily around the problem, avoiding the sponsorship issue while promising to do all that it could "to stimulate the development of medical society plans, and extend the area of coverage so that the whole United States may be covered by such plans." From published reports and correspondence, however, leaders of the AAIP&S soon came to the justifiable conclusion that the AMA—though ready to promote the right kind of national medical service plan—would not see fit to take the initiative in establishing it or the responsibility of administering it.

"We need no longer wait for the AMA," said Edward P. Heller, of Kansas City, at an AAIP&S directors' meeting in June, 1945, "and we will not be infringing in any way on their rights or prerogatives. . . . They want somebody to do it, but they have no great inclination to do it themselves."

"They said they would approve the plan, if somebody else did it," commented Holmblad.

"That is their way of turning it down," replied Slobe. "They said that the council could not approve what was not yet in effect, and the details of which had not yet been wholly worked out. The intimation here is that the council might have approved it, but they don't want to approve anything before it is set up."

If not the AMA, then who would undertake the job of correlating medical care plans nationally? Directors of the AAIP&S carefully canvassed the possibilities, at this same meeting. The urgent need for action was reiterated by speaker after speaker.

Hammond reported: "Industry is not only requesting, but demanding a package plan, a contract that would cover their employees and their families for both medical and hospital expense, at least beginning with the in-hospital expense." He predicted: "Unless the medical profession, some national body, begins now, today, to organize a central coordinating agency, it is going to be done by somebody else, and you know who it is—either federal or state government, with compulsory insurance for which the rates will be much higher and which will be much more expensive for the American people."

Here, indeed, was a many-sided problem. The contemplated new organization must conform with approved medical standards and procedures. It must meet the requirements of employers and be acceptable to labor. It must not violate sound insurance practice nor work to the detriment of medical service plans already in successful operation. As matters stood, Blue Cross could offer adequate benefits for hospitalization, but labor was demanding comparable coverage for costs of medical care. And there remained the difficult task of operating both hospital and medical service plans on a national basis.

Speaking of labor's growing interest in health plans, Richard O. Schofield, of Sacramento, described to the AAIP&S Board of Directors what he called a period of "red hot" compulsory insurance activity in the California legislature. Two bills, he said, both providing for a form of compulsory insurance, were presented at the 1945 session. One of them was sponsored and actively supported by the CIO. "Labor," he said, "is the one element that is directing everything in the state of California from the standpoint of prepaid medical care, and the legislature was divided not on party lines but on the issue of compulsion." Because of strong opposition from the California Medical Association and insurance companies, he explained, neither bill came to a vote on the floor, though the question was still what he called "very much of a live issue."

"In our section [Michigan], as in California," said Frank T. McCormick, of Detroit, "labor is of course very strong, and I wonder whether there has been any serious threat that the CIO and the AFL might take over."

"There is a threat," replied Hammond, "but my impression is, and you folks ought to know, that there is more to favor the Hospital Service Plan than any other, because the benefits are greater and the cost is less."

"I should like to supplement that," interjected Alfred Whittaker, "by saying that there is a great deal of dissatisfaction in the CIO with the present Michigan plan because they don't regard it as comprehensive enough. This dissatisfaction has grown to such an extent that they have withdrawn some large groups from the plan. "I should like to say further, since these plans depend so much on payroll deduction, that the industrial physicians are in a strategic position to make this plan nationally a great success by the advice we can give employers. Of all medical groups in the country, including even the AMA, this is the group which can best act in an advisory capacity."

It will be noted that in all discussions of prepayment insurance plans at AAIP&S meetings, there was general agreement that the Blue Cross system of hospital care had operated successfully and satisfactorily throughout the country. On the other hand, there was recognition of the fact that complete coverage of medical costs involved other and more serious difficulties.

Earlier in these 1945 discussions Whittaker had reported to the Board: "The Michigan (Blue Cross) plan went $415,000 in the red during the first two years of its operation because it was an all-inclusive plan. By eliminating *medical care*, they gradually worked it out." The problem of organization and finance, obviously, was as important as that of sponsorship. It was, as President-elect Melvin Newquist pointed out, "an insurance problem on a national scale."

The experience of Michigan—whose hospitalization and medical service plans were both among the oldest and largest in the nation—served as a convincing example of the inadequacy of a health insurance system limited by state lines. "The number of men covered by medical services [in 1945]," said Whittaker, "is pathetically small in this country."

As a matter of record, Michigan's knowledge of medical service plans was probably backed by longer experience than that of any other state. Whittaker's personal participation in such planning dated back to September 1931, when he introduced at a meeting of the Michigan State Medical Society's House of Delegates in Pontiac a resolution calling for a survey of health problems and a study of existing health services. It asked for a committee of five to make this investigation.[5]

In July 1932, the house directed the committee to continue its study and to prepare a plan for health insurance which would include, among others, these policy provisions: free choice of physician, control of medical service by the profession, exclusion of individuals or organizations that might engage in health insurance for profit.

Years of study, consultations and decisions followed before the Michigan legislature, in March, 1939, passed, by an overwhelming majority, a bill "establishing a nonprofit corporation" to operate the medical service plan as it was set up. And, when the agency opened its offices in February 1940, the ninth year had elapsed since the original proposal.

In Whittaker's opinion, an opinion shared by others who had observed such operations at close range, the weakness of local groups sponsoring medical-surgical services at that time was that most of them were "working on a shoestring," and the resultant insurance setup could not in good conscience be recommended to large employers. On the other hand, a national organization, well financed, would provide a solid actuarial base and could be endorsed to any employer for the insurance of his working force.

Executive heads of the Blue Cross evidently were well aware of the difficulties and dangers of the situation. Hammond reported to the directors of the AAIP&S:

> For about five years the Hospital Service Plan Commission, that is, eighty-four hospital service plans, have been urged to see the necessity of adding medical care.
>
> Gentlemen, they have done everything possible to avoid putting in their own insurance company. Why? Because of the underground suspicion in the minds of the doctors that the hospital people want to assume prerogatives and control of the medical profession. It has come to be such a momentous problem that rather than put in one themselves they have considered having two or three or four commercial companies come in to write the insurance.

Outstanding among the research projects of the middle forties was a study by Louis Reed and Henry F. Vaughan, of Ann Arbor, Michigan, financed by the American Public Health Association and titled "The Coordination of Medical and Blue Cross Plans."[6] Vaughan and Reed toured the country gathering data on all medical service plans. These they divided into four types, one of which they recommended as best suited to the current situation. Reading the report to the AAIP&S directors, Whittaker commented: "It is the solution to which the plans will probably come ultimately." A rapid-fire dialogue followed:

Whittaker: "Under this arrangement, the hospital plan as such ceases to exist. The medical plan as such ceases to exist. Instead, there is a combined medical and hospital plan, a health plan for the whole country."

Chairman Slobe: "There was a very similar report by Perry in the *Journal of the American Medical Association,* February 10, 1945. He comes to the same conclusion."

B. L. Vosburgh (General Electric Company): "So did the National Physicians' Committee in its report."

In this planning stage of national medical services the life insurance companies were, in a sense, relegated to the role of observers, deeply interested observers, it is true, but avoiding commitments to any specific group. On the whole they were reported to be much in favor of any plan operated and sponsored by doctors, because they were so strongly opposed to any form of compulsory insurance on a federal or state level.

A current pamphlet dealing with social security, published by the Life Insurance Division of the American National Association of Life Underwriters, expressed this policy as follows: "The importance of the role of the doctor in new developments is self-evident. Hence, our cooperation is essential in plans for a better distribution of medical care. In addition, the receptive field for voluntary and government action should be carefully worked out through cautious experimentation, utilizing existing machinery as far as possible."

Dr. Newquist commented: "The insurance companies, of course, are very interested in seeing the government stay out of this picture as much as possible. The casualty companies are all busy and have all decided now to go into the hospital and medical insurance business."

There had been a widespread belief in some circles that the Blue Cross Hospital and Blue Shield Medical plans, as they gained momentum, would be competing directly with private insurance. Events proved the exact opposite; their success greatly stimulated the demand for private insurance, a fact soon realized by both the insurance and the medical professions.

Newquist (in 1945) pictured the possibilities of that trend in these words: "Today the total annual premiums for medical and hospital insurance are far greater than the total annual premiums in the entire nation for workmen's compensation. That is big business. . . . And they can thank the Blue Cross and the rest of them for getting the people insurance minded and ready to buy."

With demands for a nationwide system of health care becoming more and more insistent, with pressure for compulsory government-controlled insurance mounting steadily, with the AMA and Blue Cross hesitating to assume sponsorship, it seemed to many that events were pushing organized industrial medicine into a position that called for decisive action. "Somebody should do it, some medical group," said Slobe. "The point is, nobody is doing it." Whittaker remarked: "Even though every state in the Union should form an organization, there would still be need for a national coordinating group."

It is safe to say that in all top-level discussions the officers, directors and committeemen were in full accord with that basic thinking. The AAIP&S was the medical group closest to the great mass of the nation's workers, and its cooperation was essential in plans for the better distribution of medical care. There was, however, a strong feeling that the association should not assume responsibility for an insurance program. C. O. Sappington, editor of *Industrial Medicine,* believed a national medical care plan, well administered, would be a boon to the insurance companies, but expressed the hope that the AAIP&S would limit itself to acting as coordinator. "It ought," he said, "to avoid all semblance of going into the insurance business."

Stripped of ramifications and unimportant detail, a national coordinating agency was precisely what Hammond's committee proposed. Such an organization would not interfere with existing medical service programs. It would follow, in the main, New York's United Medical Service plan, with the exception that it would pay indemnity benefits in cash instead of in services. It would operate a central office, supply financial data, provide actuarial service, and coordinate state and local plans on a national basis.

Slobe announced that large medical service agencies in several states had offered, collectively, to advance approximately $250,000 to launch the proposed corporation, if the association would sponsor it. The money was to be repaid out of earnings. A belief was freely expressed that the plan as a whole met all important specifications and that it could ultimately be broadened to include complete medical, dental and nursing care.

Ending many months of study and discussion, the Board of Directors of the AAIP&S took final action on the proposal at its June, 1945, meeting, approving the committee report by unanimous vote, including the recommendation that the offer of financial aid for a new corporation be accepted.

It was, however, neither the AMA nor the AAIP&S which, in the long run, took over official responsibility for coordinating the medical-care insurance plans to operate nationally. Instead, with the counsel and help of the medical and hospital organizations of the country, a plan was worked out which preserved the identity and autonomy of the state and local medical care groups yet made it possible to extend benefits to out-of-state employees of national employers.

Morris Fishbein is authority for the fact that the AMA Council on Industrial Health at one point in its planning definitely decided to establish a Division of Medical Care Insurance. He wrote:

> This was done, because it seemed that stimulation of the formation and extension of medical society plans could be greatly helped by active participation on the part of the AMA.
>
> The House [of Delegates] directed the council in December 1945 to endeavor to effect national coverage by these plans. Conferences were held with medical care plan directors, and finally it was decided not to start a separate national plan but to form an independent organization.[7]

As a result of this decision the medical care plans themselves were banded together to establish a new coordinating body—Associated Medical Care Plans, Inc. From its inception this group worked closely with the Council on Industrial Health, three of whose members were seated on the Board of Trustees of the new organization. And it was from this beginning that the national structure of the Blue Shield Medical Care Plans finally emerged.

The form of organization and method of operation of both the Blue Cross and the Blue Shield are a matter of public record and need no detailed comment here. Though distinct and separate agencies, they have followed parallel courses. Both are nonprofit organizations. Both are administered, nationally, by commissions. Both have set up special corporations[8] to provide a means of enrollment that enables organizations with national coverage to obtain uniform rates, benefits and payments. Both, too, require the rigid maintenance of high professional standards; each Blue Cross plan is approved by the American Hospital Association, and all Blue Shield plans must have the approval of the medical societies in their areas.

At the distance of a decade or more it seems fortunate that all this planning turned out as it did. The chief aim of the AMA, the IMA and other medical and surgical groups has been to get a workable program of insured health services in operation nationally. None of these organizations has shown any real desire to sit in the driver's seat.

Nor were the months of time and labor spent by these planners wasted. They were, after all, members of the state, county and city societies sponsoring the medical-care plans. They knew, better than anyone else, the requirements to be met. And all their specialized knowledge and experience went, through various channels, into the national plans as finally established.

In his report as secretary of the AAIP&S in March, 1948, Slobe voiced the thinking of the Board of Directors when he said: "The proposed organization two years ago of a national medical service insurance plan to be sponsored by our association, although it did not reach fruition, was a worthwhile step. . . . It is interesting to note that virtually all the measures advocated by our association have either been put into effect or are in the process of being developed."

Judged by the degree to which they met basic requirements, the standards set up for operation of the national hospitalization and medical care plans were indeed remarkably comprehensive. They kept medical services under medical control. They did not interfere with the operations of other existing plans and agencies. Far from penalizing insurance companies, they greatly broadened the field of commercial carriers. They answered satisfactorily the demand of national employers for a standard "package" program.

To just what extent agitation for compulsory, government-sponsored health insurance influenced the growth of voluntary plans is a matter of conjecture. Certainly voluntary hospital and medical service programs were inspired by a sincere and humane desire for a broader and better distribution of medical care. But just as certainly, the activities of private agencies were stimulated by the strength and persistence of the campaign for what has conveniently been called "government medicine."

The answer to the question of motives is not, after all, particularly important. Compulsory insurance had its day (or rather, its days) in Congress. A perennial succession of bills, covering essentially the same plan, was introduced during the forties. Professional men, business and labor leaders, and lobbyists appeared at committee hearings. One labor representative, at a hearing in 1944, told a committee: "The real answer is to take Joe Worker by the hand and lead him into a modern hospital or clinic and say to him, 'Here is health for you, Joe. You pay for it according to your income, and, if you can't pay, you get it anyway.'" Such opinions reflected a more or less common misconception of health. To many it was a commodity that could be sold like cigarettes—from a vending machine.

Actually, issues in the compulsory-versus-voluntary insurance controversy were many, complex, and open to sharp differences of opinion. As early as 1921, leaders in the AAIP&S were on guard against groups that appeared to be favoring a compulsory system. Through the thirties the AMA vigorously attacked socialized medicine in any guise. Under the title, "What is Wrong with National Health Insurance?" the November 1933 issue of the *Bulletin* (official journal of the House of Delegates) abstracted with approving comment a bitter criticism of the British system by the influential English doctor, Sir Henry Brackenbury.[9]

Two years later Fishbein and R. G. Leland teamed up in a radio debate broadcast over a national network, arguing against the proposition that the various states should enact legislation providing complete medical service for all citizens at public expense.[10] Speakers for the affirmative were William T. Foster and Bower Aly. The AMA continued its war inexorably through the forties, condemning by public statement and formal resolution the compulsory insurance bills introduced in Congress.

The AAIP&S took its strongest stand against government encroachment at its business meeting in Detroit April 7, 1949. There was a dramatic moment when Benjamin Frees read to the members a resolution placing the organization on record as "against any form of compulsory health insurance or any system of political medicine designed for bureaucratic control."[11]

"I am very sorry," said Frees, "that the medical profession has to bring a resolution like this before its members, but the battle is on. Mr. President, I move the adoption of this resolution." Put to a vote, the motion was carried by acclamation. "That was a very lusty 'Aye'," commented Chairman Vonachen, outgoing president of the association. One of the earliest bits of business for the incoming administration, headed by Whittaker, was to mail a copy of the resolution to the White House, under date of April 25.

Many other organizations, medical and nonmedical, including the American Association of Industrial Nurses, took similar action urging rejection of federal insurance proposals. Voluntary plans were spreading rapidly; commercial insurance business was flourishing. And, as records show, none of the bills introduced in the Congress reached the floor of either House or Senate for a decisive vote.

* * *

During the eventful forties the AAIP&S was still fighting stubborn resistance to the recognition of industrial medicine as a specialized field. In an important report to the Board of Directors on October 3, 1944, the Committee on Policy and Plan (F. E. Poole, chairman) predicted: "These [resisting] forces will continue to find expression through social or government-social agencies, labor unions, and other lay organizations now and in the reconversion period. Strong guidance will be required by the medical profession to accomplish for industry the most efficient results, while at the same time maintaining the highest scientific and ethical standards." Pleading for a stronger public relations program, the report continued: "The AMA is showing little leadership in this field. Lay organizations such as the National Association of Manufacturers, Princeton University (Industrial Relations Research), the National Conference Board, and Chambers of Commerce are actually doing more promotion work than any medical agency."

There was no doubt even at the time of the report that organized labor was keenly aware of the vast social benefits that could result from a broad expansion of health insurance and also aware of the influence that labor might exercise in that field. Various union leaders were among the strong proponents of a federally sponsored compulsory system; and the United States Department of Labor sought by one means or another to extend its authority in matters of industrial health.

In December 1944, at the Eleventh Conference on Labor Legislation called by the Secretary of Labor, the United States Public Health Service and state health departments were bitterly attacked from the floor for their work in the field of industrial hygiene. Committee reports accused them of operating in a sphere in which they had no authority and, more specifically, of blocking federal legislation which would place industrial hygiene activities in the Labor Department.

Industrial Medicine sprang to the defense of the health services with an indignant editorial branding the charges as "preposterous" and presenting facts and figures to expose what it termed "the smear technique."[12] The legislation in question was not passed in 1944 or in 1945, but the effort persisted. Similar bills[13] were still awaiting action in 1946. Their main provision was the allocation of $5 million to state agencies administering labor laws for maintaining safe working conditions and controlling health hazards.

The AMA went on record in February 1946 as opposing this legislation. At a Board meeting of the AAIP&S on April 9, the directors approved another resolution asking that any tax project of this kind "be developed in such a manner as to provide funds ultimately for the state departments of health in cooperation with the United States Public Health Service." In presenting the resolution President Newquist pointed out that this work in industrial hygiene had always been handled by the USPHS through state health agencies, except in New York and Massachusetts, where the hygiene bureaus were part of the labor departments.

Under different circumstances, this same issue came up again in 1950. The occasion was a hearing before the Schaeffer Commission (known as the Little Hoover Commission) of Illinois on a labor-supported proposal to move the Industrial Hygiene Division from the Department of Health to the Department of Labor. Among industrial physicians testifying were J. F. McCahan (Bausch & Lomb Optical Company), J. H. Chivers (Crane Company), and M. H. Kronenberg

(Caterpillar Tractor Company), who strongly supported the opinion that matters of health should be under jurisdiction of health departments. In spite of opposition from various sources, the Illinois transfer was approved and put into effect.

There were also moves in the same direction in other states during the same period. When a report of the Schaeffer hearing was made to the directors of the AAIP&S in December 1950, members mentioned that in Michigan, without public hearings, the Labor Department was empowered to set the standards for first aid in industry and that the department had authority to go into any Michigan plant and make an inspection.

In these and similar controversies there was no implication that government agencies had no place in industrial medicine or that their functions should be unduly restricted. Medical organizations, since their beginning, have cooperated fully and wholeheartedly with public health services at every level. But they have insisted that government, as such, should not interfere with doctor-patient relations or dictate medical practices and procedures.

It is a matter of record that, at mid-century, there were twenty-five federal health agencies performing nine different types of service; at the state level, sixteen major types of agency and many miscellaneous categories; and a host of city, county, and city-county agencies engaged in health service and supervisory activities.[14] Rarely has there been anything that could be underscored as conflict between organized medicine and this multitude of governmental groups.

Moreover—although federal compulsory insurance projects have been stead-fastly opposed, and the transfer of medical authority to government labor units has been strongly resisted—it is significant that organized labor has been neither stifled nor impeded in the constructive promotion of health plans for the benefit of the working force and society as a whole.

It is obvious that no one program, formula or panacea can meet all the health needs of the nation, and, as should be the case in this free economy, a vast number of different medical care plans have become operative within the memory of men still living. A few of these, typical of many, are described briefly here:

Union Health Center, New York City, famous as the first experiment in medical service sponsored by the workers in an industry. Founded in 1913 by Dr. George Price and directed since his death in 1942 by his son, Dr. Leo Price, it presently provides a wide range of preventive and medical care to more than 200,000 members of the International Ladies' Garment Workers' Union and limited services to their dependents. In its first forty years of operation, the total number of individual services rendered annually grew from slightly over 1,200 to well above 5.5 million. Most of the medical services, through collective bargaining, have been paid for by the union's health and welfare fund since 1946.

Railroad Retirement Program, authorized by the federal Railroad Insurance Act of 1936 and administered by the Railroad Retirement Board in coordination with unemployment insurance. All railroad workers covered by unemployment insurance are eligible for sickness benefits, which were first made available July 1, 1946. Benefits and services are financed by employer contributions with no additional contribution for temporary disability insurance. The size and scope of the program are indicated by figures for a typical year (1948–49), which show that benefits for sickness were paid to 151,200 employees, after adjustment for recoveries; and that the average amount per beneficiary was $188.

Medical Research Institute, Detroit, another type of union-sponsored medical enterprise, launched by the United Auto Workers in 1944. An ambitious project serving a large membership, it maintains clinical services and carries on an educational and promotional program covering hygiene and safety in industry. Its most significant activity has been to advance health, group insurance and compensation clauses for inclusion in union contracts.[15]

Federal Employee Health Program, a medical care plan roughly paralleling private industrial plans. According to Dr. Anthony J. Lanza (director, Institute of Industrial Medicine, New York University), the federal government lagged far behind industry in this respect until World War II. Measures then introduced included treatment of on-the-job illness and dental treatment in emergencies, pre-placement and other examinations, and preventive programs related to health. All federal employees (with specific exceptions) are eligible for such services.

Kaiser Foundation Health Plan, a prototype of large industrial-prepaid-group plans; founded by Dr. Sidney R. Garfield in 1942 for workers at the Kaiser San Francisco Bay (Permanente) shipyards. Garfield was an active member of the Western component society of the AAIP&S. During and after the war boom this initial enterprise expanded into a chain of Kaiser hospitals in California, Oregon, and Washington, giving widely varied service for one basic fee to a group estimated (in 1953) at 350,000.

Health Insurance Plan of Greater New York, another large group-project differing from the Kaiser plan mainly in that it is community-sponsored. Founded in 1947, HIP also has grown into a chain of clinics, large and small, dotting the New York area. Through organized groups of physicians, these centers serve union and civil service units on a monthly fee basis, a large majority of its subscribers being city employees.

Philadelphia Medical Service Plan, again emphasizing the wide differences among medical programs, even within labor organizations. The Philadelphia project was proposed in 1946 by the Central Labor Union of the American Federation of Labor, but little was done until the Luggage Workers, Local 61, advanced $20,000 toward establishment of a health center. Other funds were procured through loans, and the center opened in 1951, serving three unions with a total of 3,000 members. By the end of its second year it boasted a membership of 18,000, representing seventeen Philadelphia locals. Funds for operating costs were provided from a per capita amount assessed against each member, and in most cases the assessment was paid from health and welfare funds secured by collective bargaining contracts.

The Tennessee Plan, developed by insurance companies in cooperation with the medical profession and cited at the annual Congress on Industrial Health, in February, 1950, as "an outstanding example of what is being done to ease the burden of catastrophic illness." The Tennessee State Medical Association worked out a surgical schedule and enlisted 1,600 doctors as participants in the plan. All insurance companies and associations licensed in the state were invited to design policies, and although most of them had been active in the program eighteen months or less, more than 70,000 policyholders and dependents had been insured by 1950.

Akron Medical Insurance Plan, providing company-paid hospital and surgical insurance for some 100,000 rubber and aircraft workers in the Akron area. Established in 1953 through labor negotiations, it was the first plan fully financed by employers to cover all the top companies in one industry, as opposed to the steel plan in which the employee as well as the employer contributes.

These examples do not even begin to suggest the almost infinite variety of organization and procedure to be found in existing medical care plans. They are intended, rather, to indicate essential differences in the concept of prepaid health insurance, and in methods of operation, among a few of the better known ones.

Nor are we by any means justified in assuming that any type of prepayment plan has had the unqualified blessing of the medical fraternity, or of employers, or of organized labor. In some quarters the Akron Plan was hailed as "a glimpse of the future of medical insurance"; on the other hand, some doctors and some employers complained of "socialized medicine"; some union chiefs were dissatisfied; some surgical fees were disputed. Extensive programs (of the type of HIP and the Kaiser enterprise) were condemned as "supermarket" and "assemblyline" medicine, exploiting the physician and compromising standards; yet advocates praised them as "guideposts for many new plans now in the formative stages."

These evidences of controversy, however, should be tempered by a reminder that this is democracy in action, free enterprise at work. Prepayment health insurance, fortunately, is in an extremely fluid stage, fortunately since that circumstance permits exploration of many channels, making it possible to select the best and reject the unproved and unsuccessful. If medical care plans were cast into a rigid mold by legislation, there could be no such freedom of choice and no such continued evolution.

XXXI

IMA—SYMBOL OF AN EPOCH

No ONE who has traced the history of occupational medicine in America since 1900 can fail to marvel not only at the extent of its progress, but also at the few years that were required for such gains in position, influence and accomplishment.

Since 1900, medical science as a whole has also undergone sweeping changes. But the basic principles and practices of general medicine were already well established at the turn of the century. The profession was fortified by a rich tradition, and was held in high regard. Its central organization, the American Medical Association, had been building steadily and wisely for more than fifty years. Many state and county societies were much older.

But not until after the first World War was there much in industrial health procedures that resembled occupational medicine as it is now defined. The "specialty" did not exist in this country, except in embryo, and a whole new lexicon of occupational ailments was still to be compiled. Regardless of their medical and surgical skill, doctors doing industrial work were more often regarded as pariahs than as pioneers. We must remember that for many years after World War I, comparatively few plant medical departments were well equipped and well operated. The great majority were actually First Aid stations, staffed, at their worst, by partially trained personnel that could improvise with bandages and home medicaments, and at their best, by qualified nurses, with surgical and medical services available on call as needed.

When the American Association of Industrial Physicians & Surgeons was founded in 1916, it received little recognition and less acceptance in either medical or business circles. It had no body of precedent to follow, no reliable guideposts to mark the path ahead. Nor was there any hint of formidable occupational health problems that were to come in the wake of modern industrial technology. Industrial medicine today is as distant in concept and practice from that of 1920 as the motor car of today is from the horse and buggy. Yet the complete metamorphosis has covered a span of approximately forty years.

The association, as we have seen, made haste slowly in its early life. Beset by money troubles and membership crises, it was forced to fight desperately for mere survival. But what may be considered its severest test and its greatest triumph came at a time of comparatively smooth sailing, when management was more favorably disposed toward enlightened health programs than ever before, when able young doctors were turning to the industrial field in larger numbers, and when the specialty appeared to be on its way to the realization of long-cherished hopes.

In the middle 1940's it became evident that the little association of the past had, suddenly, become a big association. It had doubled its membership in something like five years and was growing steadily. It had, moreover, passed from relative obscurity to a position of considerable importance. The resulting problems were problems not only of mere size, but of organization and activity. Association leaders were quick to see the immediate need for big thinking, broader viewpoint, new planning.

There was the medical challenge of problems associated with the remarkable developments in industry. As the editors of *Industrial Medicine and Surgery* wrote, of that period: "Henceforth [industrial medicine] must keep abreast of both medicine and technology."[1] And employers, extending and modernizing their health and welfare programs, rightly expected commensurate services in return for their investment.

There was the educational challenge to be met, the provision of special undergraduate and graduate courses in the medical schools, as preparation for industrial practice. Occupational medicine surely was not entitled to full certification as a specialty unless candidates were uniformly qualified by specialized training and experience.

There was also an administrative challenge to the organization, a rapid expansion of its sphere of activity, a much broader program of professional and public relations, and multiplication of services to members. It was a primary responsibility of the association to further, in every possible way, knowledge and understanding of modern occupational health hazards and the means for their control.

Seemingly, there was no end to the pressing problems that crowded in upon the association after the war; yet difficult transitions in policy and action were accomplished smoothly and with due deliberation. Though all issues were debated in infinite detail, many major decisions received almost no publicity even within the profession. Among these were several that have had a vital bearing on the progress of occupational medicine, and for that reason are worthy of summary here.

One precedent-making step came from a chance remark by Loyal A. Shoudy at a critical point in World War II. As general chairman of the association's Convention Committee for the 1944 meeting, Shoudy suggested to President Harvey Bartle that the organization was big enough to divide itself into sections for the discussion of selected subjects. Thus, he said, a member could devote his time to topics of greatest interest to him instead of getting "part of what he wants and part of what he doesn't want" at large, unwieldly general sessions.

The idea, of course, was not new; sectional meetings were standard procedure with such organizations as the AMA and the American College of Surgeons. Membership of the AAIP&S at the time was nearly 1,600, enough, certainly, to make sectional meetings feasible. Yet opinion was sharply divided. Queries were sent to prominent members, asking what they wanted in the way of a meeting. The returns likewise indicated a wide range of preference. Members, it seemed, wanted discussions on eyes, heart, chest, mental troubles, deformities, loss of limbs, and so on and so on.

"That list," Shoudy reported to the directors, "reminded me of the old topic that has been a pet of mine: Who can work? Where can they work? What can they do?" The Board, after some debate, voted to include in the program "two group meetings, running concurrently." They were held as scheduled: one on the subject of welding and noise hazards, the other on medical care in small plants and the over-all topic, Who Can Work? There was no mention of sections.

Probably, no more constructive subjects could have been assigned than these. Small plant problems were of great concern to health authorities, and the rehabilitation, reconditioning and placement of the disabled and handicapped in useful employment was of paramount importance to the nation, as it still is.

Congratulating Shoudy on his persuasiveness, at the annual meeting (in May 1944), President Bartle commented: "No one could refuse you a request. Some of the rest of us, perhaps, would refuse."

"We did send out some orders," replied Shoudy.

Unfortunately, there was a considerable lapse of time before sectional meetings were developed to fulfill their original promise. Travel restrictions prevented an annual meeting in 1945. In 1946 and 1947 a good deal of organizational business was deferred to provide time for dealing with acute postwar problems.

Late in December 1947, President Henry S. Brown carefully reviewed various proposals for sectional meetings organized along industrial lines, and as a result a plan to hold seminar discussions with oil, steel, chemical and other similar groups was introduced at the January, 1948, directors' meeting. The idea was well received, but the complex arrangements for such joint sessions could not be made in time for the spring convention. In a state-of-the-association report at that meeting, however, Secretary Slobe praised the medical-industrial conference plan as a highly constructive step, adding: "And of course we all know how greatly the scope of our convention has increased each year."

Detailed development of this new program feature got under way in June 1948 when Dr. Adolph Kammer (Carbide and Chemicals Corporation) submitted to the directors a code of rules governing the "what, where and how" of section procedures, important because they represented a radical departure from convention precedent. The reasoning behind the change, as he expressed it, was simple and cogent:

"As a member who goes to these conventions on the chemical industry's expense account, I like to learn something about the technology of industrial medicine in the chemical industry. I don't think I should attend the convention every year and hear extolled year after year the virtues of pre-employment examinations. I am prepared to consider that I am somewhat technically advanced, and I should like to meet with a group of people similarly technically advanced and get down to a serious discussion."

There was nothing timid or tentative about the first scheduling of sectional meetings as such, at the Detroit convention on April 5, 1949. Time was provided on the same day for sessions of four different groups, each with a varied program of subjects of common interest in special industrial fields. With Dr. M. W. Jocz (Chrysler Corporation) presiding, a Section of General Manufacturing heard and discussed five papers presented by automobile company personnel and faculty members of medical schools. A Section on Steel and Heavy Industries, headed by Paul Bamberger (Bethlehem Steel Company), listened to seven technical papers on respiratory diseases and their control, given by authorities in various aspects of that field. The speakers then sat as a panel for a discussion period. A meeting of the Section on Petroleum and Chemicals, with Robert C. Page (Standard Oil Company, of New Jersey) as chairman, followed a similar pattern, with a series of professional papers and a panel discussion covering the interpretation of medical information to company personnel. In a meeting of the Section on Mining Industry, with G. W. Easley of Williamson, West Virginia, presiding, the Association of Mine Physicians, then a component society of the AAIP&S, discussed the disease and accident hazards of the coal fields.

Later in the day, Edward Holmblad reported success for the trial balloon of section meetings. The rooms that had been reserved, he told the directors, proved to be too small; meetings had to be moved to larger quarters. Adolph Kammer commented: "I think the sections can become a very important force in the growth of this organization and in the ever increasing number and quality of the people who will attend such meetings."

One great advantage of this type of program was its flexibility. Enlarged and improved in later years, the plan has been used to focus attention on any topic or combination of topics requiring special emphasis. There have been meetings of medical sections and surgical sections; sections for various industrial groups; sections devoted to certain disease categories or to special problems ranging from alcoholism to workmen's compensation.

Of such stuff is medical progress made. Sectional meetings, so employed, have enabled the association to cover a vastly wider range of subject matter in one fast-moving convention program. Beyond that, they have given management executives a special interest in attending and participating in chamber sessions at which problems related to their own industries are freely debated.

The interchange of ideas made possible by this and other mid-century innovations is responsible for a conviction, shared by the various participating associations, to the effect that there is no finer forum for discussion of occupational medical subjects than that provided by the (now) Industrial Medical Association health conferences.

The selection of Detroit as the 1949 convention city was a happy one. It seemed fitting that the association, in a cycle of great expansion, should return to the place where the founding fathers had gathered in 1916, with high hopes, to launch their organization. Vivid was the contrast between that small, unobtrusive meeting and the modern convention at the same site. The handful of men who attended both could look back with pride upon the accomplishments of the intervening thirty-three years.

Following precedent, President-elect Whittaker served as chairman of the 1949 Convention Committee. He and his committeemen (E. A. Irvin, Earl F. Lutz, A. L. Brooks, H. L. Krieger, J. J. Prendergast, F. B. MacMillan) developed a program in keeping with the broadened scope of the association's interests and influence. It included assignments for 200 speakers, whereas the total attendance at the organizing (1916) meeting was only about 125.

Detroit, like the association, had grown up. From an easy gaited manufacturing city, it had expanded into a giant center of industry, ideally equipped for the role of host to visitors interested in the problems of occupational medicine. During the convention week the faculties of the University of Michigan College of Medicine and Wayne University College of Medicine made panel presentations of industrial medical subjects. There were impressive clinics at Harper and Henry Ford hospitals. The great automobile companies and a score of other plants opened their doors that the guests might see modern mass production at close range and inspect medical departments.

Closing a year of fine achievement, H. A. Vonachen relinquished the presidency at the business meeting in Detroit, and Alfred Whittaker was installed as his successor. Other officers were Edward H. Carleton as president-elect, Adolph G. Kammer, first vice-president, E. A. Irvin, second vice-president, with Secretary Slobe and Treasurer-Managing Director Holmblad continuing in office. Newly elected as directors were a group of men representing varied industrial interests and widespread geographical areas: V. C. Baird (Humble Oil & Refining Company), Texas, Harley L. Krieger (Ford Motor Company), Dearborn, C. O. Sappington (industrial health consultant), Chicago, Jerome W. Shilling (Pacific Telephone & Telegraph), Los Angeles, James H. Sterner (Eastman Kodak), Rochester, New York, C. Richard Walmer (Mellon Institute), Pittsburgh.

The incoming president, Alfred H. Whittaker, was born in Ohio and attended

404

Ohio State University College of Medicine from 1913 to 1918, his medical education having been interrupted by service in the Medical Corps, United States Army. Upon graduation he became house surgeon at the Roosevelt Hospital, New York, where medical services had been established for industries in the northwestern section of the city. He then served as a resident surgeon in Bellevue Hospital (1919) and the Detroit Industrial Hospital (1920). In the following year he was junior attending surgeon at Bellevue but returned to Detroit in 1922 and two years later started building his present practice as an industrial surgeon and consultant.

Whittaker's decision to enter industrial practice is an interesting example of the way careers may be shaped by circumstance and chance contacts. While he was in his senior medical year at Ohio State, the Jeffry Manufacturing Company, of Columbus, asked the College of Medicine to supervise the medical care of its employees. It was one of the very first companies in the country to establish such a university connection. W. J. Means, dean of medicine, assigned young Whittaker to this work, and until his graduation he made daily trips to the plant to care for current cases.

It happened that Dean Means, some two years previously, had been greatly impressed by Emery R. Hayhurst's monumental survey of industrial health in Ohio,[2] and it was he who persuaded Hayhurst to teach industrial hygiene at the College of Medicine. Among his students was Whittaker, and the combination of in-plant training and instruction by one of the leading authorities on occupational health opened a whole new world of medicine to him. "Here," he comments, "were men dedicated to and responsible for the medical and surgical care of great groups of workers, rather than individuals." It may be noted that at the time of this incident Hayhurst was already writing, in collaboration with Kober, his master work on industrial health.[3]

A man of many diverse interests, Whittaker has been continuously active in organized medicine at the city, county, state and national levels. He has also been a frequent contributor of professional papers and sketches appearing in the medical press. Joining the AAIP&S at the time of his earliest industrial practice, he served as a director and vice-president of the organization and as a member of many committees.

The association, at mid-century, was embarked upon a new and higher plane of activity. A great deal of unfinished business awaited its turn. There were continuing projects to be carried on. As a result of growth, the functions of the presiding officer changed radically in the late forties. The Executive Committee took over some decisions formerly made by the directors. More work was assigned to committees; and Board members assumed a more active part in the supervision of committee projects. The later history of the association thus becomes a story of the accomplishments of administrations rather than of individuals. Regrettably, a great many well known names have had to be omitted in the interests of brevity.

In the stimulating atmosphere of postwar thinking, it was to be expected that some long-standing precedents in organized industrial medicine should come under fire, and among the convenient targets was the name which the association had borne honorably for more than four decades, despite periodical attacks. As early as June 1922, when the AAIP&S was exactly six years old, "Tom" Crowder wrote to William Sawyer placing himself on record as favoring a change. There is nothing to indicate that the question was even put to a vote.

Similar proposals were made in the thirties, but at no time did they win enough support to press the issue to a decision. At a Board meeting in October 1948, however, E. A. Irvin, then medical director of the Cadillac Division of General Motors, formally suggested that the association change its name by the simple expedient of lopping off the "& Surgeons." Rank and file members were agreed that the original name was too long and cumbersome. Nor was it looked upon with particular favor by other established organizations of physicians and of surgeons. Apparently, however, most members were reluctant to make a change. They felt much as did Loyal Shoudy, who wrote of the 1948 proposal: "I agree the name is long, but everyone has grown used to it, and it is so well known, expecially the word 'Industrial.' My reaction is *let it alone.*" Nevertheless, Irvin's suggestion found considerable favor among directors. Secretary Slobe expressed the opinion that "American Association of Industrial Physicians" was as inclusive as the old name. President Vonachen polled the Board, which voted to refer the proposal to the Committee on Public Relations for recommendation.

By that action the issue became unfinished business for the Whittaker administration. In a report on the program planned for the 1949 convention, Whittaker discussed the proposal and urged members to come prepared to "help us select the very best possible new name." Records show there was no lack of suggestions, most of which were built around the words "industrial," "occupational," "medicine" and "health," in one combination or another. All were referred to the same committee.

The turning point in this search actually came in October 1949. At that time Irvin, after months of further consideration, presented the name "Industrial Medical Association" for approval by the Board. It, too, was referred, without discussion, to the Public Relations Committee, headed by Charles E. Dutchess (medical director, Schenley Laboratories).

Sentiment was rapidly crystallizing in favor of this new proposal. The name, as Irvin pointed out, was short, easy to say, easy to remember, simple but conclusive, easily abbreviated, and it did not confine activities to the American continent. A great deal of work, however, remained to be done before the change could become effective. A constitutional amendment was required, calling for approval by a two-thirds vote of the membership.

Ultimately the name, "Industrial Medical Association," with the blessing of officers and directors, was turned over to the important Committee on Constitution and Bylaws, to be handled along with other organizational changes. This committee (consisting of Chairman E. A. Irvin, Henry S. Brown, E. C. Holmblad, J. D.

Miller, F. E. Shaffer, Jerome W. Shilling, and James H. Sterner) was engaged in an extensive revision of that basic document, a formidable task. Recommendations were exhaustively reviewed at a directors' meeting in December 1950.

Not until the annual business meeting on April 26, 1951—at the close of E. H. Carleton's term as president—were the combined returns from floor- and proxy-balloting announced. The name change was approved by a vote of 598 to 277. The American Association of Industrial Physicians & Surgeons became, at long last, the Industrial Medical Association, but by a surprisingly small margin above the two-thirds required.

At the time Dutchess' committee took over the task of sifting association names, some members thought the organization ought to go further and compound a new name for the speciality itself, something akin to "pediatrics," "geriatrics," or the various "-ologies." Several suggestions were submitted by mail, and the doctor obligingly explored them all. Most of the names proposed were coined by combining the suffix "-iatrics," from the Greek work *iatrikos* (art of healing), with suffixes also of Greek derivation. Examples: "emporiatrics" or "poriatrics," from *emporia* (commerce, trade); "ergiatrics," from *ergatis* (workman); "poniatrics," from *ponos* (work, labor).

Replying to a letter from Dutchess, the G. & C. Merriam Company, publishers of Webster dictionaries, found no fault with the selections with respect to Greek usage. But when it came to choosing a name and campaigning for it, member enthusiasm cooled quickly. The general reaction: We've found it hard enough to teach people what industrial or occupational medicine is, without trying to popularize a foreign compound of our own invention.

Among noteworthy developments in the mid-century years has been the building of a closely knit, active group of district counselors, functioning in front-line positions throughout the country. The need for such field representatives was first recognized officially in 1942, when the component societies were in their formative stage. The counselors had been ambassadors without portfolio, carrying no title, guided by no uniform policies, doing what they could to bring association, components and industrial employers into closer harmony of ideas and effort.

Early in 1948, at the request of Whittaker, the Board of Directors approved a plan calling for a series of meetings, attended by representatives of the Executive Committee, component societies and district counselors, to improve this liaison. The counselor organization had been officially established two years before, but there were still only six districts and six appointees to cover the entire country.

At a meeting in October 1948, Whittaker, then president-elect and also a district counselor, told the Board: "We have not carried out the possibilities; haven't even begun to carry them out. . . . I think we have reached a stage in our development where we might proceed in the next few months with a very real effort to promote a formal organization and make it function."

The plan met with immediate approval by President Vonachen and the directors;

and, strongly supported by successive administrations, the district counselor organization began to measure its progress in giant strides. It was apparent to all that without open lines of communication, and constant contact between central office and field, the association could be little more than a loose federation, lacking vitality and falling far short of its potential in services to industry.

During 1948 a new counselor district was created in Canada, and through the following year encouraging reports were read into the minutes of directors' meetings, indicating increased interest and activity. Counselors were welcomed at meetings of component societies and attended them *ex officio* as guests. Individually, they began to acquire an intimate familiarity with the problems of components and the health needs of local industries. The practical, and measurable, results of this type of contact have been of incalculable value to industrial medicine.

Between 1950 and 1951 the counselor organization made its greatest gain, emerging as a network of twenty-one well staffed districts. And in 1952 George F. Wilkins, president-elect, produced a carefully worked-out code of standards and a memorandum of procedures for the guidance of component societies and district counselors, crystallizing objectives and stabilizing operations. By that time the re-drawing of district lines had increased the number of districts to twenty-nine, and by 1954 further splitting of territories brought the total to a peak of thirty-two.

Signalizing their new importance, the counselors gathered at the Atlantic City convention in 1951 for their first breakfast meeting and discussed their common problems in great detail. So successful was the affair that it was repeated at Cincinnati in 1952. Outlining the program at that time, President-elect E. A. Irvin commented: "Cooperation from all the district counselors has been most unusual in the past year." And after the breakfast President Kammer reported: "It was one of the most inspiring of meetings, with thirty-one present." Productive from a professional viewpoint, and socially pleasant, the counselors' breakfast has become a fixture at annual meetings, growing in popularity and attendance. The counselor organization has proved to be a potent factor in attracting membership and stimulating members to constructive activity.

As if voicing a consensus on that point, Jerome Shilling expressed this opinion to President Robert C. Page and the directors at the 1955 convention: "To me our meeting with the district counselors is the most important meeting in this whole conference. It is the grass-roots—it is the life's blood—of our organization."

While the annual conventions, at the mid-century mark, were gaining steadily in size, range of interest, and prestige, they still bore no label that did justice to the objectives sought and the services rendered. They were programmed as annual meetings of the industrial physicians and surgeons, and as the annual meetings of the four participating organizations of hygienists, nurses, and dentists. A name was needed to describe the entire enterprise as a united effort.

That need was met, in 1951, by a very simple expedient. And thereby hangs an anecdote that dates back many years.

The American Industrial Hygiene Association, having completed its organization in 1939, was seeking an affiliation of one kind or another with some established group in the field of industrial health. An agreement was soon reached that the hygienists should hold their first annual meeting in June, 1940, jointly with the twenty-fifth convention of the AAIP&S. At a meeting on the eve of that convention Secretary Volney Cheney told the directors he was disturbed by the possibility that the hygienists might decide to admit as members the nurses, technicians, sanitary engineers, and even medical men, a move that would cause a confused and difficult situation.

"I have thought it over," he said, "and have made up a plan. . . . It would be a means of getting together all the agencies that are interested in industrial health." And with that remark he passed out copies of a proposal to form a new organization, to be known as the American Conference on Industrial Health.

"Do you really want to organize this thing?" asked Clarence Selby. Cheney did, and in the end he had his way. "We are interested only in people who are interested in industrial health," he told the Board. "There may be other agencies that are trying to do the same thing, but it is for us to do. We don't want industrial medicine to get away from us."

So the new conference was launched, with Cheney as president, and Holmblad, Slobe, Vonachen and Sappington among the officers. Its stated purpose was "to pool information from all kinds of persons, both medical and non-medical, with reference to industrial health problems." Under sponsorship of the AAIP&S it conducted an elaborate symposium in Chicago in November 1940 and held its second annual meeting a year later.[4] Little more was heard of the Conference during the war or in the immediate postwar period. The foreword of the 1950 convention program of the association, however, referred to the meeting as an "industrial health conference," and in 1951 at Atlantic City all activities were officially grouped under the aegis of the "1951 Industrial Health Conference." Thus was Cheney's dream realized, and the purpose of his original organization fulfilled. The Industrial Hygiene Association, as we know, has continued to meet annually with the Industrial Medical Association, and has been joined by the American Conference of Governmental Industrial Hygienists, the American Association of Industrial Nurses, and the American Association of Industrial Dentists as participants.

To promote efficiency in the conduct of the association's internal affairs, and to further the effectiveness of its field work, Alfred Whittaker's administration (1949–1950) speeded plans for national coverage by the network of district counselors and better integration of their activities with those of the component societies. The committee structure of the association also was expanded; duties and personnel were realigned to meet new needs. Of great importance in the same year was the introduction of a modern system of budget control and other basic accounting reforms.

Nowhere did the burden of a growing public relations program fall more heavily than upon the shoulders of the managing director, Edward Holmblad. In one seven-week period at the end of 1948 he attended no less than nine major meetings, at widely separated points and including such items as a lecture to industrial nurses, a conference on civil defense, a symposium on alcoholism and the annual dinner of the American Association of Railway Surgeons. Nor was there any prospect of less exacting schedules; on the contrary, the load grew steadily, pointing the need for more district counselors and the division of field work among them.

Early 1949 brought glowing reports from the thriving Territorial Association of Plantation Physicians in Hawaii and from other component societies. Though great distances and thinly scattered manufacture hampered industrial medicine in Canada, the 1949 convention in Detroit was well attended by Canadian industrial doctors and nurses. In the autumn of that year Holmblad was delegated to attend the annual meeting of the Hawaiian association. It was a highly successful mission. After a visit to Quebec in the same period Frank R. Griffin, district counselor for Canada, and E. A. Irvin reported increasing activity among industrial medical organizations in leading Canadian cities.

The fruits of these early contacts between the central office and the field were not long in ripening. Interest in occupational medicine was quickening. The phenomenal growth of industry in the south and west brought a corresponding increase in the number of industrial doctors and presaged the addition of component societies in Texas and the Northwest.

The success of the thirty-fourth annual meeting of the association in Detroit stimulated further efforts to enhance the prestige of these conventions. The 1950 meeting in Chicago, at which Whittaker presided, outshone its predecessor in attendance, in interest, in activities, and in brilliance. The association had indeed reached maturity.

Opening the directors' meeting on that occasion, Whittaker as outgoing president said: "I am impressed more and more each year by the tremendous stature which this organization is attaining. The all-day session of about 150 General Motors men here yesterday and all these groups meetings today, with the rooms overcrowded, are some indication of the importance in medicine which our association is assuming." A gavel was presented to Whittaker by the Sherman Hotel management "as a souvenir by which to remember this convention," and the Board settled down to business.

Among group meetings at the 1950 meeting the annual luncheon of past presidents of the association was again an event of importance. Two years before, in Boston, the retiring president, Henry Brown, had a set a precedent by entertaining the group at lunch. At Detroit in 1949 sixteen of the nineteen living ex-presidents were present as guests of H. A. Vonachen. Among them were three founding members—Mock, Geier and Shoudy. Following precedent, Whittaker was host to the group at the Chicago University Club in 1950, an occasion marked by the first display of portraits of all past presidents, painted by a Chicago artist. This series, originally proposed by Whittaker, has been continued down to the present.

The banquet at the close of the convention was a gala affair, carefully planned to reflect the size and dignity of the association. It attracted a record-breaking attendance. An imposing array of prominent medical men and local dignitaries filled the head table, and the guest speaker was Rear Admiral Clifford A. Swanson, surgeon-general, United States Navy. The importance of the occasion, the Convention Committee had concluded, called for a fair amount of formality.

It so happened that on the same day, April 27, Otto Geier celebrated his 76th birthday. His thoughts, on that anniversary, could well have run parallel to those of Daniel Lynch, who, from retirement in Connecticut, had written to Whittaker a few days before: "How the little army of despised 'company doctors' has grown, and what a grand job they are doing!"

At the business session the association followed traditional procedure in its choice of executive officers. As president-elect, Edward Carleton automatically moved into the presidency; Adolph Kammer was named president-elect, E. A. Irvin, first vice-president, and George Wilkins, second vice-president.

Reporting for the Nominating Committee, Henry Brown paused in his reading of the list of candidates to announce, regretfully, the resignation of Secretary Slobe because of the press of professional duties. He had served the association with distinction for nearly five years after completing his term in the presidency (1944–45). As new secretary the membership elected Arthur K. Peterson, medical director of the R. R. Donnelley and Sons Company, Chicago.

In November, 1949, the association had been shocked by the sudden death of Clarence O. Sappington. Editorial consultant for the association's official journal from its inception, he was named chairman of the first Committee on Publications and Editorial Policy in 1939 and became editor-in-chief of the magazine in 1940. Sappington's loss not only necessitated changes in the staff of the journal but created a vacancy on the Board of Directors. To fill the unexpired term on the Board, the members endorsed Carey P. McCord, then medical adviser to the Chrysler Corporation and consulting editor of *Industrial Medicine and Surgery*. It was a significant choice, in view of the part he was soon to play in shaping the subsequent progress of the journal.

New directors elected for 1950–52 were James M. Carlisle (Merck & Company), Robert C. Page (Standard Oil Company, New Jersey), Max Burnell (General Motors Corporation), Floyd Shaffer (Bethlehem Steel Company), Russell Birrell (Imperial Oil Company of Canada), and Daniel Braun (Consolidated Coal Company).

The incoming president, Edward H. Carleton, was born in Massachusetts but received his higher education at the University of Louisville and its medical school, from which he was graduated in 1932. After two years in general practice and two more in orthopedic surgery he made, in 1937, his first and only industrial affiliation with the Inland Steel Company, which he has served since 1957 as general medical director.

411

Carleton took over the presidency with a conviction that members, by and large, were not adequately represented in the affairs of the association and that they should participate much more widely in its activities. He also believed that further steps should be taken to improve the status of industrial medicine and the association in the eyes of the medical profession and public.

From its start the Carleton regime gave strong support to plans that would increase quantity and maintain quality of membership. To that end it sought out means of reactivating the interest of delinquent members and pushed to conclusion a long awaited revision of the association's bylaws. Completion of this laborious task, among other things, solved an old problem, for the revised document altered and clarified provisions that had theretofore hampered the healthy growth of membership through the component societies.

Under Carleton's administration, too, the expanded district-counselor program was placed in operation on a truly national basis by the appointment of added counselors, in old and new districts, which tripled the force available for liaison work in the field. Further strengthening outside activities and enhancing association prestige, a Speakers' Bureau was started in September 1950 and announced two months later in *Industrial Medicine and Surgery*. At a directors' meeting in December Edward Holmblad reported that thirty well known members had registered with the bureau and expressed their willingness to speak on a combined total of thirty-one different subjects.

"We could possibly conceive of multiplying that by thirty," commented Carleton. "We certainly would be spreading the gospel if we could get speakers all over the country carrying the message we would like to carry to the public and interested groups." The activity has remained an integral part of association service, supplying speakers wherever possible to organizations planning industrial health conferences in various areas.

On the very day on which Carleton took over the presidency (April 26, 1950) an acute problem of inter-association relations flared up at the business session, after the managing director had read into the record a report filed by Margaret S. Hargreaves, R.N., on behalf of the American Association of Industrial Nurses. There was absolutely nothing controversial in the report itself. The document was a simple statement of progress made by a joint committee studying the so-called "Standing Orders" for nurses in industry, and it expressed the hope that an amicable agreement could be reached as to their content and wording. Nevertheless, it was to have widespread repercussions.

The joint committee had been formed in the summer of 1949. It consisted of Slobe, Carleton, and Holmblad, representing the AAIP&S; Carl M. Peterson of the AMA Council on Industrial Health; and Mrs. Hargreaves and two other representatives of the AAIN. The AMA, long interested in industrial nursing procedures, had previously published a compilation of Standing Orders, but it did not meet the needs of the new industrial age, and a revised edition was contemplated.

There was almost no discussion of Mrs. Hargreaves' AAIN report at the 1950 business meeting. Delegates promptly approved the nurses' statement but kept the underlying issues very much alive by referring the entire matter back to the association "for intensive study." Given high priority by the Carleton administration, the project was ardently debated at every meeting of the IMA directors for more than a year and a half.

Exploratory work by the joint committee had quickly shown that the problem faced by the industrial nurses was much broader, and far more complex, than that of Standing Orders and that it could not be solved by a revision of old text. "We know," said they, "that Standing Orders cannot be considered a substitute for medical directions." They also knew that Standing Orders, as a blanketing code of instructions, had no legality in courts of law.

More disturbing were reports that industrial nurses in some states had become involved in lawsuits charging them with illegal practice of medicine. The core of the problem, as the AAIN saw it, lay in the question of *what constitutes medical direction for nurses in industry.* It was an acute, even critical, problem in small plants, which were in the majority and which for the most part did not have full-time medical directors.

What was really needed was a comprehensive and unequivocal statement of guiding principles covering the duties and responsibilities of management, the doctor and the nurse with respect to industrial health services. Each of the three associations (AMA, IMA and AAIN) set forth its ideas as to the content of such a code. There were areas of agreement, but they were offset by areas of disagreement, resulting largely from the legal implications of any action taken by a professional group or groups. Seemingly, complete accord was remote if not impossible, yet the nurses became more and more insistent that their status be clarified by policy and/or by law.

J. F. McCahan, in his April 1951 proposal[5] listed in some detail the conditons under which a nurse in industry could "render her services with ethical and legal impunity." Apparently, however, this document did not meet AMA specifications, for soon afterward Carl Peterson, secretary of the Council on Industrial Health, introduced a drastically abbreviated version which he indicated would be acceptable to the council and the Board of Trustees. This new suggestion was duly submitted to the IMA for action at a directors' meeting in October 1951, over which President Kammer presided.

Presenting the proposed text as chairman of the Committee on Policy, Paul J. Bamberger (Bethlehem Steel Company) severely criticized its "bare outline form," its vague tone, and its sins of omission in content. "It is innocuous," he said, "and therefore is perfectly all right." In its formal report the committee summarized the document as "a confusing disavowal of realistic practices, which we cannot endorse for your approval either in principle or in fact."

Viewing the situation objectively, the Board of Directors found itself in a dilemma. The AMA would publish the outline version with or without IMA endorsement. If approval were denied the association could be accused, with some justice, of unwillingness to cooperate. If approval were given, it would be construed as unqualified agreement on all points of policy and the form in which they were presented. On the other hand, as Board members pointed out, the statement was "what the nurses wanted." For all its shortcomings, it was legally correct. And, as a preface to a more thorough handling later, it was at least a step in the right direction. With an expressed hope that further work would be done on the basic problem, the Board voted to approve the statement "as submitted."

Under the title "Essentials of Medical-Nursing Services in Industry," the abbreviated version of this much-discussed text was published in the AMA *Journal* of June 7, 1952.[6] It occupied less than a column. More than three years later the *Journal* published an exhaustive report, a full five pages in length, which it described as "a revision of the Council's previous publication titled 'Standing Orders for Nurses in Industry.' "[7] It is interesting to note that on the committee in charge of this revision were Emmett B. Lamb, representing the IMA, and George F. Wilkins, serving as a member-at-large.

This sequence of events has been examined in some detail, not to indicate discord and controversy in the ranks of medicine, but as an example of what Whittaker has called "problems in partnership," illustrating the difficulty of reconciling differences in viewpoint, which in this instance, if hurriedly or intemperately handled, could have consigned the industrial nurse to a routine of elementary tasks, unattractive, and unrewarding.

There were many such differences of policy and opinion to be resolved in the period under discussion. The IMA's activities were branching out in every direction, its professional relations growing steadily more complex. It is to the credit of all organizations involved that problems, small and large, were approached and worked out with patience and understanding.

The number of interassociation contacts calling for cooperative effort was surprisingly large, and the projects involved varied widely. A few are mentioned briefly here, as a record for the future.

Typical of these contacts was the association's participation in the work of an organization wordily but descriptively named the International Association of Industrial Accident Boards and Commissions. This group, though small, was very influential in the field of workmen's compensation. Represented in its membership were forty states, three territories and three federal bureaus, as well as other agencies interested in industrial health problems. In the fall of 1947 Slobe and Holmblad were delegated to attend the IAIABC meeting in Toronto, and two years later Carl T. Olson was sent to its thirty-fifth annual convention in St. Louis, at which there was a long discussion of the ethics and standards of practice in compensation medicine and the responsibilities of industrial management and medical departments in that connection. On his return Olson reported the proceedings in full detail. Such a contact yielded two important benefits: it gave organized industrial medicine a listening post in the councils of compensation officials, and it kept the industrial doctors posted on developments of vital importance to them.

Needless to say, industrial physicians and surgeons have followed closely, as both observers and participants, the activities of the annual AMA Congress on Industrial Health since its inception in 1941. The IMA has also maintained its interest in the medical meetings of General Motors Corporation and has strongly supported conferences sponsored by local industrial health agencies.

During the same period the association took every opportunity to extend its contacts on an international scale. In 1949 it was represented at the first American Congress of Industrial Medicine, in Buenos Aires, by Colonel Wesley Cox, who was also the United States Army delegate. Some four hundred delegates, from twenty-two countries, attended the sessions. Colonel Cox was one of the speakers and for the excellence of his address was decorated by President Juan Peron, whose star was then still ascendant.

Two years later the association named Carey McCord and J. M. Carlisle as its official representatives at the famed International Conference on Industrial Health in Lisbon in 1951. Robert T. Legge was delegated to deliver the official invitation to the conference to hold its next meeting in the United States, in honor of the tenth anniversary of the conference. But it was not until 1960 that the conference was held on this side of the Atlantic.

Noting these broad international contacts and considering the magnitude of America's occupational health programs, one may look back with some satisfaction to the Brussells congress attended by Dr. Alice Hamilton in 1910, at which a Belgian official dismissed industrial hygiene in the United States with a contemptuous "*Ça n'existe pas.*"[8]

The association story in what we may, for convenience, call "the mid-century period" tends to support the old belief that the way to get work done is to assign it to a busy man. A more or less random listing indicates the many directions in which affiliations and activities were developed during that period by the IMA officially and by too-busy members individually.

By the end of the war the work of the Railroad Retirement Board (under the Act of 1937) had reached substantial proportions, and in 1947 the board asked the association to help in the selection of medical examiners to evaluate disability and to make other examinations in problem cases. From its own membership the association was able to provide a list of thoroughly qualified doctors in nearly a dozen specified cities.

Since 1950 the IMA has performed substantial services in the scientific attack on the common cold and other chest diseases. Its interest in these started with the passage of a simple resolution of approval and encouragement, at the request of the American College of Chest Surgeons. Lip service to the cause, however, soon developed into active support and participation.

Formulation of a vigorous and effective program was hampered at the start by the fact that two separate organizations, the American Research and Education Foundation for Chest Diseases and the Common Cold Institute, were at work on the same problems, seeking the same goals by different routes. This duplication was corrected in 1951 by a merger of the two into the Common Cold Foundation, with William A. Sawyer as its first director. Serving on the Board of Directors and the Medical Advisory Committee of the foundation were representative groups of members of the IMA.

To stimulate interest in the scientific study of chest diseases, the IMA and College of Chest Physicians participated jointly at Atlantic City in June 1951 in a symposium on these diseases. It was a great success, holding an enthusiastic audience of eight hundred in the meeting room for more than two hours. Representatives of the IMA on that occasion included E. C. Holmblad, Leo Price, D. C. Braun, A. W. Vorwald, F. R. Ferlaino.

In the same year the association undertook new working arrangements with several other national health agencies, in recognition of their common interests. The Aero-Medical Association, dealing with the formidable physiological and psychological problems of modern flight, was invited to participate in the annual IMA conventions. Representatives of the IMA and the American Public Health Association discussed steps by which duplication of effort and overlapping of functions could be avoided in the field of industrial hygiene. And there was consultation with a committee of the American Industrial Hygiene Association which was considering a year of in-plant postgraduate training as a requirement for hygiene engineers.

In the midst of these programs to strengthen the internal organization and improve the outside relationships of the association, the Carleton administration took decisive action on plans to reorganize the American Foundation of Occupational Health as a fund-raising agency and to develop a basically new method of surveying and certifying medical services in industry. These activities are further discussed in the following chapter.

For all their preoccupation with urgent professional business the Board of Directors found time, over a period of several years, to discuss the possibility of buying or building a national home to house the central offices of the association and to provide facilities "in keeping with its size and importance and the scope of its activities."

This project was first submitted for official consideration at a Board meeting in October 1948 by Alfred Whittaker, then president-elect of the association. With Holmblad he had toured Chicago's medical center and studied plans for future development along the lake shore. There were conferences with city planners and real estate brokers, prices were obtained, and costs estimated.

The idea was favorably received by this and succeeding Boards. Reports and discussions continued at meetings through the next four years. There was general agreement that the proposed building would meet a real need and would be a wise investment. Costs, however, were rising rapidly, and in 1952 a committee headed by E. S. Jones advised against commitments at that time. The national-home idea is still

416

a dream, but, the association periodically reminds itself, the dream will one day become a plan, and the plan a reality.

Carleton ended his term in 1951 with the unique distinction of having been elected president of one organization, the AAIP&S, and of stepping out of office as president of another, the IMA. For the last official act of his administration, at the business meeting of April 26, was to announce the result of the balloting that authorized the change of name.

The 1951 election at Atlantic City brought to the presidency another able executive and administrative head, A. G. Kammer. Other officers chosen were E. A. Irvin, president-elect, George F. Wilkins, first vice-president, Robert Collier Page, second vice-president, with A. K. Peterson continuing as secretary and E. C. Holmblad as treasurer and managing director. As directors for the 1951–52 term, the members endorsed Carey P. McCord, Leo Price (International Ladies Garment Workers), C. Richard Walmer (Industrial Hygiene Foundation), Carl T. Olson (Liberty Mutual Insurance Company), Milton Kronenberg (Caterpillar Tractor Company), E. P. Luongo (General Petroleum Corporation), and, to fill Page's unexpired term, James H. Sterner (Eastman Kodak Company).

Adolph G. Kammer received bachelor's and master's degrees from the University of Wisconsin in 1925 and 1926, respectively, and his M.D. from the University of Pennsylvania. His earliest industrial affiliation was made in 1934, and since 1949 he has served as professor and chairman of the Department of Occupational Health, University of Pittsburgh, and as consultant medical director of the Carbide and Carbon Chemicals Corporation. Aside from his university connection, he has served the association as chairman of the Committee on Education and Training and was a member of the Atomic Energy Commission Committee on Industrial Medicine. His background and experience fitted him well for a period in which one of the most conspicuous problems was that of industrial medical education.

From the beginning of his term Kammer worked zealously to develop a strong and responsible Executive Committee and to transfer certain presidential duties to junior officers, some of whom would eventually succeed to the presidency. Time, on the whole, had dealt kindly with the past presidents of the association; the majority of those living were still active, and fourteen of them attended their annual lunch at Atlantic City in 1951. In those seasoned veterans was a source of experience and judgment that could be used to great advantage. Having perpetuated their informal organization and retained their interest in association affairs, they have in latter years performed invaluable services as district counselors and on important committee assignments.

As for administrative procedures, he cast some light on his philosophy in commenting to the Board of Directors at an October, 1951, meeting: "The whole team is working on the problems of the association. We are not a Damon and Pythias group; we have our fights. I should say we 'scrap clean' and we usually come out all the better for having had some differences and having argued them out."

XXXII

OBJECTIVES ACHIEVED!

O F ALL organized activities of the Industrial Medical Association over the years, none has aroused more partisan zeal than the campaign for certification of occupational medicine as a specialty. Without certification the association could not possibly expect to reach its one central objective: namely, the development —with the cooperation of allied agencies—of occupational medicine, hygiene, and safety to maximum effectiveness and the extension of their benefits to the largest possible number of workers and employers. That, of course, is the purpose for which industrial health services exist. It is the end that justifies all expenditures of thought, time and effort.

With its status on a par with that of other medical and surgical specialties, it was certain that a much larger number of able young doctors would be attracted to the industrial field, where they were urgently needed. With American Medical Association board control it would be possible to set and enforce the highest standards of medical practice in industry.

It is not hard to understand why the membership of the IMA felt that they had not only a priority of interest but a good deal of seniority in their chosen field. The founding fathers had regarded industrial practice as a specialty long before they talked of organizing. The infant association cut its teeth on the problem of recognition by employers and by other medical groups, in particular, the AMA. In those early times the doctor who talked of ambitious in-plant programs was as likely to be greeted by indifference as by outright opposition. A common rejoinder was, "Industrial medicine! What is that?"

The American Association of Industrial Physicians & Surgeons had been spreading its gospel for six years before the AMA amended (in 1922) the name of its Section on Preventive Medicine and Public Health to include the word "Industrial."

The AMA Council on Industrial Health did not start full-scale operation until the end of 1937. The industrial doctors had been discussing certification of their specialty since 1935, only two years after the first American boards were approved, and they started to campaign in earnest when the council was only a few months old.

How often must it have seemed discouragingly like a tilt with windmills or the pursuit of a will-o'-the-wisp!

Very early it became apparent that priority of interest and length of experience in the field carried little or no weight. No medical organization could win board status by a solo effort. The process of certification, seemingly simple, was hedged about with an intricate web of safeguards and requirements even in its first years of operation.

The validity of the AMA's activities in the industrial field, as in other fields, was not to be questioned. As "the voice of American medicine," and its recognized leader, the AMA was (and is) a guardian of the public interest and the interests of any medical group within its membership. It was then, as now, responsible for maintenance of medical ethics and standards of practice both public and private.

Actually, of course, membership in the AMA is a prerequisite to membership in the IMA. But though the two organizations have usually agreed on questions of basic policy, there was no such harmony in assigning a place for industrial practice in the medical scheme of things. Negotiations were disturbed by wide differences of opinion, a good deal of distrust, and criticism which at times bordered on open controversy.

In the 1940's the "whether and how" of certification became the biggest and most fundamental of all interassociation issues. Widespread professional, business, and socio-political interests were involved at every step, as a timetable story of events reveals.

The first official step toward certification of occupational medicine took the form of a friendly call at the Chicago headquarters of the AMA in 1935, when Edward Holmblad and Volney Cheney spent a pleasant half-day with Morris Fishbein, R. G. Leland, and Ernest Brown, discussing the procedures to be followed.

"We were told," Holmblad reported, "that there was no such thing as a specialty of industrial medicine and surgery. We were led to believe that this was simply one of the sub-topics under general medicine, and were advised orally not to try to make it a specialized field at that time."

In August, 1938, less than a year after the AMA's new Council on Industrial Health launched its own ambitious program, the AAIP&S tried again. Secretary Cheney wrote a letter of inquiry, tantamount to an application, to Dr. Paul Titus, then secretary of the AMA Advisory Board for Medical Specialties. He received a prompt and cordial reply. "The board you propose," said Titus, "overlaps in both medicine and surgery, and, therefore, in all probability would need to be an affiliate of one of these boards." He enclosed a booklet spelling out the requirements for certification and explained the procedures in some detail.

To the industrial doctors, however, a compromise of this kind was definitely unsatisfactory. As Holmblad reasoned: "When you speak to interns, when you speak to residents, when you speak to the younger men in medicine, they look to the board of surgery, or one of the others for their requirements. If we do not offer these young men in medicine an equal basis and an equal footing in the specialty of industrial medicine and surgery, the better men will go into the specialties that offer recognition, and we will take what is left."

In 1939 the association, through its Certification Committee, consisting of Slobe, Cheney, and Holmblad, again sounded the possibility of board status under the regular form of the AMA and was met with a variation of the same answer. "We were told," the committee reported, "that there was no place at this time for a specialty of industrial medicine and surgery."

Balked in this exchange of words, the association decided to organize a board of its own, which was duly incorporated on April 22, 1941, as the American Board of Industrial Medicine and Surgery, with Holmblad, Slobe, Cheney, Sappington and Hazlett listed as members. Actually, the charter did not improve, or even alter, the official status of industrial medicine, but it served the purposes of a declaration of independence, and it provided useful bargaining points for future negotiation.

It is at this point in the story of occupational medicine that the problem of certification became inseparably linked with the problem of education, and in subsequent discussions of the one topic, we find mention of the other. It was obvious to any thinking member of the profession that unless enough of the right kind of industrial medical courses were available to enough students in enough schools, there could be no certification of the specialty in the accepted sense.

During 1940, committees gave what time they could to setting up an outline of such courses, which would meet board requirements and which they hoped could be incorporated into already crowded medical school curricula. Armed with this outline, Vonachan, Slobe and Holmblad paid another visit to AMA headquarters early in 1941. They were cordially received and discussed the ins and outs of special graduate training with three representatives of the Council on Industrial Health: S. J. Seeger (chairman), Carl M. Peterson (secretary), and A. J. Lanza, who was prominent in the activities of both associations.

Encouraged by this reception, the committee dispatched another letter to Paul Titus in April 1941 suggesting that since the attitude of the AMA toward industrial medicine had changed considerably, the Advisory Board's opinion about certification might also have changed. The doctor (who was no longer secretary of that body) was cooperative but noncommittal. He recognized the AAIP&S as the *one* national organization in its special field but pointed out that several other agencies had to be consulted before a new certification board could be formally set up.

The association promptly changed its strategy to fit the circumstances. At its annual business meeting in the same month, it passed a resolution calling attention to the increasing number of physicians and surgeons in industrial practice and the diversified activities of the AMA Council on Industrial Health in that field. It also requested of the AMA the appointment of a joint committee of three from each of the associations "to further the establishment of an American Board of Industrial Medicine and Surgery" and to seek its approval by the Advisory Board of Medical Specialties. In June 1941 this resolution was introduced at a meeting of the AMA Section of Preventive and Industrial Medicine and Public Health by Robert T. Legge. On the following day the request was approved and a committee appointed to represent the AMA in interassociation conferences. It should be noted that all three appointees, Leverett D. Bristol, of New York, William A. Sawyer, of Rochester, New York, and R. T. Legge, of Berkeley, California, were members of the AAIP&S as well as of the AMA.

Surely this was progress! The association's journal, in a gay editorial, reported jubilantly: "Thus industrial medicine, which only a little while ago was pretty generally thought about as of possible specialty status only in the remote future, is well on its way toward full recognition *now.*"[1]

The road to certification, however, was not destined to become a rosy path. Disappointment followed disappointment. Negotiations were slowed by successive disagreements as to what should be done and how and when it should be done. And war was soon to change every perspective and affect every phase of medical service.

There was solid accomplishment to report, nevertheless, on the educational front. T. Lyle Hazlett had established a Department of Industrial Hygiene at the University of Pittsburgh Medical School and was blazing new academic trails in that field. As incoming president of the association in 1941, he urged the Board of Directors to accelerate action on a concrete program. "I hope," he said, "we may formulate a plan that can be presented to the senior class of each medical school in the country. I think it is most important that we guide that education. If we don't guide it, I don't know who will."

The association's Committee on Medical Education, headed by Milton H. Kronenberg, eagerly took up this challenge. It was ready in October 1941 with specific recommendations for undergraduate and graduate courses in industrial medicine. By the end of the year, in conferences with a corresponding committee of the AMA, a complete program had been worked out, and a joint report for study by the deans of medical schools was published in February 1942.[2]

Meanwhile, the Committee on Certification was beset by new difficulties. The corresponding group in the AMA did not like the name proposed for the new board, American Board of Industrial Medicine and Surgery. There was a feeling that the word "surgery" might lead the public or doctors to confuse certificates from the Industrial Board with those issued by the existing American Board of Surgery. The identities of the Board of Surgery and of the American College of Surgeons, it was argued, should be protected from any possible chance of conflict or misunderstanding. As a substitute, the AMA committee submitted the name American Board of Industrial Practice, but the industrial doctors would have none of that. It mentioned neither medicine nor surgery and could as well be associated with industrial production. A bit nonplused, the Certification Committee went back to work. It inserted a change of name, American Board of Physicians and Surgeons in Industry, in a ten-page plan for organization of the proposed board and distributed copies at a meeting of the Committee on Standards and Examinations of the AMA Advisory Board for Medical Specialties in February 1943.

Slobe reported back to the Board of Directors that the AMA representatives at that session included one radiologist, one pathologist, one internal medical consultant, and one dermatologist, C. Guy Lane (secretary). "I don't think any of them," Slobe added, "had any conception of what this specialty really means."

Nothing was heard from the influential AMA group for three months, but the answer, when it came, was brief and to the point. The application for a new specialty board had been rejected, for three expressed reasons: standards of the proposed Founders' Group were not clearly defined; adequate facilities for graduate training were not available; and the existence of industrial medicine as a specialty was still questioned. For the first and third of these objections, the industrial doctors had ready answers. The size and character of the founders' group could easily be adjusted to meet any requirements. And the important work being done by the AMA Council on Industrial Health was itself sufficient recognition of industrial medicine as a special field. There was general agreement, however, that the second objection was valid at the time. Facilities for three years of graduate training for career candidates simply did not exist. It was obvious that an enormous amount of educational planning remained to be done, and with dogged determination the association set about doing it.

During the next few years the organization dipped deeply into its membership for personnel, old and new, to man necessary projects. Existing committees were enlarged, new committees formed. Past presidents, former officers and directors gave invaluable services. An incredible volume of study, analysis and detailed planning was handled by groups assigned to certification, medical education, graduate fellowships, qualifications, policies and practice.

During 1943, Hazlett and Kronenberg outlined a comprehensive three-year program of basic classroom courses and in-plant training. Word came that a growing number of medical schools were laying the groundwork for special graduate instruction in occupational medicine, the list including Pittsburgh, Buffalo, Long Island, Columbia, Harvard, Johns Hopkins, California. Slobe reported: "We have established a beachhead and I think we can hold it, but that is about as far as it has gone at the present time."

As time went on, the need for substantial aid to graduate students became more and more apparent. Very few had the means to extend their formal training for two or three extra years, and, recognizing this, the association decided to set up a fund-raising organization to operate in conjunction with the educational program. Officers and directors were thinking, roughly, in terms of courses covering from eighteen to twenty-seven consecutive months, depending on the amount of in-plant training included to meet certification requirements. The cost of fellowship aid per student was estimated at about $3,000 for a course of minimum length to $6,000 or $7,500 for a three-year period.

There was no delusion among the directors that these objectives could be reached either quickly or easily, but they were in a mood for action. Reporting in October 1944, the Committee on Policy and Plan, with F. E. Poole as chairman, sounded a militant note in tune with their thinking.

Strong guidance will be required by the medical profession to accomplish for industry the most efficient results, while at the same time maintaining the highest scientific and ethical standards.

The AMA is showing little leadership in this field. Lay organizations such as the National Association of Manufacturers, Princeton University [Industrial Relations Research], the National Conference Board, and Chambers of Commerce are actually doing more promotion work than any medical agency.

In summary the report expressed the belief that "this association, representing industrial medicine in the United States, should take the initiative and make itself the recognized authority in industrial medicine" and urged it to "become the active and dominant agent" in promoting undergraduate and graduate training, organizing and financing fellowships, and developing a standardizing and accrediting agency for industrial medical services.

In 1945 the association wrote one of the most important pages in its entire history, with the establishment of the American Foundation of Occupational Health (now the Occupational Health Institute). In its original form this foundation was a tax-exempt trust set up by the officers of the association and administered by a Board of Trustees (consisting originally of incorporators Slobe, Cheney, and Holmblad) for the purpose of promoting the program summarized above.

From a financial viewpoint at least, the fellowship plan was the most ambitious project yet undertaken by the association. Its annual cost, for pilot operations of optimum size, was estimated at $50,000 to $60,000. How and where to seek the required funds? Within that single problem there were many problems.

Employers were the most logical source of contributions. By and large they were receptive to the development of practical medical programs in their plants and recognized that effective control of health hazards was reflected directly in less absenteeism and greater production. Yet employers wanted to know exactly how the money was to be spent, and many expected to see graduate training plans in full operation before committing themselves to any substantial support.

Labor, too, was interested in industrial health plans but could not be regarded as a source of funds for the education or in-plant training of physicians and surgeons. Unions, through their accredited spokesmen, were more prone to endorse federal aid proposals and insofar as possible to administer their own programs.

At times it seemed as though the foundation were destined to travel in an endless circle—there could be no certification without specialized education, no adequate graduate instruction without fellowships, no fellowships without financial support—and few contributions without proof that the fellowship plan was workable and would provide trained men in the numbers required.

During the formative stage of the foundation, the association's Committee on Medical Education was in close contact with the deans of medical colleges. "Their cry," committee Chairman Kronenberg reported, "is that they need time to bring the industrial courses into their curriculum, which they hope to do after the war."

As chairman of the Committee on Graduate Fellowships in 1945, Hazlett filed a detailed report listing proposed minimum requirements for a graduate program in industrial medicine, setting up criteria for the selection of candidates, and outlining basic classroom and clinical courses. It also specified laboratory or in-plant medical department training acceptable to certifying boards. This material was made available to the deans of medical schools; and Hazlett stimulated further interest with a compact text titled *Introduction to Industrial Medicine*[3] which was distributed to all graduates of the course at Pittsburgh.

In the same period came a report from Kronenberg that of fifty-two medical schools in the United States and Canada which had replied to a mail inquiry, only three were giving no instruction in industrial medicine. Among schools mentioned as doing particularly good work were Stanford, Colorado, and Illinois; and Yale and Wayne were projecting plans on an ambitious scale. "The seed," commented President Newquist, "is beginning to take hold in those medical schools."

Across the nation, as the war drew to a close, there were signs of growing enthusiasm not only for formal education in occupational medicine but for practical training in industry. *Medical Economics* cited on-the-job plans carried out by eastern utilities "in lieu of formal residencies."[4] Said J. J. Wittmer (Consolidated Edison, New York): "We are constantly teaching by plant symposium and conference." The American Telephone and Telegraph Company had a similar plan.

True to hopes and promises, medical deans in every section of the country were adding special industrial courses to their curricula. Long Island College of Medicine offered a refresher course for men who had been in war service, and it planned to expand both its undergraduate and its graduate courses. In industrial Detroit Raymond Hussey, dean of Wayne University's School of Occupational Medicine, gave a fifteen-week orientation course as the "testing out of a pattern" for industrial instruction.

Another straw in this favorable wind was a substantial increase in publicity relating to occupational medicine. The AFOH published a timely brochure outlining the association's educational views and plans. The Wayne program, which included a continuing series of outstanding conferences on industrial medical relations, was described in an article in *The Detroiter,* the journal of the Detroit Board of Commerce.[5]

Of national interest was a radio round table sponsored by the University of Chicago, in cooperation with the National Broadcasting Company, in April 1946.

The topic, management's responsibility for the medical care of its employees, was discussed by a panel of five prominent doctors, four of whom were active in the AAIP&S. The text was widely distributed in booklet form.

In spite of such encouragement, the association found itself seriously handicapped by the lack of action on certification. Slobe pictured the dilemma in a paragraph: "Men who take residencies have to point toward something. If they don't have certification to point to, as other specialties do, they won't have the incentive, and I'm afraid it is going to be difficult to get applicants for fellowships."

In this peculiar situation the association did about the only practical thing it could do, proceed on an independent course. Through its chairman, Henry S. Brown, the Committee on Certification recommended formation of a founders' group "that would be nationally recognized and acceptable"; presentation of definite evidence of the establishment of occupational courses in outstanding medical schools; and "reaffirmation of our faith in the premise that industrial medicine in its component branches is a definite specialty."

This recommendation was followed to the letter, and the resulting proposal was discussed and approved in 1947 by the joint committee of the two associations. Then came what was described as "an epoch-making development." The entire plan, including detailed provisions for graduate instruction, residencies and fellowships, was approved by the House of Delegates and by the all-important AMA Council on Medical Education and Hospitals (created in 1933 to formulate standards of administration and to recognize new boards meeting those standards).

There were other favorable signs in the same year, most notable among them a conference on industrial medical education sponsored by the Council on Medical Education and the Council on Industrial Health of the AMA. Stanley Seeger (chairman of the Council on Industrial Health) reportedly had withdrawn his objection to certification, and in his address of welcome he spoke freely of "specialists in the field of occupational medicine." Carl Peterson (council secretary) discussed the essentials of a residency in the same specialty.

Significant, too, was the fact that Raymond Hussey presided over the conference and that William A. Sawyer (then editor of AMA's war-born publication, *Occupational Medicine*) was one of the principal speakers. Other industrial physicians and surgeons taking an active part were Woody, McCord, Sander, Holmblad, Kronenberg, Sappington, Whittaker, J. M. Carlisle, L. J. Goldwater, and Colonel W. C. Cox.

Further emphasizing its changed attitude toward "the specialty," the Council on Industrial Health was working closely with Kronenberg's Committee on Medical Education in a canvass of activities among Western universities, a dozen of which showed definite interest in industrial curricula, although programs were not uniform and planning was in varied stages of development.

In October 1948, President Vonachan and other association personnel attended a meeting in Chicago with a delegation from the AMA for an important discussion of postgraduate education in industrial medicine. The American Academy of Occupational Medicine was represented by J. M. Carlisle. Also present were the medical deans of several schools doing outstanding work in that field, including Hazlett (Pittsburgh), Princi (Colorado), Lanza (New York University), Goldwater (Columbia), Ashe (Cincinnati), Meigs and Willard (Yale), Seeler (Harvard), and Hussey (Wayne).

The discussion of industrial curricula was both thorough and practical, but the action taken was even more significant. For the joint committee had decided definitely that the American Board of Occupational Medicine be incorporated (a necessary step in the process of certification) and had approved as groups representing the specialty in certification the AAIP&S, the related section of the AMA, the American Academy of Occupational Medicine, and a representative of schools teaching the subject at the graduate level. The public health group was also included on an undergraduate basis.

Never before had the outcome of the ten-year battle for specialty status appeared so promising. It was not a battle *won,* but it was a victory *in the making.* And a satisfactory expansion of educational facilities seemed to be on the way. Nevertheless, while continued contacts with the heads of medical schools were doing much to activate comprehensive industrial courses, many medical deans at the time did not yet understand the highly specialized needs of such instruction. As Dr. Whittaker commented: "I have talked with some who thought they were doing a great deal in the teaching of industrial medicine but who were not even scratching the surface."

At the same meeting President Vonachan told the Board of Directors that many men, particularly in the East, seemed to regard public health as occupational medicine, whereas they were "two separate and distinct entities." He added: "I think we are going to have to assert ourselves with this particular group. I personally never want to see us become a sub-board under public health, and I don't think any of us do."

Early in 1949 the AMA put itself unequivocally on record regarding both education and certification, formally recognizing the need for postgraduate instruction in industrial medicine and for "a certifying program or appropriate modification thereof."[6]

At this point, the initiative in both of these key activities passed to a large extent out of the hands of the IMA and into the hands of the AMA. Details concerning certification had to be cleared through various councils and sections, and the criteria governing in-plant training presented problems that called for considerable study and discussion.

Actual fund-raising for postgraduate fellowships had proved, since 1945, the least productive activity in the association's educational program. This was to be expected, for the project had to be built up from nothing, and there was a basic job of promotion to be done. Even the preliminary work was handicapped by lack of money. Many employers, though anxious to improve medical services in their plants, still doubted the efficacy of the average medical school programs. Curricula, it seemed to them, placed too much emphasis on public health courses, as though industrial medicine were something for general practitioners to handle on a part-time basis.

During Vonachan's administration (1948–49), Edward H. Carleton and his Foundation Fund Committee made a direct appeal for help from the membership of the association. Its objective was the establishment of a $5,000 fellowship sponsored by the AFOH itself—to set a good example and to stimulate similar activities. Supporting the appeal President Vonachan wrote: "Certification will come if we in the field will prove that young men will have the opportunity and facilities for proper training. For this, fellowships must be available."

The money was raised through small contributions from members and was used to finance a two-year postgraduate fellowship in industrial medicine at the University of Pittsburgh, the first to be established for this specific purpose. Carleton remained a constant worker for the foundation in the following years, promoting its activities through his own and other presidential administrations.

In 1949 Melvin Newquist reported that the Texas Company had approved the establishment of a two-year fellowship in industrial medicine at the University of Cincinnati, with a year of training in one or more industrial plants. Reported too was a General Motors plan for ten such combination courses. Within the association, the help of the district counselors was enlisted to encourage similar action by other progressive organizations. So the principle of in-plant training to supplement postgraduate instruction slowly gathered momentum.

At the annual convention in Chicago in April 1950, the foundation took another long step toward completion of its long-range program. C. R. Walmer, chairman of the Committee on Health Achievement, had reported that in the course of its field work his committee was frequently asked: "Is our company eligible for American College of Surgeons certification?"

The college had done fine work, said Walmer, but he believed the association now was in a better position to evaluate medical departments, including administration and ramifications, than the ACS. Such a change had been under consideration, and he wondered why steps had not been taken in that direction. Steps *were* taken at the Chicago convention in 1950.

In the final directors' meeting at that time Walmer was asked to comment further on the question of in-plant medical services. He reminded the Board that the ACS had initiated its program of inspection and evaluation some twenty years before as a public service. At that time the chief requirement for approval of a department was that it meet emergency standards.

Procedures and standards, however, had changed radically. Surgical approval had become relatively less important; medical administration, with its program of preplacement and periodic examinations, was involved. Costs had risen; the annual expense of surveys had become a considerable burden. In brief, occupational medicine itself was so broad in scope that a board of surgery could not be expected to deal with all its complex activities.

Little time was lost in reaching a satisfactory settlement of this problem of evaluation. With strong support from the incoming administration, headed by President Carleton, the association promptly agreed to assume responsibility for the evaluation and accreditation of medical services in industry. And on July 1, with a vote of thanks to the ACS, the AFOH took over the responsibility. Between 1932 and 1950, the ACS had made nearly 2,300 surveys and issued some 1,500 certificates of approval.

There was no doubt that this change of sponsorship greatly strengthened the position of the association in its battle for board status. In the final analysis the right of occupational medicine to be ranked as a specialty would be judged by the quality and extent of the services it rendered to industry. And with the accrediting program under its wing, the association had an opportunity to improve as well as to expand those services. Moreover, since the new project required substantial financing, the foundation was in a position to demonstrate to industrial management not only how the funds were to be used but the practical benefits that would accrue to contributors.

At best, this process of education and solicitation was slow and laborious, but generous contributions by several member firms of the American Iron and Steel Institute tided the foundation over the transition period, and the actual work of inspection and evaluation got under way by May 1, 1951.

Soon after succeeding to the presidency, Adolph Kammer (1951–52) wrote: "No president of the association has begun his term of office under more auspicious circumstances."[7] The newly named Industrial Medical Association was operating under revised bylaws that greatly broadened the scope of its work. Important progress had been made in the three-point program of industrial medical education, accreditation of medical services, and certification of the specialty.

Earlier in the year Carleton had started organization of an advisory committee of twenty to twenty-five members, thoroughly representative of industrial medicine and hygiene and related fields.[8] This group, headed by the immediate past president of the IMA, was to act as a board of governors for the AFOH in matters concerning the medical services program. To assist during the changeover period the association also retained Gaylord Hess, who had been a key figure in ACS administration.

The Kammer administration concentrated its efforts upon these key activities, at the same time working to improve relations with other associations in the Industrial Health Conference. The district counsellors and component societies lent vigor and vitality to the entire program and, through their nationwide field contacts, contributed substantially to its success.

So important was the Foundation in this over-all program that Kammer, in July 1951, delegated supervisory powers to a special Committee on Foundation

Activities, with Robert C. Page as general chairman, and seven sub-chairmen assigned to administrative duties: E. A. Irvin and G. H. Wilkins (administrative), E. H. Carleton and J. H. Sterner (fund raising), E. F. Lutz (fellowships), Robert O'Connor and Joseph T. Noe (program evaluation).

This committee was both equipped and empowered to correlate all Foundation functions and procedures into an orderly working program, which it immediately set out to do. Its first report to the directors (October 1951) covered past activities and blueprinted plans for the future. And, thanks to an earlier fund-raising campaign among industrial corporations, Foundation finances at the time permitted this work to go forward without delay.

At the 1952 Industrial Health Conference in Cincinnati, marking the thirty-seventh annual meeting of the IMA, E. A. Irvin succeeded Kammer in the presidency. At the same election George F. Wilkins (New England Telephone & Telegraph Company) became president-elect, Robert Collier Page (Standard Oil Company, New York) first vice-president, Eli S. Jones, second vice-president, with Secretary A. K. Peterson and Managing Director E. C. Holmblad continuing in office. New directors for the 1952–54 term, were R. G. Birrell (Imperial Oil Ltd., Toronto), Kieffer Davis (Phillips Petroleum Company), H. Glenn Gardiner (Inland Steel Co.), Earl F. Lutz (General Motors Corp.), Gradie R. Rowntree (Fawcett-Dearing Printing Company), L. Holland Whitney (New Jersey Bell Telephone Company).

Earle A. Irvin entered industrial practice by way of the automobile business and depression times, and his rise in its ranks was rapid. Receiving his M.D. degree from the University of Michigan in 1933, he interned at Hurley Hospital in Flint. His first industrial affiliation was with the Fisher Body Company and all subsequent connections have been automotive, for he has served successively the B. F. Goodrich Company, the Cadillac Division of General Motors (as medical director at the time of his IMA election), and since July 1, 1954 the Ford Motor Company (as medical director).

In the IMA Irvin had done outstanding work as a committeeman and chairman, notably in membership drives, in the revision of bylaws at mid-century, and in certification and AFOH activities. His presidential administration, like others in the 1950's, gave priority to the educational, certification, and medical service programs. Other stated objectives were larger membership for the IMA, improved relations with local medical societies and private practitioners, and closer cooperation with industrial management in working out medical department policies.

Starting in 1950 there had been several significant developments in industrial medical education which had a direct bearing on certification of the specialty. One milestone of importance was the conferment, for the first time in the history of American industrial institutions, of the degree of Doctor of Industrial Medicine upon medical graduates. The ceremony took place at a special University of Pittsburgh convocation in February 1950, the three recipients of the degree (D. John Lauer, H. S. Gibbs, J. H. McDonough) being the first to complete the special industrial course established by T. Lyle Hazlett. Among the invited guests on this occasion was Alfred Whittaker, then president of the IMA.

What this precedent might have accomplished in the way of a trend will never be known. For also in 1950, the University of Pittsburgh announced the establishment of a new graduate school of public health, headed by Thomas Parran, former surgeon-general of the USPHS. This project was made possible by a $13,600,000 gift from the A. W. Mellon Educational and Charitable Trust; and the only industrial degrees granted were those of Doctor and Master of Public Health.

In 1950 also there was further recognition of industrial practice from the AMA. Early in the year the Council on Medical Education and Hospitals approved the establishment of residencies in occupational medicine at the Saginaw (Michigan) General Hospital, the first such residencies of record. They carried a fellowship stipend of $75 per month.

Then there were nineteen specialty boards operating with AMA approval, of which two, the Board of Internal Medicine and Board of Pediatrics, were certifying candidates in sub-specialties. Neither of these being particularly pertinent to industrial practice, interest and discussion turned to four other boards which were certifying candidates in special divisions of specialties, among them the American Board of Preventive Medicine and Public Health. This board, established in 1948, had grown rapidly and within two years had certified 780 physicians. An affiliation with it seemed, in 1950, at least a definite possibility.

The IMA, however, had worked long and hard for specialty status; in fact April 1951 marked the tenth anniversary of the incorporation of the proposed Board of Industrial Medicine and Surgery, an occasion that led Slobe to remark: "Certification has been on the calendar so long that I can almost reminisce about it." The association had its heart set upon an independent board, and members were vocal in their rejection of "second-class certification."

In its stand on this issue the IMA received welcome support from a respected and influential ally, the American Academy of Occupational Medicine. An organization of full-time physicians in the occupational field, the academy was founded in 1946 and has enjoyed a steady growth since that time. Its charter members were predominantly members of the IMA. Its main objective has been improvement in the practice of industrial medicine and the greatest possible improvement in the health of industrial workers. It is active also in the education of medical, nursing and technical personnel.

There had been a meeting of a committee of the academy with the joint committees of the IMA and AMA. Bylaws had been drawn up and proposed incorporators selected for an interim American Board of Occupational Medicine. In the eyes of IMA leaders, the one ingredient needed to give the board equal status with others was graduate training of comparable duration and quality, and on this point there was a basic difference of opinion.

The chief difficulty was to get credits for postgraduate training in plant medical departments. For the AMA, while approving industrial residencies (as in the Saginaw General Hospital), made it perfectly clear that it did not consider a like period of in-plant training comparable to the hospital experience required in other specialties.

Although this difficulty necessitated long discussion and ultimate compromise, the march toward certification moved at a swifter pace than in any previous period. In the summer of 1951 the IMA Executive Committee provisionally appointed four members to serve on its American Board of Occupational Medicine for various terms: Robert C. Page (six years), A. G. Kammer (five years), J. H. Sterner (four years), F. W. Slobe (three years), with G. F. Wilkins and H. S. Brown as alternates. At its next meeting the Board of Directors approved these appointments, and also sanctioned representation on the American Board by four members of the AMA Section on Preventive and Industrial Medicine and Public Health and one member of the Academy of Occupational Medicine.

There were objections, however. In the opinion of many, the AMA section with the long and often-amended name covered altogether too much ground. Public health people did not like its domination by industrial medical men, and the industrial doctors were only mildly enthusiastic because it was so closely identified with public health. The IMA suggested that it be split into two sections, but the AMA said no.

After due consideration the parent association countered with a somewhat vague proposal that the interim Board of Occupational Medicine become a part of the American Board of Preventive Medicine and Public Health. A majority of the IMA directors, and industrial doctors, almost unanimously opposed this proposal. Again the cry was: "We want no halfway certification."

Early in 1952, at an interassociation committee meeting, the AMA group made a further concession, proposing that the name of the certifying board be changed to the American Board of Preventive Medicine, which would serve as a "canopy" covering two or more specialties whose central interest might be termed "preventive medicine." This board would include occupational medicine, public health, and other specialties which might be considered later. This new basis for organization was a definite improvement from the IMA viewpoint, because each divisional specialty was to have self-determination as to training requirements and because of the "very considerable component of preventive medicine within the field of occupational medicine."[9] This latter fact applied equally to public health and to aviation medicine, which at the time was negotiating, through the Aero-Medical Association, for similar status. The date of this proposal, February 9, 1952, could well be recorded as the date on which industrial medicine won its long fight for recognition as a specialty. In substantially the same form it was a blueprint for the program finally ratified, though not until two more years had passed.

A noteworthy characteristic of these eventful 1950's is the extent to which team activity had replaced individual performance. It belittles no man's ability to find that he works well with others. And the late history of the IMA provides many fine examples.

Immediately upon its appointment (in 1951) the special Committee on Foundation Activities plunged into work. During the remainder of President Kammer's term, and through Irvin's administration, it compiled a remarkable record of accomplishment. At the end of that period, in May 1953, came a detailed report from the trustees, which is briefly summed up here.

A critical survey of 161 leading industrial medical services, representing thirty-two types of industrial activity and employing more than a million persons, was completed and published.

A symposium on medical services in industry was conducted at the 1952 Industrial Health Conference,[10] and copies of the proceedings in booklet form were distributed to medical schools and universities and to organizations with approved medical services.

The number of trustees of the American Foundation of Occupational Health was increased from three to six, to include the entire IMA Executive Committee.

An advisory board was established, representing recognized associations and including top executives in basic types of industry.

Finally, minimal standards were set up for medical services in organizations having 100 to 2,500, and 2,500 to 25,000 employees. Here was the measuring stick for appraisal and approval of industrial medical departments.

In the spring of 1953 an impressive illustrated brochure on medical services was mailed, with a covering letter, to 6,500 management executives in important industries across the nation.[11]

At the 1953 Health Conference in Los Angeles, a skilled administrative officer succeeded to the IMA presidency, George F. Wilkins. On the supporting ticket were other familiar names: Robert Collier Page (Standard Oil Company, New Jersey), president-elect, Kieffer Davis (Phillips Petroleum Company), first vice-president, E. S. Jones (Hammond, Indiana), second vice-president, and, as new directors, Edwin DeJongh (General Motors Company), J. E. Kirkpatrick (San Francisco), H. W. Lawrence (Procter & Gamble Co.), J. L. Norris (Eastman Kodak Company), Charles F. Shook (Owens-Illinois Glass Company), R. Lomax Wells (Chesapeake and Potomac Companies).

George Wilkins, medical director of the New England Telephone and Telegraph Company, received his medical degree from Harvard in 1932, and joined the telephone company as staff physician five years later. He has done significant work in medical education, serving as assistant and instructor in surgery at Harvard and as a lecturer in industrial medicine in the School of Public Health.

The policies of the Wilkins administration followed the distinctive trends that have marked IMA activities through the 1950's. In his first statement of objectives[12] he promised continuance of the membership campaign initiated by Irvin; advancement of the quality and quantity of medical services; promotion of facilities for industrial medical education; and, above all, a concerted effort to establish a mutually productive rapport with industrial management in matters of health.

In the fall of 1953, in his capacity as chairman of the Board of Trustees, President Wilkins announced that the mail campaign conducted earlier in the year had brought more than $22,000 in contributions from industrial concerns for the Medical Service in Industry Fund.

Since the start of the 1950's there had been growing criticism of the name of the American Foundation of Occupational Health and of its fiscal organization. The word "foundation" implied a trust with money to *give* for worthy causes, rather than a trust that *solicits* funds for its own purposes. As President Wilkins commented: "It is somewhat incongruous for one foundation to approach another foundation for financial support." There also was a strong conviction that non-professional personnel should be well represented in such an organization, to assure satisfactory results from a fund-raising program. Both the advisory board of the AFOH and the Board of Directors of the association concurred in this thinking, and the trustees were authorized to proceed with the reorganization.

As for certification, it was apparent by 1953 that the AMA had no intention of establishing any more specialty boards in the foreseeable future. President Wilkins expressed to the IMA directors his belief that occupational medicine had "not a prayer" of getting a separate board; and a great many members had arrived at the belief that specialty status under the "canopy" of preventive medicine was better than no board status at all. At a meeting in February 1954, the directors voted unanimously that "our four representatives on the provisional board be instructed to proceed with speed to establish an affiliate Board of Occupational Medicine with the American Board of Preventive Medicine, Incorporated."

Throughout the 1950's the administration laid great emphasis upon the quality of industrial physicians who were to represent the association as certified specialists. There were constant warnings that standards should be kept beyond criticism. And it was with that goal in mind that members of the provisional board submitted 325 names, from which about 100 were to be chosen as a "grandfather group."

When the 1954 Industrial Health Conference opened in Chicago, the campaign for certification was within a few legal and executive steps of consummation. And the American Foundation of Occupational Health was in the final stages of reorganization as the Occupational Health Institute. It was only natural that these two activities should dominate the administrative program at the convention and in the months to come.

At the business session (April 28) Robert Collier Page succeeded to the presidency of the association; Kieffer Davis was advanced to the post of president-elect; Eli S. Jones was elected first vice-president; and Jerome W. Shilling (Pacific Telephone & Telegraph Company), second vice-president. The new Board of Directors included Leonard Arling, of Minneapolis, Paul J. Bamberger (Bethlehem Steel Company), R. E. Eckardt (Esso Research & Engineering Company), D. John

Lauer (Jones & Laughlin Steel Corporation), E. P. Luongo (General Petroleum Corporation), and E. J. Showalter (Western Electric Company).

One other important change was made in the executive roster. After five years of exacting duty as secretary, Arthur K. Peterson asked to be relieved, and H. Glenn Gardiner (Inland Steel Company, East Chicago) was elected to fill the post. Gardiner entered industrial practice in 1936 and, prior to his affiliation with Inland Steel, had served as medical director of Foote Brothers Gear & Machine Company and of Sears, Roebuck & Company.

The incoming president, Robert Collier Page, was born in England but received his higher education in the United States. Graduating from Northwestern University Medical School in 1934, he did postgraduate work in England at the University of Leeds, then returned to serve as resident physician and surgeon at the Philadelphia Presbyterian Hospital. His most important industrial work was done during his long association with the Standard Oil Company. He came to that organization in 1939 from the staff at Northwestern Medical School, where he was clinical assistant in medicine. In 1946 (after his discharge from military service) he was appointed general medical director of the company, and for ten years was charged with medical coordination and administration of its world-wide empire.

As a director (1950–52) and an officer of the IMA Page plunged into certification and foundation activities and assumed important responsibilities in the promotion of both programs. During his administration he also continued the trend toward decentralization of functions and duties within the association and worked closely with agencies studying the problems of industrial alcoholism.[13]

At the 1954 annual meeting in Chicago, outgoing President Wilkins and Kieffer Davis (as secretary of the foundation) presented a complete summary of recommendations to effect the conversion of that organization into the Occupational Health Institute. The Board of Directors unanimously approved the program. Davis' report included the information that 190 medical services had been certified "in the past year or two." Salient features of the plan, beyond the change of name, were incorporation of the OHI under the laws of New York state, re-endorsement of the foundation's trust agreement, in its original form, organization of a Board of Trustees of not less than ten or more than thirty-four members, and establishment of a Board of Industrial Advisers.

These boards were so set up as to leave professional activities of the OHI under control of the IMA. At least half of the trustees were to be professionally trained personnel, including the medical profession, industrial hygiene and nursing. There was a provision that the number of trustees who were *not* medical doctors should not exceed one-half of the total. The president and president-elect of the IMA were to be ex-officio trustees, *with full voting power,* and the president was to be responsible for the development, maintenance and approval of medical standards involved in the Institute's activities.

Completion of the OHI structure proceeded rapidly from this point. In December

1954, its incorporation was approved by the New York Supreme Court and the state Department of Education, and its tax-free status was confirmed by the Commissioner of Internal Revenue. Only action by the IMA Board of Directors remained.

Final steps to launch the Institute into actual operation were taken at the association's annual meeting in Buffalo in April 1955. An enormous amount of work had been done by the special OHI committee (composed of President-elect Davis, Shilling, Wilkins, and Gehrmann) and by the Standards Committee with James Hughes of Ohio State University as chairman. The in-plant program of inspection and certification had been laid out in minute detail, largely under the supervision of Drs. Lawrence and Lauer, representing the Board of Directors. The entire plan, as recommended, was approved by the Board with a vote of commendation.

At the same convention the OHI formally organized its Board of Trustees, in the first meeting of the group ever attended by individuals other than doctors. It consisted of five representatives of the IMA (Page, Davis, Carleton, Wilkins, and Gehrmann), three members from medical school faculties, one from the American Association of Industrial Nurses, two from insurance companies, one from the pharmaceutical field, and one representative of *Industrial Medicine and Surgery.* Page was elected chairman of the institute, S. G. Halos vice-chairman, and Miss Catherine Dempsey (AAIN) secretary. The Board then proceeded to elect five highly ranked management executives as the nucleus of a new Board of Industrial Advisers and established a Board of Regional Consultants composed of the thirty-two IMA regional counselors, who had performed invaluable services in the survey and liaison work of the former foundation.

To IMA members at the annual business meeting, outgoing President Page was able to announce: "The Occupational Health Institute can well be looked upon as a 100 percent affiliate of the Industrial Medical Association." And he added: "It provides the yardstick which industry needs in planning effective health services. It helps industry meet accepted standards. It makes available a well of knowledge gained by experienced men and women who carry out effective industrial health programs of their own."

This meeting saw Kieffer Davis take office as president, at the head of a ticket that included E. S. Jones, president-elect, Jerome W. Shilling, first vice-president, H. W. Lawrence, second vice-president, and Secretary Gardiner and Treasurer Holmblad continuing in office.

Davis, medical director of the Phillips Petroleum Company, Bartlesville, Oklahoma, received his medical education at Missouri University Medical School and the University of Louisville School of Medicine and did his post-graduate work at the St. Louis City Hospital. He joined the Phillips Company in 1947.

Along with sound industrial experience Davis brought to the IMA presidency the ability to chart a practical course of action, the tenacity to follow it through, and a personality that won support from his associates. The chief problems of his administration were the further development of medical services of value to industry, and the vigorous promotion of certification and educational programs already maturing.

In the autumn of 1954 the AMA had cleared away the last real obstacle to certification of the specialty, with the announcement that the American Board of Preventive Medicine had approved a sub-specialty status for the American Board of Occupational Medicine, on an equal basis with the Board of Public Health and the Board of Aviation Medicine. This action, in short, authorized the interim board to become the American Board of Occupational Medicine, as a division in the category of preventive medicine. Through the following winter the work of board organization and discussion of standards and requirements continued. At the April meeting in 1955 President Page reported: "As far as I know, the specialty board is a certainty. It requires one more 'go-around' by an AMA committee, but there are no complications."

Under the plan finally adopted, occupational medicine was allotted three members on the American Board of Preventive Medicine, Incorporated, two of them representing the IMA and the third, the Academy of Occupational Medicine. In line with a decision reached in June 1955, the Board of Preventive Medicine issued a bulletin outlining the requirements for certification, based on approved standards of education, training and experience. It also listed the board's sponsoring organizations[14] and its administrative personnel. Among the vice-chairmen was Robert H. Kehoe (active in both the Academy of Occupational Medicine and the IMA), and the members included A. G. Kammer and J. H. Sterner, representing the IMA.

As had been predicted, the certification requirements were stringent, and justified the IMA's insistence on men of outstanding caliber in the founders' group and the highest standards of eligibility for fellowships. It was also apparent that a great number of good industrial doctors could not expect to be certified with the charter member group. Many of these doctors by training and by experience in the surgery of occupational medicine were advised to secure certification under the American Board of Surgery.

This brief outline indicates a few of the main conditions surrounding the certification of physicians by the Board of Preventive Medicine for special knowledge and competence in the field of occupational medicine. Details of policy and procedure are a matter of record, readily available for reference.[15]

It cannot be said that the settlement of this controversial issue met with unanimous approval by the membership of the IMA. Reactions ranged from moderate enthusiasm to outspoken dissatisfaction. Nevertheless, majority opinion prevailed, and time and experience have altered some earlier viewpoints.

It will be remembered that preventive medicine has been an undertone in all discussions of health activities for many years. There has been, in a like period, growing emphasis on the prevention of disease associated with employment. And in this final certification program we find the occupational specialty recognized as a distinct division of preventive medicine, as are public health and the fascinating newcomer, space medicine.

Perhaps the comment of President Kieffer Davis, at the last meeting of the Board of Directors in 1955, may be taken as reflecting a realistic and typical attitude: "I don't believe there is any need for us to speculate on this board situation. It will take its course in due time . . . and some of us will be disappointed and others will be elated."

As 1955 drew to a close, problems of importance also awaited solution by the Occupational Health Institute. A new administrative plan had been in operation since June of that year, when Dr. Frank Calderone was elected president of the institute. A man of broad experience in the field of preventive medicine and active in the development of the World Health Organization, he faced the difficult task of putting the OHI fund-raising program on a sound basis and of correlating other diverse activities.

Summing up his estimate of the institute's functions, he told the directors: "The OHI has much more to do than to conduct a purely certification (of services) program. It is your academy of medicine. It is your educational force if you support it." Thus, *education* has emerged as a dominant factor in the success of institute activities, as it has in the final recognition of occupational medicine as a major medical specialty.

Education, of course, is the sum of many things; even the simplest discussion of its functions and ramifications is a task not for volumes but for entire libraries. In the single field of occupational medicine, it includes the formal education of medical students and the postgraduate training of specialists, and the education, in a broader sense, of physicians in the fields of industrial management, of labor, and the general public.

Medical organizations and their affiliates in other health agencies have recognized that fact, and prodigious progress has been made in meeting the need in the 1940's and, more particularly, in the 1950's. Periodic conferences under auspices of the National Fund for Medical Education, for example, have brought together the finest minds in many professions "to explore ways and means of strengthening the link between academic and environmental medicine, to the end that medicine can better serve the needs of industry and the public."

This fund, started in 1949, is a non-profit central fund for the nation's medical schools. Its regional conferences have been co-sponsored by great universities, by various councils of the AMA, by the Mellon Institute and similar related agencies. The fund is also served by a large Committee of American Industry, and a Medical Advisory Committee on which the IMA has been frequently represented. Members of the IMA have also participated actively in the fund's panel programs.

Another powerful stimulus to industrial health education has stemmed from such endowed enterprises as the General Motors Institute for Industrial Health, established at the University of Michigan in Ann Arbor, late in 1950. This $1.5 million agency has as its broad objectives research, education, and service in industrial medicine, health and safety. Carey P. McCord served as its director during its formative period and early years of operation.

In still another category of industrial medical education are projects exemplified by the intensive program on occupational skin problems held at the Kettering Laboratory in October 1955, a joint presentation by the University of Cincinnati and the Occupational Health Division of the USPHS. Robert A. Kehoe was one of the major contributors to this program, which embraced every aspect of occupational skin disease. The program brought together two-score physicians, the majority of whom were likely candidates for specialty certification at the time. Commenting on its significance, Editor McCord stressed the fact that this country was "confronted with a stark shortage of qualified industrial physicians" and suggested that many practicing physicians might "drop their activities and undertake one or more years in precise academic training in occupational health."

Too numerous, too varied to recount are the institutes, seminars, and panel discussions held by medical schools and other health agencies in the *renaissance* of medical education and the *naissance* of training in occupational medicine. References are legion, and the bibliography of the subject is enormous.

One of the most fruitful, but least publicized, channels of industrial medical education is the IMA's monthly journal. Editorially it has always spoken forthrightly, without fear or favor, on controversial medical issues. It has castigated quackery in any form yet has been moderate in its appraisal of the so-called "cults," from the old-time electro-magnetic "cures" to faith healing in various forms. Its opinions on the later developments in the fields of osteopathy and the chiropractic have usually been voiced in terms of the formal medical education available to students.

The journal, of course, has prior right and first access to professional papers delivered at IMA conferences and is in a position to obtain much other authoritative medical and surgical material. Its content offers a refresher course for the veteran industrial physician and an introduction to the latest developments for the younger practitioner.

Since the founding of the association journal in 1932, the membership has been aware that its editorial policies are largely responsible for keeping industry and industrial doctors informed on potential health hazards and their control. As early as 1939 the association had strong committees on Publications and Editorial Policy. And through the editorships of C. O. Sappington, Jean S. Felton, and Carey McCord there has been insistence on constant improvement of editorial material, and maintenance of highest ethical standards in both advertising and professional papers.

Interest in formal education in industrial medicine spread rapidly through the late 1940's and reached a new peak in the early 1950's. There was particular emphasis on medical school curricula and procedures during the administrations of Presidents Carleton and Kammer, to a large extent the result of industry's growing demand for qualified medical personnel.

438

At that time there was increasing criticism of the failure of medical schools, uniformly, to inaugurate full-scale undergraduate and graduate curricula for candidates in the field of occupational health. This failure had been largely responsible for industry's reluctance to establish industrial medical fellowships. From the opposite viewpoint it was apparent that medical education had been patched and repatched since the days of the Flexner report, and, as one university head attested, there was the danger of fragmentation of teaching time, caused by a multiplicity of special courses.

Of interest in this connection is the judgment of Arthur J. Vorwald, chairman of the Department of Industrial Medicine and Hygiene at Wayne State University College of Medicine, a pathologist, former director of the Trudeau Foundation and formerly the director of the Saranac Laboratory. Says Doctor Vorwald:

> The deans of medical schools and/or the committes determining medical school curricula are fully aware of the problems, and all medical educators are seeking a solution.
>
> The central problem, in essence, is that of introducing industrial courses in our overcrowded curricula. This involves sub-problems of time, teaching personnel and facilities—and money. The first responsibility of medical schools is to make good doctors in a department or division of occupational medicine; it is then our duty to stimulate the student at undergraduate level to an understanding of the opportunities in industrial practice. Our third responsibility is to give him the best possible preparation for that practice.
>
> One conclusion is obvious at this stage: industrial education, as a province of our medical schools, has emerged from its cocoon. Its final form and importance, in my opinion, will be determined by a gradual process of evolution—not settled as a single issue.

* * *

The annual Industrial Health Conferences have now become big business in a professional sense, meetings planned with scrupulous care and at great labor, for the discussion of matters that profoundly affect the strength of the nation. And in the same professional sense the IMA, with its components and participating agencies, has become a large and influential organization, accepting and discharging responsibility for the health of millions of workers.

Comparing the "cigar-box" First Aid stations of half a century ago with the superbly equipped and expertly administered departments of this latter day, one may wonder: "What miracle is this?" There has been none, unless to combine the highest of practical ideals with the hardest of hard work may be called a miracle.

Modern occupational medicine is a specialty that brings together all specialties—physiology, pathology, bacteriology—of an environmental, psychological and social nature. It has translated tools created by the other specialties into health conservation for masses of people in business and industry as well as for individuals.

In the process, occupational medicine has attracted to its inner circle a great many of the best minds trained in other special disciplines. The association has ever prized quality above quantity. It could echo the comment of President Dodd of Princeton, who once said of the university: "We have no illusions of grandeur which size will satisfy." Beyond question, its membership policy has added substantially to the prestige of the association and increased respect for its professional standards. This fact is a reminder that men of outstanding attainment in industrial practice are to be *weighed,* not *counted.*

After more than a decade of concentrated effort, occupational medicine has won certification by the American Board of Preventive Medicine. And in what other category of specialized practice could the IMA devote its activities to better purpose? Preventive medicine can accomplish what remedial medicine alone cannot. True preventive practice has long been considered a goal of greater importance than more immediate objectives.

Within a few years the association has seen formal education in occupational medicine develop from a few academic courses in scattered medical schools to practical undergraduate and postgraduate curricula in many schools. There is much still to be done, but the pace of progress is steadily quickening.

The association itself has exerted a powerful educational influence not only through its national health conferences but in a journal of superlative excellence, *Industrial Medicine and Surgery.* This publication—now under the editorial direction of Dr. Carey P. McCord—is looking forward to the thirtieth anniversary of its founding in 1932. In the late 1950's the association decided to supplement coverage of this field with a journal of its own. The result was establishment of the *Journal of Occupational Medicine,* edited by Dr. Adolph G. Kammer—the first issue appearing in January, 1959.

The IMA, over the years, has continued development of the Occupational Health Institute—as a fund-raising body to further education, and as the agency certifying medical departments that meet the requirements for approval. It has also influenced a growing recognition by business management of its obligations in the matter of employee health and the wisdom of supporting medical fellowships and providing in-plant training for medical personnel.

These are among the *objectives achieved*—the culmination of the long and difficult struggle recorded in this book. They are the outward symbols of what occupational medicine has come to mean within a few recent years. And it may be that history, one day, will regard medical and surgical progress in those years as the greatest ever made in a comparable period of time. Yet this is the beginning, not the end, the beginning of an era that promises for occupational medicine an opportunity of service matched by few other medical specialties.

Is our science at its zenith, or near it? Our grandchildren will have some answers to that question. But it is safe to say that whatever the triumphs of chemical therapy, whatever miracles are wrought in the war on ailments that scourge society and whatever feats man may perform in the conquest of space, organized occupational medicine, and the Industrial Medical Association, will play a vital role in their accomplishment.

The American dream hurries on, eager for tomorrow. Man, the Worker, moves with it—as does industry and the medicine of industry—each to keep a date with destiny. That destiny will be the fulfillment of the inspired dreaming of Paracelsus and Ramazzini centuries ago—and the reward of the flaming faith of Andrew Harvey, Loyal Shoudy, Harry Mock, Otto Geier and Robert Legge in our time.

441

Appendix 1

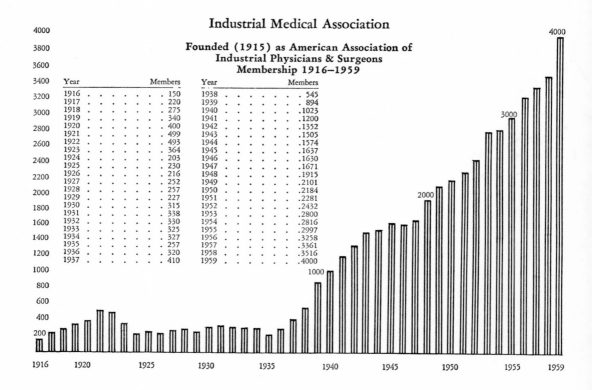

Industrial Medical Association

Founded (1915) as American Association of Industrial Physicians & Surgeons
Membership 1916–1959

Year	Members	Year	Members
1916	 150	1938	 545
1917	 220	1939	 894
1918	 275	1940	1023
1919	 340	1941	1200
1920	 400	1942	1352
1921	 499	1943	1505
1922	 493	1944	1574
1923	 364	1945	1637
1924	 203	1946	1630
1925	 230	1947	1671
1926	 216	1948	1915
1927	 252	1949	2101
1928	 257	1950	2184
1929	 227	1951	2281
1930	 315	1952	2432
1931	 338	1953	2800
1932	 330	1954	2816
1933	 325	1955	2997
1934	 327	1956	3258
1935	 257	1957	3361
1936	 320	1958	3516
1937	 410	1959	4000

Appendix 2

INDUSTRIAL MEDICAL ASSOCIATION
ANNUAL MEETINGS AND
PAST PRESIDENTS

No.	Meeting at	Date	President Elected	Term
1	Detroit, Mich. Cadillac Hotel	1916 June 12	*J. W. Schereschewsky, M.D.	1916–17
2	New York, N.Y. McAlpin Hotel	1917 June 4	(Re-elected)	1917–18
3	Chicago, Ill. Congress Hotel	1918 June 10	*Harry E. Mock, M.D.	1918–19
4	Atlantic City, N.J. Breakers Hotel	1919 June 9	(Re-elected)	1919–20
5	New Orleans, La. Hotel Grunewald	1920 April 26–27	*Otto P. Geier, M.D.	1920–21
6	Boston, Mass. Copley Plaza	1921 June 6–7	*C. E. Ford, M.D.	1921–22
7	St. Louis, Mo. Hotel Statler	1922 May 23–23	(Re-elected)	1922–23
8	Buffalo, N.Y. Hotel Statler	1923 October 1–3	*Loyal A. Shoudy, M.D.	1923–24
9	Chicago, Ill. Auditorium Hotel	1924 June 9–10	(Re-elected)	1924–25
10	Atlantic City, N.J. Traymore Hotel	1925 May 25–26	*William B. Fisk, M.D.	1925–26
11	Philadelphia, Pa. Univ. of Pennsylvania Hospital	1926 May 24–26	William A. Sawyer, M.D. Rochester, N.Y.	1926–27
12	Baltimore, Md. Hotel Belvidere	1927 May 16–17	*Thomas R. Crowder, M.D.	1927–27
13	Rochester and Minneapolis, Minn. Radison Hotel	1928 June 11–12	*Guy L. Kiefer, M.D.	1928–29

* Deceased.

443

No.	Meeting at	Date	President Elected	Term
14	Detroit, Mich. Hotel Statler	1929 May 10–11	*C. F. N. Schram, M.D.	1929–30
15	Detroit, Mich. Hotel Statler	1930 June 23–24	Cassius H. Watson, M.D. Brookfield Center, Conn.	1930–31
16	Philadelphia, Pa. Normandie Hotel	1931 June 8–9	*Don B. Lowe, M.D.	1931–32
17	No meeting	1932	(Lowe term extended)	1932–33
18	No meeting	1933	(Lowe term extended)	1933–34
19	Cleveland, Ohio Hotel Statler	1934 June 11–12	Edward C. Holmblad, M.D. Chicago, Ill.	1934–35
20	Philadelphia, Pa. Univ. of Pennsylvania Hospital	1935 June 10–11	Floyd E. Shaffer, M.D. Bethlehem Steel Co. Bethlehem, Pa.	1935–36
21	Atlantic City, N.J. Traymore Hotel	1936 October 7–9	*Robert P. Knapp, M.D.	1936–37
22	Detroit, Mich. Hotel Statler	1937 May 6–7	Royd R. Sayers, M.D. Washington, D.C.	1937–38
23	Chicago, Ill. Palmer House	1938 June 6–9	Clarence D. Selby, M.D. Port Huron, Mich.	1938–39
24	Cleveland, Ohio Hotel Statler	1939 June 5–8	McIver Woody, M.D. Elizabeth, N.J.	1939–40
25	New York, N.Y. Pennsylvania Hotel	1940 June 4–7	*Daniel L. Lynch, M.D.	1940–41
26	Pittsburgh, Pa. William Penn Hotel	1941 May 5–9	T. Lyle Hazlett, M.D. Coral Gables, Fla.	1941–42
27	Cincinnati, Ohio Gibson Hotel	1942 April 13–17	*John J. Wittmer, M.D.	1942–43
28	Rochester, N.Y. Seneca Hotel	1943 May 24–27	Harvey Bartle, M.D. Roxboro, Philadelphia, Pa.	1943–44
29	St. Louis, Mo. Jefferson Hotel	1944 May 9–14	Frederick W. Slobe, M.D. Blue Cross-Blue Shield Chicago, Ill.	1944–45
30	Cancelled (Proxy meeting)	1945 June 22	Melvin N. Newquist, M.D. The Texas Company New York, N.Y.	1945–46
31	Chicago, Ill. Sherman Hotel	1946 April 7–13	*Loyal A. Shoudy, M.D.	1946–47
32	Buffalo, N.Y. Hotel Statler	1947 April 26–May 4	Henry S. Brown, M.D. Detroit, Mich.	1947–48
33	Boston, Mass. Hotel Statler	1948 March 27–April 4	Harold A. Vonachen, M.D. Caterpillar Tractor Co. Peoria, Ill.	1948–49

* Deceased.

No.	Meeting at	Date	President Elected	Term
34	Detroit, Mich. Book Cadillac and Hotel Statler	1949 April 2–8	Alfred H. Whittaker, M.D. Detroit, Mich.	1949–50
35	Chicago, Ill. Hotel Sherman	1950 April 22–29	Edward H. Carleton, M.D. Inland Steel Company Chicago, Ill.	1950–51
36	Atlantic City, N.J. Chalfonte-Haddon Hall	1951 April 21–28	A. G. Kammer, M.D. University of Pittsburgh Pittsburgh, Pa.	1951–52
37	Cincinnati, Ohio Netherland Plaza Hotel	1952 April 19–25	E. A. Irvin, M.D. Ford Motor Company Dearborn, Mich.	1952–53
38	Los Angeles, Calif. Hotel Statler	1953 April 18–25	George F. Wilkins, M.D. New England Telephone & Telegraph Co., Boston, Mass.	1953–54
39	Chicago, Ill. Hotel Sherman	1954 April 24–30	Robert Collier Page, M.D. Carmel, N.Y.	1954–55
40	Buffalo, N.Y. Memorial Auditorium	1955 April 23–29	Kieffer Davis, M.D. Phillips Petroleum Co. Bartlesville, Okla.	1955–56
41	Philadelphia, Pa. Convention Hall	1956 April 21–27	E. S. Jones, M.D. Hammond, Ind.	1956–57
42	St. Louis, Mo. Kiel Auditorium	1957 April 20–26	Jerome W. Shilling, M.D. Los Angeles, Calif.	1957–58
43	Atlantic City, N.J. Convention Hall	1958 April 19–26	H. W. Lawrence, M.D. Cincinnati, Ohio	1958–59
44	Chicago, Ill. Hotel Sherman	1959 April 25–May 1	D. John Lauer, M.D. Pittsburgh, Penna.	1959–60

Appendix 3

OFFICERS, DIRECTORS, DISTRICT COUNSELORS*
INDUSTRIAL MEDICAL ASSOCIATION

OFFICERS
1959–1960

President:
D. JOHN LAUER, M.D., Jones & Laughlin Steel Corporation, Pittsburgh 30, Pa.

President-Elect:
R. E. ECKARDT, M.D., Esso Research & Engineering Co., Linden, N.J.

First Vice President:
GRADIE R. ROWNTREE, M.D., Fawcett-Dearing Printing Co., Louisville 1, Ky.

Second Vice President:
H. GLENN GARDINER, M.D., Inland Steel Company, East Chicago, Ind.

Secretary:
LEONARD ARLING, M.D., Northwest Industrial Clinic, Minneapolis 14, Minn.

Treasurer:
JOHN L. NORRIS, M.D., Eastman Kodak Co., Rochester 4, N.Y.

DIRECTORS
1958–1961

DONALD C. BEWS, M.D., Bell Telephone Company of Canada, Montreal, Que.

ALLAN J. FLEMING, M.D., E. I. du Pont de Nemours & Co., Wilmington 98, Del.

S. CHARLES FRANCO, M.D., Consolidated Edison Co. of N.Y., New York 3, N.Y.

O. TOD MALLERY, M.D., Employers Mutuals of Wausau, Wausau, Wis.

EMMETT B. LAMB, M.D. International Harvester Co., Indianapolis 4, Ind.

1959–1962

EDWIN DEJONGH, M.D., Pontiac Motor Division, General Motors Corp., Pontiac 11, Mich.

JAMES P. HUGHES, M.D., Kaiser Aluminum & Chemical Corp., Oakland 12, Calif.

LOGAN T. ROBERTSON, M.D., Consultant Occupational Health, Asheville, N.C.

RICHARD C. SWAN, M.D., Delco Remy Division, General Motors Corp., Anderson, Ind.

L. HOLLAND WHITNEY, M.D., American Telephone & Telegraph Co., New York 7, N.Y.

EXECUTIVE OFFICES,
Chicago, Ill.:

Director
CLARK D. BRIDGES

Assistant Director
RITA KIRTLEY PACKER

DISTRICT COUNSELORS*

ALABAMA
William G. Thuss, Jr., M.D., Birmingham 3

ARIZONA
Carl H. Gans, M.D., Morenci Hospital, Morenci

ARKANSAS
Philip T. Cullen, M.D., Little Rock

* For further data on district counselors, see Chapter XXXI.

CALIFORNIA—Northern
John H. Leimbach, M.D., San Francisco 2

CALIFORNIA—Southern
Clarence Lee Lloyd, M.D., North American Aviation, Inc., Los Angeles 45

COLORADO
Lewis C. Benesh, M.D., United Air Lines, Denver 5

CONNECTICUT
C. Fred Yeager, M.D., Bridgeport

DELAWARE
Howard L. Reed, M.D., Hercules Powder Company, Wilmington 99

FLORIDA
Homer A. Reese, M.D., Miami

GEORGIA
Joe M. Bosworth, M.D., Liberty Mutual Insurance Co., Atlanta

HAWAII
William H. Wilkinson, M.D., Wahiawa, Oahu

IDAHO
George L. Voelz M.D., Atomic Energy Commission, Idaho Falls

ILLINOIS
Eugene L. Walsh, M.D., International Harvester Co., Chicago 1

INDIANA
David Joe Smith, M.D., L. S. Ayres & Co., Indianapolis 9

IOWA
C. Harlan Johnston, M.D., Des Moines 12

KANSAS
Raymond F. Holden, Jr., M.D., Wichita 7

KENTUCKY
E. H. Kremer, Jr., M.D., Louisville 2

LOUISIANA
A. N. (Sam) Houston, M.D., New Orleans 12

MAINE
Niles L. Perkins, Jr., M.D., Oxford Paper Company, Rumford

MARYLAND
Walter E. Fleischer, M.D., Armco Steel Corporation, Baltimore 13

MASSACHUSETTS
Robert C. Thompson, M.D., General Electric Company, West Lynn 3

MICHIGAN
Otto J. Preston, M.D., Flint

MINNESOTA
John F. Shronts, M.D., General Mills, Inc., Minneapolis 26

MISSISSIPPI
William J. Witt, M.D., Jackson 2

MISSOURI
William L. Macon, Jr., M.D., St. Louis 17

MONTANA
Russell B. Richardson, M.D., Great Falls Clinic, Great Falls

NEBRASKA
G. Prentiss McArdle, M.D., Omaha 2

NEVADA
Lorne M. Phillips, M.D. The Henderson Clinic, Henderson

NEW HAMPSHIRE
Robert Flanders, M.D., Manchester

NEW JERSEY
C. Scott McKinley, M.D., Union Carbide Plastic Co., Bound Brook

NEW MEXICO
Lewis M. Overton, M.D., Albuquerque

NEW YORK—Metropolitan and Upper
Harold Brandaleone, M.D., New York 21

NEW YORK—Niagara Frontier
Reeve M. Brown, M.D., Chevrolet-Tonawanda Div., GMC, Buffalo 7

NORTH CAROLINA
MacRoy Gasque, M.D., Olin Mathieson Chemical Corp., Pisgah Forest

NORTH DAKOTA
Henry A. Norum, M.D., Fargo

OHIO—Eastern
Paul A. Davis, M.D. Akron 4

OHIO—Western
Edward F. Buyniski, M.D., General Electric Co., Lockland

OKLAHOMA
Tom Hall Mitchell, M.D., Carter Oil Company, Tulsa

OREGON
Ralph R. Sullivan, M.D., Oregon State Board of Health, Portland 1

PENNSYLVANIA—Eastern
Gilbert B. Meyers, M.D., Oreland

PENNSYLVANIA—Western
Albert J. Blair, M.D., Consolidated Natural Gas Co., Pittsburgh 30

RHODE ISLAND
Stanley Sprague, M.D., Pawtucket

SOUTH CAROLINA
John M. Perry, Jr., M.D., Sonoco Products Company, Hartsville

SOUTH DAKOTA
Edward E. Greenough, M.D., Sioux Falls

TENNESSEE—Eastern
C. R. Sullivan, Jr., M.D., Union Carbide Nuclear Co. Oak Ridge

TENNESSEE—Western
Edward C. Segerson, M.D., Memphis 12

TEXAS—Northern
Robert J. Potts, M.D., Magnolia Petroleum Company, Dallas 21

TEXAS—Southern
Robert A. Wise, M.D., Humble Oil & Refining Co., Houston 1

UTAH
Harold C. Jenkins, M.D., Bingham Canyon

VERMONT
John F. Lynch, M.D., Burlington

VIRGINIA
Mallory S. Andrews, M.D., Norfolk 10

WASHINGTON
Sherman M. Williamson, M.D., Boeing Airplane Co., Seattle 14

WEST VIRGINIA
Richard J. Sexton, M.D., Carbide & Carbon Chem. Corp., Charleston 30

WISCONSIN
George H. Peterson, M.D., Fisher Body Div., G.M.C. Janesville

WYOMING
R. H. Reeve, M.D., Casper

CANADA

ALBERTA
Stanley Greenhill, M.D.,
Edmonton

BRITISH COLUMBIA
A. John Nelson, M.D.,
B. C. Electric Company,
Ltd., Vancouver 1

MANITOBA
Paul K. Tisdale, M.D.,
Winnipeg 1

ONTARIO
A. J. Denne, Toronto 2

QUEBEC & NEWFOUNDLAND
Edwin A. Turcot, M.D.,
Imperial Oil Limited, Mon-
treal East 5

SASKATCHEWAN
Norman Williams, M.B.,
B.S., Saskatchewan Dept.
of Public Health, Regina

CUBA

Rafael Penalver Ballina,
M.D., Habana

PUERTO RICO

H. Vazquez-Milan, M.D.,
San Juan

Appendix 4

INDUSTRIAL MEDICAL ASSOCIATION

STANDING COMMITTEES
1959

COMMITTEE ON ORGANIZATION

Edward J. Schowalter, M.D.,* Western Electric Co., New York, N.Y.

W. Harvey Cruickshank, M.D., J. C. Duffy, M.D., Paul J. Whitaker, M.D., Wilbur J. Harley, M.D.

A.S.A. LIAISON

Kenneth C. Peacock, M.D.,* New York 17, N.Y.

Frank J. Borrelli, M.D.

BY-LAWS

Duane L. Block, M.D.* Ford Motor Co. Dearborn Mich.

George F. Wilkins, M.D., Merle Bundy, M.D., Ralph F. Schneider, M.D., Edward J. Zaik, M.D., Harold Y. Allen, M.D.

CARDIOVASCULAR DISEASES

C. A. D'Alonzo, M.D.,* E. I. du Pont de Nemours & Co., Wilmington 98, Del.

Paul J. Bamberger, M.D., Glenn S. Everts, M.D., Gerald J. Friedman, M.D., L. J. Goldwater, M.D., Robert J. Halen, M.D., W. F. Lienhard, M.D., George R. Lovell, M.D., Arthur M. Master, M.D., Sidney Pell, Ph.D., John J. Thorpe, M.D., John M. Trapnell, M.D., Neill K. Weaver, M.D.

CHEST DISEASES

Harry E. Tebrock, M.D.,* Sylvania Electric Products Inc., New York 17, N.Y.

CHEST DISEASES— *Continued*

Martin F. Bruton, M.D., Jan Lieben, M.D., O. A. Sander, M.D., Arthur J. Vorwald, M.D., E. L. Walsh, M.D., George W. Wright, M.D.

DERMATOLOGY

Raymond R. Suskind, M.D.,* The Kettering Laboratory, University of Cincinnati Cincinnati 19, Ohio

Donald J. Birmingham, M.D., William R. Buckley, M.D., Harold H. Golz, M.D., Joseph V. Klauder, M.D., Earl D. Osborne, M.D., M. Harriss Samitz, M.D.

EDUCATION AND TRAINING

Jean S. Felton, M.D.,* University of California, Division of Occupational Health, Los Angeles 24, Calif.

Rodney R. Beard, M.D., Bernard Behrend, M.D., Bertram D. Dinman, M.D., John C. Duffy, M.D., David H. Goldstein, M.D., Hallett A. Lewis, M.D., Lemuel C. McGee, M.D., J. Wister Meigs, M.D.

EMERGENCY AND DISASTER PLANNING

Max N. Howard, M.D.,* Socony Mobil Oil Co., Inc., Brooklyn 22. N.Y.

Herman J. Bennett, M.D., John W. Borino, M.D., Nor-

EMERGENCY AND DISASTER PLANNING— *Continued*

vin C. Kiefer, M.D., William N. Young, M.D.

FINANCE

John L. Norris, M.D.,* Eastman Kodak Co., Rochester 4, N.Y.

Allan J. Fleming, M.D., Richard C. Swan, M.D.

GERIATRICS AND RETIREMENT

Edward C. Holmblad, M.D.,* Illinois Public Aid Commission, Chicago 1, Ill.

Carl W. Gatter, M.D., Melvin N. Newquist, M.D., William A. Sawyer, M.D., Frederick W. Slobe, M.D.

GROUP INSURANCE

George J. Cooper, M.D.,* Chicago 3, Ill.

Richard J. Bennett, M.D., Clem Martin, M.D., John A. Palese, M.D., Walter Prusait, M.D., Bryce B. Reeve, M.D.

HEALTH ACHIEVEMENT IN INDUSTRY AWARD

Richard A. Sutter, M.D.,* St. Louis 1, Mo.

Joe M. Bosworth, M.D., Jean S. Felton, M.D., Lloyd E. Hamlin, M.D., C. Scott McKinley, M.D.

HISTORY

Alfred H. Whittaker, M.D.,* Detroit 7, Mich.

Robert T. Legge, M.D., James I. Roberts, M.D., McIver Woody M.D.

* Committee chairmen are designated by asterisks.

449

INDUSTRIAL MEDICAL PRACTICE

Preston N. Barton, M.D.,* Meriden, Conn.

Lawrence S. Cannon, M.D., John H. Ganschow, M.D., MacRoy Gasque, M.D., John M. Lynch, M.D., Bernard A. McAleer, M.D., Robert L. Quimby, M.D., C. F. Shook, M.D.

JOURNAL

Arthur K. Peterson, M.D.,* R. R. Donnelley & Sons Co., Chicago 16, Ill.

H. W. Lawrence, M.D., J. L. Norris, M.D., J. W. Shilling, M.D., S.D. Steiner, M.D., Clark D. Bridges,† A. G. Kammer, M.D.†

KNUDSEN AWARD

Kieffer Davis, M.D.,* Phillips Petroleum Co., Bartlesville, Okla.

Lemuel C. McGee, M.D., James H. Sterner, M.D.

MEDICAL CARE

Asa Barnes, M.D.,* Louisville 2, Ky.

Herbert K. Abrams, M.D., Frank P. Guidotti, M.D., Kenneth E. Markuson, M.D., Anthony A. Mira, M.D., Frederick D. Mott, M.D., Leo Price, M.D., William A. Sawyer, M.D., John D. Winebrenner, M.D.

MEMBERSHIP

Allan K. Harcourt, M.D.,* Indianapolis Industrial clinic, Indianapolis 4, Ind.

Glenn S. Everts, M.D., D. D. Holaday, M.D., E. M. Kline, M.D., Bryce Reeve, M.D., Wilfred N. Sisk, M.D.

MENTAL HEALTH

D. W. Caldwell, M.D.,* Esso Research & Eng. Co., Linden, N.J.

John H. Beatty, M.D., Ralph T. Collins, M.D., Leonard E. Himler, M.D., William Lee, M.D., John M. Lynch, M.D., Donald G. Mackay, M.D., Joseph C. Placak, M.D., John Scott, M.D.

MERIT IN AUTHORSHIP AWARD

William F. Ashe, M.D.,* Medical Center, Ohio State University, Columbus 10, Ohio

Allan J. Fleming, M.D., Lloyd E. Hamlin, M.D., James P. Hughes, M.D., N. J. Roberts, M.D.

MERITORIOUS SERVICE AWARD

James H. McDonough, M.D.,* Rome Cable Company, Rome, N.Y.

NATIONAL SAFETY COUNCIL MEDICAL ADVISORY

J. F. McCahan, M.D.,* Western Electric Co., Chicago 23, Ill.

G. H. Collings, M.D., H. G. Gardiner, M.D., N. Gillmor Long, M.D., H. I. Meyer, M.D., J. A. Palese, M.D., B. B. Reeve, M.D., E. L. Walsh, M.D., P. J. Whitaker, M.D.

PROBLEM DRINKING

John F. Jellema, M.D.,* Fisher Body Plant No. 2, Grand Rapids, Mich.

Edward F. Buyniski, M.D., Raymond A. Mezera, M.D., James I. Roberts, M.D., John F. Shronts, M.D.

PUBLIC RELATIONS

Thomas G. Rigney, M.D.,* Standard Oil Co. (N.J.), New York 20, N.Y.

Reeve M. Brown, M.D., James R. Fox, M.D., David H. Goldstein, M.D., Lemuel C. McGee, M.D., Douglas D. McKinnon, M.D., Wilfred N. Sisk, M.D.

RADIATION

W. D. Norwood, M.D.,* General Electric Co., Richland, Wash.

Charles T. Disney, M.D., Thomas S. Ely, M.D., Lt. Col. Francis W. Lanard, Thomas L. Shipman, M.D., W. L. Sutton, M.D., Albert A. Spritzer,

M.D., Irving H. Tabershaw, M.D., Mitchell R. Zavon, M.D.

SMALL PLANT SERVICES

Logan T. Robertson, M.D.,* Asheville, N.C.

Joe M. Bosworth, M.D., Bert W. Brooks, M.D., William W. Dickinson, M.D., Paul L. Gradolph, M.D., Harry Lamb, M.D., James H. McDonough, M.D., Daniel M. Murphy, M.D., William G. Thuss, Jr., M.D., Leon J. Warshaw, M.D.

STANDARDS

Carl U. Dernehl, M.D.,* Union Carbide Corporation, New York 17, N.Y.

D. C. Braun, M.D., B. W. Goodman, M.D., Lt. Col. Lee B. Grant, MC, James P. Hughes, M.D., Clark R. Miller, M.D., E. A. Turcot, M.D., Charles E. Work, M.D.

STANDARDS FOR VEHICLE DRIVING

Harold Brandaleone, M.D.,* New York 21, N.Y.

Lamson Blaney, M.D., Gerald J. Friedman, M.D., Gerald Gordon, M.D., George H. Irwin, M.D., Hedwig S. Kuhn, M.D., Seward E. Miller, M.D., Rafael Penalver, M.D., Forrest E. Rieke, M.D., Robert P. Sim, M.D.

SURGERY

Joseph M. Dziob, M.D.,* Lackawanna 18, N.Y.

Joseph T. Andrews, M.D.

CLINICAL TOXICOLOGY

Frank Princi, M.D.,* The Kettering Laboratory, University of Cincinnati, Cincinnati 19, Ohio

Robert T. P. deTreville, M.D., John H. Foulger, M.D., Leonard J. Goldwater, M.D., Harriet L. Hardy, M.D., Rutherford T. Johnstone, M.D., Charles E. Lewis, M.D., Lemuel C. McGee, M.D., J. H. Wolfsie, M.D.

* Committee chairmen are designated by asterisks.

† Ex-officio

WORKMEN'S COMPEN-
SATION

N. Gillmor Long, M.D.,*
Lumbermen's Mutual Cas-
ualty Co., Chicago 6, Ill.
Thornton I. Boileau, M.D.,
J. Van Donaldson, M.D.,

Robert J. Goldson, M.D.,
Ralph W. Haswell, M.D.,
John R. Merriman, M.D.,
Carl E. Nemethi, M.D.,
Joseph H. Schiff, M.D.,

Earl C. Steele, M.D., W. G.
Thuss, Sr., M.D., John L.
Tyler, M.D., Willis M.
Weeden, M.D.

* Committee chairmen are designated by asterisks.

Appendix 5

Industrial Medical Association

Chart shows division of duties and responsibilities in IMA organization

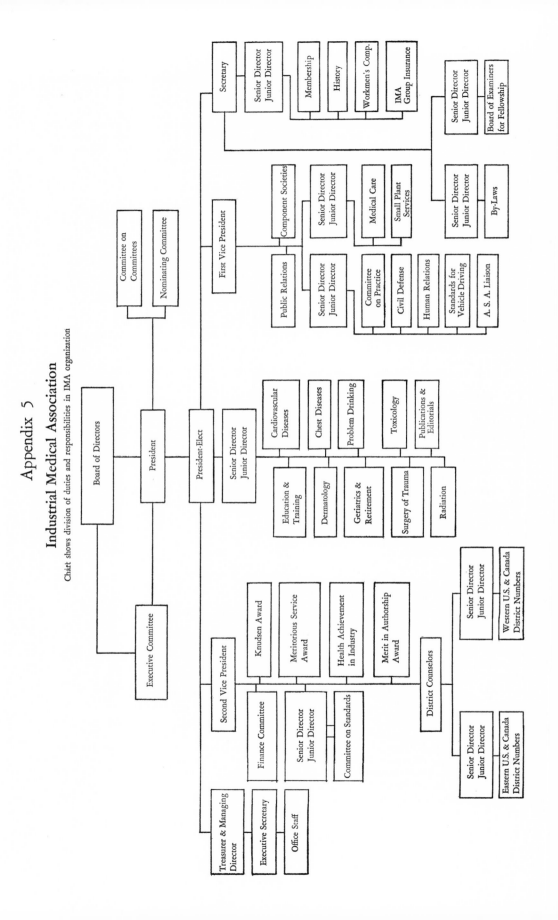

Appendix 6

INDUSTRIAL MEDICAL ASSOCIATION

COMPONENT SOCIETIES (1959)*

CENTRAL STATES SOCIETY OF INDUSTRIAL MEDICINE AND SURGERY

President: Richard A. Sutter, M.D.
President-Elect: Paul J. Whitaker, M.D.
Vice-President: Eugene L. Walsh, M.D.
Secretary-Treasurer: Allan P. Skoog, M.D., 28 East Jackson Blvd., Chicago 4.

HAWAII ASSOCIATION OF PLANTATION PHYSICIANS

President: Richard Y. Noda, M.D.
Vice-President: Patrick Cockett, M.D.
Secretary-Treasurer: Garton E. Wall, M.D.
Executive Secretary: Mrs. Betty Arnott, 1527 Keeaumoku St., Honolulu, Hawaii

INDUSTRIAL MEDICAL ASSOCIATION OF NEW JERSEY

President: Ralph M. L. Buchanan, M.D.
Vice-President: F. H. DeGrace, M.D.
Secretary: M. R. Vaschak, M.D., E. R. Squibb & Sons, New Brunswick, N.J.
Treasurer: Thomas F. Nevins, M.D.

INDUSTRIAL MEDICAL ASSOCIATION OF PHILADELPHIA

President: Walter Vernon, M.D.
President-Elect: Howard J. Johnson, Jr., M.D.
Secretary: Charles E. Rigby, M.D., Sun Oil Company, Marcus Hook, Pa.
Treasurer: Saverio F. Brunetti, M.D.

INDUSTRIAL MEDICAL ASSOCIATION OF PITTSBURGH

President: Daniel V. Dougherty, M.D.
President-Elect: Daniel C. Braun, M.D.
Vice-President: J. L. Thompson, M.D.
Secretary-Treasurer: Merle Bundy, M.D., U.S. Steel Corporation, Pittsburgh 30.

KANSAS CITY INDUSTRIAL MEDICAL ASSOCIATION

President: James R. McVay Jr., M.D.
President-Elect: Arthur B. Rhoades, M.D.
Secretary: Albert J. Clarke, M.D., Phillips Petroleum Co., Box 268, Kansas City 17, Kansas
Treasurer: William H. Duncan, M.D.

MICHIGAN INDUSTRIAL MEDICAL ASSOCIATION

President: Harold H. Gay, M.D.
President-Elect: Duane L. Block, M.D.
Vice-President: Richard D. Mudd, M.D.
Secretary-Treasurer: Henry J. Kreulen, M.D., Fisher Body Plant No. 1, General Motors Corporation, Grand Rapids, Mich.

MINNESOTA ACADEMY OF OCCUPATIONAL MEDICINE AND SURGERY

President: John A. Williams, M.D.
Vice-President: Robert W. Goltz, M.D.
Secretary: Earl T. Opstad, M.D., 430 Oakgrove, Minneapolis 3.
Treasurer: B. I. Derauf, M.D.
Recorder: Davitt Felder, M.D.

NEW ENGLAND INDUSTRIAL MEDICAL ASSOCIATION

President: Norman White, M.D.
Vice-President: Francis LeBaron, M.D.
Secretary-Treasurer: James I. Roberts, M.D., 441 Stuart Street, Boston 16.

THE NEW YORK STATE SOCIETY OF INDUSTRIAL MEDICINE, INC.

President: David H. Goldstein, M.D.
Vice-President: Harry E. Tebrock, M.D.
Secretary-Treasurer: Gerald J. Friedman, M.D.
Corresponding Secretary: Frank M. Dua, 30 Rockefeller Plaza, Room 2400, New York 20.

* For a detailed account of the component societies and their functions, see Chapter XXVIII.

NORTHWEST ASSOCIATION OF OCCUPATIONAL MEDICINE

President: Charles M. McGill, M.D.
Vice-President: Forrest E. Rieke, M.D.
Secretary-Treasurer: W. J. Sittner, M.D., 919 Taylor Street Bldg., Suite 410, Portland 5, Ore.
Asst. Secy.: Mrs. Lorna Crosgrove.

TEXAS INDUSTRIAL MEDICAL ASSOCIATION

President: Max E. Johnson, M.D.
President-Elect: Noble B. Daniel, M.D.
Vice-President: Carl A. Nau, M.D.
Secretary-Treasurer: J. G. Burdick, M.D., Ethyl Corp., P.O. Box 472, Pasadena, Calif.

WESTERN INDUSTRIAL MEDICAL ASSOCIATION

President: Verne G. Ghormley, M.D.
Vice-President: Clarence L. Lloyd, M.D.
Secretary: Richard M. Brundage, M.D., Rocketdyne, 6633 Canoga Ave., Canoga Park, Calif.
Treasurer: Clark R. Miller, M.D.

WESTERN NEW YORK SOCIETY OF INDUSTRIAL MEDICINE AND SURGERY

President: Joseph T. Andrews, M.D.
President-Elect: James H. McDonough, M.D.
Secretary: George A. Hardie, M.D., Eastman Kodak Co., 343 State St., Rochester 4, N. Y.
Treasurer: Elsa K. Chaffee, M.D.

Appendix 7

C. O. SAPPINGTON MEMORIAL

LECTURE

This series of lectures, delivered at annual meetings of the Industrial Medical Association, was established as a memorial to Clarence Olds Sappington, physician, author and editor, in recognition of his many significant contributions to occupational medicine. At the time of his sudden death in November 1949, Dr. Sappington had been editor-in-chief of the journal *Industrial Medicine and Surgery* for nearly ten years.

The memorial fund, built up by contributions from association members, was originally intended to finance a postgraduate scholarship in occupational medicine. It was later decided, however, that the Sappington Memorial could be used to even better advantage as part of the human relations program of the Occupational Health Institute, which was charged with administration of the fund. Since the inception of this program, outstanding speakers selected for the award have delivered lectures on aspects of occupational medicine that are of special interest and concern to industrial management.

1953
REESE TAYLOR, President, Union Oil Company, Los Angeles

"Industrial Medicine As It Looks to Management"

1954
EDWARD J. STIEGLITZ, M.D., F.A.C.P., Washington, D.C.

"Constructive Health—Management's Stake in Industrial Health Programs"

1955
E. DWIGHT BARNETT, M.D., Professor of Administrative Medicine, Columbia University Medical School, New York City

"Administrative Medicine —A Necessary Component of Industrial Health"

1956
EDWARD L. BERNEYS, B.S., Counsel on Public Relations, New York City

"The Engineering of Consent"

1957
FRANK CURTIS, Vice-President, Monsanto Chemical Company, St. Louis

"The Problem of Producing Executives"

1958
C. W. SHILLING, M.D., Deputy Director, Division of Biology and Medicine, Atomic Energy Commission, Washington, D.C.

"Everybody's Business— The Problem of Fallout and Radiation"

1959
CAREY P. MCCORD, M.D., Consultant, School of Public Health, University of Michigan, Ann Arbor, Michigan

"Scurvy as an Occupational Disease"

Appendix 8

WILLIAM S. KNUDSEN AWARD

This coveted citation, an annual award for "the most outstanding contribution to industrial medicine" during the preceding year, was announced in June 1938 by William S. Knudsen, then president of the General Motors Corporation.

1939 *DR. C. O. SAPPINGTON, Chicago, Ill.
1940 *DR. L. U. GARDNER, Saranac Lake, N.Y.
1941 DR. ROYD R. SAYERS, Washington, D.C.
1942 DR. C. D. SELBY, Detroit, Mich.
1943 DR. WILLIAM A. SAWYER, Rochester, N.Y.
1944 DR. HAROLD A. VONACHEN, Peoria, Ill.
1945 No award
1946 DR. ANTHONY J. LANZA, New York City
1947 DR. CAREY P. MCCORD, Detroit, Mich.
1948 DR. T. LYLE HAZLETT, Pittsburgh, Pa.
1949 DR. ROBERT A. KEHOE, Cincinnati, Ohio.
1950 DR. EDWARD C. HOLMBLAD, Chicago, Ill.
1951 *DR. ROBERT T. LEGGE, Berkeley, Calif.
1952 DR. MAX R. BURNELL, Detroit, Mich.
1953 DR. ALICE HAMILTON, Hadlyme, Conn.
1954 DR. NILS PAUL LARSEN, Honolulu, Oahu.
1955 DR. GEORGE H. GEHRMANN, Wilmington, Del.
1956 DR. RUTHERFORD T. JOHNSTONE, Los Angeles, Calif.
1957 DR. JAMES H. STERNER, Rochester, N.Y.
1958 DR. A. G. KAMMER, Pittsburgh, Pa.
1959 DR. LEMUEL C. MCGEE, Wilmington, Del.

* Deceased.

Appendix 9

MERITORIOUS SERVICE AWARD

An award presented since 1946 by the Industrial Medical Association, at annual banquets, to the individual who has, in the opinion of the committee making the selection, rendered the most distinguished service to the association and to industrial medicine during the preceding year.

1946 *DR. LOYAL A. SHOUDY, Bethlehem, Pa.
1947 *DR. OTTO P. GEIER, Cincinnati, Ohio.
1948 DR. DANIEL LAWRENCE LYNCH, Boston, Mass.
1949 DR. FREDERICK W. SLOBE, Chicago, Ill.
1950 MR. ARTHUR DAVID CLOUD, Chicago, Ill.
1951 DR. HENRY SEABURY BROWN, Detroit, Mich.
1952 DR. EDWARD H. CARLETON, East Chicago, Ind.
1953 DR. EDWIN DEJONGH, Detroit, Mich.
1954 DR. CARL T. OLSON, Chicago, Ill.
1955 DR. JAMES P. HUGHES, Columbus, Ohio.
1956 DR. GLENN S. EVERTS, Philadelphia, Pa.
1957 DR. CHARLES F. SHOOK, Toledo, Ohio.
1958 DR. ALFRED HEACOCK WHITTAKER, Detroit, Mich.
1959 DR. LOGAN T. ROBERTSON, Asheville, N.C.

* Deceased

Appendix 10

MERIT IN AUTHORSHIP AWARD

A citation presented annually by the Industrial Medical Association, at its convention banquet, to the author (or authors) of an article or other publication of outstanding significance and value in the field of occupational medicine.

1948 JAMES M. CARLISLE AND AUGUSTUS GIBSON
    for "Need for Scientific Research in Industrial Medicine," in *Occupational Medicine*, August 1947, *4*:185–88.
    JEAN SPENCER FELTON
    for "Orientating the New Employee in the Services of the Industrial Health Department," in *Industrial Medicine*, November 1947, *16*:519–25.
    NATHAN MILLMAN
    for "Medical Departments in Small Plants—Layout, Equipment, and Costs," in *Industrial Medicine*, April 1947, *16*:174–80.

1949 REX H. WILSON, GLENN V. HOUGH, AND WILLIAM E. MCCORMICK
    for "Medical Problems Encountered in the Manufacture of American-Made Rubber," in *Industrial Medicine*, June 1948, *17*:199–207. Award presented to Dr. Wilson, senior author.

1950 R. T. JOHNSTONE
    for "Occupational Medicine: Its Role in the Social World," in *Industrial Medicine*, November 1949, *18*:451.

1951 A. J. VORWALD, THOMAS M. DURKEN AND PHILIP C. PRATT
    for "Experimental Studies of Asbestosis," in *Archives of Industrial Hygiene and Occupational Medicine*, 1951, *3*:1. Award presented to Dr. Vorwald, senior author.

1952 JAMES H. STERNER AND MERRIL EISENBUD
    for "Epidemiology of Beryllium Intoxication," in *Archives of Industrial Hygiene and Occupational Medicine*, August 1951, *4*:123–151.

1953 LOUIS H. HEMPELMANN, HERMAN LISCO AND JOSEPH G. HOFFMAN
    for, "The Acute Radiation Syndrome," in *Annals of Internal Medicine*, February 1952, *36*:279–510.

1954 JOSEPH M. DENARDI, H. S. VAN ORDSTRAND, GEORGE H. CURTIS, AND JOHN ZIELINSKI
    for "Berylliosis," in *Archives of Industrial Hygiene and Occupational Medicine*, July 1953, *8*:1–24.

1955 J. RICHARD DURHAM AND LEMUEL E. MCGEE
    for "The Electrocardiogram in the Examination of the Industrial Worker," in *Annals of Internal Medicine*, November 1954, *41*:918–934.

1956 THEODORE HATCH AND KENNETH COOK

for "Patitional Respirometry" in *Archives of Industrial Health,"* February 1955, *12:*142–158.

1957 LEO J. WADE

for "Needed: A Closer Look at Industrial Medical Programs," in *Harvard Business Review,* March–April 1956, 34, No. 2; reprinted in *Industrial Medicine and Surgery,* April 1956, *25:*167.

1958 H. RICHARD BLACKWELL

for "Quantitative Relationships of Illumination and Vision," in the *Archives of Industrial Health,* August 1957, *16:*108–124.

1959 WILLIAM J. FULTON

for "Medical Department Layout and Design," in *Industrial Medicine and Surgery,* 1958, *27:*1–14, 85–104, 123–138, 179–198.

Appendix 11

HEALTH ACHIEVEMENT IN
INDUSTRY AWARD

The Award for Health Achievement in Industry has been given annually since 1949 by the Industrial Medical Association in recognition of the inauguration and improvement *by the management of a company* of a comprehensive medical service for its employees. The significance of this award is that it is bestowed upon a *company,* because of its medical department, rather than upon the department itself. Thus it recognizes the improvement factor in a medical situation and management's responsibility in bringing it about. Selection of companies for this award is entrusted to a special committee of the association.

1949   ROME CABLE COMPANY, Rome, N.Y.

1950   BRADLEY MINING COMPANY, Stibnite, Ida.

1951   C. T. DEARING PRINTING COMPANY, Louisville, Ky.
           (name changed in 1952 to Fawcett-Dearing Printing Company)

1952   EAST LIVERPOOL DISTRICT POTTERIES, East Liverpool, Ohio.

1953   IMPERIAL OIL LIMITED, Toronto, Ontario, Can.

1954 (a) THE R. R. DONNELLEY AND SONS COMPANY, Chicago, Ill.
      (b) THE INLAND STEEL COMPANY (INDIANA HARBOR WORKS), East Chicago, Ind.

1955   SONOCO PRODUCTS COMPANY, Harsville, S.C.

1956   PENNSYLVANIA RAILROAD COMPANY, Philadelphia, Pa.

1957   HUMBLE OIL AND REFINING COMPANY, Houston, Texas

1958   FORD MOTOR COMPANY, Dearborn, Mich.

1959   KAISER STEEL CORPORATION, Fontana, Calif.

Appendix 12

Exhibits

Exhibits at industrial health conferences reflect the growth of occupational medicine and progress in the development of medical department equipment and supplies.

Few chronicles of modern industrial safety fail to mention the introduction, in 1897, of goggles to protect the eyes of factory workers from flying splinters. Crude equipment of that type has come to be regarded as symbolic of early efforts to reduce accident hazards in American plants, at a time when little thought was given to safeguarding the general health and well being of employees. Only during the latest great upswing in science and technology has the development of special hygienic safeguards, pharmaceutical aids, and many other types of protective equipment, kept pace with the changing conditions of a modern world.

Thus, it was to be expected that the value of exhibits, both scientific and commercial, in the special field of industrial medicine should be slow to win recognition. In March 1922, answering an inquiry from a St. Louis laboratory, Dr. William A. Sawyer, secretary-treasurer of the American Association of Industrial Physicians & Surgeons, wrote as follows:

"It will not be possible for us to arrange any display to the members of our association. I would suggest that you get in touch with the local committee of the American Medical Association and possibly secure space in their exhibition."

About six years later the AAIP&S decided that a scientific exhibit at the annual AMA meeting might do much "toward putting industrial medicine before the profession in general." Accordingly, a questionnaire was mailed to members, asking whether they had any special apparatus, any dispensary arrangement, any short-cuts in examinations, any special forms of treatment, any studies of health hazards, any statistical or printed matter that would be of scientific interest to other doctors. In reply, the association received a discouragingly high percentage of unqualified "noes" and very few exhibit ideas of any promise. As a matter of fact, neither scientific nor commercial exhibits assumed much importance in number or quality until the late thirties.

Since 1938, scientific exhibits at the annual conventions of the association have followed an irregular pattern as to number but have been of uniformly superior quality and effectiveness. They have continued to attract intense interest over the years.

The history of the commercial or technical exhibits is a quite different story. From the viewpoint of the Industrial Medical Association these exhibits must fulfill the primary purpose of acquainting employers and medical directors with the latest and best in equipment and supplies for industrial and business use. Appearance, interest and educational value are criteria by which they are judged.

Obviously, an annual IMA health conference could not, under any circustances, be utilized for the competitive selling of any product or service. Exhibitors, in the main, are not looking for orders at these meetings. The value of a display to its sponsor is measured by the attendance and interest shown at his booth. His is a long-range promotion of good will and patronage.

461

The association, on the other hand, can reasonably expect some financial return for its own efforts and assistance. The entire activity is a cooperative venture, profiting everyone concerned.

In the early years, both the association and the suppliers to the profession were apathetic toward such a venture. The association, small in membership and limited in scope, could offer medical exhibitors few advantages that would warrant a substantial investment in space, materials and time. But when in the booming economy of the forties and fifties the growth of occupational medicine was paralleled by the development of services, equipment, and pharmaceutical aids for industrial medical departments and the IMA was recognized as representing this specialty, the technical exhibit section of its annual conferences became a lusty young giant.

From the first date of record for which detailed figures are available, the chart curve for technical exhibits has followed an upward trend in number and importance. In 1938, at one end of the scale, there were twenty-six commercial exhibitors; at the other end, in the mid-fifties, the number totaled close to a hundred. Sales executives of important equipment and drug supply firms recall that in the early years of this two-decade span they found it difficult to convince their management officials that the expense of representation at an exclusively industrial medical meeting could be justified. Many a potential exhibitor, in that formative period, cautiously agreed to a trial display—for the most part with encouraging results. Over the years manufacturers for this specialty came to realize that while industrial physicians and surgeons were not, as individuals, particularly large buyers of medical equipment and supplies, employers relied largely upon their knowledge of departmental needs and their judgment of available products. In total size, it was apparent, industry represented a great and growing medical market. Today, the blue book of American industry is represented among technical exhibitors and registrants at the annual industrial health conferences.

Manufacturers have shown remarkable vision and ingenuity in devising new processes, creating new products, and designing new equipment to meet the special needs of industrial physicians, hygienists, nurses and dentists.

An observant nurse noticed that a man with an injured arm sat astride his chair, facing the rear and resting his arm on the back. From this idea evolved a dressing chair with work shelf and dressing basin, at which the nurse works facing the back of the chair.

There was need for a sterile dressing that was also waterproof, transparent and flexible—the result, a liquid plastic sprayed from a self-contained dispenser on wounds, burns and abrasions.

Taking their cue from fashionable interior decoration, designers of medical department equipment specified pastel colors in the latest mode, imparting an air of beauty and quality in otherwise drab surroundings.

The principle so successfully used in the sectional bookcases and filing cabinets was adapted to the production of sectional steel dispensary and laboratory equipment which can be expanded or contracted as space needs dictate.

The following list can do no more than suggest the number and variety of products with which the medical supply houses have responded to the in-plant needs of industry, large and small:

Electronic instruments which count red and white blood cells, tirelessly, far more accurately than by human visual methods and in one-tenth the time. Automation in medicine:

New and improved designs for gas analyzers, oxygen breathing apparatus, dust and sampling instruments, face filters and dust respirators, audiometers and apparatus for vision screening.

A variety of hydro-, electro-, and thermotherapy apparatus for the treatment of industrial injuries and for rehabilitation, and new chemical tests for intoxication, useful in dealing with problem drinking.

Lotions to protect the skin against industrial dermatoses, an adjustable stretcher that requires no lifting of the patient, a surgical light with a powerful built-in magnifier.

A variety of adhesive bandages specially designed for industrial use and a revolutionary tubular gauze-applicator that simplifies the task of applying gauze to any part of the body.

Industry itself has also pioneered many valuable improvements in medical department procedures—either constructing its own equipment or apparatus, or having it built to specifications.

Realizing the value of health conference exhibits to American industry, to medical suppliers and to the medical fraternity in any type of practice, the IMA has kept the entire program under constant study, with an eye to its improvement. At Board meetings, directors have spent many hours each year in reviewing and discussing the commercial exhibit program. They have been scrupulous in their examination of products and services featured in displays and have insisted on the same high ethical standards that are required of advertisers in the association journal.

As for the exhibiting companies, each representative sends to his home office an evaluation report based on attendance and interest in his display. The exhibitors have an association of their own, which sends evaluators to each meeting to compile a summary report for the guidance of its members.

Because they add life and interest to large and unspectacular meetings, because they serve many constructive purposes, exhibits are today a solid and thriving institution in American business and professional life. When this was written more than 360 medical and surgical meetings were being held in this country every year, a fact that insures top-level planning and programs of broad interest from any association.*

* For much of the material in this review of medical exhibits we are indebted to Henry J. Scherck, vice-president of the A. S. Aloe Company, of St. Louis, and to Stephen G. Halos, president, Industrial Medical Publishing Company. For his work in developing the exhibit section of the IMA annual health conferences, the Board of Directors in 1953 awarded Halos a special certificate of merit.

Appendix 13

The IMA and Compulsory Health Insurance

Despite its frequent differences and difficulties with the American Medical Association, the Industrial Medical Association has, with practically no exceptions, strongly supported the parent organization in matters of national and governmental policy affecting health care in the United States. The text of the resolution printed below is evidence of that fact. This resolution was passed by acclamation at the annual meeting of the American Association of Industrial Physicians and Surgeons in Detroit, April 7, 1949. For context bearing on this action, see Chapter XXX.

WHEREAS, under a system of free enterprise the American medical profession has established the world's highest standard of medical care, thereby helping the United States to become the healthiest major nation in the world; and,

WHEREAS, the benefits of American medicine now are available to the majority of the people of this country and can be extended to every American through budget-basis voluntary health insurance; and,

WHEREAS, the experience of all countries where government has assumed control of medical services has shown that there has been a gradual erosion of free enterprise and a progressive deterioration of medical standards and medical care to the detriment of the health of the people; and,

WHEREAS, the great advances which have been made in our own specialty under the stimulus of private enterprise would be impeded by any form of Federal control of medicine, NOW, THEREFORE,

BE IT RESOLVED, that the American Association of Industrial Physicians & Surgeons does hereby go on record against any form of compulsory health insurance or any system of political medicine designed for bureaucratic control; and that a copy of this resolution be forwarded to the President of the United States, and to each Senator and Representative in the Congress of the United States, and that the said Senators and Representatives be and hereby requested to use every effort at their command to prevent the enactment of such legislation.

Appendix 14

Certification of Services

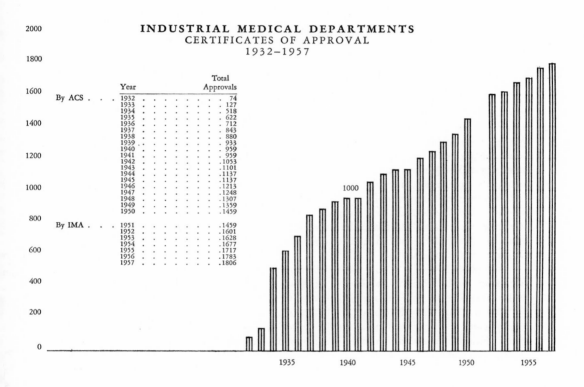

INDUSTRIAL MEDICAL DEPARTMENTS
CERTIFICATES OF APPROVAL
1932–1957

	Year	Total Approvals
By ACS . . .	1932	74
	1933	127
	1934	518
	1935	622
	1936	712
	1937	843
	1938	880
	1939	933
	1940	959
	1941	959
	1942	1053
	1943	1101
	1944	1137
	1945	1137
	1946	1213
	1947	1248
	1948	1307
	1949	1359
	1950	1459
By IMA . . .	1951	1459
	1952	1601
	1953	1628
	1954	1677
	1955	1717
	1956	1783
	1957	1806

465

Appendix 15

Graduate Education in Occupational Medicine

Lack of uniformity in the plans and procedures of American medical schools has been a conspicuous characteristic of graduate education in occupational medicine, during the mid-century phase of its development. So wide is the range of variation—in curricula, in degrees granted, and even in nomenclature—that an accurate statistical comparison is virtually impossible.

One of the most thorough studies of available training facilities was reported in 1953 by the Committee on Education of the Industrial Medical Association, under the chairmanship of Dr. A. G. Kammer, University of Pittsburgh School of Public Health.* This committee, while acknowledging that its information might be incomplete, summarized in some detail the programs of nine medical schools doing outstanding work in this field. We list these schools, with the degrees offered in industrial and public health and the basic requirements for candidates, in extremely condensed form, as reported by Kammer's committee:

University of Cincinnati Institute of Industrial Health (part of the Graduate School of the university, but located in the College of Medicine). The degree of Doctor of Industrial Medicine offered after three calendar years of study, the third year being devoted to training in an industrial plant under adequate supervision. The course was designed to produce medical directors for industry.

Columbia University School of Public Health. Offers degrees of Doctor of Public Health, Master in Public Health, and Master of Science. Special graduate courses in occupational health available to physicians who have "suitable professional qualifications."

Harvard University School of Public Health. Course covering one academic year offered to physicians wanting graduate study for degree of Master of Industrial Health or Master in Public Health. Candidates must be graduates of acceptable medical schools, with a year's internship in approved hospitals.

Johns Hopkins University School of Public Health. Advanced study in the field of occupational health offered to physicians, in the Department of Environmental Medicine, leading to degrees of Master in Public Health, Doctor of Public Health, Master of Science and Doctor of Science. Students working for degrees may do part-time work. Curriculum includes advanced courses in industrial and public health, and original research into problems. Seminars and field studies also available.

University of Michigan School of Public Health. Degrees of Master in Public Health (one year) and Master of Occupational Medicine offered for physicians. A wide variety of short courses (non-credit) available in the occupational field. Clinical training offered in the University Hospital, with opportunities for field experience in General Motors and other plants.

---

* "Graduate Training in Occupational Medicine," *Industrial Medicine and Surgery*, April 1953, pp. 149–152. Other members of the committee were: Harriet L. Hardy (Harvard University), L. G. McGee (Hercules Powder Company), J. Wister Meigs (Yale University), I. R. Tabershaw (Columbia University), and H. A. Vonachen (Caterpillar Tractor Company).

New York University. Degree of Master of Science in Industrial Health offered in the postgraduate school of the institute established as a partnership between New York University—Bellevue Medical Center and the College of Engineering.

University of Pittsburgh School of Public Health. Degrees of Master in Public Health, Doctor of Public Health, and Doctor of Philosophy offered for graduate students in the field of occupational health. All applicants must be graduates of a Class A medical school, with at least one year of hospital internship. Courses provide for considerable clinical training, lectures and seminars, and individual programs of practical in-plant training.

University of Rochester. Candidates with the degree of M.D. from recognized medical schools, with at least one year of internship, are accepted in the graduate school of the university for work toward the degree of Master of Science in Industrial Medicine. The majority of courses are given in and by the School of Medicine. Curriculum includes a broad program of lectures, substantial clinical training in Rochester hospitals, and required work in the medical departments of local industries.

Yale University Department of Public Health. Degrees of Master in Public Health (two years), Doctor of Public Health (four years), Master of Science, and Doctor of Philosophy are offered for graduate study in the field of occupational health. Physicians seeking the degree of M.P.H. must be graduates of accredited medical schools. Basic courses in occupational and public health are supplemented by clinical training in local hospitals; clinical work in industrial medicine is arranged with individual industries.

In addition to these facilities we cite two other important programs as representative of recent developments:

The Ohio State University Department of Preventive Medicine, College of Medicine. This department was established in its present form in 1954, with William F. Ashe, M.D., as professor and chairman. It offers graduate education in the fields of occupational and aviation medicine through two three-year programs, both of which have met the academic requirements of the American Medical Association for specialty certification. Two years are spent on basic courses, for which a Master of Science degree is given; the third year is devoted to preceptorial in-plant training. A fourth year is provided for selected applicants seeking a Ph.D.

Wayne State University College of Medicine, Department of Industrial Medicine and Hygiene. This department, headed by Arthur H. Vorwald, M.D., was established in 1954 with a broadly based program of study pointing toward the degrees of Master of Science in Industrial Hygiene (one year), and Doctor of Philosophy in Industrial Medicine (three years).

Appendix 16

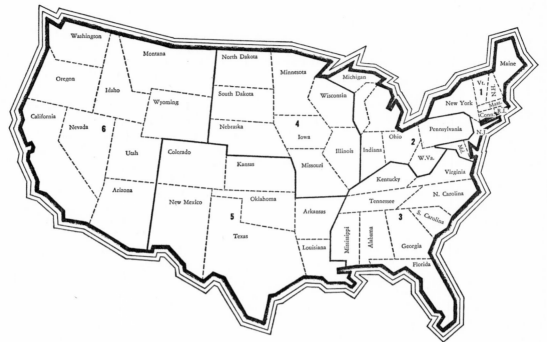

Industrial Medical Association Counselor Districts, about 1944

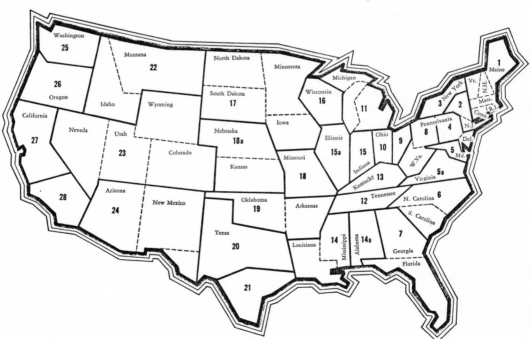

Industrial Medical Association Counselor Districts, April, 1958
(*Hawaiian, Eastern, Middle, and Western Canadian districts not shown.*)

NOTES

Chapter I

1. Stuart Chase, *The Proper Study of Mankind* (New York: Harper & Brothers, 1948), p. 115.
2. Edgar L. Collis and Major Greenwood, *Health of the Industrial Worker* (London: J. & A. Churchill, 1921), p. 2.
3. Herbert Butterfield, *The Origins of Modern Science* (London: G. Bell & Sons, 1949), p. viii.
4. Collis, *op. cit.,* p. 5.
5. George M. Kober and Emery R. Hayhurst, *Industrial Health* (Philadelphia: P. Blakiston's Son & Company, 1924), p. ix.
6. *Ibid.,* p. viii.
7. W. E. H. Lecky, *History of England in the Eighteenth Century,* Ch. XXI, as quoted in Collis and Greenwood, *op. cit.,* pp. 10–11.
8. Sir Thomas Oliver, *Occupations* (London: Cambridge University Press, 1916), p. 3.
9. Quoted from *History of England in the Eighteenth Century,* in Collis and Greenwood, *op. cit.,* p. 10.
10. Philip Gaskell, *The Manufacturing Population of England* (London, 1833), p. 216.
11. F. A. Hayek, *Capitalism and the Historians* (Chicago: University of Chicago Press, 1954), pp. 9–10.
12. *Ibid.,* pp. 18–25.
13. W. Hunt, *Political History of England* (New York: Longmans, Green & Company, 1905), X, 278.
14. J. L. and B. Hammond, *The Town Labourer—1760–1832* (New York: Longmans, Green & Company, 1917), p. 149.
15. Kober and Hayhurst, *op. cit.,* p. ix.
16. Oliver, *op. cit.,* p. 7.

Chapter II

1. Bernardino Ramazzini, *De morbis artificum* (Diseases of Workers), 1713, trans., Wilmer Gave Wright (Chicago: University of Chicago Press, 1940), p. 7.
2. Quoted in Stuart Chase, *The Proper Study of Mankind* (New York: Harper & Brothers, 1948), p. 21.
3. Henry E. Sigerist, *A History of Medicine* (London: Oxford University Press, 1951), Vol. I, Intro. to section on paleopathology.
4. Arthur Selwyn-Brown, *Physicians Through the Ages* (New York: Capehart-Brown, 1928), p. 9.
5. Henry E. Sigerist, "Historical Background of Industrial and Occupational Diseases" (A Wesley M. Carter Lecture), *Bull. N.Y. Acad. Med.,* Nov., 1936, 2nd ser., *12:*599.
6. Quoted in Alfred H. Whittaker and David J. Sobin, "Biographical Sketch of Ulrich

Ellenbog," *Ind. Med.,* May 1941, *10:*203–05. Original text printed in Augsburg, Germany, 1523–1524.

7. Ramazzini, *op. cit.,* p. 5.

8. *Ibid.,* p. 27.

9. Robert T. Legge, "First Oration Before Ramazzini Society" (May 17, 1946, St. Clair, Michigan), *Occ. Med.,* July 1946, *2:*22.

10. Robert T. Legge, "Relapsing Fever: A New Etiological Observation." Leaflet reprinted from *Cal. & West. Med.,* May 1933, Vol. 38.

11. Edgar L. Collis and Major Greenwood, *Health of the Industrial Worker* (London: J. & A. Churchill, 1921), p. 7.

12. Quoted in T. S. Ashton, *Capitalism and the Historians* (Chicago: University of Chicago Press, 1954), p. 131.

13. Galen, "On Anatomical Procedure." Quoted in Logan Glendenning, *Source Book of Medical History* (New York: Harper & Brothers, 1942), pp. 48–49.

14. Robert T. Legge, "Tanquerel des Planches: A Historical Review of His Classic Masterpieces on Lead Diseases," 1954. MS.

15. Sir Thomas Oliver, *Occupations* (Cambridge: Cambridge University Press, 1916), p. 9.

16. *Ibid.,* p. 71.

17. Neville K. Moss, *Gases, Dust and Heat in Mines* (London: Charles Griffin & Company, Ltd., 1927), p. 1.

18. *Ibid.,* p. 3.

19. Robert Legge, "Biographical Sketch of Thomas Morison Legge, 1954." MS.

20. Oliver, *op. cit.,* p. 53.

21. *Ibid.,* p. 54.

Chapter III

1. W. E. Woodward, *The Way Our People Lived* (New York: E. P. Dutton & Company, Inc., 1944), p. 51.

2. *Ibid.,* p. 23.

3. *Ibid.,* p. 33.

4. *Ibid.,* p. 46.

5. *Ibid.,* p. 56.

6. Carroll D. Wright, *The Industrial Evolution of the United States* (Meadville, Pa.: Chatauqua-Century Press, 1895), p. 47.

7. *Ibid.,* pp. 11–12.

8. Woodward, *op. cit.,* pp. 190–91.

9. Wright, *op. cit.,* pp. 119–23.

10. Matthew Josephson, *The Robber Barons* (New York: Harcourt, Brace & Company, 1934), p. 75.

11. Quoted in *ibid.,* p. 75.

12. *Ibid.,* pp. 51–52.

13. "The Workers' Story (1913–1953)," *Labor Yearbook No. II, 1953* (Washington: Bureau of Labor Statistics, Department of Labor, 1953), p. 7.

14. Abstracted from a speech given by William T. Gossett, vice-president, Ford Motor Company, to the Chicago Bar Association, June 15, 1950.

15. *Ibid.*

16. Wright, *op. cit.,* p. 283.

17. *Ibid.,* p. 239.

18. *Ibid.,* p. 345.

19. *Ibid.,* p. 347.
20. *Ibid.,* p. 291.

Chapter IV

1. Dr. McCord's articles on "Lead and Lead Poisoning in Early America" appeared in seven installments in *Ind. Med. & Surg.,* Vols. 22, 23; Sept., Nov., Dec. 1953; Jan., Feb., Mar., Apr. 1954.
2. See George M. Price, *The Modern Factory* (New York: J. Wiley & Sons, 1914). This is the first important book of its time on factory medical inspection.
3. Curt Proskauer, "A Civil Ordinance of the Year 1846 to Combat Phosphorus Necrosis," *Bull. Hist. Med.,* May 1942, *11:*562.
4. *Ibid.,* p. 563.
5. *Ibid.,* p. 563.
6. Sir Thomas Oliver, *Dangerous Trades* (London: John Murray, 1902), Ch. XXVII.
7. Alice Hamilton, *Industrial Poisons in the United States* (New York: The Macmillan Company, 1925), p. 308.
8. Alice Hamilton, *Exploring the Dangerous Trades* (Boston: Little, Brown & Company, 1943), p. 116.
9. John B. Andrews, *Phosphorus Poisoning in the Manufacture of Matches* (American Association for Labor Legislation, Publication No. 10, June 10, 1910), p. 16.
10. Hamilton, *Exploring the Dangerous Trades,* p. 115.
11. *Ibid.,* p. 119.
12. *Ibid.,* pp. 127–28.
13. Carey P. McCord "Occupational Health Publications in the United States Prior to 1809," *Ind. Med. & Surg.,* Aug. 1955, *24:*363.
14. As cited by McCord in *ibid.:* K. Ryland, "Necrosis of Maxillary Bone, *St. Louis Med. & Surg. Jour.,* 1854, *12:*28; James R. Wood, "Description, Removal of Jaw." *N.Y. Jour. Med.,* 1856, *16:*31.
15. As cited by McCord in *ibid.:* W. Detmold, *N.Y. Jour. Med.,* 1843, *1:*185.
16. Robert T. Legge, "Chronological Events in Industrial Medicine, 1900–1916." MS. in possession of Dr. Legge.
17. Titles in this list are chiefly from *Proceedings of Second National Conference on Industrial Diseases, Atlantic City Sessions of 1912.* Long-term trends of common industrial hazards are discussed more fully in a later section of this volume.
18. David L. Edsal, "Industrial Poisoning," *Am. Labor Legis. Rev.,* 1912, *2:*281.
19. Sir William Osler, *Principles and Practice of Medicine* (New York: D. Appleton & Company, 1892).
20. George M. Kober and William C. Hanson, *Diseases of Occupation and Vocational Hygiene* (Philadelphia: P. Blakiston's Son & Company, 1916).
21. George M. Kober and Emery R. Hayhurst, *Industrial Health* (Philadelphia: P. Blakiston's Son & Company, 1924).
22. Henry W. Farnham, in opening address, *Proceedings of First National Conference on Industrial Diseases* (American Association for Labor Legislation, Publication No. 10, 1910), p. 6.

Chapter V

1. Sir Thomas Oliver, *Dangerous Trades* (London: John Murray, 1902), p. 1.
2. Early figures and 1954 estimates from Automobile Manufacturers Association. Labor forces includes manufacture of materials, parts, cars; petroleum production; truck drivers and employers; insurance sales and service.

3. United States Manufacturing Corporations, *Quarterly Report, Federal Trade Commission and Security Exchange Commission,* 1953 (Fourth quarter).

4. Robert T. Legge, "Progress of American Industrial Medicine in the First Half of the Twentieth Century," *Am. Jour. Public Health,* Aug. 1952, 40:906.

5. Harry E. Mock, *Industrial Medicine and Surgery* (Philadelphia: W. B. Saunders Company, 1919), pp. 772–75; quoted from *The Immigration Problem* (Washington: United States Immigration Commission, 1917), pp. 201, 477–79.

6. *Labor Yearbook No. II, 1953* (Washington: Bureau of Labor Statistics, Department of Labor, 1953), pp. 19–20.

7. Frederick L. Hoffman, "Problem and Extent of Industrial Diseases," *Proceedings of First National Conference on Industrial Diseases* (American Association for Labor Legislation, Publication No. 10, 1910), p. 35. See also p. 49.

8. Gaylord R. Hess, *Medical Service in Industry and Workmen's Compensation Laws* (Chicago: American College of Surgeons, 1946), p. 1.

9. Union Health Center, founded by Dr. George M. Price. Continued after his death by his son, Dr. Leo Price. A detailed history of the Union may be found in *Ind. Med. & Surg.,* Oct. 1953, 22:489–97.

10. For chronology of legislation by states, see Hess, *op. cit.,* p. 63.

11. Detailed analyses of compensation laws will be found in *ibid.,* Ch. VIII, and in Mock, *op. cit.,* Part V, Ch. XLI.

12. Hess, *op. cit.,* Preface, p. x.

Chapter VI

1. Gaylord R. Hess, *Medical Service in Industry and Workmen's Compensation* (Chicago: American College of Surgeons, 1946), p. 1.

2. "The Workers' Story (1913–1953)," *Labor Yearbook No. II, 1953* (Washington: Bureau of Labor Statistics, Department of Labor, 1953), p. 53, 54.

3. Alice Hamilton, *Exploring the Dangerous Trades* (Boston: Little, Brown & Company, 1943), p. 3.

4. See *Ind. Med.,* June 1943, 12:396.

5. J. W. Schereschewsky, "Industrial Insurance," *USPHS Bull. No. 197* June 5, 1914.

6. J. W. Schereschewsky, *Industrial Hygiene,* a USPHS Report, Reprint No. 302, Oct. 1, 1915.

Chapter VII

1. *Jour. Am. Med. Assoc.,* May 6, 1916, 66:1514.

2. From the report of Dr. Shoudy's speech as retiring president, Buffalo, May 1, 1947.

3. *The Detroit News,* June 13, 1916, p. 1.

4. Quoted in *The Detroit Free Press,* June 17, 1916, p. 1.

Chapter VIII

1. Alice Hamilton, *Exploring the Dangerous Trades* (Boston: Little, Brown & Company, 1943), p. 187.

2. *Ibid.,* p. 185.

3. *Ibid.,* p. 195–96.

4. Robert T. Legge, "Progress of Industrial Medicine," *Am. Jour. Public Health,* Aug. 1952, 40:909.

5. Otto P. Geier, "The Human Potential in Industry." Address to American Society Mechanical Engineers, Cincinnati, May 1917.

6. Surgeon General William C. Gorgas (Army), 1916–1918; Admiral William C. Braisted (Navy), 1914–1920; Rupert Blue (Chief, Federal Health Services), 1912–1920.

7. Clarence D. Selby, *Studies of the Medical and Surgical Care of Industrial Workers, USPHS Bulletin No. 99,* 1919.

8. Harry E. Mock, *Industrial Medicine and Surgery* (Philadelphia: W. B. Saunders Company, 1919), p. 130.

Chapter IX

1. Alice Hamilton, *Exploring the Dangerous Trades* (Boston: Little, Brown & Company, 1943), p. 4.

2. Otto P. Geier, "The Physician and Surgeon in the Industrial Crisis." Paper read at the ninth annual meeting, Clinical Congress, American College of Surgeons, Oct. 20–24, 1919.

3. *Ibid.*

4. Harry E. Mock, "The Application of Physical Reconstruction Methods to Peace-time Civilian Practice." Paper read at Third Interallied Conference for Assistance to the Disabled of the War, Rome, Italy, 1919.

Chapter X

1. Carey P. McCord, *Industrial Hygiene for Engineers and Managers* (New York: Harper & Brothers, 1931), p. 53.

2. C. O. Sappington, *Medicolegal Phases of Occupational Diseases* (Chicago: Industrial Health Book Company, 1939), p. 105.

3. Emery R. Hayhurst, "Occupational Disease Considerations," *Ind. Med.,* July 1943, *12:443.*

4. Michigan Department of Labor and Industry, *Amendments Workmen's Compensation Law Passed During 1935 and 1937 Sessions of the Michigan Legislature.* Pamphlet, 1937, p. 2.

5. Council on Industrial Health (E. S. Jones, chairman), "Guiding Principles of Occupational Medicine," *Jour. Am. Med. Assoc.,* 1954, *155:364.*

6. Clarence D. Selby, "Studies of the Medical and Surgical Care of Industrial Workers," *USPHS Bulletin No. 99,* 1919, p. 5.

7. Otto P. Geier, "Human Potential in Industry." Address to American Society Mechanical Engineers, Cincinnati, May 1917.

8. Stuart Chase, *The Proper Study of Mankind* (New York: Harper & Brothers, 1948), p. 10.

9. Harry E. Mock, *Industrial Medicine and Surgery* (Philadelphia: W. B. Saunders and Company, 1919), p. 87.

10. Selby, *op. cit.,* p. 15.

11. *Ibid.,* p. 5.

12. R. B. O'Connor, "The Industrial Team Completes Itself," *Proceedings, Fourth Discussional on Industrial Health Programs* (Ann Arbor: University of Michigan School of Public Health and Institute of Industrial Health, 1953), p. 15.

Chapter XI

1. Otto P. Geier, "Industrial Medical Service of the Future," *American Industries,* July 1917, p. 13.

2. Otto P. Geier, "The New Era and Modern Medicine," *Med. & Ind.* May 1919, p. 33.

3. Clarence D. Selby, "Studies of the Medical and Surgical Care of Industrial Workers," *USPHS Bull. No. 99,* 1919, p. 36.

4. Harry E. Mock, *Industrial Medicine and Surgery* (Philadelphia: W. B. Saunders Company, 1919), p. 125.

5. William R. Bradley, "An Industrial Hygiene Analysis," *Proceedings, Fourth Discussional on Industrial Health Programs,* p. 10.

6. Adolph G. Kammer, "The Industrial Health Team Analyzes Itself," *Proceedings, Fourth Discussional on Industrial Health Programs,* p. 9.

7. Joseph W. Mountin and Evelyn Flook, *Guide to Health Organization in the United States* (Washington: Federal Security Agency, USPHS, 1951), p. 5.

8. Otto P. Geier, "Physician and Surgeon in the Industrial Crisis." Paper given before Clinical Congress, American College of Surgeons, October 20–24, 1919; MS.

9. Mountin and Flook, *op. cit.,* pp. 68–69.

10. C. O. Sappington, *Essentials of Industrial Health* (Philadelphia: J. B. Lippincott Company, 1943), p. 105.

11. "Outline of Procedure for Physicians in Industry," *Jour. Am. Med. Assoc.,* 1942, *118:* 895–96.

12. Michael Fooner, "Company and Private M.D.'s—Must They Feud?" *Medical Economics,* March 1954, pp. 152 ff.

13. Earl F. Lutz, "Relationship Between the General Practitioner and the Industrial Physician," *AMA Arch. Ind. Hyg. & Occ. Med.,* 1953, 8:299–306.

Chapter XII

1. Clarence D. Selby, "Studies of the Medical Surgical Care of Industrial Workers," *USPHS Bull. No. 99,* 1919, p. 6.

2. T. Lyle Hazlett, "Fundamentals of Industrial Hygiene." Paper delivered at Annual Congress on Medical Education and Licensure, Feb. 13–14, 1939.

3. Stuart Chase, *The Proper Study of Mankind* (New York: Harper & Brothers, 1948), Ch. XI.

4. Alexander Meiklejohn, Graduating Class Address, *Brown Alumni Monthly,* July 1953, pp. 15–16.

5. Harry E. Mock, *Industrial Medicine and Surgery* (Philadelphia: W. B. Saunders Company, 1919), p. 7.

6. Selby, *op. cit.,* p. 9.

7. *Ibid.,* p. 112.

8. Earl F. Lutz, "Relationship Between the General Practitioner and the Industrial Physician," *AMA Arch. Ind. Hyg. & Occ. Med.,* Oct. 1953, 8:299–306.

9. C. O. Sappington, *Essentials of Industrial Health* (Philadelphia: J. B. Lippincott Company, 1953), p. 69.

10. Clarence D. Selby, "The Physician's Responsibility in Industrial Hygiene," *Ind. Med.,* Aug. 1938, 7:519.

11. Clarence D. Selby, *USPHS Bull. No. 99,* 1919, p. 28.

12. Otto P. Geier, "Health of the Working Force," *Factory and Industrial Management,* Oct. 1917, 54:14–15.

13. Otto P. Geier, "Physician and Surgeon in the Industrial Crisis." Paper read before Clinical Congress, American College of Surgeons, Oct. 20–24, 1919.

14. Otto P. Geier, Address before AAIP&S, Sept. 29, 1920. MS. in possession of Geier family.

Chapter XIII

1. Editorial comment in *Ind. Med. & Surg.,* Oct. 1953, 22:502–03.

Chapter XIV

1. "The Industrial Physician." A General Motors Corporation documentary film, produced in 1944.

2. Carroll D. Wright, *The Industrial Evolution of the United States* (New York: Flood and Vincent, 1895).

3. Friedrich Esmarch, *Handbuch der Kriegschirurgischen Technik* (Hanover: Carl Rumpler, 1877).

4. Baron Dominique-Jean Larrey, *Surgical Memoirs of the Campaigns of Russia, Germany and France,* trans., John C. Mercer (Philadelphia: Carey and Lee, 1832).

5. George A. Otis, *A Report on Amputations at the Hip Joint,* War Department Circular No. 7 (Washington: Government Printing Office, 1867).

6. Roy Meredith, *Matthew B. Brady (1823–1896) Mr. Lincoln's Camera Man* (New York: Charles Scribner's Sons, 1946).

7. Joseph K. Barnes, *The Medical and Surgical History of the War of the Rebellion* (Washington: Government Printing Office, 1870).

8. Joseph Lister, "On a New Method of Treating Compound Fractures, Abscess, etc.," *Lancet,* 1867, Vols. 1 and 2.

9. Pierre Paul Emile Roux, "Louis Pasteur: L'oeuvre medicale de Pasteur," *Agenda du chimiste* (Paris: Pasteur Institute, 1896), p. 528.

10. James T. Whittaker, *The Theory and Practice of Medicine* (New York: William Wood & Company, 1893).

11. "Industrial Health and Medical Programs," *USPHS Bull. No. 15,* 1950, p. 50.

12. *Management and Union Health and Medical Programs,* a USPHS Publication, No. 329, 1953, p. 3.

13. See Andrew Magee Harvey in *Ind. Med. & Surg.,* Oct. 1953, *22:*440.

14. See A. D. Cloud, "Who's Who in Industrial Medicine: Robert Thomas Legge," *Ind. Med. & Surg.,* May 1957, *26:*236–40.

15. Earl Chapin May, *Principio to Wheeling, 1715–1945—A Pageant of Iron and Steel* (New York: Harper & Brothers, 1945), pp. 244–46.

16. *AAIP&S Bull.,* May 1929, 3:1.

17. Harry E. Mock, *Industrial Medicine and Surgery* (Philadelphia: W. B. Saunders Company, 1919).

18. George M. Kober, "Progress and Tendency of Hygiene and Sanitary Science in the Nineteenth Century," *N.Y. Jour. Med.* June 8, 1901, *73:*991–1001.

19. George M. Kober, *Industrial and Personal Hygiene—A Report of the Committee on Social Betterment* (Washington: President's Homes Commission, 1908).

20. W. Gilman Thompson, *The Occupational Diseases* (New York: D. Appleton & Company, 1914).

21. E. R. Hayhurst, *Industrial Health Hazards and Occupational Diseases in Ohio* (Columbus: Ohio State Board of Health, 1915).

22. George M. Kober and Emery R. Hayhurst, *Industrial Health* (Philadelphia: P. Blakiston's Son & Company, 1924).

23. Willis W. Lasher, *Industrial Surgery* (New York: Paul B. Hoeber, Inc., 1938).

24. Jose Luis Sert, *Can Our Cities Survive?* (Cambridge: Harvard University Press, 1944), p. 130.

25. Leon Losseau, *De la reparation des accidents de travail* (Bruxelles, 1897).

26. Packard Thurber, Sr., *Evaluation of Industrial Disability* (New York: Oxford University Press, 1950) and "A Guide to the Evaluation of Permanent Impairment of the Extremities and Back," *Jour. Am. Med. Assoc.,* special edition, Feb. 15, 1958, pp. 1–109.

27. A. H. Whittaker, "Disability Evaluation," *Am. Jour. Surg.,* Apr. 1956, *91:*708–10.

28. C. C. Schneider, "Disability Evaluation," *Wisc. Med. Jour.,* Jan. 1954, Vol. 53.

29. Ambroise Paré, *Cinq livres de chirurgie* (Chez André Wechel à Paris, 1572).

30. Thomas P. Teale, *On Amputations* (London, 1858).

31. Valeda von Steinberg, "The Doctors Who Rebuild Living Hands," *Saturday Evening Post* CCXXVII (Jan. 8, 1955), 36.

32. Edwin Morris, *A Practical Treatise on Shock After Surgical Operation and Injuries* (Philadelphia: J. P. Lippincott & Company, 1868).

33. C. B. Stemen, *Railway Surgery* (St. Louis: J. H. Chambers & Company, 1890).

34. Herbert W. Page, *Railway Injuries* (Philadelphia: P. Blakiston's Son & Company, 1891).

35. J. T. Eskridge, "Mutual Relations of the Railroad Surgeon and the Neurologist," *Jour. Am. Med. Assoc.,* Apr. 23, 1898, *30:*959–61.

36. Royal Whitman, *A Treatise on Orthopedic Surgery* (Philadelphia: Lea & Febiger, 1917).

37. For example, see *N.Y. Med. Jour.,* 1855, *14:*70. See also Albert Lewis Sayre, "History of Orthopaedy," *N.Y. Med. Jour.,* 1883, *37:*116; Albert Lewis Sayre, *Excision of the Hip Joint* (Transactions of the American Orthopedic Association, Philadelphia, 1889).

38. H. Helferich, *Atlas of Traumatic Fractures and Luxations* (New York: William Wood & Company, 1896).

39. W. L. Estes, *The Treatment of Fractures* (New York: International Journal of Surgery, 1900).

40. H. J. Bigelow, *The Mechanism of Dislocations and Fracture of the Hip* (Boston: Little, Brown & Company, 1900); Charles L. Scudder, *The Treatment of Fractures* (Philadelphia: W. B. Saunders Company, 1900).

41. Frederick J. Cotton, *Dislocations and Joint-fractures* (Philadelphia: W. B. Saunders Company, 1910).

42. Hugh Owen Thomas, *Diseases of the Hip, Knee and Ankle Joints with their Deformities, Treated by a New and Efficient Method* (Liverpool: T. Dobb and Company, 1875).

43. Geoffrey Jefferson, "Head Wounds and Infection in Two Wars," *Brit. Jour. Surg.,* War Surgery Supplement No. 1, 1941, pp. 3–8.

44. A. Carrell and G. Dehelly, *Treatment of Infected Wounds* (New York: P. B. Hoeber, 1917).

45. R. Whitaker, "Gunshot Wounds of the Cranium," *Brit. Jour. Surg.,* 1916, *3:*708.

46. Jefferson, *op. cit.,* p. 5.

47. See Maurice Schnitker, *Sulphanilamide Compounds in the Treatment of Infection* (New York: Oxford Medical Press, 1940).

48. See F. Hawking and J. S. Lawrence, *The Sulphonamides* (London: H. K. Lewis & Company, Ltd., 1950).

49. See Boris Sokoloff, *The Story of Penicillin* (New York: Ziff-Davis Publishing Company, 1945).

Chapter XV

1. Alfred Blalock, *Principles of Surgical Care* (St. Louis: C. V. Mosby Company, 1940).

2. H. A. Davis, *Shock and Allied Forms of Failure of the Circulation* (New York: Grune and Stratton, 1949).

3. W. B. Cannon, *Traumatic Shock* (New York: D. Appleton & Company, 1923).

4. C. J. France and E. R. Jennings, "Recent Advances in the Understanding and Treatment of Shock," *Surg. Clin. of N.A.,* Aug. 1953, Vol. 33, No. 4.

5. C. J. Wiggers and J. M. Werk, "Cardiac and Peripheral Resistance Factors, Determinants of Circulatory Failure," *Am. Jour. Phys.,* 1942, *136:*421.

6. See the important study by Robert Chambers and B. W. Zweifach, "Typography and Function of the Mesenteric Capillary Circulation," *Am. Jour. Anat.,* 1944, *75:*173.

7. Jacob Fine, *The Bacterial Factor in Traumatic Shock* (Springfield, Illinois: Charles C Thomas, 1954).

8. E. Shorr, B. W. Zweifach and R. F. Furchgott, "On the Occurrence, Sites and Modes of Origin and Destruction of Principles Affecting the Compensatory Mechanisms in Experimental Shock," *Science,* 1945, *102:*489.

9. France and Jennings, *op. cit.*

10. E. I. Evans, M. J. Hoover, G. W. Janos III, and T. Alm, "Studies on Traumatic Shock," *Am. Surg.,* 1944, *119:*64.

11. Francis D. Moore, *The Harvey Lectures* (New York: Academic Press, Inc., 1958), p. 75.

12. George W. Crile, "The Kinetic Theory of Shock and its Prevention through Anoci-association [shockless operation]," *Lancet,* 1913, *2:*7–16.

13. See Moore, *op. cit.*

14. See Francis D. Moore, "Endocrine Changes after Anesthesia, Surgery, and Unanesthetized Trauma, in Man," *Recent Progress in Hormone Research,* 1957, *13:*511–82.

15. See *ibid.*

16. G. R. Hess, "Influences of War on Medical Service in Industry," *Bull. Am. Coll. Surg.,* June 1944.

17. Figures cited from Dwight H. Murray, "Accidental Deaths Cut Thirty Per Cent by Medical Programs in Industry," *Scope Weekly,* Feb. 27, 1958, p. 13. *Scope Weekly* is published for the Upjohn Company by Physicians News Service, Inc., New York.

18. Howard Whitman, "The Amazing New Science of Love," *Jour. Lifetime Living,* Aug. 1955, p. 76.

19. M. S. Schulzinger, *The Accident Syndrome* (Springfield, Illinois: Charles C Thomas, 1956).

20. See Ernest Baldwin, "Energy Changes and Chemical Cycles," *The Listener,* London, Feb. 14, 1957.

21. C. N. Callander, *The Attitude of the Traumatic Surgeon to the Industrial Triad—the Employer, the Employee, and the Employer's Insurance Carrier.* Pamphlet in the Engeln Reprint Series, No. 116, 1924.

22. G. C. Penberthy, "The Surgeon's Responsibility in the Readjustment of the Injured to Work," *Jour. Am. Med. Assoc.,* Oct. 8, 1932, *30:*1213–15.

23. Notably, work at the University of Michigan, under Dr. F. A. Coller, starting in 1932. See H. T. Johnson, J. W. Conn, V. Iob, and F. A. Coller, "Postoperative Salt Retention and its Relation to Increased Adrenal Cortical Function," *Annals Surg.,* Sept. 1950, *132:*374–85.

24. Anon., *Fluid and Electrolytes* (Chicago: Abbott Laboratories, 1957).

25. See Felix Wroblewski, *Biochemical Biopsy Via Body Fluids* (New York: Sloan-Kettering Institute for Cancer Research, 1957).

26. See J. D. Hardy, H. G. Wolff, and H. Goodell, "Studies on Pain," *Jour. Clin. Invest.,* Nov. 1957, *26:*1152.

27. See E. T. Morch, "The Critically Injured Chest," *Bull. of Instruments,* 1957, Vol. 11, No. 7, and M. S. Sadove, "Cardiac Arrest," *Bull. of Instruments,* 1955, Vol. 2, No. 5.

28. George M. Curtis, "Blast Injuries of the Lungs," *Wisc. Med. Jour.,* Apr. 1944, *43:*413.

29. United States Civil Defense Administration, *Civil Defense in Industry and Institutions,*

Handbook AG–16–1 (Washington: Government Printing Office, 1951). Developed from the Civil Defense Conference of May 7, 1951.

30. United States Civil Defense Administration, *Health Services and Special Weapons of Defense,* Handbook AG–11–1 (Washington: Government Printing Office, 1950).

31. For example, see mimeographed pamphlet of the Michigan Office of Civil Defense, based on a symposium on the medical aspects of civil defense, held in Detroit, Nov. 16, 1955.

32. E. L. Compere, "Research, Serendipity and Orthopedic Surgery," *Jour. Am. Med. Assoc.,* Dec. 21, 1957, *165:*2070–73.

33. See J. T. McCarthy and C. T. Nelson, "Common Bacterial Infections of the Skin," *Pediat. Clin. of N.A.,* Aug. 1956, *3:*499.

34. See A. L. Garnes and R. D. Barnard, "Histologic and Pharmacologic Studies on Non-healing Dermal Wounds," *Angiology,* Feb. 1957, Vol. 8, No. 1.

35. Arthritis and Rheumatism Foundation, "Keeping Rheumatic Patients Employable," *Ind. Med. & Surg.,* July 1953, *22:*2. See R. J. Joplin and George J. Baer, "Treatment of Arthritic Joints," *Jour. Am. Med. Assoc.,* May 10, 1958, *118:*937–44.

36. H. F. Forsyth, "Methocarbomol (Robaxin) in Orthopedic Conditions," *Jour. Am. Med. Assoc.,* May 10, 1958, *167:*163–67.

37. Detroit Industrial First Aid Advisory Committee, *First Aid Guide for the Small Plant* (Chicago: February Publishers, 1952).

38. J. G. Allen *et al.,* "Irradiation Damage and Blood Transfusion," *Science,* May 9, 1952, *115:*523.

39. Gordon W. Packer, *Handbook of Physical Fitness and Play Equipment* (Litchfield, Michigan: n.p., 1957).

40. See Rudolf Nissen and Ernst Bergmann, *Cineplastic Operations on Stumps of the Upper Extremity* (New York: Grune and Stratton, 1942).

41. See Altha Thomas and C. C. Haddan, *Amputation Prosthesis* (Philadelphia: J. B. Lippincott Company, 1945). See also Veterans Administration Pamphlet 10–37, *Handbook for the Leg Amputee* (Washington: Veterans Administration, 1951).

42. Sterling Bunnell, D. R. Pratt and L. D. Howard, Jr., "Mallet Finger," *Am. Jour. Surg.,* Apr. 1957, *93:*573–79;
F. E. Hillman, "New Techniques for Treatment of Mallet Fingers," *Jour. Am. Med. Assoc.,* July 21, 1956, *161:*1135–38;
A. H. Whittaker, "Hands," *Jour. Am. Assoc. Ind. Nurses,* Oct. 1953, *1:*4–7, 14, 15.

43. L. D. Howard, "Contracture of the Thumb Web," *Jour. B. & J. Surg.,* Apr. 1950, *32–A:* 267–73.

44. William B. Coley, "Traumatic and Industrial Hernia," *Annals Surg.,* Apr. 1922, *75:*467.

45. Max Thorek, "Lumbar Hernia," *Jour. I. C. S.,* Oct. 1950, *14:*367.

46. A. H. Whittaker and D. J. Sobin, "Interinnomino-abdominal Amputation," *Annals Surg.,* Mar. 1942, *115:*435–40; A. H. Whittaker, "Interinnomino-abdominal Amputation, *Ind. Med.,* Jan. 1942, *11:*1–3; W. H. Bickel and R. C. Lewis, "Hemipelvectomy for Malignant Disease," *Jour. Am. Med. Assoc.,* Sept. 7, 1957, *165:*8.

47. Leslie V. Rush, *Atlas of Rush Pin Technics* (Meridian, Miss.: Berivon Company, 1951).

48. A. H. Whittaker, "Fractures of the Os Calcis," *Am. Jour. Surg.,* Oct. 1954, *74:*378–79.

49. A. H. Whittaker, "Open Reduction Treatment of Fractures of the Os Calcis," *Ind. Med. & Surg.,* Oct. 1954, *23:*439–42.

50. E. G. Grantham and L. H. Segerberg, "Hypothermia in Severe Head Injuries," *Med. Science,* Sept. 10, 1958, *44:*263–67.

51. H. D. Adams, "Surgery of the Major Blood Vessels," *Texas State Jour. Med.*, May 1948, *44:*10–14.

52. W. S. Edwards and S. S. Tapp, "Chemically Treated Nylon Tubes as Arterial Grafts, *Surgery*, 1955, *38:*61.

53. A. H. Whittaker and W. D. Butt, "Some Observations On the Treatment of Burns," *Jour. I. C. S.*, Mar. 1953, *19:*349–55.

54. See A. H. Whittaker, "Treatment of Burns by Excision and Immediate Skin Grafting," *Am. Jour. Surg.*, Mar. 1953, *85:*411–17.

Chapter XVI

1. John J. McCloy, "Ten Years From Now," *Atlantic Monthly*, CXCIII (May 1954), 26–30.

2. Now *Industrial Medicine & Surgery*, official journal of the Industrial Medical Association.

3. Membership figures are from official records in *Ind. Med. & Surg.*, Oct. 1953, *22:*422. They fluctuated during calendar years, and did not always correspond exactly with interim reports.

Chapter XVII

1. William A. Sawyer, "Nurses in the Guise of Industrial Physicians," *The Nation's Health*, Oct. 1921, *3:*566–68.

2. Eugene L. Fisk, "Periodic Physical Examinations—a National Need," *The Nation's Health*, May 1921, *2:*286.

3. George M. Price, "Physical Examinations of 50,000 Garment Workers." Address at the annual meeting of AAIP&S in Buffalo, Oct. 3, 1923. Reported by W. A. Sawyer, secretary.

4. Daniel C. O'Neil, "The Endicott-Johnson Medical Service." Included in Sawyer's report of AAIP&S meeting, Buffalo, Oct. 3, 1923.

5. George M. Piersol, "Problems of Industrial Medicine," *AAIP&S Bull.*, Aug. 1926, pp. 5–8.

6. C. F. N. Schram, Presidential Address, Detroit, May 1929. See *AAIP&S Bull.*, Sept. 1929.

7. Robert T. Legge, "Progress of Industrial Medicine," *Am. Jour. Public Health*, Aug. 1952, *42:*909–11.

8. Frederick L. Hoffman, *Analysis of Deaths from Chronic Lead Poisoning*, Bulletin No. 426 (Washington: Bureau of Labor Statistics, Department of Labor, 1927). Condensed in *AAIP&S Bull.*, Apr. 1927, p. 4.

9. Bernardino Ramazzini, *De morbis artificum*, 1713, trans. William Cave Wright (Chicago: University of Chicago Press, 1940), p. 253.

10. John McManus, *The Detroit News*, July 29, 1954, p. 42.

11. Eve Curie, *Madame Curie* (New York: Doubleday, Doran & Company, 1938), p. 186.

12. *Ibid.*, p. 384.

13. Frederick L. Hoffman, "Radium Necrosis," *Jour. Am. Med. Assoc.*, Sept. 26, 1925, *85:*961–65.

14. H. S. Martland, Philip Conlon and J. P. Knep, "Some Unrecognized Dangers in Use and Handling Radioactive Substances," *Jour. Am. Med. Assoc.*, Dec. 5, 1925, *85:* 1769–76.

15. James T. Whittaker, *Theory and Practice of Medicine* (New York: William Wood & Company, 1893).

16. See Chap. XII.

17. Louis I. Dublin, "Occupational Hazards and Diagnostic Signs," *The Nation's Health,* Jan. 1921, *3:20–21.*

18. See Chap. XVI.

Chapter XVIII

1. Paul D. White, "The Heart Disease Problem in Industry," *The Nation's Health,* Sept. 1922, *4:553–56.*

2. Edward F. Humphrey, *An Economic History of the United States* (New York: Century Company, 1931), p. 539.

3. *Jour. Am. Med. Assoc.,* Nov. 26, 1927, *89:1891.*

4. The committee was headed by C. W. Hopkins, chief surgeon, Chicago & North Western Railway, and a founding member of AAIP&S. See *Annals Surg.,* Apr. 1922, *75: 467–77.*

5. Arthur B. Emmons II, *Health Control in Mercantile Life* (New York: Harper & Brothers, 1926).

6. "Growth of Group Insurance," *AAIP&S Bull.,* Aug. 1927, p. 3.

7. Data from report in *AAIP&S Bull.,* Feb. 1927, p. 4.

8. *AAIP&S Bull.,* Sept. 1928, p. 1.

Chapter XIX

1. Edward F. Humphrey, *An Economic History of the United States* (New York: Century Company, 1931), p. 512.

2. *Ibid.*

3. Figures from the 1930 Census in *National Encyclopedia* (New York: P. F. Collier and Son, 1937), X, 187.

4. *Ward's Automotive Yearbook* (Detroit: Ward's Reports, Inc., 1953), p. 43.

5. Humphrey, *op. cit.,* pp. 561–562.

6. *Ibid.,* p. 561.

7. *Ward's Automotive Yearbook,* p. 43.

8. Carroll D. Wright, *Industrial Evolution of the United States* (New York: Chautauqua-Century Press, 1895), p. 325.

9. Humphrey, *op. cit.,* p. 512.

10. *Ibid.,* p. 513.

11. American Federation of Labor estimates, *National Encyclopedia Revision Service for 1940,* p. 108.

Chapter XX

1. *The United States Census, 1930,* showed only 38,350,266 nonagricultural workers in the country, and only 14,317,535 in manufacturing and mechanical industries.

2. "Silicosis," *Ind. Med.,* Jan. 1936, *5:43–44.* Reprint from *Time Magazine,* Jan. 6, 1936.

3. These and other medical papers will be mentioned in greater detail in Chapter XXII.

4. Lewis Gregory Cole and William Gregory Cole, *Pneumoconiosis (Silicosis), Story of Dusty Lungs,* Preliminary Report (New York: John B. Pierce Foundation, 1940), p. 3.

5. "Silicosis and Allied Disorders," in *Bull. No. 1 of Medical Series,* 1937, p. 79, issued by the Medical Committee of the Air Hygiene Foundation, Pittsburgh.

6. George G. Davis, *Pneumoconiosis (Silicosis), Literature and Laws of 1934* (Chicago: Chicago Medical Press, 1935), p. 404.

7. *Ibid.*

8. *Ibid.,* p. 368; figures from *Rock Products,* April 1934.

9. *Ibid.;* figure from *Engineering & Mining Jour.,* June 1934.

10. C. O. Sappington, "Some Medical Phases of Silicosis, *Ind. Med.,* Feb. 1935, 4:67.

11. James W. Ferguson, "Pneumoconiosis and Its Social Effects," *Ind. Med.,* Jan. 1936, 5:31.

12. "Silicosis," *Ind. Med.,* Jan. 1936, 5:43. Reprinted from *Time Magazine,* Jan. 6, 1936.

13. Andrew J. Farrell, "Silicosis—in Certain of Its Legal Aspects," *Ind. Med.,* Oct. 1932, 1:35–37.

14. Andrew J. Farrell, "The Silicosis Situation," *Ind. Med.,* Apr. 1934, 3:247–50.

15. Davis, *op. cit.,* p. 33.

16. *Ibid.,* p. 33. Abstracted from *Rock Products,* May 1934.

17. See report in *Ind. Med.,* June 1935, 4:328–33.

18. "New York Silicosis Bill Vetoed." See *Ind. Med.,* June 1935, 4:342.

19. Ferguson, *op. cit.,* p. 32.

20. George G. Davis, "Pneumoconiosis Problem in Industry," *Ind. Med.,* Mar. 1936, 5:124.

21. George G. Davis, *Pneumoconiosis (Silicosis) Literature & Laws of 1937,* p. 13. Abstracted from *Ceramic Industry,* Feb. 1936.

22. See *Ibid.,* p. 40. Abstracted from *Jour. Am. Insurance,* Jan. 1936.

23. "Dust Diseases and Workman's Compensation Legislation," *Ind. Med.,* Feb. 1937, 6:90 ff. Reprinted from *Columbia Law Rev.,* Nov. 1936.

24. C. O. Sappington, *op. cit.,* pp. 67 ff.

25. "Dust Diseases and Workmen's Compensation Legislation," reprinted in *Ind. Med.,* Feb. 1937, 6:90 ff.

26. William B. Given, Jr., "A Better Place to Work," *Ind. Med.,* Dec. 1947, 16:592 ff. Reprinted from *Ind. Hyg. Digest,* Nov. 1947.

Chapter XXI

1. *Sickness and the Economic Depression,* a USPHS Report, No. 1598, 1933.

2. Dean K. Brundage, *Sickness Among Male Employees During Second Quarter of 1935,* a USPHS Report, No. 39. Cited in *Ind. Med.,* Jan. 1936, 5:44.

3. *AAIP&S Bull.,* Sept. 1930, p. 4.

4. V. S. Cheney, "Secretary's Report," *AAIP&S Bull.,* Sept. 1930, p. 2.

5. *AAIP&S Bull.,* Apr. 1930, p. 2.

6. *AAIP&S Bull.,* Oct. 1931, p. 3.

7. The word "sectional" in this case was undoubtedly intended as a reference to groups representing various other "sections" in the field of medicine, rather than to geographically sectional organizations.

8. *AAIP&S Bull.,* Sept. 1930, p. 1.

9. *Ibid.,* p. 3.

10. "Blue Book of Industry," *Ind. Med.,* Mar. 1938, 7:131 ff.

11. *Ibid.,* pp. 131, 132.

12. *Ibid.,* p. 141.

Chapter XXII

1. Name changed to *Industrial Medicine & Surgery* in Sept. 1949 issue.

2. "A New Career at 78," *Medical Economics,* Aug. 1952, p. 99.

3. "Twenty-one Years," *Ind. Med. & Surg.,* Oct. 1953, 22:417.

4. "Silicosis Committees," *Ind. Med.,* May 1936, Vol. 5.

5. *Ind. Med.,* Feb. 1935, pp. 67 ff.

6. *Ibid.,* Mar. 1936, *5:*134 ff.
7. *Ibid.,* Jan. 1937, *6:*19 ff.
8. *Ibid.,* Oct. 1936, *5:*501 ff.

Chapter XXIII
1. From speech at AAIP&S annual banquet, Buffalo, May 1, 1947.
2. J. Rollin French, "The Industrial Physician and Surgeon of the Future," *AAIP&S Bull.,* Jan. 1930.
3. *AAIP&S Bull.,* Oct. 1931.
4. W. Irving Clark, "Control of Occupational Diseases," *Ind. Med.,* Feb. 1934, *3:*123–44. Reprinted from *National Safety News,* July 1933.
5. *AAIP&S Bull.,* Sept. 1930, p. 2.
6. "Industrial Medicine," *Jour. Am. Med. Assoc.,* Jan. 4, 1930, *94:*33–34.
7. "A Medical Aid Contract," *Ind. Med.,* Oct. 1932, *1:*33, 49.
8. Michael M. Davis' address of Feb. 7, 1934, was printed in *Transactions of College of Physicians of Philadelphia, 4th Series,* 1934, *2:*65.
9. "Evils of Contract Practice," *Jour. Am. Med. Assoc.,* Oct. 10, 1936, *107:*1227.
10. *Ind. Med.,* Nov. 1936, *5:*583.
11. Robert T. Legge, "Industrial Medicine of Tomorrow," *Jour. Am. Med. Assoc.,* July 23, 1938, *111:*291–93.
12. Twenty-first Anniversary Issue, *Ind. Med., & Surg.,* Oct. 1953, *22:*447.
13. Editorial, *Ind. Med.,* Jan. 1936, *5:*39–50.
14. R. C. Johnston, "Regional Ileitis," *Ind. Med.,* Feb. 1937, *6:*67–70.
15. Program published in *Ind. Med.,* Apr. 1937, *6:*202–23.
16. "General Motors Corporation Medical Conference," *Ind. Med.,* Aug. 1938, *7:*469–516.
17. *Ibid.,* p. 517.
18. Curricula at Ohio State University and the University of Michigan are outlined and described in *Ind. Med.,* Apr. 1938, *7:*194–99.
19. See Appendix 15.
20. See the abstracted program in *Ind. Med.,* Feb. 1939, *8:*64 ff.
21. Reviewed in *Ind. Med.,* July 1939, *8:*311.

Chapter XXIV
1. See "Industrial Health and Medical Programs," *USPHS Bull. No. 15,* Sept. 1950, p. 57.
2. Leveret D. Bristol, "Industrial Health and National Defense," *Jour. Am. Med. Assoc.,* Oct. 12, 1940, *115:*1235.
3. From a paper read at Conference on Industrial Medicine and Hygiene, Ann Arbor, Michigan, Jan. 12, 1940. See *Ind. Med.,* Apr. 1940, *9:*193 ff.
4. "Preliminary Survey of the Industrial Hygiene Problem in the United States," *USPHS Bull. No. 259,* 1940.
5. "Medical and Health Programs in Industry," *Studies in Personnel Policy, No. 17* (Washington: National Industrial Board, 1940).
6. *Ind. Med.,* Mar. 1941, *10:*107.
7. For details of over-all AMA war program, see Morris Fishbein, *A History of the American Medical Association* (Philadelphia: W. B. Saunders Company, 1947).

Chapter XXV
1. Excerpts from president's address, June 6, 1940, *Ind. Med.,* July 1940, *9:*349 ff.
2. Lowell S. Selling, "Industrial Psychiatry in Wartime—Employability of Certain Mental

Cases," *Ind. Med.*, Sept. 1942, *11:*407. From the Psychopathic Clinic, Detroit Recorder's Court, Ser. I, No. 1.

3. William S. Knudsen, "Human Relations in Industry," *Ind. Med.*, July 1939, *8:*307 ff.
4. "Studies on Absenteeism," *Ind. Med.*, Sept. 1940, *9:*450.
5. D. L. Lynch and H. S. Brown, "Emergency Preparedness," *Ind. Med.*, Mar. 1940, *9:*121.
6. "Health Problems of Workers," *Ind. Med.*, Mar. 1940, *9:*121.
7. "Stop This Senseless Killing," *Saturday Evening Post*, CCXXVIII (May 12, 1956), 23.
8. See report of presentation at annual meeting AAIP&S, Pittsburgh, May 7, 1941, in *Ind. Med.*, July 1941, *10:*306.
9. Figures from General Motors Statistical Department. Supplied by W. J. Fulton, Jr., medical director, Central Office.
10. Milton H. Kronenberg, "Women in Industry," *Ind. Med.*, Dec. 1942, *11:*589 ff.
11. "New Diseases for Old," *Ind. Med. & Surg.*, Sept. 1953, *22:*413.
12. Thomas W. Nale, "Current Methods of Determining Safety in the Application of New Chemicals," *Ind. Med. & Surg.*, Nov. 1951, *20:*501 ff.
13. *Ind. Med.*, June 1942, *11:*285–86.
14. See Chap. VIII.
15. Ludwig Teleky, "Occupational Diseases of Bones and Joints, *Ind. Med.*, Apr. 1942, *11:*165.
16. John M. McDonald, "Metallic Poisons," *Ind. Med.*, Oct. 1941, *10:*447 ff.
17. Carey P. McCord, "Titanium Metal Fume Fever," *Ind. Med. & Surg.*, Dec. 1953, *22:*595.
18. Forrest E. Rieke, "Health Aspects of Aluminum Ponton Work," *Ind. Med.*, Nov. 1945, *14:*896–911.
19. McDonald, *op. cit.*
20. D. L. Lynch, "Industrial Health and the War," *New Eng. Jour. Med.*, Aug. 6, 1942, *227:*209–16.
21. Morris Fishbein, *A History of the American Medical Association* (Philadelphia: W. B. Saunders Company, 1947), p. 964.

Chapter XXVI
1. Official figure in 1931 was 338.
2. *Ind. Med.*, Mar. 1940, *9:*156–58.
3. "Industrial Health Practices," *Ind. Med.*, Sept. 1941, *10:*388–97.
4. *Ind. Med.*, July 1941, *10:*282–84.
5. See Chap. XXV.
6. See Chap. XVI.

Chapter XXVII
1. Speaking of the financial situation at that time, Shoudy said that the papers and proceedings of the New Orleans meeting were printed at the expense of the State of Pennsylvania as a public service, through the efforts of Dr. Patterson. The program of the meeting bears the imprint of the Franklin Printing Company, Philadelphia.
2. See Appendix 15.

Chapter XXVIII
1. *Ind. Med.*, May 1945, *14:*397–99.
2. Names of these components were later changed to Western Industrial Medical Association and New England Industrial Medical Association, to conform with name change of the parent organization to Industrial Medical Association.

3. *AAIP&S Bull.,* Sept. 1928, p. 3.
4. Bethel J. McGrath, *Nursing in Commerce and Industry* (Cambridge: Harvard University Press, 1946), p. 1.
5. *Ibid.*
6. Nursing Information Bureau, ANA, *Facts About Nursing* (New York: National Organization of Public Health Nurses, 1944).
7. McGrath, *op. cit.,* preface.
8. Katherine M. Holmes, *History of Industrial Nursing Up to Date* (Detroit: Privately printed, 1931), p. 5.
9. *AAIN Quarterly Newsletter,* February 1948.
10. *Ibid.*
11. Evelyn M. Johnson, "Duties and Responsibilities of the Professional Nurse in Industrial Medical Service," *Jour. Am. Assoc. Ind. Nursing,* Sept. 1956, 4:36.
12. Sara P. Wagner, "President's Annual Report," *Jour. Am. Assoc. Ind. Nursing,* July 1956, Vol. 4.
13. *Jour. Am. Dent. Assoc.,* Jan. 1, 1943, p. 143.
14. Edward R. Aston, "A Report of Dental Health Studies in 19 Selected Industries," *Ind. Med. & Surg.,* Feb. 1951, 20:74 ff.
15. *Ind. Med.,* Mar. 1940, 9:122.
16. *Ibid.,* Mar. 1941, 10:104.
17. *Ibid.,* Oct. 1944, 13:777.
18. Reprinted in *ibid.,* Mar. 1947, 16:140–41.
19. *Ibid.,* Apr. 1942, 11:158.
20. *Ibid.,* Sept. 1952, 11:43.
21. Quoted from *Tic* (published by the Ticonium Laboratories), Mar. 1953, p. 10.
22. Edward R. Aston, *op. cit.,* p. 78.
23. *Tic,* Apr. 1953, p. 11.
24. *Ibid.,* Mar. 1953.
25. Grant MacKenzie, "Dentistry at the Ford Motor Company," *Ind. Med. & Surg.,* July 1951, 20:331–32.
26. *Ibid.*
27. *Jour. Am. Dent. Assoc.,* Feb. 1942, p. 299.

Chapter XXIX

1. Quoted from a cycle of Adams letters in Van Wyck Brooks, *New England: Indian Summer* (New York: E. P. Dutton & Company, Inc., 1940), p. 103 n.
2. Report in *Ind. Med.,* July 1940, 9:336.
3. For National Research Council figures cited by Maurice Holland in *Industrial Explorers* (1929) and *Tested Practice in Industrial Research* (1931), see *National Encyclopedia* (New York: P. F. Collier and Son, 1937), 5:445.
4. Sumner H. Slichter, "Prospects Are Bright," *Atlantic Monthly,* CXCIII (June 1954), 31–33.
5. "The Big Surge . . . the New America," *Newsweek,* XLVI (Dec. 12, 1955), 84.
6. Results of special study reported by United States Department of Commerce, Joint Committee for the Study of the Economic Situation of the United States, November 22, 1953.
7. See *Newsweek,* XLVII (Mar. 26, 1956), 81.
8. Slichter, *op. cit.,* p. 32.
9. G. W. Bachman and Associates, *Health Resources in the United States* (Washington: The Brookings Institution, 1952).

10. Forrest E. Rieke, "Health Aspects of Aluminum Ponton Work," *Ind. Med.,* Nov. 1945, *14:896.*

11. Gerald Gruman, "Introduction to Literature on the History of Gerontology," *Bull. Hist. Med.,* Jan.–Feb. 1957, *31:78.*

12. See Chap. XIII.

13. "Trial by Ordeal," *Ind. Med.,* Sept. 1945, *14:698.*

14. W. J. Fulton, "Industrial Medical Potentials," *Ind. Med.,* July 1949, *18:270–82.*

15. *Ind. Med. & Surg.,* Oct. 1953, *22:51.*

16. Otto P. Geier, "The Future of Industrial Medicine in a Labor Policy." MS. in possession of the Geier family.

17. "The Workers' Story (1913–1953), *Labor Yearbook No. II, 1953* (Washington: Bureau of Labor Statistics, Department of Labor, 1953), p. 80.

18. Extensively revised in the Labor Management Relations Act (Taft-Hartley) of 1947.

19. Henry Ford II, "Challenge of Human Engineering." See *New York Times,* Jan. 10. 1946, p. 1, col. 6.

20. *Ibid.*

21. "Horsepower and Horse Sense." Abstracted in *Detroit Free Press,* Apr. 29, 1955.

Chapter XXX

1. Read at the annual meeting, American Association of the History of Medicine, Detroit, May 12, 1955. See *Bull. Hist. Med.,* Mar.–Apr. 1956, *30:124.*

2. "Management and Union Health and Medical Programs," *USPHS Pub. No. 329* (U.S. Dept. of Health, Education, and Welfare, 1953), p. 216.

3. Morris Fishbein, *History of the American Medical Association* (Philadelphia: W. B. Saunders Company, 1947), p. 433.

4. *Ibid.*

5. *Jour. Mich. St. Med. Assoc.,* Oct. 1931, *30:883.*

6. Research reported in *Jour. Am. Med. Assoc.,* May 1945, *128:22–25.*

7. Fishbein, *op. cit.,* p. 475.

8. (Blue Cross) Health Services, Inc., an Illinois corporation; (Blue Shield) Medical Indemnity of America, Inc., an Ohio corporation.

9. See also *Jour. Am. Med. Assoc.,* Nov. 1933, *105:1988.*

10. Reported in full in *Am. Med. Assoc. Bull.,* Nov. 1935, *28:113.*

11. For complete text, see Appendix 13.

12. "Let's Look at the Record," *Ind. Med.,* Apr. 1945, *14:288.*

13. Resolutions introduced in 79 Cong., HR 525 and SR1271.

14. See *Guide to Health Organizations in the United States, 1951,* a Federal Security Agency publication.

15. Frederick S. Mallette, "The Role of Industrial Hygiene in Labor Relations," *Ind. Med.,* Oct. 1944, *13:775.*

Chapter XXXI

1. See *Ind. Med. & Surg.,* 21st Anniversary Issue, Oct. 1953, *22:417.*

2. Emery Roe Hayhurst, *Industrial Health-Hazards & Occupational Diseases* in Ohio (Columbus: F. J. Heer Printing Company, 1915).

3. George M. Kober and Emery R. Hayhurst, *Industrial Health* (Philadelphia: P. Blakiston's Son & Company, 1924).

4. See *Ind. Med.,* Nov. 1940, *9:572;* and Aug. 1941, *10:359.*

5. Report and proposal by J. F. McCahan to AMA Council on Industrial Health, Apr. 1951.

6. *Jour. Am. Med. Assoc.,* June 7, 1952, *149:*597.
7. See "Guiding Principles and Procedures for Industrial Nurses, *Jour. Am. Med. Assoc.,* Nov. 5, 1955, *159:*1028–34.
8. See Chap. IV.

Chapter XXXII
1. *Ind. Med.,* Aug. 1941, *10:*360.
2. *Jour. Am. Med. Assoc.,* Feb. 28, 1942, *118:*731.
3. Published by courtesy Westinghouse Electric Corporation.
4. "Preparing for Industrial Practice," *Medical Economics,* Nov. 1946, *24:*131.
5. Alfred H. Whittaker, "Medical Education in Occupational Diseases," *The Detroiter,* Mar. 18, 1946.
6. Supplementary report (mimeographed), Council on Industrial Health of AMA, Ninth Annual Congress, Jan. 1949.
7. "President's Page," *Ind. Med. & Surg.,* July 1951, Vol. 20.
8. Representing the American Medical Association, the Industrial Medical Association, the American College of Surgeons, the American College of Physicians, the American Academy of Occupational Medicine, the Association of American Medical Colleges, the Industrial Hygiene Foundation, the American Association of Industrial Nurses, and industrial and business management.
9. American Foundation for Occupational Health, "Trustee's Report of Status." Originally printed in *Ind. Med. & Surg.,* May 1953, Vol. 22; reprinted in pamphlet form.
10. Reported in *Ind. Med. & Surg.,* June 1952, *21:*282.
11. Printed by courtesy of Fawcett-Dearing Printing Company, Louisville.
12. "President's Page," *Ind. Med. & Surg.,* May 1953, Vol. 22.
13. See Robert Collier Page, "Alcoholism and Industrial Health," *Ind. Med. & Surg.,* Apr. 1954, *23:*145.
14. American Medical Association, American Pharmaceutical Association, Association of Schools of Public Health, Canadian Pharmaceutical Association, Southern Medical Association, Aero-Medical Association, American Academy of Occupational Medicine, Industrial Medical Association.
15. See Ernest L. Stebbins, "Present Status of Certification in Industrial Medicine," *Ind. Med. & Surg.,* Nov. 1955, *24:*503.

PATRONS

Alfred H. Whittaker, M.D.
1427 E. Jefferson Ave.
Detroit 7, Mich.

Stephen F. Halos
605 N. Michigan Ave.
Chicago 11, Ill.

Emmett B. Lamb, M.D.
23 E. Ohio St.
Indianapolis, Ind.

J. W. Shilling, M.D.
740 S. Olive St.
Los Angeles 55, Calif.

Wilfred N. Sisk
Upjohn Co.
Kalamazoo, Mich.

Dr. Mostafa El Batawi
Graduate School of Public
Health
University of Pittsburgh
Pittsburgh, Pa.

James I. Roberts, M.D.
441 Stuart St.
Boston, Mass.

Kenneth C. Peacock, M.D.
Owens-Illinois Glass Co.
400 Madison Ave.
New York 17, N.Y.

Rafael Peñalver, M.D.
2,60S, Vedado
Havana, Cuba

John H. Ganschow, M.D.
10025 Nadine Ave.
Huntington Woods, Mich.

A. A. Mira, M.D.
New York State Medical
Society
386 Fourth Ave.
New York 16, N.Y.

Joseph D. Solomayer
18599 Lake Shore Blvd.
Cleveland 19, Ohio

Stephen G. Halos
5301 S.W. 76th St.
Miami, Fla.

Homer S. Elmquist, M.D.
629 S. Westlake Ave.
Los Angeles 57, Calif.

Eli S. Jones, M.D.
30 Douglas St.
Hammond, Ind.

Hans W. Lawrence
Procter & Gamble Co.
Cincinnati 17, Ohio

A. J. Blair, M.D.
Consolidated Natural Gas
Co.
No. 2 Gateway Center
Pittsburgh 22, Pa.

Robert E. Eckardt, M.D.
Esso Research & Engineering Co.
Linden, N.J.

M. N. Newquist, M.D.
135 E. 42nd St.
New York 17, N.Y.

Glenn S. Everts, M.D.
Curtis Publishing Co.
Philadelphia 5, Pa.

Burton S. Shook, M.D.
101 Benet Circle
Huntsville, Ala.

Preston N. Barton, M.D.
290 Pratt St.
Meriden, Conn.

Jean Spencer Felton, M.D.
University of Oklahoma
School of Medicine
Oklahoma City 4, Okla.

F. P. Guidotti, M.D.
Hotel Health Center
501 W. 50th St.
New York City, N.Y.

H. Glenn Gardiner, M.D.
Inland Steel Co.
East Chicago, Ind.

N. L. Claybourn, M.D.
3210 Watling St.
East Chicago, Ind.

Inland Steel Company
East Chicago, Ind.

Richard D. Mudd, M.D.
1629 N. Washington St
Saginaw, Mich.

Charles E. Work, M.D.
Procter & Gamble Co.
Cincinnati 17, Ohio

John Kimmich, M.D.
Campbell Soup Co.
Camden, N.J.

Joseph C. Laue, M.D.
Long Island Lighting Co.
Hicksville, N.Y.

L. F. Fagnano, M.D.
Republic Steel Corp.
Youngstown, Ohio

D. John Lauer, M.D.
1311 Terrace Dr.
Pittsburgh 28, Pa.

R. Lomax Wells, M.D.
725 13th St., N.W.
Washington 5, D.C.

Manfred Bowditch
60 E. 42nd St.
New York 17, N.Y.

R. B. O'Connor, M.D.
United States Steel Corp.
Pittsburgh, Pa.

R. G. Birrell
Imperial Oil Limited
111 St. Clair Ave., W.
Toronto, Ontario, Can.

Harold A. Vonachen, M.D.
Caterpillar Tractor Co.
Peoria, Ill.

E. H. Carleton, M.D.
Inland Steel Co.
East Chicago, Ind.

Hugh A. Vore, M.D.
Inland Steel Co.
East Chicago, Ind.

Clarence Lee Lloyd, M.D.
North American Aviation Inc.
Los Angeles 40, Calif.

H. W. Lawrence, M.D.
Procter & Gamble Co.
Cincinnati 17, Ohio

George J. Curry
346 S. Saginaw St.
Flint 3, Mich.

Robert T. Legge
6 Roble Rd.
Berkeley, Calif.

W. N. Dawson, M.D.
Aluminum Co. of America
Alcoa, Tenn.

A. M. Puled, M.D.
18599 Lake Shore Blvd.
Cleveland 19, Ohio

Gradie R. Rowntree, M.D.
1100 W. Broadway Ave.
Louisville, Ky.

R. F. Brace, M.D.
Lago Oil & Transport Co., Ltd.
Aruba, Netherlands Antilles

MacRoy Gasque, M.D.
Pisgah Forest, N.C.

T. E. Barber, M.D.
Hormel & Co.
Austin, Minn.

Arthur J. Vorwald, M.D.
College of Medicine
Wayne State Univ.
Detroit, Mich.

Henry S. Brown, M.D.
18101 Jas. Couzens Hwy.
Detroit 35, Mich.

David Joe Smith, M.D.
L. S. Ayres & Co.
Indianapolis, Ind.

James W. Salomon, M.D.
Ford Motor Co. Aircraft Engine Division
Chicago 29, Ill.

J. G. Samuels, M.D.
Hickman, Ky.

McIver Woody, M.D.
552 Westminster Ave.
Elizabeth, N.J.

A. Landinez, M.D.
Colombian Petroleum Co.
Cucuta, Colombia, S.A.

Jacques C. Presner, M.D.
30 W. 54th St.
New York 19, N.Y.

E. Kern Linder, M.D.
260 S. Broad St.
Philadelphia, Pa.

Lt. Col. Philip M. Bourland
U.S. Army Hospital
Aberdeen Proving Ground, Md.

Douglas B. Wilson, M.D.
839 Equitable Building
Baltimore 2, Md.

L. Holland Whitney
A.T.&T. Co.
195 Broadway Ave.
New York 7, N.Y.

Forrest E. Rieke, M.D.
1313 N.W. 19th St.
Portland 9, Ore.

Walter Gillogley, M.D.
1016 6th Ave.
Belmont, Calif.

A. R. Sirna, M.D.
Chevrelot Engineering & Stamp Div.
General Motors Corp.
Flint 1, Mich.

Allan J. Fleming, M.D.
11400 Nemous Bldg.
Wilmington 98, Del.

Niel E. Eckelberry, M.D.
Consolidated Edison Co. of New York Inc.
New York 3, N.Y.

Angel R. L. Reyes, M.D.
R-204 Alcazar Bldg.
Manila, Philippines

Floyd E. Shaffer
701 E. 3rd St.
Bethlehem, Pa.

James H. McDonough
Rome Cable Corp.
Rome, N.Y.

Harry D. Riddle
Box 349
Gastonia, N.C.

Duncan G. Kilgour, M.D.
195 Broadway Ave.
New York 7, N.Y.

J. W. Crookshank, M.D.
210 S. Ryan St.
Lake Charles, La.

W. A. Meadows
900 State St.
Lockport, Ill.

Henry B. Nachtigall, M.D.
130 E. 67th St.
New York 21, N.Y.

F. W. Barden, M.D.
Saco-Lowell Shops
Biddeford, Me.

R. W. Podorsky, M.D.
5548 W. 65th St.
Chicago, Ill.

C. H. Hine, M.D.
School of Medicine
University of California
San Francisco, Calif.

Earl F. Lutz, M.D.
General Motors Corp.
13–211 General Motors Bldg.
Detroit 2, Mich.

Thomas W. Nale, M.D.
Union Carbide Corp.
30 E. 42nd St.
New York 17, N.Y.

Volney S. Cheney, M.D.
500 Gold Ave., S.W.
Albuquerque, N.Mex.

A. D. Cloud
162 Greenbay Rd.
Winnetka, Ill.

T. Lyle Hazlett
1809 Granada Blvd.
Coral Gables, Fla.

Richard A. Sutter, M.D.
915 Olive St.
St. Louis 1, Mo.

Marion W. Jocz
Chrysler Corp. Medical Adm.
Detroit 31, Mich.

E. C. Holmblad, M.D.
1350 N. Lake Shore Dr.
Chicago, Ill.

Col. John R. Hall, Jr., M.C.
Surgeon, U.S. Army Corps
APO 79, New York, N.Y.

C. D. Selby, M.D.
1916 Military Ave.
Port Huron, Mich.

N. Gilmore Long, M.D.
20 N. Wacker Dr.
Chicago 6, Ill.

Leonard Arling, M.D.
Northwest Industrial Clinic
3101 University Ave., S.E.
Minneapolis 14, Minn.

William L. Macon, Jr., M.D.
7200 Manchester Ave.
St. Louis 17, Mo.

Ralph L. Schneider, M.D.
Standard Oil Co. (N.J.)
30 Rockefeller Plaza
New York, N.Y.

D. John Lauer, M.D.
1311 Terrace Dr.
Pittsburgh 28, Pa.

R. R. Sayers, M.D.
2540 Mass. Ave., N.W.
Washington 8, D.C.

Industrial Medical Association
28 E. Jackson Blvd.
Chicago 4, Ill.

INDEX

This manuscript was edited by Esther Ellen Jacoby and Alexander Brede. The book was designed by S. R. Tenenbaum, Richard Kinney, and Richard Berube. The type face for text and display is Garamond based on a face probably cut by Jean Jannon in 1615; the design is a variation of the original design by Claude Garamond.

The book is printed on Warren's Olde Style Antique White Wove and Warren's Offset Enamel made by the S. D. Warren Paper Company. The standard edition is bound in Holliston Mills' Roxite vellum; the deluxe edition is bound in genuine cowhide and Elephant Hide paper from the Fromson Orban Company. Manufactured in the United States of America.

This is book number 299 of the half-leather bound deluxe edition.